ENCYCLOPEDIA OF COMPLEMENTARY HEALTH PRACTICE

ENCYCLOPEDIA

OF COMPLEMENTARY

HEALTH PRACTICE

Carolyn Chambers Clark
EdD, RN, ARNP, FAAN, HNC
Editor-in-Chief

Rena J. Gordon, PhD
Contributing Editor

Barbara Harris, RN, LMT, HNC, and
Carl O. Helvie, RN, DrPH
Advisory Contributing Editors

S Springer Publishing Company

Earlier versions of the following entries were published in the journal *Alternative Health Practitioner,* © Springer Publishing Company: Acupuncture in Gynecological Disease (IV), *Alternative Health Practitioner* 1996;2(2):123–130. Bioacoustics (IV), *Alternative Health Practitioner* 1996;2(3):169–175. Centering: The Path to Healing Presence (IV), *Alternative Health Practitioner* 1995;1(3):191–194. Diarrhea, Acute Childhood (II), *Alternative Health Practitioner,* 1996;2(1):11–14. Healing Retreat for People with HIV (IV), *Alternative Health Practitioner* 1995;1(2):131–137. Homeopathy: Dosage Forms (IV), *Alternative Health Practitioner* 1996;2(3):211–212. Homeopathy: Miasm (IV), *Alternative Health Practitioner* 1996;2(2):143–144. Homeopathy: Potency (IV), *Alternatiave Health Practitioner* 1995; 1(3):179–180. Ketogenic Diet (IV), *Alternative Health Practitioner* 1996;2(1):45–48. Massage for Cancer Patients (IV), *Alternative Health Practitioner* 1996;2(2):101–104.

Springer Publishing Company, Inc.
536 Broadway
New York, NY 10012-3955

Acquisitions Editor: Sheri W. Sussman
Production Editor: Helen Song
Consulting Editor: Faye Zucker
Cover design by Janet Joachim

99 00 01 02 03 / 5 4 3 2

Library of Congress Cataloging-in-Publication Data

Encyclopedia of complementary health practice / Carolyn Chambers
  Clark, editor in chief ; Rena J. Gordon, contributing editor;
  Barbara Harris, Carl O. Helvie, advisory contributing editors.
      p.   cm.
    Includes bibliographical references and index.
    ISBN 0-8261-1239-0 (softcover). — ISBN 0-8261-1237-4 (hardcover)
    1. Alternative medicine Encyclopedias.   I. Clark, Carolyn
  Chambers.   II. Gordon, Rena J.
    [DNLM: 1. Alternative Medicine Encyclopedias—English.   WB 13
  E56279 1999]
  R733.E525   1999
  615.5'03—dc21
  DNLM/DLC
  for Library of Congress   99-25832
                                                                       CIP

Printed in the United States of America

CONTENTS

Part III

Influential Substances

Part IV

Practices and Treatments   **279**

Editor-in-Chief

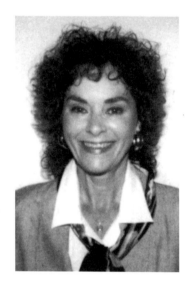**Carolyn Chambers Clark**, EdD, ARNP, FAAN, HNC, is on the Doctoral Faculty at Walden University, and on the graduate health promotion faculty at Schiller International University. Dr. Clark is Founder, the Wellness Institute, and Founding Editor, *Alternative Health Practitioner: The Journal of Complementary and Natural Care.* Her book, *Wellness Practitioner: Concepts, Research, and Strategies, 2nd Edition* (Springer, 1996), won an American Journal of Nursing Book-of-the-Year-Award. She has published widely on complementary health topics and is author of *Integrating Complementary Procedures Into Practice* (Springer, 1999). Dr. Clark is certified as an holistic practitioner by the American Holistic Nurses Association and has been a member of the American Academy of Nursing since 1980. She serves as a research grant reviewer for Sigma Theta Tau International.

Contributing Editor

Rena J. Gordon, PhD, is Research Lecturer in family and community medicine, College of Medicine, University of Arizona, and Visiting Professor, Arizona State University East. Dr. Gordon was lead editor (with B. C. Nienstedt and W. M. Gesler) of *Alternative Therapies: Expanding Options in Health Care* (Springer, 1998) and is Editor of *Alternative Health Practitioner: The Journal of Complementary and Natural Care*. Committed to improving health care services for special populations, her research has assisted the delivery of health care in Hispanic and American Indian communities. Her book, *Arizona Rural Health Provider Atlas* (1984, 1987), was selected by the U.S. Department of State for distribution to overseas organizations involved in epidemiological studies, and it served as a model for Florida's health care atlas. She has published widely on intraurban physician location, malpractice and rural obstetric service, maternal and child health, long-term care and elder services, primary care services in underserved areas, health policy issues, and health services delivery and healing practices in Cuba.

Advisory Contributing Editors

Barbara (Bobbi) Harris, RN, LMT, BA, HNC, is a Registered Nurse who is nationally certified in Holistic Nursing. She is also a Certified Natural Health Care Practitioner and Licensed Massage Therapist in the state of Florida. She received her Bachelors Degree in Psychology (magna cum laude) and has studied Counseling, Mental Health, and Transpersonal Psychology at the graduate level. Her holistic studies include receiving certification as a Reiki Master/Teacher. She is author of *Conversations with Mary: Modern Miracles in an Everyday Life* (1999). Correspondence can be sent to her at P.O. Box 1449, Osprey, FL 34229.

Carl O. Helvie, RN, DrPH, is Professor of Nursing at Old Dominion University, and teaches graduate and undergraduate courses in community health nursing and on homelessness in developed countries. He has over 35 publications in nursing and health journals and has given 30 presentations at national and international conferences in the past 5 years. Two of his latest books are *Advanced Practice Nursing in the Community* (1998) and Homelessness in the United States, Europe, and Russia (1999). He has been active with national nursing and homeless organizations and with national journals. In 1996 he was awarded a grant from the Division of Nursing, HHS, to open a nursing center for the homeless and low income of his community. He has applied for funding to continue this center into the next century. He was awarded the Ruth B. Freeman Distinguished career award in public health from the Public Health Nursing section of the American Public Health Association in 1998.

PREFACE

The *Encyclopedia of Complementary Health Practice* responds to a need for comprehensive, authoritative, and concise information concerning the application of complementary health practices that supplement traditional medical procedures. The compilation of this Encyclopedia was a challenge because many of the complementary practices presented are recent health care developments, while others are ancient practices. Recently, medical practitioners have shown interest in complementary health practices and have begun to offer courses in some of the methods. At the urging of several U.S. senators who have benefited from complementary approaches, the Office of Alternative Medicine in the National Institutes of Health was established in 1992. As a result, research on complementary methods has burgeoned, encouraging an in-depth examination of practices from a scientific viewpoint. A highly accessible resource, this encyclopedia offers work from the most competent practitioners in this progressive area of health care. All of these factors make this Encyclopedia timely.

Conceptual Framework

The conceptual framework for the book is based on a health-care approach, not a medical one. Complementary practices are not envisioned as part of medical care, but complementary to it. In keeping with this view, every effort has been made to use the terms consistent with this framework: complementary, client, and health care.

Interdisciplinary Nature of the Encyclopedia

The Encyclopedia is a vehicle for communication across traditional and complementary disciplines. For this reason we have tried to avoid using terms specific to one discipline, and made every effort to define what is meant if particular terms must be used. For practitioners, the Encyclopedia can bring new meaning to the term interdisciplinary. Hopefully, it will encourage practitioners to think about how a given practice will affect, interrelate with, and complement other health-care practices. Some questions that may be answered in this process are: What do other practitioners do that is similar to and different from what I do? Whom do I refer my clients to, when, and for what purposes, based on my knowledge of other practitioners' specialties? How and when can complementary practices combine with traditional ones?

Complementary practitioners and consumers are characteristically open to maintaining lines of communication and advocating active exploration of positive health interventions and practice. To facilitate communication between practitioners and practitioners and consumers, a directory of contributors and addresses is included at the end of the Encyclopedia. It should promote networking with experts and other practitioners about issues of importance.

Primary Audience

The primary audience for this Encyclopedia is the educated inquirer who needs a brief, authoritative introduction to the key topics and issues of complementary health-care approaches. Educated inquirers may include students who are contemplating careers in one or another specialization as well as experienced practitioners, both medical and complementary, who want to know more about practice outside their area of expertise. Other readers may include legislators, organizational, educational and foundation personnel, and all persons with a particular interest in complementary modes of treatment. Model sources of discipline information and treatments are provided in the text and referenced at the end of the volume.

How to Use the Encyclopedia

The Encyclopedia is divided into four parts.

   I.   Contemporary Issues in Complementary Health Practices
  II.   Conditions
 III.   Influential Substances
 IV.   Practices and Treatments

I.) *Contemporary Issues* contains a broad-based overview of concepts and issues that influence and affect health-care consumers and providers. Included are economic and practice concerns; education and research issues; legal, legislative, and health policy trends as well as historical perspectives.

II.) *Conditions* provides a list of disorders and research-based treatment. Because there is so much information available on the treatment of conditions, it was decided to include only research-based treatments. Research in complementary approaches is still in its infancy and many practices are based on a holistic framework that does not readily conform to the more typical double-blind research models. For these reasons, recent research, even if not currently evidence-based, is included.

III.) *Influential Substances* includes constituents such as herbs, that are powerful or effective, either in a negative or positive way.

IV.) *Practices and Treatments* describes complementary treatments and disciplines.

- Cross Referencing. Extensive use of cross references to other entries has been made. Rather than repeating key information in related entries, cross-referenced entries are listed. "See" directs the reader to relevant *Practices and Treatments* articles. "See also" directs the reader to relevant *Conditions* or *Influential Substances* entries.
- A Contributor Directory allows for networking and communication in regard to complementary health practices.
- A Resource Directory appears in the back of the Encyclopedia to assist further with referral and networking for specific practices.

- Extensive References provide the most comprehensive and up-to-date coverage of complementary publications currently available.
- The Subject Index provides additional assistance in locating topics and issues of interest that cannot be identified by the title of the article.
- A Contributor Index assists the reader in locating a specific contributor's work in specialized areas.

What the Encyclopedia Is Not

The Encyclopedia does not provide in-depth treatment of topics. It is not a textbook on complementary health practice, nor does it provide information on how to perform a specific procedure. For that, readers will need to turn to specialized publications, such as *Integrating Complementary Procedures into Practice* (Springer, 1999), designed to accompany this Encyclopedia. The extensive reference list to this volume is another useful place to start.

Development of the Encyclopedia

This project began in the summer of 1997. The enormous interest in complementary practices by academics, practitioners, clients, legislators, managed care personnel, and health consumers has made this volume almost mandatory. Following on the heels of the popular Springer publication, *Alternative Health Practitioner: The Journal of Complementary and Natural Care*, its development seemed a natural next step.

The launching of an encyclopedia requires the help of many people. I am indebted to the many authors who made this volume happen. My many complementary health colleagues who took time out of their busy practices to contribute deserve a loud chorus of kudos. Two of them even took on the task of being Advisory Contributing Editors. Carl Helvie and Barbara Harris provided contacts with potential authors and organizations, and were generally supportive and helpful. I much appreciate their cooperation. At the suggestion of publisher Ursula Springer, Rena Gordon became a Contributing Editor, bringing with her many contributing authors who add depth and breadth to this volume. Dr. Springer deserves praise for having proposed that there was a need for the Encyclopedia and for providing the positive energy and resources for the task. Others at Springer also deserve thanks: Sheri W. Sussman, Editor, Svetlana Katz, Editorial Assistant, and Helen Song, Production Editor, have helped me move forward with this project in many ways. Finally, my assistant, Jennifer Vozne, has been incredibly efficient, helpful, and unfailingly good humored through all phases of this complex project. I am exceedingly grateful to her.

Carolyn Chambers Clark

Carolyn Chambers Clark
Editor-in-Chief
St. Petersburg, Florida

PUBLISHER'S FOREWORD

Complementary health practice—or "alternative medicine" as it is still called in many places—has come of age, after some decades of growth. Actually, many of the practices and non-pharmaceutical medicines are centuries old and were transmitted as folk customs and family recipes. Since the 1960s the appeal of alternative health practice has been growing. Articles about alternative medicine appeared in popular magazines. Doctors became curious; finally in 1992 the Federal Government Office of Alternative Medicine (now the National Center for Complementary and Alternative Medicine) was established (with a low budget) to explore this health practice that seemed to attract more and more interest. Obviously, time is ripe for a comprehensive source of knowledge in this field. And this Encyclopedia has been designed to fill the need.

It was an enormous project—from the initial broad vision to the final decisions where to draw the limits of materials to be included. Moreover, we had to decide how to present the relations of treatments and practices to the conditions or "problems." The editor-in-chief did not merely want to list explanations of all items in alphabetical order, as it would be done in a dictionary.

The person who undertook this very taxing project measured up to its challenges with unparalleled energy, clear ideas and hard work. Dr. Carolyn Chambers Clark deserves highest respect for envisioning the final product and designing the dimensions and limits of the work, where needed consulting with the publisher and editors. Dr. Clark enlisted associates and contributors to plan and present the content of the entries. The main criterion for including a practice or treatment was that it was research based. Only a few very recent practices were included without the seal of research evidence.

The readers—nurses, doctors, health and social-service workers, and general reference-seekers—should be aware that this volume provides information primarily. As a guide to practical applications in complementary health care practices, Dr. Clark wrote a supplementary, smaller volume, to be published in the fall of 1999.

As the publisher of the Encyclopedia of Complementary Health Practice, I am proud of this pioneering compendium. It may seem different from our usual publications, but carrying the "Springer Seal of Approval," the book will have a successful sail into the vast world of our health care literature.

Part I

Contemporary Issues in Complementary Health Practices

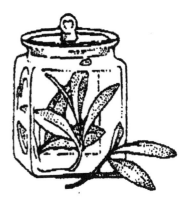

Section 1

Concepts and Issues

A THEORY FOR COMPLEMENTARY HEALTH PRACTITIONERS

What are complementary health practices? Under this umbrella is found a wide range of therapies. These include such practices as massage, homeopathy, biofeedback, acupuncture, yoga, chiropractic, breathing, and therapeutic touch. These may or may not be used in combination with traditional treatments.

What do all of these therapies have in common? They all involve some aspect of energy. For example, those who practice acupuncture say there are energy channels that run through the body that may become blocked and they work with these channels, and those who practice therapeutic touch say the universe has unlimited energy that can be channeled to clients to overcome an imbalance of energy. In addition, the intake of such substances as food, oxygen, medications, and love can be considered to be energy. These are assessed and/or prescribed by health professionals when appropriate. Whether therapy is directed toward removing blockages so energy can flow through the body, or whether it is to correct an imbalance (treatment) or maintain a balance (prevention), all treatments used by health practitioners involve energy.

Helvie's Energy Theory is a useful theory for complementary health practitioners. This theory uses a systems approach and is organized around the concept of energy. The systems approach requires the practitioner to assess the family and community as well as the individual when

*Reprinted from *Alternative Health Practitioner*, *1*(1) (1995, Spring).

working with individual clients. Organizing the theory around the concept of energy facilitates learning and practice use because every aspect of the theory relates to the concept of energy.

Riehl and Roy (1990) and Meleis (1991) say that *theory* can be a set of sentences that conceptualize a practice area. The purpose of these sentences is to describe and predict health care. The Helvie Energy Theory follows this definition.

Helvie Energy/The Theory

The theory can be outlined as follows:

1. Individuals are open energy systems.
2. The individual's environment is energy.
3. Individuals exchange energy with the environment.
4. Individuals continually attempt to adapt holistically to energy exchanges.
5. Individual energy needs vary with time and situation.
6. Adaptation to energy exchanges determines the individual's level of health.
7. As individuals move toward the illness end of a health/illness continuum, they often require assistance from others.
8. Health practitioners assist high-risk individuals (actual, potential, poor adapters) to maintain or regain efficient adaptation to energies.

Individuals Are Open Energy Systems

Individuals are open energy systems composed of three types of energy: bound, kinetic, and potential. These constitute the internal environment. *Bound energy* is organized energy, or mass, and includes cells, organs, or the whole body. *Kinetic energy* is energy in motion that assists in meeting the needs of the bound energy and maintaining a homeodynamic balance. Kinetic energy relates to such processes as maintaining a steady blood sugar level, stable vital signs, or movement of nerve impulses to and from the brain. Kinetic energy also includes the energy that flows through the body in meridian pathways discussed by acupuncturists, or through the zones discussed by reflexologists. *Potential energy* is stored energy on which work has been done and which is available for future use. This includes such energies as stored glycogen in the liver and stored knowledge, attitudes, role behaviors, and defense mechanisms in the brain. All individuals are open systems because they exchange energy with the environment.

The Environment Is Energy

The environment of individuals is energy, which can be internal or external. The internal environment was discussed earlier. The external environment is all energy beyond the individual's bound energy (body) or energy field around the body. This can be subdivided for purposes of study into chemical, physical, biological, or psychosocial. In reality these are interrelated and overlapping. In addition, some *environmental energies* such as humans, plants, and animals can be seen with the eye, whereas other energy forms, such as bacteria, can only be seen with the microscope. Other types of environmental energy cannot be seen, but register on other senses. For example, sound and heat register on our auditory organs and skin, whereas energy generated by prayer and laying-on-

of-hands is in a grey area but can be felt by the sensitive individual.

Chemical energies include objects such as food, oxygen, air pollutants, cigarettes, and medications. *Physical energies* include color, heat, light, sound, radiation, and others. *Biological energies* include bacteria, fungus, virus, rabid animals, allergens, plants, and insect bites. *Psychosocial energies* include anger, fear, love, and hate, as well as nonverbal expressions, sociocultural values, prayer, healing, and physical closeness or distance. Many of the psychosocial energies are supplied through the family.

Another level of environmental energies exists in the community and can be conceptualized as the services and resources available to individuals by economic, health, education, legal, recreation, and sociocultural subsystems. For example, economic services include employment availability, and health services include all health services in the community.

Individuals Exchange Energy with the Environment

From the chemical environment, individuals select food and give off waste products or breathe oxygen and exhale carbon dioxide. In addition, society has learned to convert energy for future use (potential) in such forms as pesticides, antibiotics, and fuel for automobiles. These affect exchanges and have both positive and negative consequences for society. Exchanges between an individual and a bacterium (biological input) might include an infection, symptoms of illness, and possible changes in the urine, vital signs, and other measurable body indicators as output. For community exchanges, the individual may pay taxes or a fee, and in return receive an education from the educational subsystem or health care from the health subsystem. There are also exchanges between the individual and sociocultural subsystem that influences values and attitudes.

Input varies from person to person and some input is more controllable than others. For example, the oxygen-carbon dioxide and other autonomic exchanges are not under the control of individuals, and unless there is damage to the bound energy resulting from past energy exchanges, they usually remain fairly consistent from person to person. On the other hand, food intake may vary from individual to individual in relation to amount, type, and frequency. Individuals also make decisions about whether or not to smoke, take drugs, eat candy, or drink alcohol.

Output may also vary from individual to individual. Input is transformed and the byproduct of what is used or stored is discarded. *Physiological output* is usually fairly consistent from person to person unless there are changes in the body resulting from past energy excesses or deprivations. Thus, these outputs can be compared with standards to determine normality. For example, normal feces have a certain consistency, color, and frequency whereas normal urine has a certain specific gravity, volume, and color and is free from sugar, acetone, blood, and other abnormalities. Output for the chiropractor, acupuncturist, or massage therapist (in response to tension or disease in clients) may be in the form of energy blockage or disrupted patterns of energy flow. Output in the form of behavior is less consistent from person to person because of the transformation that combines the input with potential energy (knowledge, values, attitudes). For exam-

ple, one person who has a sore throat and fever as a result of an exchange with a disease agent (biological energy) may consult a physician, whereas another with the same symptoms may consult a nurse practitioner, herbalist, chiropractor, or no one (Helvie, 1991).

Although the practitioner cannot always predict input and output, there are standards with which to compare assessment data. These data in combination with an assessment of the basis for the observed behavior determine interventions.

Excesses and deprivations of energy from exchanges may lead to damage to the bound, kinetic, and/or potential energies of the body. (See the discussion of entropy below.)

Individuals Continually Attempt to Adapt

The ongoing exchanges (input, output) between the individual and the environment that are necessary for life and growth require the individual to continually adapt. *Adaptation* is the homeodynamic adjustment of the individual as the parts work together to keep the parts and the whole system in balance when faced with internal and external energy forces against this balance (Helvie, 1991, p. 13). Within the internal environment the interrelated parts such as the heart, liver, and muscles work interdependently using kinetic and potential energy to maintain the individual's balance and purposeful direction. For example, a reduction in blood sugar will trigger a conversion of glycogen (potential energy) in the liver to glucose to maintain the blood sugar level. Likewise, a change in environmental temperature will bring into play interrelated mechanisms to maintain a steady body temperature. In addition, the brain assists in maintaining balance by reasoning, problem-solving, and using knowledge (potential energy) to influence exchanges, such as eating when hungry, or putting on a coat when cold. These and other processes that tend to maintain a steady physiological state are known as *negative feedback.* The other type of feedback is *positive feedback,* which tends to amplify change from a steady state, and leads to growth and learning.

Change that requires adaptation may be introduced by any variation in external environmental energies. For example, a loss of health care, job, or spouse will all require adjustment.

As change is introduced there is a need to reestablish a temporary balance. For example, when individuals lose a job, there is no exchange with the economic subsystem and they must look for another job, use savings, and/or apply to social services for assistance. During this period they may have less money for food, shelter, recreation, and other necessities. The ramifications of these changes will lead to a new temporary balance that may move them toward or away from health.

Although responding to change (nonautomatic response) may vary from individual to individual, it usually follows a specific pattern for an individual based on learned behaviors (potential energies of knowledge, attitudes, values). For example, we learn what to do and what is acceptable in our group when we lose a job. We also learn what to eat, when to eat, whom to love, and so forth for nonautomatic behaviors. Responses to change may also involve such concepts as bargaining, pressuring, and voting to arrive at a consensus among factions such as family members who are for or against a specific change.

Entropy is the energy lost during transformation and not available for use. An example would be the loss of some energy when food is converted to a usable form by the body. The subsystems (circulatory, nervous, respiratory) continually lose some energy as they adjust to and transform external energies. This loss is not detrimental to the individual when all parts are working efficiently and there is enough additional energy to meet needs for growth and movement toward a higher form of organization (*negentropy*).

Harmful entropy results from a defect in a part of the system (bound, kinetic, potential) usually resulting from previous excesses or deprivations of energy. This breakdown of a part of the system will affect other parts and consequently decrease the efficiency of the system. For example, emphysema, which may result from excess chemical energy (cigarette smoking or polluted air), will affect the oxygen-carbon dioxide exchange (because of the decreased lung capacity), and will subsequently affect the circulatory and nervous subsystems, which will accommodate, but function at a less efficient level. This makes it more difficult for the system to meet its goal of maintenance and growth. Other examples include cancer, cardiovascular disease, and allergies.

All behavior is considered adaptive, but there is a range (*efficient adaptation*) beyond which there may be irreversible changes in the energy system (bound, kinetic, potential) resulting from excessive or deprivation of energy. *Efficient adaptation* has been defined as the "genetically/environmentally determined range of adaptability for the specific individual in which changes in the bound, kinetic, and/or potential energies may take place but are easily reversible and maintain the efficient functioning of the system" (Helvie, 1991, p. 18). An example of efficient adaptation would be normal weight loss. It is important to distinguish between reversible and irreversible changes because they may dictate the need for outside assistance (see below). For example, the loss of body protein when there is an inadequate intake of food is adaptive behavior by the body but this change is probably not easily reversible.

Individual Needs Vary

Energy needs of individuals vary as they move through time depending upon such factors as the rate of growth and the energy used for activities and with negative feelings (worry, hate). The elderly person needs less chemical energy in the form of food than a young active person, but may need more chemical energy in the form of medicines or herbs. A pregnant woman may need different energies than a woman of the same age who is not pregnant. Developmental and situational changes such as these have been studied and the energy needs documented. Thus, it is possible to compare a specific individual's needs with standards established using concepts and tools such as the Denver Developmental Screening Test (Frankenburg, Goldstein, & Camp, 1971), Piaget's stages of cognitive development (Piaget, 1963), or Erikson's stages of psychosocial development (Erikson, 1959).

Adaptation Determines Level of Health

Health is "the adaptation of humans to the changing energies in the environment" (Helvie, 1991, p. 22). It can be conceptual-

ized on a continuum from an optimum balance of energies (high-level wellness) to a dissipation of energy (death). At the optimum balance of energies end of the continuum are individuals who are within an efficient range of adaptability regarding the intake and output of energies appropriate for the age, condition, and so forth. It also includes a balance in biopsychosocial and spiritual dimensions.

As individuals experience excesses and deprivations of energies over a period of time and move outside the range of adaptability, they move down the continuum. This movement may be temporary or more permanent, depending whether or not the changes from the energy excesses or deprivations are reversible. For example, the effect of an excess of biological energy resulting in the common cold or influenza may move individuals down the continuum temporarily until they recover from the illness. However, a common cold or influenza in a person who has had previous excesses and deprivations of energy that have led to structural or process changes (bound, kinetic) may produce a more permanent movement down the continuum.

Continuum Movement Usually Requires Assistance   Although individuals can use assistance to remain within an efficient range of adaptability, when they move outside this range, they will require assistance from others: teaching about wellness behaviors, healthy chiropractic adjustments, use of herbs for health. Assistance may come from family members or from community resources (health practitioners, social workers, or others), depending upon the results of an assessment.

Health Practitioners Assist High-Risk Individuals   Health practitioners help high-risk individuals maximize their efficient adaptation, that is, they help individuals stay within the efficient range of adaptability by altering or maintaining energy exchanges or help clients return as closely as possible to the efficient range of adaptability by altering energy exchanges and/or working with the effects of past energies on the bound, kinetic, or potential energies. All interventions are based upon an adequate assessment or health history that may focus on all or selected aspects of current energy exchanges and/or the effects of past energy exchanges.

High-risk individuals are those individuals who are experiencing, have experienced, or are likely to experience a developmental or situational change and who are deemed least likely to adapt based upon epidemiological data about groups. These groups of individuals comprise all who have experienced the effects of past excesses or deprivations of energy, or who are currently experiencing or may experience excess or deprivation of energies and thus may be considered to have actual or potential health problems as a result of the energy exchanges.

Process and Theory Model

The process used to apply this theory is known by various names. Nurses call it the *nursing process,* consisting of assessing, planning, implementing, and evaluating. Physicians have not named the process but identify components of taking a health or medical history, developing a treatment plan, carrying out the plan, and evaluation. Others call it the *scientific method, problem-solving process, research process*, or some other name. Each discipline, however, seems to include the four components identified above.

In practice the theory of energy can be applied through the process identified above. First, assess the effects of past energies on the bound, kinetic, and/or potential energies of the individual. If there have been excesses or deprivations of energy exchanges in the past, there may be changes in the bound or other energies of the individual and often movement outside the efficient range of adaptability. These changes are usually the basis for an individual seeking assistance from a health practitioner. Some practitioners such as the herbalist, massage therapist, acupuncturist, chiropractor, hospital nurses, and physicians may work primarily with the effect of these past energy exchanges and will obtain a health history as a basis for treatment.

The next step in the model is to assess the current energy exchanges between the individual and environment. Here the practitioner assesses the chemical, physical, biological, and psychosocial exchanges (including the family) and also exchanges with the community subsystems such as health, social services, education, economic, and others. Current exchanges will be compared with standards as a basis for identifying excesses and deprivations that have the potential for causing changes in the bound, kinetic, or potential energies of the individual.

Assessment tools specific to a discipline will be used, but all practitioners will consider the person's energy needs dependent upon time and situation. In addition, some disciplines will assess a part of the exchanges whereas others may assess all exchanges as a basis for treatment. For example, social workers may be more interested in the exchanges with the economic or social subsystems of the community, whereas community health nurses more often use a holistic approach to meet their goals. Other practitioners may be less interested in assessing current exchanges than in assessing the effects of past energy exchanges.

From the assessment of exchanges compared with standards, the practitioner makes a determination about the energy exchanges. They may be adequate, excessive, or deprived. The practitioner also determines the basis for the observed exchanges before planning. For example, is the food deficit a result of a lack of knowledge, a lack of income, a desire to lose weight, or some other factors? Different causal factors will require different interventions.

A *diagnosis* is written in relation to the energy terminology. For example, inadequate food intake could be written: "A deficit in the chemical energy input of food (specify) due to a lack of knowledge of proper nutrition." A diagnosis related to the effects of past energies on the body might be "blockage or imbalance of energies in bound energy (specify area, e.g., neck) due to stress."

After writing an energy diagnosis, a treatment plan is developed. Treatments will involve some aspect of energy related to the diagnosis. Goals, objectives, and planned treatments may be identified in part or whole. *Goals* are broad and usually relate to an increase, decrease, or *maintenance* of energy exchanges for exchanges between the individual and environment. Goals for past energy exchanges that have affected the bound or kinetic energy of the body may be written in terms of increasing, decreasing, removing, or rebalancing energies. For example, a goal for the diagnosis

above related to nutrition might be "increase chemical energies of food (specify)"; and a goal for the blockage identified above might be "remove the blockage of energies."

Objectives relate to the expectations for the client in meeting the goal. These usually have at least three components: *Who* is to carry out the activity (usually the client); *what* activity is to be carried out; and *when* the activity is to be completed. For example, an objective to meet the goal of increasing the chemical energy of food might be: "Client will eat three green leafy vegetables a day beginning 12/21/94" (if these vegetables had been identified as the deficit energy in the diagnosis). Other related objectives would also be written to meet the goal. A goal for the blockage diagnosis might be "Client will practice stress management exercises for 10 minutes nightly beginning 12/12/94." This would supplement the manipulations of the massage therapist or chiropractor and would help prevent further blockage.

Treatments are identified and direct the interventions of the practitioner. These may take many forms: increasing physical energy through such activities as manipulation by the chiropractor or osteopath, massage therapy, giving a bath, or providing for other activities of daily living. They might involve increasing chemical energy by altering the diet, providing oxygen therapy, teaching deep breathing exercises, or prescribing medications, herbs, or other oral preparations. They might involve increasing sound energy by teaching specific to the problem, increasing light energy through the use of ultraviolet light, or decreasing these energies in a quiet, dark hospital room.

After planning is completed, the practitioner and client implement the plan, and with the client's assistance, the practitioner evaluates the effect of the treatment. Reassessment and development of new plans or the end of treatment follows.

CARL O. HELVIE

See
Acupuncture and Chinese Medicine (IV)
Biofeedback (IV)
Chiropractic: Definition, History, and Theory (IV)
Herbal Therapies (IV)
Homeopathy: The Molecular Basis (IV)
Reflexology (IV)
Therapeutic Touch: Definition, History, and Theory (IV)
Yoga (IV)

THE ROLE OF SCIENCE IN COMPLEMENTARY HEALTH CARE

Critics of complementary health care claim that there is no scientific evidence to indicate that these therapeutic approaches work. As recent developments indicate, this criticism is increasingly outdated. It was a review of the scientific data that led the Food and Drug Administration (FDA) to reclassify the acupuncture needle from an experimental to a therapeutic device. The agency acted because of evidence indicating that this treatment provided significant relief to those suffering from chronic pain and asthma for example. In a related development, which surprised many people, the U.S. Agency for Health Care Policy and Research concluded that spinal

manual adjustment as practiced by chiropractors, osteopathic physicians, and others constitutes a more effective and cost-effective treatment for lower back pain than drugs or surgery. This decision was based on the kind of outcomes-based research that advocates and critics alike of complementary health care have long called for.

In fact, so many units of the federal government are currently researching different aspects of complementary medical approaches that U.S. Senator Arlen Specter (R–Pennsylvania) has requested a government-wide survey documenting these efforts.

One problem, which complicates the current debate, is that when significant research on the efficacy of complementary approaches is published in a foreign country, the research is largely ignored in the United States. A recent case in Germany provides a clear example of this challenge. For much of the last 200 years, German research set the standard for scientists around the world. When a commission established by the German government (known as Commission E) issued reports on the efficacy of hundreds of natural medicines, its work attracted little attention in the United States. A private, nonprofit group, the American Botanical Council published English translations of these monographs in the fall of 1997. They have provided this information to legislators and health policymakers. Other nations, in Asia, Africa, and Latin America have also published research on natural medicines.

Conducting clinical trials or outcome-based research is a very expensive process, but guidelines may be developed to help to save both the federal government and potential private funders considerable time and money. It is important to make a distinction between complementary approaches that truly represent alternatives and those that are simply unusual. Most credible complementary approaches (such as Chinese acupuncture or Ayurveda—the medicine of India) have been passed down from generation to generation for thousands of years. They have been used by thousands of practitioners on millions of patients. From a cultural historical perspective, approaches that have no value probably would have died out a long time ago. Conversely, unusual therapies have no cultural traditions. Typically, such approaches are associated with a few individuals who are unable or unwilling to scientifically replicate their results. To date, complementary approaches, which have been validated by contemporary science, are generally those with long cultural histories.

Scientific validation of complementary approaches is important because physicians use any ethical treatment that has been proven to work. Contemporary physicians depend on clinical evidence when making decisions about appropriate treatments. While we have decades of experience in doing clinical trials, the financial resources needed to do complementary research are not easy to obtain.

If the federal offices doing the research continue to be hampered by small budgets, information that could help to save lives might be delayed for years. Some experts believe a joint public-private initiative involving the government, foundations, universities, and corporations should help initiate the kind of comprehensive research program needed to determine which complementary therapies may benefit health.

MARC S. MICOZZI

See
Acupuncture and Chinese Medicine (IV)
Ayurveda (IV)
Chiropractic: Definition, History, and Theory (IV)

COMPLEMENTARY HEALTH PRACTICE: A NEW PARADIGM

Modern physicians diagnose and treat diseases (abnormalities in the structure and function of body organs and systems), whereas clients suffer illnesses (experiences of undesirable changes in states of being and in social function; the human experience of sickness) (Kleinman, Eisenberg, & Good, 1978). Pain is the essential experience of illness because it defies all the diagnostic tests of modern medicine, yet it produces its ravages of disability and dysfunction.

Complementary practitioners must define physical illness differently from conventional medicine. This is accomplished by reversing common conceptualizations of conventional medicine. Suffering then, presents with physical symptoms, emotional symptoms or social symptoms. Physical illness is suffering expressed through the language of the body. As suffering continues, tissue changes accrue until damage is eventually irreversible. Mental illness is suffering expressed through the language of the mind. Social illness is suffering expressed in the relationships among people.

From a complementary point of view, no illness is purely physical. Rather, suffering manifests in multiple dimensions: physical, emotional, social, or spiritual. What is of concern is how suffering becomes physicalized. How does suffering result in body symptoms, some of which are so severe as to be associated with changes in tissue structure and function?

Take, for example, cancer. How does cancer begin? We know that immune deficiency is important. Abnormal cells are continually appearing, but our body possesses the wisdom to eliminate them. What happens to allow a nidus of such cells to take hold? We know that emotions contribute to cancer. Depression suppresses immunity and leads to decreased cellular function. We know that watching a tragic movie suppresses immune parameters in the laboratory. We know that poor nutrition interferes with immune function. We know that some families carry genes that make them easier targets for cancer. What then sparks the flame that establishes the cancer? Toxic exposures are one candidate. Agent Orange exposure in Vietnam increased the likelihood of cancer. Toxic wastes as in the infamous Love Canal in New York increase the likelihood of cancer. But not all exposed persons develop cancer. Some are stronger than their exposure. What confers this strength is another unanswered question confronting complementary practitioners. What makes some people stay healthy among conditions that lead to disease for others?

The Black Plague of the 14th century exemplified this. Even in same families who were theoretically similarly exposed to the plague, not everyone became ill. Members of families were mysteriously spared. Some communities were mysteriously spared. Homeopaths argue that this sparing was related to microinoculations of the plague agent. Was it that, or was it simply an optimum health for those who were spared vis-a-vis that infectious agent? It could not be simply optimum health, for those who were spared were not all the most healthy, and those who contracted the illness were not necessarily the weakest.

We need a new science of resiliency, of hardiness, of survival. If we know what keeps people healthy, even in the face of adversity, we could improve our treatments for those who are ill.

Spiritual factors are certainly important. " . . . [T]he oldest mind-body effect [is] the relationship between spirituality and medicine" (Friedman & Benson, 1997).

Even the power of the mind is discounted in the allopathic understanding of resiliency from disease. "The scientifically oriented biomedical community tend[s] to discount the importance of psychological and behavioral variables as important etiological and exacerbational factors in pathogenesis. This community tend[s] to devalue or even demean the significance of these factors in treatment" (Angell, 1985). This despite the widely reported therapeutic value of addressing psychology and behavior in the study of disease (Lehrer, Carr, Sargunaraj, & Woolfolk, 1993).

It is generally accepted that an individual's psychosocial characteristics and behavior patterns need to be considered when the development and treatment of most of the major health problems confronting our society are discussed (National Institutes of Health, 1996). An individual's spiritual or religious belief system clearly influences psychosocial and behavioral variables (Friedman & Benson, 1997). Most Americans feel that psychosocial and behavioral variables should be more integrated with health care (*USA Weekend*, 1996).

Here is an example from the internet of a conceptualization of disease within complementary practice circles from the old paradigm. Then we will see how this could be re-conceptualized from a new paradigm. One correspondent wrote on the paracelsus mailing list:

If the wisdom teeth have been pulled, there may be hidden osteonecrosis of the extraction socket, which may also affect distal sites via acupuncture meridians. I learned a fascinating lesson from a patient yesterday. We had been treating him for chronic never-ending every day migraine headaches for months, using everything—Chinese herbs, acupuncture, bodywork, nutrition, thyroid supplementation, detoxification—with zilch results. Our secretary suggested he contact her dentist, who has helped some people with migraines. The dentist checked him, and found nothing wrong, but then referred him to his teacher, who has some sort of expensive machine that measures electrical flow through the teeth somehow (he didn't understand it). This found a tooth with an abnormality, and, lo and behold, when it was opened, a large pocket of putrid tissue was found, and cleaned accordingly. His headaches worsened for two days, then began to disappear. I'm a believer. (Tillotson, 1997)

What comes from this old paradigm is the implicit belief that a physical cause exists for every symptom or illness. Here the hidden cause was putrid tissue within a root canal. A natural scientific point of view, however, which is not how modern allopathic medicine is conceptualized or practiced, except in rare circles, would recognize that no evidence is provided in the above passage that necessarily implicates the cleaning out of the putrid tissue in the tooth with the disappearance of the illness. Many other explanations are possible. For instance, (1) on that day, the cumulative effect of all the other therapies surpassed a threshold and healing happened; (2) the patient became so convinced that the procedure would help, that it did (Mind-body healing; probably responsible for 70% of patient improvement; also known as the placebo response rate when both patient and practitioner believe in the therapy); (3) a major life change occurred around the time of the dental procedure, which then became inculcated into the dental procedure as ceremony to mark the end of the illness (surgery can be as important a ceremony as any machinations of a shaman); (4) The Angel Gabriel happened to be passing by and remembered that he had neglected to answer the patient's prayers for healing and took that moment to do so; (5) it was coincidental: and more of course. As many more as can be imagined.

How would a 21st century conceptualization of complementary practice view the above? First, that the cause of illness is multiple and somewhat indeterminate. Second, that the treatment which will help need have no relation to the cause of the illness in space or time or physicality. Third, that an element of mystery remains about how individuals get well. This mystery defies logical analysis, and prevents us from saying that one specific treatment definitely cured the illness.

Other clients have undergone the same dental procedure and not noticed a change in symptoms. One case should not make a believer out of anyone.

In summary, a new conceptualization of physical illness needs to recognize that (1) illness is an expression of suffering—social, political, emotional, biological. It is an expression of lack of harmony amidst all the aspects of a person's life. This lack of harmony leads to the formation of a nidus of illness or disharmony within the person's life. Once disharmony exists, then the illness begins to develop itself in a self-organizing manner. Once organized, at a certain level of relationships to the rest of the body and the person's life, the illness becomes its own entity. It creates itself. Once created, the illness finds ways to shape the person's destiny to maintain itself. The body, life, family, and emotions are codirected with the illness to maintain the illness. This process obscures the original cause.

Once established, an illness has a life of its own. Native Americans and other cultures describe this by saying that the illness has a spirit and that the spirit of the illness must be addressed for the illness to be cured. How we transform a person/family/community so that it no longer contains the illness may bear no relation to how the illness arose. Once an illness is created, how it maintains itself is more important, usually, than how it arose. The Quebecoises say, "Qu'est-ce que se mange en hiver?" about things they do not understand. This means, what does it eat in the winter? To rid the person of an illness, we need to know what the illness eats, how it supports itself, how it survives within the economy of the person/family/community. Then conditions can be transformed so as to no longer support the illness.

Once we introduce the concept of self-organization, illness can never be viewed the same as it is in the allopathic paradigm. This is what makes complementary health care unique.

LEWIS MEHL-MADRONA

See
Native American Medicine (IV)

COMPLEMENTARY HEALTH CARE RESEARCH BASE

Complementary and alternative health practices are becoming increasingly popular in the United States. These practices have been used extensively in other countries for some time. The amount of scientific research on these health practices is very limited and generally related to case studies or anecdotal records. Part of the reason for this has been insufficient research funds available for complementary and alternative research and a lack of legitimacy as scientific research in the view of allopathic medicine. Until 1992, when the National Institutes of Health established the Office of Alternative Medicine, which became the National Center for Complementary and Alternative Medicine (NCCAM) in 1998, there was no central group or organization directed to either fund or evaluate research (Dossey, Keegan, Guzzetti, & Kolkmeier, 1995).

The literature on clinical and scientific research on alternative health care practices is widely scattered, and background information is sparse. The literature in some instances is available only in other countries and therefore hard to access in the United States. In other instances, it has been handed down as oral tradition and is not available in print.

A compounding problem relating to health foods and supplements is that these substances are not regulated, and there is no consistency in potency, equivalency, or efficacy between and among compounds from different companies. It is therefore difficult for the health care provider and the client to know exactly what is in a herbal supplement.

In the United States, we refer to "alternative therapy"; Europeans prefer to call it "complementary therapy." These therapies are considered an adjunct to allopathic medicine. The ultimate goal of investigation of complementary therapies is to integrate validated therapies with current conventional medical practices (Micozzi, 1996).

Quantitative research is a systematic, formal, objective process in which numerical data are used to obtain information about a subject. This is the most commonly used and respected method of scientific inquiry and involves description of variables, study of relationships among variables, and determination of cause-and-effect interaction between variables. A key issue in quantitative research is the ability to predict and control variables and rigor. Rigor is the striving for excellence and involves discipline, scrupulous adherence to detail, and strict accuracy. Logistic and deductive reasoning are essential to the process of quantitative research. Quantitative research is usually classified into four categories: (1) descriptive research, exploring and defining phenomena in real-life situations; (2) correlational research, examining the relationships between two or more variables and the type and degree of the relationships; (3) quasi-experimental research, examining the cause-and-effect relationships between selected independent and dependent variables; and (4) experimental research, examining the cause-and-effect relationships between selected independent and dependent variables under very controlled conditions. With this type of research, it is possible to generalize the results in one study to similar client populations and to replicate the results in similar studies. This type of research has been deemed necessary to identify cures for illnesses.

Research designs have been ranked by the United States Preventive Services Task Force (1996) in descending order of importance as they relate to clinical studies. The task force was particularly interested in studies least subject to bias and misinterpretation. The ranked order was (1) randomized controlled trials, (2) nonrandomized controlled trials, (3) cohort studies, (4) case-controlled studies, (5) comparisons between time and place, (6) uncontrolled experiments, (7) descriptive studies, and (8) expert opinion. Some researchers also have conducted meta-analysis or decision analysis of several research studies to synthesize the results of several studies.

Few randomized controlled trials, cohort studies, or even case-controlled studies are available regarding research on complementary and alternative health practices. Since federal funding became available from the National Center for Complementary and Alternative Medicine in 1993, more of these types of studies are being reported.

In addition to quantitative research, there is a need for qualitative research to study patterns and the meaning and context of observed patterns. A holistic approach helps to describe all possible explanations. Qualitative research focuses on understanding the whole. There are six types of qualitative research: (1) phenomenological research, examining lived experiences; (2) grounded theory research, examining theory on the basis of the data from which it was derived; (3) ethnographic research, examining the culture; (4) historical research, examining the events of the past; (5) philosophical inquiry, using intellectual analysis to clarify meanings, make values manifest, identify ethics, and study the nature of knowledge; and (6) critical social theory, examining how people communicate and develop symbolic meaning. Qualitative research has not always been valued. As qualitative research is published, discussed, and analyzed, it will continue to gain respectability.

In the area of complementary and alternative therapies, there is a place for both quantitative and qualitative research. There is a need to obtain data on which complementary therapy is the treatment of choice, for which clients, and for which clinical problems. The provider of care is barraged with a multitude of conventional and nonconventional practices: Which one should be selected for the client? How do I evaluate?

Instruments to measure the holistic effect of therapies are many times minimal or nonexistent. Instruments must be developed that facilitate assessment, diagnosis, and selection of interventions, as well as measure the effectiveness of interventions.

Most complementary health practices will continue to remain unaccepted by allopathic medicine until large-scale randomized placebo controlled trials have been conducted validating their efficacy. Complementary health practices place greater emphasis on the validity of individual therapeutic experience.

MARY E. HAZZARD

ETHICS AND COMPLEMENTARY MODALITIES

Every modern society has formal, semiformal, and informal systems of health care. The vast majority of health activity takes place informally; over 80% of treatment in the United States happens in the home, as people treat themselves, one another, or their children (Zola, 1972). Semiformal systems, in which practitioners cater to people outside the officially sanctioned system, include folk health care (knowledgeable elders or those with healing talents pass received wisdom on to their kin); ethnic healing (subgroups in society set up healing modalities primarily for the use of their members); and complementary care

(believers in the efficacy of a modality or system create services to provide that modality to interested clients). In most cases, those who question the ethics of care outside the formal system are targeting complementary care, and to a lesser extent ethnic and folk care; few question the legitimacy of home care. It may not be a coincidence that the degree of objection is directly proportional to the degree to which a set of practitioners challenges the formal system for clients (Wolpe, 1994).

In one sense, it is strange to speak of ethics and complementary modalities as if those ethics should differ from the ethics of conventional practitioners. Complementary practitioners confront many of the same problems as conventional practitioners—fully informing individuals of the risks and benefits of the procedure, being truthful and open, knowing one's limitations as a healer, setting a fair price, not taking advantage of the power inherent in being a healer (sexually, financially, or interpersonally), and so on. All healers have a profound and unconditional responsibility to adhere to these accepted standards of care, whether the healer is a physician, a neighborhood herbalist, or a part-time massage therapist.

Those complementary systems that are more fully developed—those with formal training institutions and at least some state licensure, such as chiropractic or acupuncture—usually have guidelines and training sessions addressing the ethical provision of care. Unfortunately, many complementary modalities do not involve licensure or involve only licensure in certain states, and many training programs (in conventional care as well), correspondence courses, or apprenticeships do not appreciate the need to discuss and teach ethical principles. One of the reasons some complementary health care advocates call for licensing of complementary practitioners in general is to provide some oversight and general guidelines for ethical behavior (Eisenberg, 1997).

In journals and news sources, discussions of the ethics of complementary health care usually take one of two directions. First, there is a common argument that the complementary system keeps individuals from seeking needed attention in the medical system (Eisenberg, 1997; Kolata, 1996). Poorly trained or unethical complementary practitioners might well retain clients who would be better off seeing a conventional physician or being hospitalized. Yet medical practitioners also can be faulted for keeping individuals from seeking needed attention in the complementary system, even when there is convincing evidence that a condition can be better treated by low-tech therapies. For nearly a century and a half, the American Medical Association considered referrals by members to nonorthodox practitioners grounds for disciplinary action. Truly ethical care can come only when there is acceptance and mutual cooperation among practitioners of all philosophies.

The second issue often seen in conventional journals is the degree to which the health care system should incorporate complementary therapies, given the claims that they have not been scientifically validated. From the turn of the century until the early 1990s, physicians routinely refused to recognize or incorporate nonorthodox therapies, painting all with the broad brush "unscientific." In the last decade of the 20th century, in contrast, there has been a profound change in attitude, most likely due to the clear and growing market share of consumer dollars that complementary therapies are claiming. Suddenly, both community and academic medical centers have been establishing clinics, in-house services, and even academic departments dedicated to complementary therapies.

Incorporating complementary treatments into the conventional health care system is both welcome and ethically problematic. It is welcome because it legitimizes complementary care, provides therapies that are preventive in philosophical outlook, can often be practiced by non-physican personnel in outpatient settings, and expands the options available to people seeking healing. However, the rush to incorporate complementary practices into the health care system also offers ethical challenges. While the health care system has often fallen short of its promise to provide quality care, it is to no one's benefit to abandon it altogether. The health care system has a responsibility to evaluate complementary modalities honestly but critically.

The developing professionalization of complementary health care practices and its flirtation with conventional health care will continue to highlight the ethical concerns that confront both systems as they try to begin a period of closer cooperation. Most medical schools now have formal, ongoing courses in medical ethics and try to incorporate ethics into clinical training and continuing physician education. Complementary systems need to take ethics education as seriously. Both systems have much to learn from and to teach each other.

PAUL ROOT WOLPE

See

Acupuncture and Chinese Medicine (IV)

Chiropractic: Definition, History, and Theory (IV)

ETHICAL ISSUES IN BIOMEDICAL PHYSICIAN LICENSURE

The cultural authority of biomedical physicians is of relatively recent origin. Through the nineteenth century health practitioners were a heterogenous group with widely divergent theories about illness. Few had formal training. They offered their services in a free market, unrestricted by regulatory licensure and unaware of most of the scientific principles that now dominate modern medicine. Outcomes were mixed. With the help of the Carnegie Foundation, the American Medical Association (AMA) successfully campaigned to establish allopathic medicine as the dominant ideology, increase the admission standards, length, and scientific rigor of medical education, while decreasing the number of schools. "Regular" physicians' emphasis on scientific knowledge and improved outcomes convinced the public of their value and their ethical, altruistic aims. As a result, they won regulatory licensure under peer control in the early part of the twentieth century. "Irregular" practitioners were absorbed, conquered, or marginalized. The new profession gained autonomy, authority, and monopoly over what it chose to define as the practice of medicine. As the twentieth century ends, the hard-won consolidation of biomedical physicians is strained by the centrifugal force of specialization and some ethical dilemmas related to the nature of medical licensure.

When demand for biomedical physicians exceeded supply in the 1950s, the Federal government funded a massive increase in medical students and opened the door to foreign medical school graduates. By 1994 there were 276 physicians for every 100,000 people[1] (U.S. Bureau of the Census, 1996:173), compared to 155 in 1965 (U.S. Bureau of the Census, 1984:102). The increased supply intensified existing financial and technological pressures to specialize within medicine.

Physicians are a far less homogeneous occupational group than they were in the middle of the century. By 1994 only 11% were general or family practitioners and only 5% were general surgeons (Randolph, Seidman, & Pasko, 1996:21–22). The American Board of Medical Specialties (ABMS) is made up of 24 member boards that offer "board certification" in a specialty. They range from allergy and immunology to urology. All require additional education and experience, as well as the successful completion of comprehensive written and oral examinations for board certification. Many of these specialties offer additional certification in "subspecialties." Obstetrics and gynecology, for example, has subspecialties in gynecologic oncology, maternal and fetal medicine, and reproductive endocrinology. Specialization is an ongoing process fueled by innovation. There are at least 130 self-designated specialty boards that are not recognized by the ABMS (Gradinger, 1995). These boards also certify competence, although the rigor of their requirements varies. Some eventually may be accepted into the ABMS, as others have in the past.

In spite of the specialties that divide the actual practice of biomedical physicians, medical licensure encompasses all areas and contains no restrictions on practice, regardless of training. The AMA opposes

---

[1]This ratio was calculated using both the number of federal and nonfederal medical doctors and the number of doctors of osteopathic medicine, who have the same licensure rights as medical doctors.

specialty licensure, fearing it would create a rigid hierarchical division of labor and prevent physicians from changing their practices, if their interests change. The AMA additionally supports physicians' right to call themselves specialists in an area of practice without certification from a corresponding specialty board. The Federal Trade Commission (FTC) also endorses free trade within medicine and filed 27 health care antitrust cases between the mid 1970s and the mid 1980s to insure it. In the absence of either professional or government restrictions, regulation of specialty practice is left to informal peer control. Informal peer control, however, has eroded, creating some ethical dilemmas.

Lack of hospital privileges no longer precludes physicians from doing any surgery; most elective surgery now takes place outside hospitals. The potential for high profit in out-of-hospital surgery attracts physicians from a variety of surgical backgrounds and some with no surgical background. Office-based surgery raises questions not only about the adequacy of practitioner training, but also about safety equipment and protocols. Seeking to reestablish peer control over office-based surgery, some physicians formed voluntary accreditation programs and lobby to make accreditation mandatory. By mid 1997 California was the only state with such legislation. Risks are rampant with voluntary accreditation. A 1992 Department of Health and Human Services inspection of 160 facilities in four states revealed that 131 were neither licensed nor accredited, including 7 of 21 performing "high risk" procedures (*Plastic Surgery News*, 1993 (5):12). Over half have no written medical emergency protocol; 80 percent have no life support or resuscitation equipment. No comprehensive data on deaths or complications exist for out-of-hospital surgery, although the media have publicized a few deaths.

Referrals from other physicians also no longer control specialty practice. In 1982 the U.S. Supreme Court upheld the FTC's charge that long-standing bans on personal advertising by the AMA, local medical societies, and specialty associations violated the Sherman Antitrust Act. In spite of initial opposition among physicians, medical advertising has proliferated. Such blatant commercialization provokes complaints among physicians of unscrupulous fellow practitioners who advertise false or deliberately misleading statements about their personal expertise, treatment risks, and probable outcomes. Only a few states regulate medical advertising and their restrictions are minimal. Arizona ambiguously states that physicians cannot advertise as specialists "when such is not the case." Texas requires those who claim to be board-certified to name their board, but makes no distinction between self-designated boards and ABMS-member boards. Five other states acknowledge certification by ABMS-member boards as sufficient evidence to support advertising claims of specialty status, but also allow their medical licensure boards to determine "equivalent" evidence.

In conclusion, changes in the scope and complexity of medicine over the twentieth century have led to a highly structured division of labor among biomedical physicians. This change in the profession has not been matched by a corresponding change in the structure of physician licensure. Nevertheless, unwary consumers continue to assume that professional and governmental regulation of biomedical practitioners protects them from unqualified and unscrupulous practitioners. Their vulnerability to exploitation, especially for elective health care such as infertility treatment, vision correction, and cosmetic surgery, has been exacerbated by the trend toward out-of-hospital surgery and legalization of advertising. As a result, people are being sold treatments they do not need by biomedical physicians who may, or may not, be adequately trained in facilities that may, or may not, be adequately equipped and staffed.

DEBORAH A. SULLIVAN

HEALTH CARE PLURALISM

In contrast to indigenous or tribal societies, state societies manifest the coexistence of an array of health care systems, or a pattern of health care pluralism. From this perspective, the health care system of a society consists of the totality of subsystems that coexist in a cooperative or competitive relationship with one another.

Various social scientists have created typologies that recognize the phenomenon of health care pluralism in complex societies. Dunn (1976) delineated three types of health care systems based on their geographical and cultural settings: (1) local, (2) regional, and (3) cosmopolitan. Local health care systems are folk or indigenous systems of small-scale foraging, horticultural, or pastoral societies, or peasant communities in state societies. Regional systems are distributed over a relatively large geographical area, such as Ayurveda and Unani in south Asia and traditional Chinese medicine. Cosmopolitan health care refers to the global system or what commonly

has been termed "Western" or "allopathic medicine." Complex societies generally contain all three types of health care systems. For example, modern Japan has a variety of east Asian health care systems, including the local system of the Ainu, the aboriginal people of the Japanese archipelago. The most popular form of complementary health care in Japan today is *kanpo*, a form of herbal treatment that was brought to Japan from China in the 6th century. In addition to prescribing herbs, *kanpo* physicians administer acupuncture, manipulative therapy, and moxibustion.

Patterns of health care pluralism tend to reflect hierarchical relations based on class, caste, racial/ethnic, regional, religious, and gender distinctions in the larger society. Plural systems may be described as "dominative" in that one system generally enjoys a preeminent status over the others. Within the modern context, allopathic medicine exerts dominance over all complementary systems.

India, the second most populated country, is an outstanding example of a complex society exhibiting a dominative health care system. Leslie (1977) delineates five levels in the Indian dominative system: (1) allopathic medicine, which relies on physicians with M.D. or Ph.D. degrees from prestigious institutions; (2) "indigenous systems," which have within their ranks practitioners who have obtained degrees from Ayurvedic, Unani, and Siddha medical colleges; (3) homeopathy, whose physicians have completed correspondence courses; (4) religious scholars or learned priests with unusual healing abilities; and (5) local folk healers, bonesetters, and midwives. While approximately 150,000 physicians practiced allopathic medicine in India in the early 1970s, they were outnumbered by an estimated 400,000 practitioners of the three principal traditional medical systems: Ayurveda, which is based on Sanskrit texts; Unani, a Greek system based on Arabic and Persian texts; and Siddha, a traditional approach in south India (Leslie & Young, 1992). In addition to 95 allopathic colleges, India has 99 Ayurvedic colleges, 15 Unani ones, and a college of Siddha medicine.

The U.S. dominative health care system consists of several levels that tend to reflect class, racial/ethnic, and gender relations in the larger society (Baer, 1989). In rank order of prestige, these include (1) allopathic medicine, which has become highly capital-intensive and specialized; (2) osteopathic medicine as a parallel medical system focusing on primary care; (3) other professionalized systems (namely, chiropractic, naturopathy, and acupuncture); (4) partially professionalized systems (e.g., homeopathy, herbalism, rolfing, and reflexology); (5) Anglo-American religious healing traditions (e.g., spiritualism, Seventh-Day Adventism, Christian Science, and evangelical faith healing); and (6) folk or ethnic approaches (e.g., southern Appalachian and Ozark herbal treatments, African-American folk medicine, *curanderismo* among Mexican-Americans, *espiritismo* among Puerto Ricans, *santeria* among Cuban-Americans, *vodun* among Haitian-Americans, traditional Chinese medicine, and various Native American healing systems).

As a result of financial backing of initially corporate-sponsored foundations and later the federal government for its research activities and educational institutions, allopathic medicine evolved into the dominant health care system. It then asserted scientific superiority and clearly established authority over other professionalized health care disciplines, such as homeopathy, eclecticism, hydropathy, osteopathy, and chiropractic. Homeopathy and eclecticism have been somewhat absorbed by allopathic medicine at both the organizational and therapeutic levels. Chiropractic evolved into the leading professionalized health care system in the United States. Osteopathy initially constituted a manual treatment system founded by Andrew Taylor Still, a disenchanted allopathic physician who viewed the spine as the key to good health. It evolved into osteopathic medicine and surgery and achieved full practice rights in all 50 states and the District of Columbia by the early 1970s. At the beginning of the 20th century, hydropathy became part of naturopathy, a highly eclectic health care system. Naturopathy declined in the 1930s but has been undergoing a rejuvenation under the rubric of the holistic health movement.

Allopathic medicine's dominance over rival health care systems has never been absolute. The state, which primarily serves the interests of the corporate class, must periodically make concessions to subordinate social groups in the interests of maintaining social order and the capitalist mode of production. As a result, certain complementary practitioners, with the backing of clients and particularly influential patrons, were able to obtain legitimization in the form of full practice rights or limited practice rights. Lower social classes, racial and ethnic minorities, and women have often utilized complementary therapies as a forum for challenging not only allopathic dominance but also, to a degree, the hegemony of the corporate class or state elites. Complementary health care systems often resist, at least subtly, the elitist, hierarchical, and bureaucratic patterns of allopathic medicine. In contrast to allopathic medicine, which is dominated ultimately by the corporate class or state elites, folk healing systems are more generally the domain of common people. Unfortunately, folk healing has been used to obfuscate and confuse native peoples and working classes (Elling, 1981). Ethnic practitioners in the modern world have shown an increasing interest in acquiring new skills and using certain allopathic-like treatments or technologies in their work. Many third world peoples receive regular treatment from "injection doctors" and advice from pharmacists who may indiscriminately sell antibiotics and other drugs over the counter. Allopathic and complementary systems, despite antagonistic relations between them, exhibit a great deal of overlap and fusion.

The growing interest of corporate and governmental elites in complementary therapies is related to the cost of high-technology medical treatment. Even in countries where explicit financial and/or legal support is absent, governments often prefer to support complementary approaches because they focus on self-limiting diseases or diseases that tend to run their natural course without treatment. Bastien (1992) presented a favorable report of the efforts to integrate allopathic medicine and folk healing systems in Bolivia. Conversely, Philip Singer (1977) views the therapeutic alliance between allopathic and folk healers as a manifestation of a "new colonialism." An emancipatory therapeutic alliance ultimately requires an egalitarian relationship between various health care systems, one that transcends the hierarchical structure of existing dominative systems associated with capitalism.

HANS A. BAER

See

Acupuncture and Chinese Medicine (IV)
Ayurveda (IV)
Chiropractic: Definition, History, and Theory (IV)
Herbal Therapies (IV)
Reflexology (IV)
Rolfing: Structural Integration (IV)

FACTORS INFLUENCING THE USE OF COMPLEMENTARY HEALTH PRACTICES

Americans in record numbers are using complementary health practices. Therapies such as homeopathy and naturopathy are not new healing approaches. They are accepted medical practices in many parts of the world, including developed countries. In the United States they are enjoying a renaissance. Why is this occurring now?

Several factors are converging to fuel this movement. First, there is dissatisfaction with elements of Western allopathic medicine that focus on intervention by surgery, pharmaceutical remedies, and sophisticated technology rather than on prevention and less invasive techniques. Second, considered by some analysts as the most significant factor encouraging complementary approaches to health care is the generation that is "remaking America," the baby boomers currently beginning to enter their 50s (McGuire, 1988; Russell, 1993). And third, Americans are becoming more diverse culturally and ethnically. Using health care practices from other countries and cultures is a natural part of this diversity.

An element of dissatisfaction with Western allopathic medicine is the fact that it is expensive. With costs increasing yearly, basic health care is becoming out of reach of many Americans. Differentials in benefits and in access to health care is reflected in the chronic gap between the health of Americans who are rich and poor and white and black (Kilborn, 1998).

Complementary therapies satisfy the consumer desire for cost control and for information and empowerment, the very elements consumers often find lacking in allopathic medicine. These complementary options are viewed by many as promoting (1) shared decision making and more time for communication in the provider-client interaction, (2) an emphasis on spirituality and on the whole person, and (3) a focus on prevention and quality of life and on less invasive and dangerous treatment modalities.

The excessive use and reliance on high tech procedures and toxic drugs can injure, even kill, patients. Starr (1982) coined the term iatrogenic (from the Greek *iatros*, meaning doctor) to refer to illnesses that are induced inadvertently by a physician or a treatment. Examples of diagnostic procedures that could cause injury include taking sample pieces of tissue, injecting dyes into arteries, exposing patients to X rays, and injecting powerful drugs. Often simpler methods that are safer, cheaper, and equally helpful can be used in their place (Weil, 1995). Furthermore, allopathic medicine often has limited success in dealing with chronic health problems, such as arthritis, allergies, and asthma. With Americans living longer than in past generations, there is a desire for prevention and for safer ways to ameliorate the chronic health problems that tend to accompany old age.

Aging baby boomers are leading the consumer quest for wellness. The 76 million Americans born from 1946 to 1964 have reshaped the country with their attitudes, values, styles, and tastes. According to the U.S. Bureau of the Census (1996a), one of the 76 million will be hitting age 50 every 7.5 seconds for the next 15 years. By the year 2020, 16.4% of the country's population is expected to be 65 or older, up from the current 12.8%. Because boomers are likely to live longer than their parents, the over-65 population will just keep growing and will comprise 20% of the population by 2030.

Increased longevity indicates that the percentage of the population comprised of "middle-aged" seniors, those who are now ages 75 to 84, is growing at a faster rate than the population as a whole. The growth rate of people age 85 and older also is increasing. There is expanding interest in complementary health practices by seniors generally (Squires, 1996), and by aging baby boomers particularly.

This age cohort is so large that it has always driven the market for goods and services, from hula hoops and Barbie dolls to rock-and-roll music. Its sheer size dominates the demographic landscape. As members of this group age, they face a myriad of health problems and, in turn, increase the demand for health care. Their mindset and values favor prevention, self-help, and less invasive healing practices.

In addition to outnumbering previous generations, this generation of aging Americans differs from those that preceded it. They are well traveled and highly educated. As youths, some of them studied in other countries, experiencing other cultures and societies and healing practices. This firsthand exposure makes them more open to cross-cultural ideas about health and healing. Also, advances in worldwide communication, including television and computer communication networks, make the baby boomers the most globally aware generation.

Baby boomers are characterized by individualism, believing that self-interest of the individual supersedes the shared interest of the community. The belief in the primacy of the individual finds them "obsessed with their own bodies" (Russell, 1993, p. 164). They form enormous markets for products and services that promise to stop or slow the aging process. Millions belong to local health clubs and are turning to anti aging remedies, including natural foods, herbs, and vitamins. Also, there is an increasing use of cosmetic surgery.

Baby boomers are interested in a spiritual quest for the meaning of life. Their interpretation of spiritual is a private expression of faith, not necessarily an institutionalized religious faith. Spiritual therapies such as meditation, hypnotherapy, and psychic and faith healing are compatible with their belief structure.

Given these characteristics, the baby boom generation is bringing about change with respect to a middle-class healing movement. McGuire's benchmark study (1988) documented this movement by depicting adherents to various forms of non-medical healing as middle class, middle aged, well educated, socially, culturally, and residentially established suburbanites who were generally female and white. Consumer studies (Emerich, 1996) report that more than members of the baby boom generation find natural health products and practices appealing. Young mothers in their 20s as well as older people in the 60s and beyond are searching for natural,

effective, and safe health care solutions and for ways to prevent illness for themselves and their families.

A nationwide *New York Times*/CBS News telephone poll that questioned men and women on health issues reported that women, especially those who are young and well educated, say they are open to complementary health practices and willing to do their own research. The popularity of alternative medicine was evident. Nearly 4 in 10 women say they have either tried alternative medicine or thought about trying it (Elder, 1997).

Another important factor fueling the use of complementary health practices is that Americans are becoming more diverse culturally and ethnically. Seventy-three percent of the total U.S. population in 1996 (265 million) was white (excluding Hispanic, which is included in a separate category). This is projected to shrink to 70% of the total in 2010 and to 52.7% in 2050 (U.S. Bureau of the Census, 1996b, Table 1). By the year 2056, the U.S. Census Bureau projects an even split in the percentage of white and non-white populations.

Data on the extent to which racial and ethnic minorities are using complementary therapies are sparse in the research literature. Two major systematic studies of patterns of usage of complementary health practices underrepresented race and ethnicity. Eisenberg and his colleagues (1993) excluded non-English speaking respondents from the survey and underrepresented certain minority groups in the sample. McGuire's (1988) suburban study area was almost exclusively white, thereby limiting the representativeness of its results to racial and ethnic minority populations. We do know that a rich cultural complex lies behind health care seeking behavior. It is known that such specific practices as *root-work*, *curanderismo*, medicinal plants, and faith healing thrive in many communities throughout the country. *Rootwork, Hoodoo,* and *Voodoo* are all terms used to refer to a wide variety of traditional African American medical, religious, and magical beliefs and practices. Root doctors practice a mixture of syncretic Christian healing, voodoo, and herbalism. They are still common in rural North Carolina. *Curanderismo*, based on the Spanish word "curar" (to heal), is the Mexican American system of folk medicine and healing that combines herbal medicines with religion. *Curanderos(as)* act as specialists in medical information and healing for Hispanic cultures in the U.S. They are still common in Arizona, Texas, and other Southwestern states (Gordon, Nienstedt, & Gesler, 1998).

In summary, many factors play a role in the increasing popularity of complementary health practices, including the high cost of allopathic medicine, its *iatrogenic* effects, and the exclusion of spirituality in healing the whole person. The overarching factor operating in this movement is the sheer number, values, and characteristics of baby boomers entering middle age. Because the demand for health services will continue to increase as this cohort ages, the use of complementary health practices also will increase. The trend toward cultural and ethnic diversity of the American population also is a likely factor in expecting cross-cultural healing practices to increase in the 21st century.

RENA J. GORDON

See
Complementary Folk or Ethnic Approaches (I)

Homeopathy: Use in Family Practice Medicine (IV)
Native American Medicine (IV)
Spiritual/Religious Approaches (IV)

MIND-BODY APPROACHES

Mind-body approaches refer to a broad range of interventions and techniques generated from research in the last 40 years (Lazar, 1996). Such strategies use mental techniques to positively affect physical and biochemical functioning.

In the United States and Europe, attention and research in mind-body approaches has been rapidly increasing. However, the roots of these investigations have been used for thousands of years in Eastern cultures. This history has generated a conceptualization of mind-body as an interactive, coinfluential process.

The mind-body response is a complex neuroendocrine interaction generated by such conditions as fear, anxiety, physical trauma, pain, fever, hypothermia, or malnutrition. The mind-body response mobilizes energy to avoid injury or to repair it. It has been most extensively studied in the hypothalamo-pituitary-adrenocortical system and the hypothalamo-sympatho-adrenomedullary system but also involves others, such as insulin, glucagon, vasopressin, growth hormone, testosterone, and interleukins. The evolutionary development of this mind-body system presumes that the source of all energy is endogenous and generated from multiple internal sources (Kessler & Whalen, 1998). Mind-body interactions in everyday life have self-regulating predictable consequences, which in the West have been viewed as health care problems or pathology.

In the 1970s, the U.S. Surgeon General presented evidence that Americans were at greater risk of dying from behavioral factors and unhealthy lifestyles than from biological pathology. Some studies find that 60% of all visits to physicians fail to result in a confirmed medical diagnosis (Sobel, 1993).

Insufficiently attended to, mind-body problems have significant consequences. Mind-body problems make up approximately 25% of visits to primary care and in some estimates half or more of hospitalizations for illness, and 50% of mind-body problems seen by health care practitioners are not identified (Friedman et al., 1996; Academy of Psychosomatic Medicine, 1996). Individuals with untreated mind-body issues make up some of the largest utilizers of health care. Mind-body issues are particularly implicated in chronic illnesses, including neurologic disorders, heart disease, and cancer.

There is considerable evidence that intervening in mind-body problems assists their resolution. Mind-body interventions have reversed coronary artery disease; mind-body preparation prior to surgery has reduced blood loss during surgery. Mind-body medicine interventions have been shown to reduce total ambulatory care visits by 17%, reduce visits for minor illnesses by 36%, reduce pediatric acute illness visits by 25%, reduce cesarean sections by 56%, and reduce epidural anesthesia in labor and delivery by 85% (Sobel, 1993).

Major Techniques

Major techniques of mind/body approaches include meditation, imagery, relaxation training, biofeedback, stress inoculation, and hypnosis.

Meditation is probably the oldest mind-body technique, and the one from which contemporary techniques draw most heavily. The goal of meditation is to shape the capacity for self-observation. Many meditative techniques consist of focusing attention on some aspect of one's experience, such as the in-and-out flow of one's breath. The focus may be active, such as focusing on a particular word or phrase, or passive, such as merely observing one's thoughts or the flow of one's experience throughout the day's activities.

Imagery may be part of meditative practice. "Guided imagery" is frequently referred to as a technique in mind-body literature. Individuals vary widely in the vividness or intensity of their imagery. Capacity to become absorbed in fantasy is one of the correlates of measured hypnotic capacity, and it may be that individuals who respond well to imagery alone are also capable of using hypnosis (Dane & Kessler, 1994).

Relaxation training combines the focused attention of meditation with conscious intent to alter physiology through the addition of instructions about specific physiological procedures. These procedures focus primarily on alterations of breathing, alterations of muscle contractions, or alterations of sensation. Physiologic relaxation is specifically targeted by these techniques, with the assumption that affective relaxation is likely to follow.

Biofeedback uses equipment to monitor and translate the physiologic experience of relaxation (e.g., muscle tension, heart rate, blood pressure, skin temperature, galvanic skin response) and to use this relaxation to assist symptom change.

Hypnosis is often confused with the use of one or more of the above techniques, particularly distraction, relaxation, and imagery. It is true that hypnosis resembles many aspects of these other techniques. Likewise, similar types of physiological outcomes are often accomplished with either hypnosis or one of the other techniques. Hypnosis is a state of highly focused attention on internal processes that results in increased receptivity to a variety of suggestions for change and healing.

RODGER KESSLER

MIND-BODY CONNECTION

The concept of a mind-body connection evolved from psychosomatic medicine. Today, the most comprehensive concept for this connection is psychoneuroimmunology (PNI), which focuses on the connection between the mind, the neuroendocrine system (nervous and hormonal system), and the immune system. PNI is defined as a "discipline that studies the relationships between psychologic states and the immune response" (*Mosby's Medical, Nursing, & Allied Health Dictionary*, 1994).

Although incomplete from a scientific point of view, PNI is currently the most unifying theory of the mind-body connection. Multiple factors in humans and the environment are associated with health and illness, such as poor nutrition; intake of excessive candy, food, or alcohol; genetic predisposition; environmental toxins; age; gender; stress; trauma; and emotions. A part of this multifactoral framework is PNI—the effect of emotions and the mind on the immune system and body as it influences health and illness. In addition to the influence of emotions on the body, individuals use their mind to make decisions that influence illnesses and health, such as what to eat and whether or not to drink alcohol.

There are three major concepts in the PNI theory: (1) psychological distress suppresses the immune system; (2) psychological distress increases the risk of illnesses; and (3) individuals can work with their mind and emotions to increase their resistance to illnesses.

Psychological Distress and Immunity

Psychological distress suppresses the immune system through the nervous system, which communicates with the immune systems using bidirectional chemical signals. Stress is an important concept in this relationship. Enlarging upon the work of Cannon (1939), Selye (1978) showed that the body currently continues to react to stress in a fight or flight manner as if it were facing a real physical threat.

Stress may be acute or chronic. During chronic stress, the immune system suppresses or becomes less active and other serious physiological changes may occur. The normal blood pressure elevation of acute stress becomes hypertension, a prolonged increase in the heart rate may increase the risk of arrhythmia, and other symptoms may lead to serious physiological changes. The immune system then becomes depressed, making the individual susceptible to acute or chronic illnesses.

Reactions to stress are governed by the autonomic nervous system, which has two branches: the sympathetic system, which regulates the arousal response to stress, and the parasympathetic, which assists the body to relax and return to a normal mode.

Psychological Distress and Illness

The effect of psychological distress can increase the risk of illness through chronic stress, which may impair the function of the immune system and play a role in a variety of illnesses. Holmes and Rahe (1967) published research and concluded that a combination of life changes was likely to lead to high-stress reactions and illness. Although further research showed that there is no simple direct relationship between life stresses and illness, some of the theories developed to account for variations in people becoming or not becoming ill following life changes showed promise of adding to the theory. These include (1) the generic disease-prone personality (depression, anger/hostility, anxiety) that may increase the risk of illness; (2) coping methods (mood, personality characteristics, coping style, hopelessness) that influence how individuals deal with stress and may influence the immune system and illness; and (3) social networks that may buffer the effect of stress and, thus, influence health and illness.

The Mind, Immunity, and Illness

People can learn to work with emotions and thoughts and thus increase their immunological resistance to diseases or to influence recovery. Stress management techniques assist individuals to activate the parasympathetic system and to lower blood pressure, heart rate, and other physiological parameters. Mind-body approaches such as relaxation, visualization, stress management, and beliefs in the healer can influence emotions and thoughts and may have a positive effect on the immune system and health (Flowers, 1993).

Research Base

The following selected studies show the influence of the mind and emotions on illness or recovery. David Spiegel and colleagues (1989) studied 86 women with ad-

vanced metastatic cancer. In addition to the standard medical treatment received by all, one half received group therapy and learned self-hypnosis for pain relief. Women in the study group lived twice as long as the control group and the three women who survived were all in the study group.

Williams and colleagues (1980) found a relationship between hostility and coronary artery disease and coronary artery blockage. Ornstein and Sobel (1988) studied a variety of lifestyle changes used with coronary heart patients. After 1 year, subjects making lifestyle changes that were a combination of mind-body approaches and a low-fat diet showed a reversal in their atherosclerosis without medications. Benson (1996) discussed research on the influence of the mind (beliefs in the healer and their treatment) on recovery from illness and the influence of the relaxation response, a mind-body approach on recovery. Kabbat-Zinn (1994) encouraged patients to use the mind to relieve pain. In his "pain clinic" at the University of Massachusetts, Kabbat-Zinn teaches meditation and yoga and has had success relieving pain. Kemeny and Solomon (1993) used hypnosis with melanoma patients and reduced the rate of recurrence. A controlled study by Cohen, Tyrell, and Smith (1991) showed that stress can increase the risk of infections (the common cold). Additional research can be found in Goleman and Gurin (1993).

CARL O. HELVIE

ENERGY AND ITS RELATIONSHIP TO DISEASE

The difference between cells, tissues, and organisms that are sick, and those that are healthy is their relative level of energy. A system that has no energy is dead. But exactly what is energy? Where does it come from? Where does it go when it is used? Energy is derived from *érgon*, a Greek word for "work," and for practical purposes, energy may be defined as the ability to do work. The prefix *en* signifies "at" and is the basis of *enérgeio*, a noun used by Aristotle to signify something that is active, or moving, which we refer to as kinetic energy. However, energy also includes the capacity for doing work, which can exist in many different forms that have no visible motion. Energy stored in a compressed spring or battery is referred to as potential energy. A roller coaster car at the top of a loop has gravitational potential energy, electrical charges possess electrostatic potential energy, and there is also the invisible potential energy stored in foods, fuels, and chemical compounds.

Heat, light, electrical, and mechanical energies can be converted back and forth into each other, or into sound. During these, as well as chemical reactions, there is either a gain or loss of heat in the systems involved due to changes in molecular or submolecular activities. This heat exchange is governed by thermodynamic laws, which state that energy can never be created or destroyed but only transformed. In addition, during the conversion of energy from one form to another, some energy is degraded, or "lost" with respect to its availability to do the work of the system. This process, called "entropy," is readily illustrated by Albert Einstein's example of energy transfers in a roller coaster. As the car ascends the first steep rise, it acquires potential energy as it progressively resists the force of gravity. After it passes over the peak, this potential energy is increasingly converted into kinetic energy as the car accelerates back toward earth. Kinetic energy is again steadily transformed into potential energy as the car climbs up the second incline, and this sequence of events is repeated over and over, with potential energy being maximal at the top of each successive loop. If this conversion back and forth between potential and kinetic energy were absolutely complete, then the car would always attain the same height on the ascending loop, and the same speed during its descent, and we would have perpetual motion. However, we all know that this does not happen, because of friction between the wheels of the car and the rails, which creates heat. Although heat is also a form of energy, it is not available to help move the car, and thus represents entropy.

Entropy also occurs in the energy transfers of chemical reactions. The energy in biologic systems comes from the process of photosynthesis, during which chlorophyll in plants utilizes light to convert carbon dioxide and water into oxygen and energy-rich chemicals that can be stored. Chlorophyll is similar in structure to hemoglobin, except that it contains magnesium instead of iron. Respiration in animals is the exact opposite of photosynthesis. During inspiration, oxygen attaches to hemoglobin and is distributed to cells along with other nutrients by the bloodstream. Waste products are picked up in exchange, and carbon dioxide and water are released into the atmosphere during expiration. The energy generated from both photosynthesis and respiration is stored in the powerful phosphate bonds of ATP (adenosine triphosphate). Chlorophyll converts solar energy into ATP that can be stored in plants to promote growth or other activities. Animals also store the energy obtained from foods in the strong phosphorus bonds of this remarkable molecule, which is found in the mitochondria of all cells.

Since biologic systems are governed by the same thermodynamic laws as machines, entropy occurs in all chemical as well as mechanical reactions. In the roller coaster, the cars keep going because electrical energy makes up for the loss of work due to entropy. Electricity can also be used to provide light and heat for the roller coaster system to use freely in any way that it chooses. Similarly, when ATP is hydrolyzed and phosphorus becomes detached, the powerful force from its bond is released for the cell to use for any of its functions. This is referred to as free energy, or the free energy of Gibbs, in honor of Josiah Willard Gibbs, who formulated the concept of chemical potential energy and who first applied the concept of entropy to living systems.

Recent research suggests that minuscule magnetic forces may increase this free energy of Gibbs, much like electricity provides energy for the roller coaster system to use for any purpose it requires. Magnetic fields have been shown to augment the buildup of ATP high-energy phosphate bonds that provide the power for all cellular functions (Sodi Pallares, 1997). Diseases due to energy deficiencies in specific cells might therefore be benefited, if this deficit could be corrected by increasing ATP or by reducing entropy. Magnetic-field therapies appear to have this potential, which may explain why they have been found to improve so many very different disorders, ranging from cancer, cardiomyopathy, and fractures that have failed to heal for years to Parkinson's disease, insomnia, and drug resistant depression (Rosch, 1998). Keiu-

chi Nakagawa and other Japanese investigators believe that many cases of chronic fatigue are due to a magnetic deficiency syndrome and report marked improvement following the application of permanent magnets (Nakagawa, 1976).

Conversely, there have been concerns that weak environmental electromagnetic energies emanating from high-power lines, cellular telephones, and household electrical appliances can cause cancer, birth defects, and other health problems. It has been clearly demonstrated that such very subtle stimuli can have profound effects on cellular growth and function that do not involve any measurable heat exchange and are thus not regulated by current laws of thermodynamics. It has been postulated that energies of a similar weak magnitude generated internally can also have biologic effects. EEG and ECG waves may not merely be a reflection of the noise of the machinery of the brain and heart, but rather signals that are being sent to specialized receptor sites elsewhere in the body (Rosch, 1994). This is consistent with an emerging paradigm that posits an electrical circulatory system (Nordenström, 1983) and could explain such widely acknowledged but poorly understood phenomena as the placebo effect, faith healing, the power of a strong faith in spontaneous remission in cancer, the salubrious effects of certain olfactory, auditory, visual, and tactile stimuli, and certain psychokinetic observations (Rosch, 1994).

The proposal that the level or orderly flow of energy in the body determines health and illness has surfaced over the years as *qi*, (*chi*), *chakras, prana, archaeus, animal magnetism, Odic force, orgone*, and various constructs in different cultures (Lawrence, Rosch, & Plowden,

1998). Acupuncture points known since antiquity have electrical properties quite different from surrounding sites, even though no distinctions can be seen with electron microscopy, and these energy characteristics can be influenced by mental processes. Energy fields emanating from healers can be readily demonstrated through various photographic techniques, but only while they are engaged in their activities. The powerful external force generated by *chi gong* masters, as well as the ability of certain renowned healers to produce voltage surges of 100 volts and more in recipients several feet away and separated by a copper wall have been well documented in scientific studies (Muehsam et al., 1993; Green, Parks, Guer, Fahrion, & Coyne, 1991).

The potential to cure disease and enhance health by harnessing such natural energies, as well as similar forces that can be artificially generated, seems enormous. Highly sophisticated technologies may now make it possible to achieve this goal and to integrate ancient Eastern and current Western concepts of health and illness.

PAUL J. ROSCH

See
Acupuncture and Chinese Medicine (IV)
Therapeutic Touch: Definition, History, and Theory (IV)

ENERGY FIELDS

The Einstein paradigm views human beings as networks of energy fields that interface with cellular systems (Gerber, 1988). In this paradigm, all cells and body tissues have electrical and magnetic characteris-

tics. Electrocardiograms and electroencephalograms (EEG) register these potentials. The placebo effect and the emission of illness through faith can be explained by energy field theory: EEG waves are not just noisy machinations of the brain, but are messages being sent to specialized receptor sites on cell walls, reinforcing health. It is not known how this electrical or energy balance is maintained and regulated, although many complementary therapists theorize that when the human energy field is out of balance, disease occurs. The concepts of qi (*chi*), *prana*, and *chakras* are all energy concepts used by complementary practitioners, based on energy flow.

CAROLYN CHAMBERS CLARK

See
Acupuncture and Chinese Medicine (IV)
Ayurveda (IV)
Magnet Therapy (IV)
Nutrition (IV)
Therapeutic Touch: Definition, History, and Theory (IV)
Vegetarianism (IV)

BIOAVAILABILITY

The absorbed portion of an ingested food or nutritional supplement mineral that is available for metabolic processes, and the promotion of enhanced tissue levels is referred to as its bioavailability. Interaction most commonly occurs at the intestinal absorption site. Minerals consumed in the same meal or supplement may compete for absorption. The bioavailability of a food or supplement is also affected negatively by illness, maldigestion, injury, surgery, drugs, alcohol, anatomical defects, and naturally occurring antinutrients.

Factors that affect the absorption of minerals include the following:

1. Unsprouted seeds and grains. These contain phytic acid, which forms a strong complex with minerals, including calcium, copper, iron, magnesium, and zinc; malting and soaking can enhance absorption of zinc and iron (Larsson, Rossander-Hulthen, Sandstrom, & Sandberg, 1996).
2. Fiber. This reduces the contact time between food and the intestines and can reduce the bioavailability of calcium, iron, and zinc.
3. Coffee and tea. Both increase urinary excretion of calcium. When coffee is consumed within an hour of a meal, it can reduce iron absorption by as much as 80%.
4. Fortified foods. Such foods are nutrient dense but, in terms of bioavailability, are nutrient poor.
5. Oxylates. Found in spinach and some other vegetables, these can reduce absorption of calcium.
6. Lactose. Milk sugar and other simple sugars may improve the bioavailability of calcium and other minerals.
7. High-protein diets. Such diets increase the excretion of calcium.
8. Vitamin C. Vitamin C improves the absorption of iron but may reduce selenium absorption.
9. Stainless steel cookware. Food prepared in stainless steel pots and pans can increase chromium intake, whereas food prepared in iron cookware increases iron intake.

Bioavailability is not the same as nutrient density. It is possible to have a food with a high density of minerals that contains other dietary factors, such as phytates or oxalates, which impair the absorption of minerals. Likewise, although fortified foods are nutrient dense, they are often poorly absorbed. In a study to identify the factors affecting absorption of copper and zinc in vegetarian men (Sandstead, 1995), the percent of absorption of copper and zinc was estimated during six metabolic experiments, each of 2 weeks' duration. Dietary factors found to enhance absorption of zinc included hemicellulose, milk protein, niacin, and cereal protein. Thiamine, phytate, oxalates, ascorbic acid, and phosphorus acted as inhibitors. Copper absorption was enhanced by dietary levels of riboflavin, cellulose, milk proteins, oxalates, and zinc, and inhibited by phosphorus, niacin, calcium, and pulse protein (Agte, Chiplowkar, Joshi, & Paknikar, 1994) and by zinc (Sandstead, 1995). Copper deficiency is related to abnormal cardiac function (Sandstead, 1995). The type of dietary fiber may also influence mineral absorption.

Other studies found that pectin and cellulose bran lowered plasma cholesterol in rats and enhanced absorption of iron, zinc, and magnesium to a greater extent than oat and wheat bran dietary fiber (Galibois, Desrosiers, Guevin, Lavigne, & Jacques, 1994); haem-iron absorption is inhibited by calcium intake (Hallberg, Rossander-Hulthen, Brune, & Gleerup, 1993); calcium transport is enhanced by polyunsaturated fatty acids, which may influence the action of vitamin D3 on calcium absorption (Coetzer et al., 1994).

Both zinc and magnesium are widely used as nutritional supplements. However, it is possible that zinc interferes with the absorption of magnesium, as it has been shown to do with calcium. To test this theory, Spencer, Norris, and Williams (1994) conducted a study of three groups of adult males in a metabolic research unit. Each was given supplemental doses of 142 mg of zinc as zinc sulfate during calcium intakes of 230, 500, and 800 mg/day. The overall effect of the high zinc intake was a highly significant decrease in magnesium absorption, regardless of calcium intake.

CAROLYN CHAMBERS CLARK

See
Nutrition (IV)

HEALING CEREMONIES

The rising popularity and efficacy of complementary therapies are testimony to the need to integrate emotional, mental, and spiritual aspects of an individual's life with physically based techniques such as medication and surgery. Whether used consciously or not, the foundation of all healing interactions is contained in the ceremonial circumstances in which healers interact with clients (Miller, 1992). The physician's prescription pad, the surgeon's knife, the acupuncturist's needles, the masseuse's touch, and the shaman's drum all rely on the careful use of objects, beliefs, and rituals that become a ceremony, directing the physical, emotional, mental, and spiritual resources of the patients toward a complete healing.

Why are *ceremonies* so important? They provide the structure by which people get in touch with feelings. Feelings rather than thoughts, beliefs, and hopes rather than certainties, can get people through difficult times. The entire science of *psychoneu-*

roimmunology now gives credence to what before were thought of as superstitions. Feelings like stress, depression, and isolation suppress the immune system's ability to fend off disease, whereas those of love, attachment, and prayer can strengthen the immune response (Hammerschlag & Silverman, 1997).

Even such simple ceremonies as shared mealtimes and holiday observances provide a connectedness that promotes healing. Studies have shown that families with few or no ritual observances have a much greater occurrence of alcoholism than families in which even these simple rituals were performed (Wolin & Bennett, 1984).

Ceremonies provide strong connections between the participants, and social support mitigates against the harmful effects of stressful life events. For example, studies have shown that women with cancer who participate in support groups live longer than those without such groups (Spiegel, 1994), divorced and widowed people (especially men) have a much higher risk of dying than married people of the same age (Hu & Goldman, 1990), and marital conflict has negative effects on the immune system (Kiecolt-Glaser et al., 1987). Social isolation is a major risk factor for mortality from widely varying causes (House, Landis, & Umberson, 1988).

Ceremonies allow people to get some control over their lives by telling their stories in a new and more functional way. Chronic negativity or pessimism directed at a child is a predictor of depressive symptoms later in life (Noen-Hoeksema, Seligman, & Girgus, 1992). One's view of the world can also predict immune system dysfunction. Researchers studying elderly men and women have found that "a pessimistic style might be an important psychological risk factor (at least among older people) in the early course of certain immune-mediated diseases" (Kamen-Siegel, Rodin, Seligman, & Dwyer, 1991, p. 229). Such diseases include cancer, asthma, and arthritis. There is also data showing that people in old age homes live longer when they have a choice about food, furniture arrangements, plants, or pets (Langer & Rodin, 1976; Rodin, 1986).

Ceremonies can be connected to family or religious traditions; however, it can often be difficult to integrate them into health care. In many cases, it is necessary to adapt an existing ceremony or to create an entirely new ritual to be part of one's care. Many complementary practitioners intuitively understand the significance of the ceremony in their treatment modalities and devise ways to enhance these elements. They may turn down the lights, play special music, light candles, use incense, and tell stories.

The steps necessary to create an effective ceremony have been summarized (Hammerschlag & Silverman, 1997). First, identify the purpose of the ceremony and communicate this purpose clearly to all who will be present. Part of the purpose of every ceremony is to separate the group from the ordinary and to invite, even to expect, something extraordinary to occur. Second, select a facilitator and define the community of people who will attend. Third, prepare the ceremonial space, objects, and processes to be used during the ceremony. Finally, the *community* comes together, and the ceremony is performed under the guidance of the facilitator. The senses are heightened by the use of *sacraments* (drums, foods, wine, tobacco, etc.). When these substances are indiscriminately used, that is, outside the appropriate ceremonial container, they are frequently subject to abuse.

Ceremonies are a powerful tool to work through expected and unexpected life transitions. They are a time when feelings are shared and new possibilities are entertained. The group moves through the experience together and emerges renewed and reenergized. When properly designed and performed, they are particularly well suited to enhance the power and beauty of traditional allopathic and complementary clinical interventions.

CARL A. HAMMERSCHLAG
HOWARD D. SILVERMAN

See
Ritual As a Creative Healing Experience (IV)

Section 2

Economic and Practice Issues

THE ECONOMICS OF COMPLEMENTARY HEALTH PRACTICES

In economics, a market is the arena in which buyers and sellers negotiate for a particular commodity. The price and quantity of the commodity are determined through this interaction of supply (i.e., producers) and demand (i.e., consumers). Microeconomics is the study of markets at the level of the individual—the individual consumer (on the demand side of the market) and the individual producer (on the supply side). If the market were a forest, microeconomics would be the study of its trees.

Increasingly, health care is looked upon as a commodity, by both individual consumers and providers. On the demand side, microeconomists study health care markets and want to know how individual consumers make their consumption decisions (i.e., what complementary health services to buy, how much to buy, and when). On the supply side, microeconomists try to understand how the providers of these health practices decide how and how much to produce.

Demand Side

If the price of a commodity goes down, consumers tend to buy more of it. If the price goes up, they buy less. Price and quantity demanded are inversely related (i.e., they move in opposite directions). In the health care marketplace, where most consumers have some form of health insurance (Cockerham, 1998), there are two prices: the price the provider charges (i.e., the market price) and the amount consumers pay (i.e., their out-of-pocket expenditure). Consumer demand for health care is determined more by out-of-pocket expenditure than by the market price. For example, if insurance coverage improves (covers more services) and out-of-pocket expenditures decline, consumers tend to buy more health care. This is the case even if health care market prices increase. As insurance coverage worsens (covers less) and consumers are forced to pay more for their health care, they tend to buy less.

Most complementary health practices have not been covered by health insurance. In this era of tightfisted budgets, few insurance companies seem willing to extend their coverage to any new group of providers, such as acupuncturists, nutritionists, and massage therapists. They believe, perhaps wrongly, that new services would not replace or have a substitution effect on existing ones, but would be an addition to them and would have an add-on effect (Weber, 1996). Ultimately, they believe that adding services would cost them more money. As a result, for the most part, only those consumers able to pay out-of-pocket for their complementary health care can buy it.

However, these consumption patterns are changing. An increasing number of state and local governments, insurance companies and managed care plans have started paying for some complementary practices, such as naturopathy, reflexology, and homeopathy. They consider these alternatives to biomedicine to be safer, cheaper, and, in many cases, customer preferred (Weber,1996). For example, the city of Seattle established a naturopathic health clinic. It is supported by tax revenues and employs both naturopaths and medical physicians. It is the country's first such clinic.

In the insurance industry, companies like Prudential, the Seattle-based Health Cooperative of Puget Sound, and Mutual of Omaha now cover acupuncture, midwife-assisted home births, and low-fat vegetarian diets for heart disease patients, respectively. Some health maintenance organizations, including one of the nation's fastest growing (Oxford Health Plans), are allowing enrollees to choose alternative healers, such as naturopaths and homeopaths, as their primary care physicians (Eisenberg, 1997). These changes are increasing the demand for complementary health care more widely across the income groups (Colt, 1996).

Supply Side

Most providers of health care seek to efficiently allocate their resources and maximize their profits. When the market is not clearly defined, as is the case for many of the complementary health practices, health care providers often use cost-benefit analysis to help them decide how much to produce (or how many services to provide) (Folland, Goodman, & Stano, 1997, p. 562). If cost exceeds benefit, production does not occur at all (services are not provided), and resources are allocated elsewhere.

Although this approach to resource allocation has many shortcomings, it is especially biased against most complementary health practices. Because these practices are primarily preventative, their full benefits are neither easily quantifiable nor immediately apparent. However, their costs are just the opposite—they are relatively easy to calculate and are immediately apparent. Consequently, cost benefit analysis, which measures everything in dollars over relatively short periods of time, systematically underestimates the benefits of complementary health care, while fully capturing all of its costs. In short, it rarely supports the production of complementary health practices. This may be changing. Recently, Mutual of Omaha calculated the costs and benefits of providing a health prevention program. It reported saving $6.50 for every dollar spent on Dr. Dean Ornish's diet and wellness plan for preventing and reversing heart disease (Gordon & Silverstein, 1998). Insurance companies that are able to capture the savings from disease prevention will likely be the ones to flourish in the dynamic health care marketplace (Caplan, 1996).

RONALD L. CAPLAN

See
Acupuncture and Chinese Medicine (IV)
Homeopathy: Molecular Basis (IV)
Midwifery (IV)
Reflexology (IV)
Vegetarianism (IV)

COMPLEMENTARY HEALTH CENTERS AND NETWORKS

In the late 1990s, a significant number of "complementary care" centers and networks have emerged as public interest has grown and third-party payers have begun to consider their inclusion. There are more than 130 such centers being planned or under way within conventional medical institutions. In addition, many are appearing as teams and networks of private practitioners join in collaborative efforts. The current scene is one of exploration and innovation, hence one cannot yet describe the optimal models or best programs. An overview map of what seems to be happening and some probable trends are described below.

Types of Centers and Networks

Three factors will be compared here: (1) what disciplines are included, (2) a view of the participant's process, and (3) how the various models are integrated; that is, how the different views of life, health, and disease that are offered by the several disciplines are recognized and related to one another.

Complementary Practices Offered in Medical Center Settings

This is a rapidly growing phenomenon. It most frequently involves acupuncture, relaxation therapies, massage and/or therapeutic touch, and psycho-emotional support work and groups.

The individual process is through physician referral within the hospital system and is almost always diagnosis-based. In other words, acupuncture may become a referral possibility for pain management; relaxation therapies, massage, and support may be offered for cancer patients, surgery recovery, or trauma rehabilitation patients. Thus, the complementary practices are seen essentially as additional technologies to be applied within the conventional medical model of diagnosis and treatment of disease, not as systems with their own organizing principles.

Frequently, there is little if any effort to integrate or explore the several models of health and healing offered by complementary practices. A tendency develops to frame them in the current managed care

model of time-limited visits and application of technique according to formalized treatment protocols. Further evidence is needed to determine whether this is an effective application of complementary practices. An ever-present risk is that ineffectiveness in this model could be generalized and the conclusion reached that complementary practices were unnecessary added costs.

Multidisciplinary Clinics

Any number of these are springing up across the country, and they follow no single model. Two of the most prominent are the clinic sponsored by Mercy Healthcare Arizona in Phoenix and the King County Center in Kent, Washington.

The Phoenix Center operates with a physician gatekeeper and refers individuals to staff practitioners of a number of complementary practices. Individuals may arrive referred to a specific practitioner. In keeping with the emerging business practice of being competitive (as compared to the historic practice in medicine of sharing the best research), the Phoenix clinic has not provided its internal rationales and practices.

The Kent clinic was established under sponsorship of the King County government, and is related to and operated by leaders from the Bastyr Naturopathic University. Hence, its general organizing process will no doubt vary from the Phoenix model, especially since it is a public institution.

All such clinics face similar organizational challenges: (1) credentialization of unconventional practitioners; (2) selection of appropriate practices to include in the center; (3) legal and liability precedents that shape our health care world; (4) issues of treatment process and how best to select appropriate interventions and in what order; and (5) data management, or how to monitor treatment progress and evaluate outcomes.

Practitioner Forums and Exchanges

Although no doubt destined to spawn some coordinated clinical services, these groups have grown out of a different interest: Practitioners wanting to learn about one another, what they do, and how they can work collaboratively. The two most visible ones so far are the Health Medicine Forum in Walnut Creek, California, and the Alliance for Holistic Health in southern Florida. Each group has more than 350 practitioners of many disciplines meeting regularly in seminars and workshops, publishes a regular newsletter, and continues to seek clearer understanding of the potential contributions of collaborative approaches.

Perhaps one of the most interesting developments from these forums is the "panel interview." In this format, an individual presents a case to a panel of several practitioners. Such a panel might include a physician, a chiropractor, a Chinese medicine/ acupuncture practitioner, a homeopath, a psychologist, and perhaps a body worker/ energy practitioner. Each member of the panel has an opportunity to do a workup prior to the open presentation, then discusses the possibilities the case offers.

One observation of this process is that it appears to immediately lift the participant's hopes, sometimes moving from a place of relative hopelessness to becoming energized and motivated that improvement can be achieved. In the first presentation of such a panel review at the Health Medicine Forum, a woman who had been on disability for more than a year experienced marked reduction in pain and was able to function within a few weeks after working with some of the panel practitioners.

A significant factor in these forums is the desire to learn how best to integrate the various practices (i.e., what factors are involved in deciding which practices would most benefit each case, and in what order). So far, the pattern that seems to be developing is to look at the factors that most overload the person's system, usually sorted by (1) physical/structural/postural (including pain), (2) biochemical/nutritional/environmental, (3) energetic/systemic, and (4) psycho-emotional/relationship/career. The most pressing of these issues are then addressed first to provide some relief and relax the system. Then system balance and support can be addressed. Hence, each case will provide its own map of the journey through to healing.

Although the panel interview appears to be a potentially expensive intake model, it may save a great deal of misapplied effort later on. This approach requires a collaborative group of practitioners who are not competing for control of the case.

Team Centers

Any number of multipractitioner centers have appeared within the past few years, usually self-standing, primarily outside the standard insurance payment system. They range from the "real estate model" (i.e., several practitioners in the same physical facility, but not necessarily sharing cases) to a team model. In the team model, a group of practitioners comes together through affinity and seeks to work together in a collaborative way, sharing cases, perhaps sharing office services, billing, and so on.

This endeavor seems to indicate the possible future of "integrated" care. There are few, if any, such centers with a long history. The Meadowlark Center in Hemet, California, was perhaps the grandfather of these, operating since the 1960s, but it is no longer functioning. The A.R.E. Clinic in Phoenix is an unusual example, since it built its rationale around the work of the psychic healer Edgar Cayce.

The trend in such centers seems to be building around two models: the interview panel system, described above, and the "health guide." In the health guide model, each incoming case is interviewed by and guided through the process by a coordinator who arranges the sequence of care with the several practitioners. This model has been discussed since the 1970s but has yet to be completely implemented. The issues, of course, are the credentials of the guide, the level of trust and acceptance such a person would have to have from each practitioner, and the allocation of costs to cover this process.

Principal Issues

As groups and networks explore these new models, these issues are in the process of being resolved:

- Credentialization and acceptance of complementary practices.
- Agreements among the several practices about how best to proceed.
- Intake procedures and coordination of information from differing intake models.
- Case process: How is it determined, and by whom?

- Data management: How is the case tracked, and how is outcome data gathered?

RICHARD B. MILES

See

Acupuncture and Chinese Medicine (IV)

Chiropractic: Definition, History, and Theory (IV)

COMPLEMENTARY HEALTH PRACTITIONER LOCATIONS

Access to health care services is affected by the location of practitioners. The number and types of services available and their distribution in an area are important in assessing whether there is a shortage or oversupply of practitioners. The imbalance in the supply of physicians between rural and urban areas, for example, has been a longstanding problem in the United States (Gordon, Meister, & Hughes, 1992). In 1990 complementary therapies were being used by 1 in 3 Americans (Eisenberg et al., 1993), yet little is systematically known about where complementary health practitioners are located and how they are distributed (Gesler, 1988).

The research that has been done has looked at the distribution of licensed professional practitioners, for example, chiropractors (Gesler, 1988), rather than traditional healers. Location and distribution of traditional healers—*curanderas*, crystal healers, and all the other "underground" health care modalities—remain important areas for further investigation, particularly as they relate to less affluent population groups. One question that has received some attention over the years is whether complementary practitioners substitute for physicians, as for example, in underserved rural areas. A central issue is whether a scarcity of physicians results in an increased number of complementary practitioners. Research has found no clear evidence that substitution occurs. In fact, the opposite appears to be true: The more physicians in an area, the more one finds complementary health practitioners (Gesler, 1988).

A regional case study to see how complementary health practitioners were distributed throughout three states—California, Oregon, and Washington—focused on catchment areas composed of aggregated county units (Osborn, 1998). Chinese medicine and related therapies, including acupuncture, acupressure, shiatsu, and reflexology; chiropractic; homeopathy; and naturopathy were selected because they had significant numbers of practitioners. Not included were many nonprofessional providers who operate outside typical medical and legal channels and who usually do not advertise their services (Perrone, Stockel, & Krueger, 1989).

As expected, results of the study indicated that the greatest numbers of professional practitioners are located in large cities. However, the highest ratios of practitioners to population are found in less heavily populated secondary urban areas. For example, most complementary practitioners in California are located in the Los Angeles, Sacramento, San Diego, and San Francisco areas. However, the highest ratio of practitioners to population is in the central coast area between Santa Barbara and Santa Cruz.

This finding is contrary to what one would predict, based on general geographic principles. Central-place theory, one of the fundamental postulates of location analysis, suggests that the larger an urban area, the greater the variety of goods and services (King, 1984). Why then are so many complementary health practitioners located outside the largest cities? The findings suggest that complementary practitioners disproportionately choose to locate in relatively high-income, high-amenity areas. This raises questions regarding access to complementary health care for the poor and the disadvantaged (Osborn, 1998). Because most complementary practices are not covered by insurance, they are paid for out-of-pocket. Thus effective demand influences practice location, considering whether the location is a place where a practitioner can make a living (Doeksen, Miller, & Howe, 1988).

Research on factors relating to complementary health practice shows a strong bicoastal pattern. For example, states with acupuncture practice acts are generally located adjacent to the Pacific and Atlantic coasts (Baer & Good, 1998). Willingness to try new approaches to health care appears to have a similar bicoastal pattern. For example, participation in managed care varies across the country. States with the highest enrollment in health maintenance organizations suggest a regional pattern, with highest enrollment in the Pacific Coast, Southwest, and the North- and Mid-Atlantic regions. America's heartland has the lowest enrollment (Gordon & Silverstein, 1998). Births attended by midwives is another example. In 1990 the largest percentage of such births occurred in the New England, South Atlantic, Mountain, and Pacific Coast states. The smallest percentage occurred in the Midwest (Schneider, 1998).

Classic studies on the diffusion of innovation (Hagerstrand, 1968) support the findings that new ideas gain a foothold in areas where people are exposed to the exchange of ideas, whether from other cultures, as in coastal areas, or from formal educational institutions, such as university towns. A measure of success of an innovation is whether it diffuses to and eventually takes hold in the Midwest.

Future changes in the legal status of complementary health practitioners will affect their location and distribution. Changes in insurance practices can also be expected to have an effect on practitioner location choice and access for consumers.

RENA J. GORDON
ALAN RICE OSBORN

See

Acupuncture and Chinese Medicine (IV)

Chiropractic: Definition, History, and Theory (IV)

Homeopathy: Use in Family Practice Medicine (IV)

Reflexology (IV)

Shiatsu (IV)

MANAGED CARE AND PROVIDER REFERRAL RELATIONSHIPS

Increasing numbers of both indemnity insurers and managed care plans are beginning to extend coverage to certain types of complementary health care services. These changes are primarily the result of two factors: attempts by insurers to reduce costs and consumer demand. The coverage of complementary health care by third-party payers has implications for the growth in use of complementary modalities and also for the way these services are delivered.

Across the nation, health care is increasingly being reshaped to focus on saving money. Savings have been achieved by employers who were paying double-digit increases in premiums for employee health care and who now provide managed care programs. Managed care plans, including health maintenance organizations (HMOs) and preferred provider organizations (PPOs), have in common the establishment of a contracted or preferred provider network. By 1994 approximately 20% of the population was covered by managed care (American Association of Health Plans, 1996). This figure is very conservative, since it counts only enrollment in HMOs and does not take into account other types of managed care arrangements, such as PPOs. It is estimated that by the year 2000, national enrollment in managed care will be over 30%, exceeding 112 million members (Marion Merrell Dow, 1995). There is wide variation across the country in participation in managed care, ranging from a high of 40% in Massachusetts to a low of 0% in Wyoming (American Association of Health Plans, 1996).

Growing consumer demand and less costly therapies are appealing to the insurance industry. Several insurers have taken pioneering steps in covering selective therapies. There are currently 15 insurance companies, including the giant Mutual of Omaha, covering Dr. Dean Ornish's diet and wellness plan for preventing and reversing heart disease. The cost of Ornish's program (approximately $5,500) may be seen as a sound investment if it enables patients to avoid $15,000 angioplasties and $40,000 bypass operations. Estimated savings from Ornish's low-tech program is

$6.50 for every $1.00 spent by Mutual of Omaha. Eventually, the company could save up to $20 for each dollar spent (Cowley, King, Hager, & Rosenberg, 1995). Another example is American Western, an insurer based in California, which covers numerous alternative therapies, including acupuncture, massage, and hypnotherapy.

It is inevitable that the availability of third-party coverage for complementary health practices will change the way services are delivered. Many alternative providers in the state of Washington, for example, which mandates coverage for any licensed provider, view the coverage as a two-edged sword. Although the availability of insurance coverage for their services promises to increase their patient volume, lend an increased air of mainstream respectability to complementary health care, and increase the reimbursement of providers, this newfound "respectability" brings complications. The incorporation of insurance payments into a medical practice requires the use of specific billing forms, coding, and possibly prior authorization of services. Billing clerks have to be hired, and the practice no longer operates on a simple cash basis. Life suddenly becomes more complicated for alternative health care providers as they join the mainstream of American medicine.

In addition to its importance as a payer, managed care is an important mechanism for patient referrals. If a provider is "in demand" by multiple managed care plans, these plans could provide enough patient referrals to meet the majority of the capacity needs of the practice. Without managed care, alternative providers are more limited in their ability to attract patients. While indemnity insurance (the stand insurance plan in which patients go to whomever they want, file a claim, and generally pay 20% to the insurer's 80%) is also extremely important as a payer for alternative health care services, this type of insurance does not provide a direct referral source for patients. In an indemnity environment, the provider still needs to market the services and maintain full responsibility for attracting patients.

The development of referral relationships between alternative health care providers and allopathic/osteopathic medical providers is inevitable as insurers begin to pay for complementary therapies. Referral relationships are traditionally a significant source of patients for specialists in the U.S. health care system. Referral relationships among allopathic and osteopathic physicians generally are developed through interaction with peers in the hospital setting or through medical associations and committees, and increasingly through contractual relationships with managed care plans. Alternative providers previously have been denied these relationships since they do not interact with allopathic and osteopathic providers in these environments. With the increasing number of managed care plans covering at least some alternative therapies, these relationships are being developed. Some referral relationships that have existed between allopathic/osteopathic and complementary providers on a very informal basis are being formalized. Certain managed care plans and insurers are developing relationships with complementary providers either by contracting with them directly or by allowing their biomedical providers to refer to complementary providers outside the network in appropriate circumstances.

There is little doubt that the availability of insurance coverage for complementary therapies will have significant impact on the delivery of complementary health care services. These therapies will be more widely accessible as a result of third-party reimbursement for the services; patients who may not have been willing to "try something new" are going to be more likely to if the expense is not out-of-pocket. This will be especially true if their primary care physician (or specialist) refers them for complementary therapies. Complementary health care providers are likely to see an increase in patient volume and reimbursement (although reimbursement may decrease on a per patient visit, since managed care plans are not going to contract for full billed charges). Complementary health care providers will be required to operate more sophisticated practices with expertise in billing and collections. Whether there is more to be gained or lost for complementary health care providers as a result of these changes will be determined as an increasing number of insurance companies and managed care plans opt to include these services in their benefit packages. However, consumers stand to gain as insurers cover complementary health practices.

GAIL SILVERSTEIN

THIRD-PARTY REIMBURSEMENT FOR COMPLEMENTARY PRACTICE

Because the biomedical view of what constitutes health care has dominated reimbursement, insurers historically have denied coverage for complementary health care. Only medically diagnosable disease was considered an insurable event, and only medical treatment was considered a reimbursable event. The system focused on disease care rather than health care.

But as notions of health evolve and include preventive choices, holistic healing, and self-care, the notion of reimbursable health losses potentially embraces a broader set of deviations from well-being. Lack of proper nutrition, stress, imbalances in vital energy, and even the emotional and spiritual crises underlying disease, such as loneliness, depression, anxiety, and unexpressed frustration and rage, all may, in the future, be viewed as precursors to disease and become appropriate foci for reimbursable health care intervention.

Coverage for Complementary Therapies

Many insurers are experimenting with coverage reimbursing various kinds of holistic care. American Western Life Insurance offers Prevention Plus, an integrated health insurance plan that offers up to 12 annual visits to complementary providers alongside a conventional medical network of over 650 hospitals. Mutual of Omaha Companies covers the Reversal Program, a prevention and behavior modification program to reduce the risk of heart disease through yoga, meditation, diet, and support groups. The Harvard Community Health Plan offers behavioral therapies, including mind-body relaxation, as preventive care; so does the Oxford Health Plan in New York, Lovelace Health Systems in Albuquerque, Kaiser Permanente in California, and American Medical Security's HealthCareChoice, in Arizona, Wisconsin, Texas, North Carolina, and Colorado.

The list of insurers and covered services and providers grows. Insurers contemplate potential cost savings, consumer demand, and a wellness approach that is attractive to employers, among others, who will pay for nutritional support, counseling, and lifestyle modifications in exchange for fewer cholesterol screenings and blood pressure checks.

Pros and Cons

Many believe that the insurance industry should stay out of complementary health care. The argument is that insurance policy coverage and exclusions, utilization review, and other insurance rules and practices already have too much influence over the quantity and quality of health care delivered. Moreover, the market and economic orientation of the insurance industry may distort the principle of complementary care. For example, such concepts as prayer and managed care seem incompatible; one may imagine a pastoral counselor visiting a hospitalized patient for an allotted number of minutes to deliver a reimbursable conversation with God.

On the other hand, for many consumers, access to complementary therapies, particularly for long-term or chronic conditions, depends on third-party payment. A constitutional or statutory right of access to health care treatments—as embodied in the Access to Medical Treatment Act, in state medical freedom acts, in other legislation, and in some of the cases—loses impact if consumers cannot afford unreimbursable therapies or if insurance reimbursement schemes skew treatment in favor of risky and potentially debilitating medical therapies, such as high-dose chemotherapy with autologous bone marrow transplant. Moreover, given the way in which insurance schemes (particularly in managed care) determine the nature and level of medical care the patient receives, including complementary medicine in insurance reim-

bursement schemes will facilitate the integration of holistic modalities into the U.S. health care system.

Some of the issues that confront insurers covering complementary practices include the role of licensing laws and scope-of-practice rules in ensuring that providers within insurance networks are properly credentialed and are offering services within their legislative authorization. Providing access to licensed providers will be more palatable than reimbursing visits to unlicensed practitioners. Even among licensed providers, services will range from Swedish massage to relax the body and improve circulation to the movement of human energy fields through noncontact therapeutic touch. Insurers also must familiarize themselves with the professional organizations, ethical codes, standards of care, and malpractice and disciplinary rules relevant to the providers within the holistic health care networks.

Insurers also should check state laws regarding the numerous insurance mandates requiring the provision of certain kinds of complementary therapies, such as chiropractic and acupuncture. Some states have "any willing provider" laws. These laws require that insurers offering preferred provider policies establish the terms and conditions governing practitioners' eligibility to be preferred providers; that such terms and conditions may not discriminate against or among health care providers; and that such policies may not exclude any preferred provider willing to meet the terms and conditions set forth.

Even when consumers are covered by private insurance policies, employee benefit plans subject to the Employee Retirement Income Security Act of 1974 (ERISA), managed care contracts, or other kinds of insurance policies, complementary providers who provide treatment sometimes find reimbursement declined because the insurer views the therapy either falling within the "experimental treatment" exclusion or as "medically unnecessary." Insurers exclude experimental treatments from coverage to avoid paying for expensive medical treatments of unknown efficacy. Frequently, insurers will exclude treatments such as acupuncture on this basis.

Insureds and providers will want to argue that a therapy is not necessarily experimental simply because it has not found general acceptance within the medical community. Complementary treatments generally are preventive and oriented toward overall health and well-being. They are often holistic in approach and aim to translate psychological, emotional, and spiritual relief into improved physiological functioning. The treatments frequently derive from systems of knowledge that have historically been foreign to conventional scientific research methodologies, are practiced largely by nonphysicians, are individualized and not research driven, and are less expensive than highly technological treatments.

Perhaps in recognition of a distinction between complementary and excludable experimental treatments, the FDA recently reclassified acupuncture needles as Class II devices, or medical devices for general use, by acupuncture practitioners, rather than as Class III investigational devices limited to research.

In a similar vein, a major purpose in limiting coverage to "medically necessary" treatment is to limit insurers' reimbursement for consumer overconsumption of care. On the whole, chiropractic, homeopathy, acupuncture and massage therapy, vitamins and minerals, and other such treatments—particularly when used on a preventative basis—present less of a financial burden to insurers than medical treatments involving hospitalization and surgery.

As providers integrate complementary treatments, notions of medical necessity may evolve to include procedures necessary for balancing *chi*, for example, and for prevention of disease and maintenance of wholeness as a component of physical health. Homeopathic remedies, nutritional therapies, and spinal manipulation may be considered necessary components of health care, as peer review panels include complementary providers to ensure that the services claimed as medically necessary include modalities outside the medical model.

Some courts have provided a foundation for this position by accepting treatments such as chiropractic and massage therapy, as well as nonstandard medical treatments, within the notion of medical necessity. These decisions suggest some judicial acceptance of reimbursement for therapies outside the traditional medical scope.

MICHAEL H. COHEN

See

Acupuncture and Chinese Medicine (IV)

Chiropractic: Definition, History, and Theory (IV)

COMPLEMENTARY FOLK OR ETHNIC APPROACHES

Despite the preeminence of allopathic medicine in modern societies, folk or ethnic approaches continue to exist and often thrive throughout the world. Given its ethnically diverse population, U.S. society exhibits a wide array of complementary folk systems. Practitioners of allopathic medicine, osteopathic medicine, chiropractic, and naturopathy tend to be drawn from the white Anglo-Saxon Protestant majority group and, to a lesser extent, from Jewish and non-Latino Catholic ethnic groups. Practitioners and clients of complementary systems, such as conjure or rootwork, *curanderismo*, *espiritismo*, *santeria*, *vodun*, traditional Chinese medicine, peyotism, and southern Appalachian and Ozark herbal medicine, are largely concentrated among African-Americans, Latinos, Asian-Americans, Native Americans, and poor rural whites.

Rather than discussing the wide array of complementary folk systems around the world, this entry focuses upon certain variants of African-American, Latino, and Native American healing traditions in the United States.

African-American Healing Systems

Ethnic approaches among African-Americans emerged within the context of North American slavery. Cross-fertilization occurred in the health beliefs and practice of African Americans, European Americans, and American Indians during the antebellum period. The terms *conjure*, *rootwork*, and *hoodoo* came to be applied to a system of health care, magic, divination, herbalism, and witchcraft widespread among slaves.

Folk practices continue to be a vital part of health care delivery for African-Americans in both the rural South and the cities of the South and the North. Many working-class African-Americans rely on home remedies of various sorts as well as on an array of folk practitioners (Snow, 1993).

Contemporary African-American folk healers can be divided into four main types: (1) independent generalists, (2) independent specialists, (3) cultic generalists, and (4) cultic specialists (Baer, 1982). Independent generalists include conjurers in rural areas and spiritualists in urban areas who address a wide variety of ailments, particularly problems of living and "unnatural" illnesses. Independent specialists include midwives, herbalists, magic vendors, and neighborhood prophets who function as local healers. Cultic generalists include spiritual advisers, voodoo priests, and Black Islamic or Hebraic healers who deal with a variety of illnesses either within the context of religious services or in private consultations. Cultic specialists include faith healers or divine healers, who tend to focus on psychosomatic ailments within a religious setting.

Latino Healing Systems

Latinos, or Hispanic-Americans, consist of various ethnic groups, including Mexican-Americans, Puerto Ricans, Cuban-Americans, Central Americans, and South Americans. While there is some overlap and cross-fertilization among the ethnic health care practices of these various groups, each one of these systems is distinct. The remainder of this section discusses folk or ethnic approaches among Mexican-Americans and Puerto Ricans.

Mexican-American Healing Systems

Mexican-Americans tend to be concentrated in the Southwest (Texas, New Mexico, Arizona, and California) but are increasingly found in other parts of the United States, including Florida, the Midwest, and the Northeast. *Curanderismo* constitutes the principal Mexican-American ethnic health care system and is a term derived from the Spanish word *curandero* or *curandera*, for curer or healer. It is a syncretic system that has incorporated aspects of ancient Mexican, medieval Hispanic-Arabic, Roman Catholic, and Native American ethnic approaches (Trotter & Chavira, 1997).

Both independent generalists and independent specialists function within the context of *curanderismo*. *Curanderas* are independent generalists who treat a wide variety of physical and emotional problems. They possess *el don* (the gift of healing), which enables them to diagnose both naturalistic and supernaturalistic illnesses, including culture-bound syndromes such as *susto* (fright), *empacho* (the clogging of the stomach and upper intestinal tract from excessive food or the wrong kinds of food), *bilis* (jaundice-like condition resulting from anger or fear), *mal ojo* (evil eye), and *mal puesto* (witchcraft). *Curanderas* often prescribe foods and/or herbs to correct imbalances caused by either being exposed to cold air or eating an excess of "hot" or "cold" foods. They also rely upon the use of magico-religious objects, such as votive candles and statues, and rituals in an effort to ward off hexes. A few *curanderos*, such as Don Pedrito Jarmillo and El Niño Fidencio, evolved into folk saints following their deaths.

Independent specialists include *parteras*, or lay midwives; *sobadores*, who treat muscle sprains and misaligned bones by massaging, rubbing, or kneading the affected part of the body; *yerberos*, or herbalists, who often operate out of a *yerberia*

or *botica*, a store that sells herbs as well as perfumes, oils, candles, and other mystical objects; and *senõras*, or middle-aged or elderly women, who read cards to inform their clients about their present, past, or future circumstances.

Puerto Rican Espiritismo

Puerto Rican *espiritismo*, or spiritism, draws upon elements from the Yoruba religion, the teachings of Allan Kardec (a French spiritist philosopher), and Roman Catholicism (Harwood, 1987). Although it first was in vogue in Puerto Rican high society, *espiritismo* evolved into a decentralized religious healing system with hundreds of *centros*, or temples, among working-class Puerto Ricans on the island and the U.S. mainland. The president of a temple and his or her mediums attempt to achieve contact with the spirit realm to cure their clients. Seances and private consultations of malevolent supernatural influences are used. *Espiritualistas*, or spiritists, are generally "wounded healers" who have rid themselves of some sort of affliction. Mediums feel their clients' ailments. They use spirit guides and manipulate religious symbols to overcome negative spiritual forces.

Native American Healing Systems

There are many different Native American ethnic groups in the United States. Despite their diversity, in general Native American healing systems consider humans as an integral part of nature. These systems are both empirical and spiritual in their approaches to restoring imbalances between individuals and their sociocultural environments. They tend to view illness as emanating from sorcery (a common belief for some Southwestern groups, such as the Zuni, Navajo, and Yaqui), taboo violation, the intrusion of a foreign object or spirit, or soul loss (a common belief among the Inuit). Native American healing techniques include the use of herbs and hallucinogens, sweat and mineral baths, contact between a shaman (healer) and the spirit realm, and even surgery in the case of some groups, such as the Aleuts. Native American medicine became popular on the North American frontier and had a strong impact on European-American and African-American folk medicine (Vogel, 1977). Over 200 Native American medicinal substances are listed in the *U.S. Pharmacopeia*.

HANS A. BAER

See
Native American Medicine (IV)

THE WOMEN'S MOVEMENT AND CHOICES IN CHILDBIRTH

At the beginning of the 20th century, the vast majority of births took place in the home. Most women were attended by a friend or family member because midwifery services were no longer readily available, except in rural areas and the ethnic immigrant sections of cities. The decline in the number of midwives resulted from a highly successful campaign waged by physicians to portray midwives as dirty, backward, and poorly trained. State legislatures responded to this campaign by passing laws restricting the practice of midwifery. In many states, licensing of midwives was required even before there was a demand for physician licensing. As the pool of midwives dried up, physicians attempted to fill the void as birth attendants,

challenging the socially accepted norm that pregnancy and childbirth were natural processes.

By 1920, physicians solidified the perception that they were the keepers of the latest in childbirth technology by offering in-hospital, painless childbirth. Women of means were admitted to maternity wards, given anesthesia to reduce the memory of childbirth, and retained in the hospital for lengthy periods to recover from the experience. Poor women and those living far from hospitals remained dependent upon home delivery and attendance by friends or relatives.

By 1950, hospital birth became the social norm for all but the poorest of women and those living in remote areas. Antibiotics to cure infections became available. Blood transfusion techniques were developed, reducing the dangers of postpartum hemorrhage. Anesthesia techniques were developed that were safer and allowed the laboring woman to be conscious during delivery. Oxytocic drugs, agents that promote rapid labor, were introduced to counteract the slowing effects of anesthetics. As a result of these technological advances, maternal mortality in the United States dropped from 70 per 10,000 births in 1930 to 7 per 10,000 births in 1955, and physicians proclaimed victory. The midwife was, for all intensive purposes, extinct. A second result of these technological advances, however, was that the miraculous event of childbirth became dehumanized.

By 1960, the laboring woman was admitted to the hospital, given an enema, and shaved of all pubic hair. She was moved to a labor room, given an analgesic and scopolamine, and when she had sufficiently progressed, moved to a delivery room where she was placed flat on her back on a table. The woman's legs were strapped into stirrups above her body in the lithotomy position, a position selected by obstetricians for ease of access to and control of the perineal area, not a position designed for the comfort of labor. A fetal monitor was attached, an intravenous line inserted, and anesthesia administered. Episiotomy, a surgical incision of the vulva to prevent tearing during delivery, became routine. If there were complications, the patient was wheeled to the operating room for a caesarean section. After delivery, the patient was sutured and transferred to a recovery room. Finally, the childbirth experience was complete when the new mother was transferred to the maternity ward. During this entire experience, fathers remained in a hospital waiting room, sometimes with a television for company. After the infant was cleaned and placed into a bassinet in the nursery, the father was allowed to view the child through a glass window. It was not uncommon for the father to hold the child for the first time only after he had taken the new family home.

With the passage of Medicaid in the 1960s, even the poorest American women had access to physician in-hospital delivery. Mainstream medicine proclaimed childbirth safer than ever because all women had access to the best technology. Women, however, were less than satisfied with the childbirth experience.

The social climate of the country changed in the late 1960s and throughout the 1970s as protest movements gained steam—for civil rights, for human rights, and against the Vietnam War. Part of this social change included the women's movement, rooted in radical feminist literature and fueled by a surge in female higher education. Feminist literature of the time encouraged women to take control, including control of their own bodies. Some feminist and holistic literature questioned whether pregnancy and childbirth required medical management and encouraged women to demand control of their birthing experiences. Traditional physicians did not react favorably to such demands.

In the United States, the movement to return to home birth began in California. A male midwife, Norman Casserly, was arrested for practicing medicine without a license in 1971. His arrest, conviction, and appeal brought publicity to home birth and led a growing number of women to rally for birthing alternatives. In response, the American College of Obstetrics and Gynecology issued a policy statement in 1975 proclaiming home birth a form of child abuse. Some physicians even suggested that women who gave birth at home by choice should be prosecuted.

The number of specialty-trained physicians rose rapidly in the 1970s, and more hospitals offered maternity services than ever before. Unfortunately, the baby boom demand for childbirth services was declining and competition for births became serious business. Physicians and hospitals knew that if they offered special services to appease the demand for childbirth alternatives, they would have a competitive edge for attracting new patients. Lamaze classes, the medical establishment equivalent of "natural childbirth" that could be adapted to hospital routine, were offered. Husbands were allowed in the delivery room and bonding between mother and child was encouraged. Some progressive physicians agreed to "try" to deliver the mother without an episiotomy. Mainstream medicine was firm, however, about keeping childbirth in the hospital.

Many, but not all, women were satisfied with the new in-hospital options. For those who remained unconvinced, a new entity, the freestanding birthing center with Certified Nurse-Midwives (CNMs) as attendants, began to spring up in the late 1970s. Rather than lose business to this new competition, some hospitals hired CNMs for their own staffs during the 1980s. Others bought out freestanding birthing facilities or, if that failed, tried to put the competition out of business by starting their own in-house birthing centers.

Longitudinal data on childbirth reflect a slow but growing acceptance of midwives as birth attendants over the past two decades, a reversal of the trend seen at the beginning of the century. The original demand by feminists for control of their childbirth experience has been addressed, primarily by economic forces. Third-party payers have recognized that childbirth options that include midwives and birthing centers help keep the costs of childbirth down (De Witt, 1993). Hospitals have recognized that they must provide women with birthing alternatives if they are to keep their obstetric beds full. As a result, the approximately 5% of American women who choose a midwife-attended birth is likely to continue to grow in the foreseeable future. Today, midwives serve as birth attendants in scores of hospitals and freestanding birthing centers. They are the only providers available to women who demand a home birth, and remain the only health care professionals serving many rural areas (Bastian, 1993; Taylor & Ricketts, 1993).

DONA SCHNEIDER

See

Midwifery (IV)

HEALTH FOOD STORES AND COMPLEMENTARY HEALTH PRACTICES

More and more Americans are going to health food stores to buy natural foods and products. For the most part, people who frequent health food stores are searching for natural, effective, and safe health care solutions, more personal control over their health, ways to prevent illness, and ways to reduce health care costs. Consumers include baby boomers who are beginning to enter middle age, older people who are looking at measures to manage chronic illnesses, and young mothers in their 20s who want healthier food and products for their families (Emerich, 1996).

Health food stores are an important component in the trend toward complementary health practices because it is in many of these stores that consumers often are first introduced to products, books, and other educational materials, as well as complementary health practices and practitioner services. Over 90% of consumers make their first visit to a natural products store because they are experiencing a health problem or crisis (Emerich, 1996, p. 22). "People go to health food stores to buy products, but they also go to become well. It would be a great mistake just to call these stores businesses. These are really a modern form of a healing temple" (Anderson, 1996, p. 52).

Given the proliferation of new natural products—vitamins, herbs, personal care items, and foods—consumers need more help to make educated decisions regarding natural products than in the past. In 1996, for example, an estimated 4,000 to 5,000 new natural products were introduced. It is estimated that 80% of the products available now were not in existence 4 years ago (Picozzi, 1996). This explosion in the number and variety of products presents a challenge for the consumer.

Consumers who are not newcomers to complementary health practices continue to frequent health food stores. They are able to purchase particular brands of vitamins, supplements, herbs, homeopathic remedies, aromatherapy oils, raw and processed foods free of antibiotics, pesticides, and hormones, and other products not available elsewhere. Individuals who have educated themselves on brands buy those that use research-grade extracts. Knowledge of natural products is important, just as it is critical to be informed about prescriptive and over-the-counter drugs. Before taking any new product, one should consider such factors as reliability of brands, side effects, interactive effects, and sun sensitivity. Frequently a new natural method for treating a specific ailment creates a demand for the product. For example, there has been an explosion of interest in the herb St. John's wort (*Hypericum perforatum*) for treating depression. After being hailed as "nature's Prozac," retail sales increased 3,900% since 1995 (Monmaney, 1998).

Not all health food stores are alike. The degree to which consumers will be given educational materials and referrals for complementary health practitioners depends generally on the type of store and to a lesser degree on personnel. Stores fall into three general categories: (1) natural food and health food stores, comprised of over 6,500 stores nationally; (2) health food chains, with over 2,500 stores nationally, that focus on vitamins, supplements, herbs, and personal care items, with very little food product; and (3) mass-market stores, comprised of 136,000 mainstream grocery and supermarket stores that carry some natural products (Emerich, 1996). Some drugstore chains and mass merchandisers also carry natural products. Not included in this discussion are multilevel marketing and mail order sales of natural products, which gain much of their sales in rural areas and through the expanding World Wide Web.

Natural food and health food stores are familiar to consumers and most frequented by them. In 1995 they contributed more than two thirds of total industry sales (Emerich, 1996). The distinction between natural food and health food stores is the percentage devoted to food. Natural food stores garner at least 40% of sales from food products. That is not the case for health food stores. According to Dr. Andrew Weil, "Many health food stores might better be called pill stores, given how little food they stock in relation to all the vitamins and supplements" (Weil, 1995, p. 211).

Consumer interest in eating foods free of harmful artificial ingredients and additives is soaring. Currently, there is no regulation of food grown and manufactured without the use of added hormones, pesticides, or synthetic fertilizers. Proposed federal rules would for the first time define which raw or processed foods can be labeled organic and would set standards for the production and handling of organically grown crops and organically raised meat and poultry. Proposed December 16, 1997, regulations for standardization of organic foods have not yet been finalized by the U.S. Department of Agriculture (Burros, 1997). Because of consumer demand, organic foods eventually will account for a higher proportion of sales in natural foods and health food stores.

Personalized services are available in natural food and health food stores more than in either health food chains or mass-market stores. Generally, a consumer will find written materials on holistic health, herbs, vitamins, supplements, and complementary health practices. There are racks, bulletin boards, file cabinets, even libraries containing a wide variety of information for interested consumers.

Although natural and health food stores often are sources of referrals to complementary health practitioners, personnel generally are careful regarding specific referrals, making no recommendations, representations, or endorsements of any individual or entity. Natural and health food stores make available a variety of opportunities for referrals. These range from bulletin boards for posting business cards or file boxes with names of practitioners to printed lists with tables of contents identifying the types of health care professionals listed. These stores are more consumer-oriented than are the health food chains or mass-market stores, which would at most direct customers who ask for referrals to listings in the telephone book.

In one California natural food store, for example, customers who request names of practitioners are given a copy of a 24-page list of local health care professionals who specialize in various areas of holistic health care. The store owner reminds patrons to do a thorough investigation of anyone they might select to use and satisfy themselves of the person's ability to perform the services desired and to interview any practitioner with whom they are considering treatment. While store owners may provide a list as a convenience to their patrons, they tend to emphasize that each individual take responsibility to fulfill his or her own health care requirements.

Health store retailers try to keep up with the vast amount of information on new products by attending annual conferences where samples, demonstrations, and product literature are available. At these conferences, leading practitioners, research scientists, and writers on complementary health care give keynote addresses and participate in forums and seminars. Health care practitioners attend the sessions, leave cards and materials at show booths, and interact with peers and attendees, all in an effort to develop referral networks.

Health food stores continue to play an important role in disseminating materials and in educating the public on the benefits of natural health care. Their role as a referral source for complementary health practitioners may be superseded by health provider panels, much like physician panels, as more insurers reimburse for selected complementary practices. Their role as an educational source may increase as quality control through accuracy and consistency in labeling of products becomes established. The herb industry is taking steps to improve standards and police itself (Monmaney, 1998). The recently established Institute for Nutraceutical Advancement is an industry-funded testing group to validate methods of analyzing botanical products. The National Nutritional Foods Association (*see* Table 1) is a trade group that randomly tests members' label claims on herbal supplements. With added quality control, a whole new niche of consumers will find their way into health food stores.

RENA J. GORDON

TABLE 1   Abbreviations Found in Literature in Natural Food Stores

ABC	American Botanical Council
AHPA	American Herbal Products Association
CANI	Consultants Association for the Natural Industry
CFH	Citizens for Health
CRN	Council for Responsible Nutrition
DSHEA	Dietary Supplement Health and Education Act of 1994
EPA	Environmental Protection Agency
FDA	Food and Drug Administration
GMP	Good Manufacturing Practice
HRF	Herb Research Foundation
NIH	National Institutes of Health
NLEA	Nutrition Labeling and Education Act
NNFA	National Nutritional Foods Association
NOSB	National Organic Standards Board
OCIA	Organic Crop Improvement Association
OFRF	Organic Farming Research Foundation
OTA	Organic Trade Association
OTC	Over the counter
RDA	Recommended Dietary Allowance
UNPA	Utah Natural Products Alliance
USDA	U.S. Department of Agriculture

Source: *Natural Foods Merchandiser* (1997, October), p. 14.

NATUROPATHY: PRACTICE ISSUES

Naturopathy is a distinct profession of primary health care, emphasizing prevention, treatment, and optimal health through the use of therapeutic methods and modalities that encourage the body's self-healing process, the *vis medicatrix naturae*. Doctors of naturopathy (N.D.s) are general practitioners trained as specialists in natural health care. They are educated in conventional medical sciences, but they are not orthodox medical doctors.

Naturopathy is defined by principles rather than by methods or modalities. These principles are based on the objective observation of the nature of health and disease and are continuously reviewed in the light of current scientific advances. The following six principles are the foundation for the education of naturopathyic physicians and the practice of naturopathy:

1. *The Healing Power of Nature*. Naturopathy recognizes an inherent self-healing process in the person that is ordered and intelligent. Naturopathic physicians act to identify and remove obstacles to healing and recovery and to facilitate and augment this inherent self-healing process.
2. *Identify and Treat the Causes*. The naturopathic physician seeks to identify and remove the underlying causes of illness, rather than to merely eliminate or suppress symptoms.
3. *First, Do No Harm*. Naturopathic physicians follow three guidelines to avoid harming the patient: (1) utilize methods and medicinal substances that minimize the risk of harmful side effects, using the least force necessary to diagnose and treat; (2) avoid when possible the harmful suppression of symptoms; and (3) acknowledge, respect, and work with the individual's self-healing process.
4. *Doctor As Teacher*. Naturopathic physicians educate their clients and encourage self-responsibility for health. They also recognize the therapeutic potential of the doctor-client relationship.
5. *Treat the Whole Person*. Naturopathic physicians treat each individual by taking into account individual physical, mental, emotional, genetic, environmental, social, and other factors. Since total health also includes

spiritual health, naturopathic physicians encourage individuals to pursue their personal spiritual development.

6. *Prevention*. Naturopathic physicians emphasize the prevention of disease—accessing risk factors, heredity, and susceptibility to disease and making appropriate interventions in partnership with their patients to prevent illness. Naturopathy is committed to the creation of a healthy world in which humanity may thrive.

Practice

Naturopathic practice includes a variety of diagnostic methods and therapeutic modalities. Methods and modalities are selected and applied based on underlying principles in relationship to the individual needs of the patient. Modalities may include nutrition, herbs, botanical medicine, naturopathic manipulative therapy, public health measures and hygiene, counseling, minor surgery, homeopathy, acupuncture, and natural childbirth. The naturopathic physician performs a wide variety of diagnostic tests, exams, laboratory testing, gynecological exams, nutritional and dietary assessments, toxicity assessments, metabolic analysis, allergy testing, and x-ray examinations. As with all physicians, naturopathic physicians refer to specialists when appropriate.

History

Naturopathy grew out of the alternative healing systems of the 18th and 19th centuries but traces its roots back to the 4th century B.C. Hippocrates, considered the father of modern medicine, said, "Let your food be your medicine and your medicine be your food." Hippocratic practitioners assumed that everything in nature had a rational basis; therefore, the physician's role was to understand and follow the laws of the intelligent universe. They viewed disease as an effect and looked for its cause in natural phenomena—air, water, and food. They used the term, *vis medicatrix naturae,* the healing power of nature, to denote the body's ability to heal itself. In the late 1800s, John Scheel coined the word "naturopathy." The name was purchased by Benedict Lust, who founded the American Naturopathic Association. In 1905, Lust incorporated the first school of naturopathy under the laws of the state of New York.

During the early 1900s, the profession grew in numbers and popularity, culminating with over 20 schools throughout North America. One of the chief advantages of training during this time was the number of inpatient facilities which flourished. These facilities provided in-depth training in clinical nature cure and natural hygiene in inpatient settings. Nature cure and natural hygiene are still at the heart of naturopathic medicine's fundamental principles and approach to health care and disease prevention. After World War II, however, "miracle" drugs such as antibiotics and advances in surgical techniques created a growing belief that medical science and technology would soon find all the answers to sickness and disease. Consequently, the naturopathic profession, with its emphasis on self-healing, declined.

Since the late 1960s, growing public interest in nutrition, exercise, and healthful living has revived the search for viable health care alternatives and natural-based medical treatment. Research and epidemiological studies continue to demonstrate the relationship between diet, lifestyle, and disease, validating the long-held principles and teaching of naturopathic medicine.

It was not until John Bastyr, N.D. (1912–1995), first teaching at National College of Naturopathic Medicine, that the naturopathic profession was challenged to reach its fullest potential. Dr. Bastyr was the prototype of the modern naturopathic doctor—that is, one who culls the latest findings from the scientific literature, applies them in ways consistent with naturopathic principles, and verifies the results with appropriate studies. Dr. Bastyr saw tremendous expansion in both allopathic and naturopathic medical knowledge during his life, and he played a major role in making sure the best of both were integrated into naturopathic medical education.

Today, naturopathic medical colleges are four-year postgraduate schools with admission requirements of conventional premedical education. The degree of Doctor of Naturopathic Medicine requires four years of graduate-level study in the medical sciences. Naturopathic medical training is a blend of contemporary science, empirical naturopathic medicine, and naturopathic philosophy. It is based on the underlying naturopathic principles and utilizes a rich mixture of scientific and empirical natural methods. Modern education of natural health practitioners emphasizes development of a thorough, up-to-date, scientific understanding of the structure and function of the human body and the disease process, balanced with a profound appreciation for and ability to activate the unique self-healing ability inherent in every human being.

During their first two years, students study anatomy (including dissection), biochemistry, cardiology, neurology, microbiology, pharmacology, radiology, physiology, embryology, histology, pathology, public health, gynecology, dermatology, obstetrics, pediatrics, minor surgery, and immunology. Beginning in the second year and intensifying in the third and fourth year, the students are trained in clinical and physical diagnosis and treatment. While the conventional diagnostic skills in recognizing and naming pathology are developed (e.g., physical laboratory, radiological, and clinical diagnosis), substantial emphasis is placed on functional diagnosis. Students develop a high level of skill in nutritional evaluation, recognition of toxic load, and lifestyle assessment. It is in the area of therapies that the greatest difference from conventional medical education is seen. Substantial training in nutrition, herbs, lifestyle, psychological counseling, and physical medicine is provided. In addition, students develop basic skills in office surgical procedures, emergency medicine, and vaccinations. Faculty typically have doctorate degrees in their subject areas.

The accrediting agency for naturopathy education is the Council on Naturopathic Medical Education (CNME). It is recognized by the U.S. Department of Education, and students at accredited and candidate-status naturopathic schools are qualified to participate in federal student loan programs. The CNME has granted accreditation to Bastyr University's Program in Naturopathic Medicine and has granted institutional accreditation to NCNM. Southwest College of Naturopathic Medicine and Health Sciences has achieved Candidate for Accreditation status. This step does not assure eventual accreditation by the CNME. Bastyr University receives its institutional accreditation through the Northwest Association of Schools and Colleges.

JOSEPH E. PIZZORNO

See

Acupuncture and Chinese Medicine (IV)
Diet and Mood (IV)
Homeopathy: Molecular Basis (IV)
Lifestyle Change (IV)
Nutrition (IV)

CHIROPRACTIC: PRACTICE ISSUES

Over the last century, chiropractic has struggled to survive in the face of stiff opposition from traditional medicine, but it has emerged as the second most utilized health care discipline in the United States. From the beginning, doctors of chiropractic (DCs) were prosecuted in the thousands for practicing medicine without a license. Slowly, however, they gained legitimacy; Kansas passed the first chiropractic license law in 1913, and since then all 50 states have passed such laws.

Chiropractic's most obvious adversary has been the American Medical Association (AMA), which fought a rearguard action against the profession for decades. In 1963, the AMA established a Committee on Quackery with the purpose of containing and eventually eliminating chiropractic. After a long period of taking a defensive posture, DCs finally took the offensive when, in 1976, practitioners in three states filed federal and state lawsuits alleging that the AMA, American Hospital Association, and other medical organizations had violated antitrust laws in their efforts to monopolize American health care. The most famous case was *Wilk et al. v. AMA et al.*, finally resolved in favor of Wilk. The state of New York filed a similar lawsuit in 1979, and the Federal Trade Commission looked into possible restraint of trade violations by orthodox medicine. As a result of the litigation, the AMA revised its code of ethics, allowing its members to associate with any legally sanctioned health care professionals; it also ceased officially to label chiropractic as unscientific.

Although counts of chiropractic health personnel are notoriously imprecise, various sources (Cowrie & Roebuck, 1975; Stanford Research Institute, 1960) demonstrate increases over the years: from 400 to 600 in 1908 to 2,000 in 1910, 7,000 in 1916, approximately 16,000 in 1930, and 23,000 in 1979. Estimates in 1990 reached 45,000 to 50,000, increasing to more than 73,000 in 1993. The highest DC-to-population ratios are in the Midwest (where chiropractic and also osteopathy originated) and Pacific regions; relatively low rates are found in New England and the south central states.

Along with other forms of alternative practices, there has been an increasing utilization of chiropractic services. By 1980, DCs were treating an estimated 8 million Americans of all ages and socioeconomic status for a variety of conditions. Research shows that chiropractic is not primarily a rural phenomenon, nor do chiropractors "fill in" in areas where medical doctors are absent or unavailable (Yesalis et al., 1980).

The role and status of chiropractic in relation to the other healing professions, traditional medicine in particular, have been a matter of continual debate. DCs have gained a measure of respect—and even prospered—in part because they did not abandon their distinctive theories of disease and health and their alternative healing practices.

WILBERT M. GESLER

See
**Chiropractic: Definition, History,
and Theory (IV)**
Chiropractic Research (IV)

OSTEOPATHIC MEDICINE: PRACTICE ISSUES

Osteopathic medicine is a complete and distinctive primary care–centered approach to medical, surgical, and other health services, founded on a philosophy embracing the importance of hands-on evaluation and treatment of the total person and dedicated to the furtherance of health care for all Americans, particularly underserved populations.

The osteopathic medical profession is the fastest growing segment of the total population of physicians and surgeons in the United States. In 1968 there were five private, freestanding colleges producing slightly more than 400 graduate D.O.s (Doctors of Osteopathic Medicine). In 1997, there are 19 colleges graduating approximately 2,000 D.O.s. Seven of the new schools are affiliated with comprehensive universities, and six new schools are state-supported institutions.

In 1968, there were 12,000 listed D.O.s. In 1997, there are approximately 40,000 D.O.s licensed as "physicians and surgeons" in all 50 states and the District of Columbia, who care for the health care needs of approximately 30 million Americans. The distribution of D.O.s across the country, however, is uneven, reflecting avoidance in the past by practitioners of states with discriminatory licensure laws and clustering of D.O.s around states with osteopathic medical schools. Twelve states currently have more than 1,000 D.O.s apiece, while 11 states have fewer than 100 each.

To enter an osteopathic medical school, matriculants must have previously earned 3 years or more college credit. They then enter a 4-year undergraduate professional curriculum followed by a 1-year internship, with the great majority of recent graduates undergoing additional residency training. Currently, there are 18 osteopathic specialty boards that certify D.O.s in such fields as family medicine, surgery, obstetrics and gynecology, internal medicine, nuclear medicine, and emergency medicine.

There are three significant differences between D.O.s and allopathic physicians (M.D.s): (1) a far greater percentage of D.O.s have historically entered primary care medical fields; (2) D.O.s have a much greater percentage of their practitioners locating in underserviced, particularly rural areas; and (3) D.O.s in their training and practice, incorporate osteopathic principles, the most visible expression of which is the use of palpatory diagnosis and manipulative therapy in the overall evaluation and treatment of the neuromusculoskeletal system, focusing in particular upon the spine.

Osteopathic medicine was founded by Andrew Taylor Still (1828–1917), a Midwestern orthodox medical practitioner trained through the apprenticeship system of the day. After losing three of his children to spinal meningitis despite the best efforts of his neighboring physicians, he sought out an essentially drugless alternative, finding inspiration from the unorthodox approaches of magnetic healing and bonesetting. He came to argue that most diseases were due to misplaced bones in the spinal column, which interfered with normal physiological processes, particularly the circulation of the blood. If these misplaced bones (originally called osteopathic lesions) were mechanically corrected, the body would be able to heal itself. Still's teaching was "find it, fix it, and leave it alone." Later investigations showed that these "lesions," now called somatic dysfunctions, were palpably detected alterations in the functions of the body framework that could be documented through electromyography and other objective instrumentation.

Establishing the first school in Kirksville, Missouri, in 1892, Still attracted thousands of patients and students to the little town, treating them almost exclusively with manipulation while at the same time removing them from their reliance upon such commonly used drugs as opium, morphine, and alcohol. Within a few years, he established a surgical sanitarium and sanctioned the use of anesthetics, antiseptics, and antidotes. All other drugs, vaccines, and serums he rejected on philosophical grounds. Some of his students established colleges elsewhere before the turn of the century; by 1904, there were 4,000 D.O.s in practice, while the number of chiropractors (D.C.s), followers of Daniel Palmer who established his school in nearby Davenport, Iowa, in the late 1890s, numbered less than two dozen. However, over the decades, as D.O.s sought an unlimited field of practice encompassing all proven diagnostic and therapeutic tools, chiropractic with its continued focus on the spine, was soon recognized by most Americans as the dominant group of manipulative practitioners.

In addition to the effort to get the American Osteopathic Association (AOA) to approve the complete integration of pharmacology into the curriculum, which occurred in 1929, D.O.s have struggled successfully to upgrade the standards maintained by their colleges, beginning in the late 1930s; grow despite the willing assimilation of most California D.O.s, who became M.D.s in that state in 1962; obtain acceptance by the federal government to have D.O.s enter armed forces as commissioned medical officers, which first occurred in 1966; and have all 50 states license D.O.s as complete physicians and surgeons, the last being Mississippi in 1973.

Since 1966, in addition to AOA internship and residency programs, D.O.s have become eligible to enter approved allopathic (M.D.) programs, and as the number of D.O. graduates has exceeded the number of quality positions in osteopathic auspices and as some allopathic programs offer training opportunities otherwise unavailable or in limited supply in the osteopathic community, an increasing number of D.O.s have taken this alternative educational pathway. The continuation of this trend toward allopathic postdoctoral opportunities weakens both the distinctiveness of the osteopathic approach to health and disease among these D.O.s and the solidarity of the osteopathic profession as a whole.

While a growing number of younger D.O.s are committed to delivering a distinctive form of health care, the profession is increasingly recognizing that osteopathic principles and practices must be fully integrated into their undergraduate and graduate programs and into their hospital and ambulatory settings, if osteopathic medicine is to have a compelling rationale for its continued independent existence. The degree to which D.O.s practice medicine, "osteopathically" will dramatically shape consumer perceptions of osteopathic medicine as a real alternative in choosing their health care practitioners.

NORMAN GEVITZ

Section 3

Education
Issues

EFFECTS OF COMPLEMENTARY HEALTH PRACTICES ON MEDICAL EDUCATION

Complementary practices have emerged over the past decade as a new curricular component in many medical and nursing schools across the United States. Now over 75 medical schools offer at least elective course work and/or rotations in this area. By 1998 a few medical schools also have developed required course work in complementary medicine, and several of the nation's research-oriented academic medical centers have begun or plan to open model complementary medicine interdisciplinary programs to conduct research, educate health professionals, and deliver integrative health care to patients. These medical schools include the University of Minnesota, the University of Iowa, the University of California Los Angeles, and the University of Arizona.

A 1996 national conference cosponsored by the National Institutes of Health Office of Alternative Medicine developed explicit recommendations about incorporating complementary practice courses into medical and nursing educational activities across the country. These recommendations included the following: (1) using a range of instructional formats, for example, didactic and experiential learning opportunities, continuing education courses, faculty development programs, and self-learning through electronic and print resources; (2) incorporating information on each complementary practice relating to the discipline's philosophical and spiritual paradigm, scientific foundation, educational preparation, practice, and evidence of efficacy and safety; and (3) developing national centers of excellence to foster collaboration among complementary practitioners, nurses, and physicians and the promotion of synergy among education, research, and clinical practice.

Recently, both a special interest group of the Association of American Medical Colleges and a national professional organization of primary care teachers (the Society of Teachers of Family Medicine) have convened working groups to develop model curriculum guidelines for medical schools and primary care residency training programs, encompassing a compendium of core attitudes, skills, and knowledge base for integrating complementary modalities into the professional education of health care practitioners in the United States. According to a recent survey of family medicine programs, instruction and offerings vary considerably in both content and format (Wetzel & Eisenberg, 1997). Educational activities within these programs appear to be more common in the Northeast and Rocky Mountain regions.

The nation's first fellowship program in complementary and alternative medicine opened in July 1997 at the University of Arizona—the Program in Integrative Medicine—to train four primary care board-certified physicians annually. These fellows participate in a comprehensive 2-year clinical and research program and will be prepared, upon graduation, to develop and lead similar fellowship programs at academic medical centers throughout the country. The fellowship conducts an integrative medicine subspecialty clinic several times weekly, staffed by the program's director, Dr. Andrew Weil, and a medical director. Complementary clinicians from the community have received clinical privileges at the university's medical center and participate in weekly patient conferences and the direct delivery of complementary therapies, such as acupuncture, manipulation, guided imagery, and bodywork.

A common driving force for the remarkable emergence and rapid dissemination of complementary medicine as a "new" curricular component throughout medical education nationally is consumer demand for a broader spectrum of diagnostic and treatment options and for integration of complementary practices into the mainstream health care delivery system. The emergence is being propelled by a research agenda established and supported by the National Center for Complementary and Alternative Medicine to create an evidence-based foundation for complementary therapies. Additionally, major health care organizations in the United States (e.g., Blue Cross, United Health Care, and Oxford Health Plans) are beginning to offer members a credentialed network of holistic providers in addition to their networks of allopathic and osteopathic physicians. Consumer and practitioner access to research studies and information on alternative modalities and remedies has been accommodated by the growth of the Internet and World Wide Web home pages emphasizing complementary medicine.

Over 70% of consumers who use complementary remedies do not share this information with their mainstream physicians. This lack of knowledge can impair and delay the healing value of integrating various modalities. With the widespread availability of complementary health practice offerings in medical education programs throughout the country, it is anticipated that at minimum, mainstream health care practitioners in the immediate future will be able to routinely assess the health beliefs and full utilization patterns of their patients. Through their exposure during medical school and residency training to complementary practices offerings, conventional allopathic-trained physicians will be more likely to refer their patients to qualified and certified complementary practitioners in their area. With additional training and experience, it is reasonable to expect that growing numbers of physicians will also integrate one or more of the complementary modalities into the care they routinely deliver to patients. These three levels of practice integration are critical toward the further evolution of evidence-based, high-quality, cost-effective health care delivery in the United States.

In addition to the growth of complementary practices in the curriculum of allopathic medical schools, there continues to be an expansion of interest in naturopathic medical schools. Naturopathic physicians are now licensed in seven states and receive broad training in complementary approaches during their medical education. Nationally, there also has been major growth in both the quality and quantity of educational training programs in massage therapy, herbal medicine, Chinese medicine, acupuncture, manipulative medicine, and homeopathy. Increasingly, mainstream physicians are participating in these programs.

EVAN W. KLIGMAN

THE EFFECTS OF COMPLEMENTARY HEALTH PRACTICES ON NURSING EDUCATION AND PRACTICE

Complementary health practices and the nursing profession have had reciprocal, mutually positive effects on each other. Nursing was one of the first health professions open to complementary practices, long before they became acceptable to mainstream medicine. Nursing facilitated the entry of complementary practices into mainstream health care, and complementary health care opened a new domain for nursing practice. This compatibility occurred because nursing has always had a philosophy of dealing with the whole person, not with his or her component parts or his or her disease. Complementary health care, with its nonreductionistic orientation, was welcomed by nursing.

Starting with the nursing theory of Martha Rogers (1970) and extending into theories such as those of Watson (1988), Newman (1994), and Dossey and colleagues (1995), nursing has had theories that treat the human holistically. This is not to say that all of nursing takes this approach; some nursing programs and practices are solidly grounded in the medical model or other scientific-based models. However, holistic nursing theory and theory underlying many complementary health practices share similar notions of the human being. Among the holistic nursing theorists, Watson (1988) sees the human being as a soul vulnerable to disharmony, of which disease may be one symptom. The nurse's task is to restore harmony, and this addresses the disease as well. Newman (1994) sees the human being as continuously expanding consciousness. The nurse in this model sees disease as a signal that the patient may be ready to move to a higher level of consciousness, and the task is to facilitate that development. Dossey and colleagues (1995) simply added a new component of spirit to an old model of the biopsychosocial being. Dossey justifies holistic thera-

peutics according to newer theories of psychoneuroimmunology, theories emerging from physiological research, and asserting new and important reciprocal linkages between mind, spirit, and body. From this Dossey arrives at a dualistic theory of nursing therapeutics: doing therapy and being therapy, the latter incorporating many complementary care practices.

Whichever of these or other emerging nursing theories one applies, each involves major reorientation to what it means to be human. The theories focus on newer, closer body-mind (or body-spirit) interconnections. Most of these orientations include the fact that thoughts have greater impact on the body (and vice versa) than was imagined earlier. Using this knowledge, nurses use techniques like meditation, guided imagery, and relaxation therapy to affect the body or, more properly, the whole person.

Many of these theories (Slater, 1995a, 1995b; Helvie, 1995) also perceive the human being as basically an energy system. This may include the Eastern belief that there are various energy layers of different vibrations extending beyond the physical body (the human aura) that may be manipulated for healing. Therapeutic touch, introduced to the nursing profession two decades ago by Krieger (1979), is the most common nursing procedure used to manipulate the human being conceived as an energy system. Older Eastern techniques such as acupuncture also have been introduced to manipulate the body's subtle energy systems. Finally, many of these theories propose that a universal energy exists throughout the universe and may be channeled for healing. Other energic systems, such as Reiki and core energetics, also have found their way into nursing as ways to harness universal energy for the sake of the client. Healing in all these theories has to do with seeing the total human being in a new way and not simply as a disease process.

Nursing has adopted complementary approaches in two distinct ways. The first is as an add-on to regular practices and traditional curricula. In practice, complementary therapies are widely disbursed among traditional nursing practices. Therapeutic touch, relaxation therapy, and guided visualization are perhaps the forms most typically inserted into regular care (i.e., the relaxation therapy and healing circles used at Beth Israel Medical Center in New York City). Additionally, many nursing entrepreneurial efforts exclusively focus on complementary care (i.e., the work by the Holistic Nursing Consultants of Sante Fe, New Mexico). The growth of this practice arena also is evidenced in the rapid growth of the American Holistic Nursing Association.

Sometimes the joining of complementary therapy and traditional nursing is awkward. For example, the nursing diagnosis of spiritual distress (obviously a holistic notion) was added to the list of diagnoses produced by the North American Nursing Diagnosis Association (NANDA) and commonly used in traditional nursing practice and education. The problem with such an addition is that the holistic context is not an appropriate fit with the reductionistic NANDA system, or, as Berggren-Thomas and Griggs (1995) note, it puts the nurse in a position that may be intrusive into the consumer's privacy at best. In practice, such a perspective also assumes that the nurse has enough spiritual savvy to be able to assess the spiritual status of others.

Second, complementary health practice has been adopted in nursing education. Many master's level curricula, usually advertised as holistic programs, provide a comprehensive complementary specialty apart from traditional nursing. These curricula can be found in schools across the United States.

Complementary health practices have become the nexus of a major new format for nursing practice and education, adding, as Schaub (1995) says, the potentials of "the range and power of the imaginal state of consciousness; the ability to self-regulate physiology; the trust in an innate desire to survive and evolve that instinctively tries to reassert itself in the face of abuse; the right uses of the body in regard to food and sex; an attitude of conscious cooperation rather than of control." In addition to this focus on complementary health practice roles, nursing has also incorporated many specific complementary beliefs and practices into its traditional patterns of education and care.

BARBARA STEVENS BARNUM

See
Acupuncture and Chinese Medicine (IV)
Imagery (IV)
Psychoneuroimmunology (IV)
Reiki (IV)
Therapeutic Touch: Definition, History, and Theory (IV)
Transcendental Meditation (IV)

PHARMACY EDUCATION AND COMPLEMENTARY PRACTICES

A review of the pharmacy literature shows an increasing demand from consumers for professional advice about herbal and homeopathic products from pharmacists (DerMarderosian, 1996; Tyler, 1996). In a 1996 national U.S. survey, most community pharmacists reported that they received inquiries about herbals, and a majority indicated that they were actually made aware of the uses of various herbal products by consumers (Bouldin et al., 1997). Almost two thirds of the pharmacists believed that commercially marketed herbal products are not well standardized and would likely recommend herbals shown to be safe and effective in clinical trials. Half of all pharmacists surveyed indicated that the federal regulations provided for herbal products in the Dietary Supplement Health & Education Act of 1994 are inadequate. Almost all reported that they did not have sufficient information about potential interactions involving herbal products but only about a third have actively sought information about them. Most thought it likely that they would seek additional information about herbals. Apparently, pharmacists recognize the need to learn more about herbal and homeopathic products but are reluctant to offer advice or recommendations to consumers because they lack information and knowledge about the safety and efficacy of these products.

Pharmacy organizations and pharmacy educators are responding to the need to educate practicing pharmacists about complementary practices primarily in the form of continuing education (CE) programs and journal articles. The American Pharmaceutical Association (APhA) has recently adopted a policy that demonstrates its commitment to educating current and future pharmacists about complementary practices (i.e., herbal products and homeopathic remedies) to facilitate effective patient counseling activities. In fact, the APhA devoted an entire session to complementary and natural products in its call for abstracts for its 1998 annual meeting. Similarly, the National Community Pharmacists Association (NCPA) offered educational sessions on natural pharmacy at its 1997 annual meeting. The Texas Pharmacy Foundation sponsored a CE program on homeopathy and, in cooperation with the American Botanical Council (ABC), offers accredited pharmacy home study CE programs in phytomedicines. Other CE programs on complementary treatments have been offered through various pharmacy journals.

Detailed papers geared toward helping pharmacists understand herbals (Tyler, 1996) and homeopathy (DerMarderosian, 1996; McDermott, Riedlinger, & Chapman, 1995) recently have been published in leading pharmacy journals. DerMarderosian and Kratz (1975) contributed a chapter on complementary healthcare in the 19th edition of *Remington: The Science and Practice of Pharmacy*. Additional papers offer brief reviews and updates on herbal and homeopathic remedies, and they present lists of excellent resources for obtaining factual information about both treatment modalities (Combest & Nemecz, 1997). One such resource is the English translation of the German Commission E monographs (Blumenthal et al., 1998) which is regarded by many as the most accurate information available on the safety and efficacy of herbs and phytomedicinals.

Pharmacy schools also are responding to the increasing use of complementary therapies among consumers. According to a 1997 survey of 77 U.S. pharmacy schools, most pharmacy schools are educating future pharmacists about complementary approaches, particularly in the area of herbals (Miller & Murray, 1997). Results revealed that 57 (74%) of the pharmacy schools surveyed offered at least one course that was either partly or totally devoted to herbal medicine. Thirteen schools indicated that herbal medicine was not addressed at all in the curriculum, and seven indicated that herbal courses would be implemented within the next year. Some pharmacy schools address the use of complementary practices by offering courses with a sociopsychological focus. These courses address social, psychological, and cultural issues related to health care and are intended to teach students how those issues affect consumer choices involving the use of complementary treatments.

Eisenberg (1997) offered an excellent step-by-step strategy for health care professionals to utilize when advising consumers on the use of complementary therapies. Pharmacists, as medication counselors, are in a unique position to evaluate and monitor the use of complementary therapies among consumers, particularly those therapies that are medicinal in nature (e.g., herbals, homeopathic remedies, nutritional supplements). Many suggest that pharmacists are responsible for learning more about complementary therapies so that they can effectively discuss their use with consumers (Miller & Murray, 1997; Tyler, 1996; DerMarderosian, 1996; McDermott, Riedlinger, & Chapman, 1995). Although the pharmacist's role in advising consumers about the use of complementary therapies has been heavily debated, particularly in regard to homeopathy, the fact remains that many people are using complementary therapies to treat a variety of medical conditions. If pharmacists are to competently

provide pharmaceutical care to consumers and monitor treatment outcomes, it is important to be able to obtain information about complementary therapies and about consumer use of these therapies. Pharmacy educators and organizations are responding to this self-care movement among consumers by educating current and future pharmacists about complementary therapies.

CAROLYN M. BROWN

See
Herbal Therapies (IV)
Homeopathy: Molecular Basis (IV)

TEACHING ABOUT COMPLEMENTARY HEALTH PRACTICES IN SCHOOLS OF PUBLIC HEALTH*

There are many courses on complementary health practices in schools of medicine in the United States (Daly, 1995), but only a few in schools of public health. This is unfortunate, because complementary health practices have implications for public health that are as profound as they are for physicians, nurses, physical and occupational therapists, counselors, and other providers of health care whose curricula offer more comprehensive coverage of the topic. Implications for public health include the epidemiology of the use of services, efficacy and safety of practices, organization and finance of the delivery of complementary services, and professional licensure, certification, and accountability of providers.

In the 1993–1994 academic year, a faculty member at Boston University's School of Public Health developed a course in response to student requests. The result,

"Public Health Perspectives on Alternative and Complementary Health Care," was the first such course offered at a North American school of public health. The course syllabus reflects comprehensive public health issues concerning complementary health practice. Topics covered included (1) the theory, philosophy, and history of major forms of complementary health practices; (2) historic perspectives on the relationship between complementary and conventional health practices in the United States; (3) the epidemiology of complementary health practice, including patterns of use and reasons for use; (4) the relationships between complementary and conventional practices; (5) professionalism and the professional status of alternative and complementary health providers, including licensure, certification, and the accreditation of professional educational and training programs, regulation of professional practice, and professional liability; (6) standards of evidence in complementary health practices; (7) reimbursement; and (8) complementary health practices, managed care, and health care reform (Meyers, 1994).

Through a combination of lectures, readings, and speakers the course has addressed some of the more prevalent forms of complementary health practices, for example, self-treatment; acupuncture; herbalism; religious healing, both indigenous (Christian Science and Seventh-Day Adventism) and immigrant (e.g., *Santeria* and *Vodun*); and complementary health professions (e.g., chiropractic and homeopathy). Class sessions are divided equally between lectures by the instructor and presentations by guest speakers, some of which are supplemented by video. In some instances, students give class presentations about practices with

which they have had considerable direct experience—usually positive, but occasionally negative. Examples are discussions on Reiki (positive), apitherapy (mixed), and aloe vera (positive) as therapeutic agents.

In 1996 the course increased from a 2- to a 4-credit format. Designed for graduate students in the masters in public health program, the class has included medical students, dental students, house officers, and physician and nurse staff and faculty. In respect to the needs of a public health (vs. clinical) curriculum, there is no effort to provide technical or clinical instruction. Rather, clinicians and practitioners are asked to provide sufficiently detailed descriptions of their respective practices so that students can address the public health concerns.

There has been a limited range of satisfactory available texts. The course used two texts to address the topics covered (Micozzi, 1996a; Payer, 1988). There also is an extensive packet of supplementary readings. All students take a midterm exam, and most write final papers.

Overall, student responses to both structured and unstructured evaluation protocols indicate that the course has been successful. In both 1996 and 1997, the first years that it was offered in a 4-credit format, the course won a teaching award. Many of the students' criticisms have to do with situational factors that bear little upon pedagogy (e.g., there was too much reading; the exams were unfair; the class sessions were too long, and particular guest speakers were dull, boring, uninformed, or inarticulate). In contrast, at least two concerns, closely related and shared by both students and the instructor, have broader implications for those who want to teach public health students about health care alternatives: (1) the choices of alternative and complementary treatments and (2) the limited selection of resources that would facilitate teaching about health care alternatives to students of public health.

The selection of complementary practices was dictated by several considerations. In some cases, reasons are epidemiologic—for example, chiropractic and acupuncture are so widely practiced and, in the case of chiropractic, their practitioners so widely licensed and reimbursed by third-party payers, that it is essential to include them. In others, the reason is more parochial—for example, the Mother Church of Christian Science is located in Boston; therefore, there is a particular need for students in Boston to learn about Christian Science and a correspondingly rich resource of speakers. Assuming the importance of discussing religious traditions of healing, the choice was relatively easy.

In still other cases—and these are the most difficult—selections reflect a combination of principled and expedient reasons. For example, although there is no compelling epidemiologic reason to discuss homeopathy, there is a considerable, although methodologically uneven, corpus of both reasonable descriptions and critical reviews. These address such topics as the epidemiology, costs, and effectiveness of homeopathy, all of which are useful to students of public health. Moreover, homeopathy has considerable historical importance. But so does Ayurveda, to name just one type of healing practice that has not been part of the curriculum. That it has not been reflects the limit of time and, more significantly, the inability to find balanced readings that are descriptive and, although partisan, devoid of extravagant or outlandish claims. Similarly, there is difficulty finding speakers who can describe and explain their beliefs and practices to public health students in credible and comprehensible ways.

There are a number of instructional approaches that could facilitate the expansion of courses on complementary health care in schools of public health. One of these is to share resources, not only bibliographies and lists of films, videotapes, and home pages, but also videotapes, audiotapes, and slides of outstanding speakers. With the speakers' permission, it may be possible to make available to colleagues a videotape of a lecture by a Christian Science nurse and practitioner, or a videotaped encounter between one or both of them and a person who comes to them for assistance. Colleagues at other institutions could provide similar tapes demonstrating or describing and explaining such topics as traditional Korean medicine and Native American healing, forms of complementary practices that are not always easily and predictably available.

None of the guest speakers queried have objected to this suggestion. After all, most of them are advocates of their ideas and practices and are quite enthusiastic about the idea. Some of them are more enthusiastic about film, tape, or photography than they are about class appearances, because of some combination of convenience, inhibitions related to language, cultural concerns about visiting a university, and legal liability. There are even greater logistic difficulties and greater reluctance to bring to class patients or other beneficiaries of services. Greater potential benefits of the use of films may address this issue. With a sufficient bank of resources, there could be an assurance of wider access to a range of interesting and instructive resources, as well as an ability to change some teaching examples from year to year.

Another suggestion is to use the Internet and such media as CD-ROM. Also, with or without CDs, there could be World Wide Web links to some of the growing number of home pages dealing with different approaches or aspects of alternative and complementary health care (Wooten, 1996).

The need for teaching public health students about complementary health practices is evident. Micozzi (1996b) argues eloquently for the inclusion of courses on complementary health care. Although he appears to speak mainly to health practitioners, there is a clear, if implicit, message to schools—and professors—of public health: Their response needs to be more complete, creative, and cooperative than it has been in the past.

ALLAN R. MEYERS

*Acknowledgment: An earlier draft of this entry was presented to a symposium on "Integrating the Teaching of Alternative and Complementary Health Practices and Conventional Medical Therapies" at the 124th Annual Meeting of the American Public Health Association, New York, November 20, 1996.

See

Acupuncture and Chinese Medicine (IV)
Chiropractic: Definition, History, and Theory (IV)
Herbal Therapies (IV)
Homeopathy: Use in Family Practice Medicine (IV)
Religious Science Practitioners (IV)

THE EDUCATION OF HOMEOPATHS

It is essential to begin a discussion of the education of homeopaths with the fact that the proper education of a homeopath is lifelong. Individuals who practice homeopathy are a mixed assortment of licensed health professionals. Also, there is a small but active group of dedicated unlicensed practitioners of homeopathy. In practice, some clinicians specialize in homeopathy and prescribe homeopathic medicines to nearly all of their patients. Other practitioners, who have not learned the elaborate system of homeopathic medicine, tend to prescribe these natural medicines for a smaller percentage of their patients. Commonly, these latter clinicians are knowledgeable of a smaller number of homeopathic medicines and usually prescribe them for acute, not chronic, ailments.

The greatest number of health professionals who specialize in homeopathy in the Western world are medical doctors. In Europe, where homeopathy is one of the leading alternative medicines, it has been estimated that over 30% of French physicians and 20% of German physicians prescribe homeopathic medicines (Fisher & Ward, 1994), that over 40% of British physicians refer patients to homeopathic doctors (Wharton & Lewith, 1986), and that 45% of Dutch physicians consider homeopathic medicines to be effective (Kleijnen, Knipschild, & ter Riet, 1991). These significant numbers suggest that it may no longer be appropriate to consider homeopathy to be an "alternative medicine" in Europe.

In the United States, licensed professionals who specialize in homeopathy, other than medical doctors, include naturopathic physicians, chiropractic doctors, acupuncturists, physician assistants, nurse practitioners, and nurses. There are also hundreds of veterinarians and dentists who utilize homeopathic medicines for large numbers of their patients.

Because homeopathy is an integral part of naturopathic education, it is common for naturopathic doctors to specialize in homeopathy. There is even a separate organization of naturopathic homeopaths (the Homeopathic Academy of Naturopathic Physicians). In comparison, chiropractors have a tendency to dabble in numerous natural therapies. Even though there may be more chiropractors who prescribe homeopathic medicines than any other health professionals in the United States, only a relatively small number of them specialize in homeopathy.

In 1990 there were three training programs in homeopathy and three naturopathic medical schools in the United States and Canada. By 1996 the number increased to over 20 training programs and five naturopathic medical schools (Ullman, 1996). Commonly, training programs in homeopathy are 3- or 4-year courses usually consisting of extended weekend (3- or 4-day) classes that meet every month or every other month. Significant amounts of homework are given and required. Homeopathic training programs include detailed instruction in homeopathic philosophy, case taking, case analysis, materia medica, and repertory. Materia medica refers to the "materials of medicines" used in homeopathy, and repertory refers to the important texts and databases that list the specific medicines and their dosages. Courses open to unlicensed practitioners generally require that students first seek out courses in anatomy, physiology, and pathology at local colleges.

Although clinical training is not a part of most homeopathic programs at present, a common part of the training is the observation on video of homeopathic case taking. Instructors start and stop the video to discuss nuances of case taking and case analysis. Also, students are required to take case histories and provide an analysis of them, with treatment plans.

Naturopathic education is considerably more structured and detailed. Similar premed requirements for admission into medical schools are required for naturopathic schools. Naturopathic medical school itself is a 4-year full-time program in which the first 2 years resemble basic science and pathology training that takes place in medical schools. Years 3 and 4 are considerably different. This is when naturopathic students are taught various natural therapies, of which homeopathy is one of the most popular. Approximately 1,000 hours of clinical training is also provided.

Some students and practitioners of homeopathy are unlicensed in any health profession. While some homeopathic training programs require that students have one of the recognized health professional licenses, the majority of homeopathic training programs provide education to anyone who is interested.

In addition to the above mentioned training programs, there are a select number of correspondence courses in homeopathy. Two of the leading correspondence courses were developed in England. They are 2-3-year programs—one for 350 hours a year, the other, 1,000 hours.

There are also mail-order naturopathic programs in which homeopathy is a part. However, these programs are not highly respected, and graduates of them are not allowed to sit for licensing examinations for naturopaths in any state, nor are they able to obtain certification from leading homeopathic certification bodies.

Homeopathic certification includes certification for allopathic and osteopathic physicians and dentists (American Board of Homeotherapeutics), for naturopathic physicians (Homeopathic Academy of Naturopathic Physicians), for any licensed health professional (Council on Homeopathic Certification), and for anyone who completes a recognized school of homeopathy (North American Society of Homeopaths).

Finally, it should be noted that interest in homeopathy among health professionals is growing, and it can be expected that there will be a significant increase in the quantity and quality of homeopathic training in the coming years. One survey of members of the American Medical Association discovered that close to 50% were interested in training in homeopathy (Berman, Hartnoll, Singh, & Singh, 1997). As homeopathy attains greater popularity and respect from the general public and the medical community, increasingly higher standards of education will be demanded.

DANA ULLMAN

See

Homeopathy: Molecular Basis (IV)
Homeopathy: Use in Family Practice Medicine (IV)

THE COMPLEMENTARY AND ALTERNATIVE MEDICINE PROGRAM AT STANFORD UNIVERSITY (CAMPS)

The Complementary and Alternative Medicine Program at Stanford University (CAMPS) is one of 10 research centers established by the Office of Alternative Medicine to investigate the therapeutic effectiveness of alternative and complementary therapies. CAMPS is housed within the Stanford Center for Research and Disease Prevention (SCRDP) and is headed by the Deputy Director of SCRDP, William Haskell. The mandate of CAMPS is to explore the factors that influence the aging process and determine those most amenable to intervention. The demographic changes (AARP, 1995) that forecast significant increases in the number of elderly people make the research of CAMPS timely and important.

The research focus at CAMPS is to help determine why and how age-related changes occur, with the ultimate goal to find ways to increase the number of people who age successfully. With this in mind, CAMPS defines "successful aging" broadly as maintaining cognitive, physical, psychosocial, and spiritual functioning until the end of life. CAMPS will design projects to evaluate the effectiveness of alternative and complementary therapies in the promotion of successful aging as measured by physical indicators, quality of life, and psychosocial measures and evaluations of spiritual well-being.

CAMPS derives much of its impetus on successful aging from the work by Rowe and Kahn (1987). The authors found that the physical declines associated with aging were not inevitable and were largely associated with disease states. They articulate that a significant percentage of people age uneventfully and maintain physical, social, and cognitive capacity until very old age. They make the clear distinction between "usual" and "successful" aging.

Other work that was important in deriving the mission of CAMPS was that of Bortz (1989), who helped explicate and crystallize the unparalleled importance of exercise in maintaining function as people age. The work of Baltes (1993) concurrently makes the case for the importance of cognitive strategies and optimal social interaction to enhance function in elderly adults.

Along with promoting healthy aging, CAMPS investigates the effect of complementary and alternative treatments on the chronic and often age-related conditions that conventional medicine has shown limited effectiveness in treating and given minimal attention to preventing. In particular, CAMPS focuses its research attention on cardiovascular and musculoskeletal disease. Conventional therapies, such as surgery and pharmaceuticals, not only have demonstrated weak utility in preventing and treating hypertension and arthritis but also often lead to great expense and disabling side effects.

The initial project CAMPS undertook was to establish review teams to conduct comprehensive and critical evaluations of the state of science in the following five domains:

1. The effect of mind/body/spirit therapies in the treatment of cardiovascular and musculoskeletal disease.
2. Nutrition/herbal medicine (vegetarianism and phytochemicals).
3. Alternative systems of medical practice (traditional Chinese medicine).
4. Manual healing/exercise (yoga, massage, Tai Chi).
5. Insurance coverage for complementary and alternative medicine (CAM). This includes the evolving influence of managed care on the availability, utilization, and reimbursement of such therapies for older adults.

The reviews served as the basis for the main purpose of CAMPS, which is the de-

sign of studies that the research reviews suggested were promising. Many of these studies will be conducted in collaboration with other divisions and departments in the Stanford School of Medicine, such as psychiatry, rheumatology, cardiology, anesthesiology, and oncology. The following specific research studies are either proposed or already under way:

- Insurance reimbursement and policy trends for CAM therapies.
- Exploring the degree of CAM utilization by older adults in California.
- Using meditation and positive emotion psychosocial treatment for elderly patients with congestive heart failure.
- Evaluating the effects of plant estrogens on health-related measures in postmenopausal women.
- Exploring the medical and psychological effects of Tai Chi practice in women 70 years and older.
- Comparing the traditional management of osteoarthritis by rheumatologists with the use of chiropractic therapy.
- Comparing hormone replacement therapy with a comprehensive lifestyle intervention in postmenopausal women on physiological, psychosocial, and quality-of-life measures.
- Evaluating the effect of mindfulness meditation on arthritis pain and disability.
- Gauging the effect of lifestyle modification (nutrition, psychospiritual practice, group support, and exercise) in the prevention of disease and the enhancement of function in older men and women.

CAMPS may also investigate the possibility of collaborating in the establishment of a mind-body clinic for the elderly. The CAMPS program hopes to provide technical assistance to alternative medical practitioners for objective assessment of their efficacy through clinical trial research.

FREDERIC LUSKIN

See

Herbal Therapies (IV)
Nutrition (IV)
T'ai Chi (IV)
Yoga (IV)

EDUCATION AND RESEARCH CONDUCTED AT CAMPS

The Complementary and Alternative Medicine Program at Stanford University (CAMPS) has an active research agenda. A variety of studies are in process or in the planning stages. The studies range from the use of nutritional supplementation for postmenopausal women to the facilitation of guided spiritual practice to the analysis of complementary and alternative medicine (CAM) use in the elderly. The research programs are also assessed via a wide range of physiological and psychological instrumentation. Two of the current studies will be examined in detail here to serve as representative of the work of the center. First is a study looking at the effect of psychospiritual practices on elderly adults with congestive heart failure. Due to better medical management of myocardial infarction, the incidence of congestive heart failure is rising. The rate of hospitalization for the disease is the highest for any diagnostic category, and the annual mortality rate is 28% to 40% (AHA, 1996). In addition, a high percentage of sufferers have comorbid depression, and manage-

ment of this aspect of the condition is routinely ignored. There are no previous research studies that have investigated the effect of comprehensive psychosocial training on this population, suggesting that this project may be the first among many.

The CAMPS study is investigating the effectiveness of randomly assigning patients into one of two comprehensive psychosocial group treatments. These psychosocial programs are provided as complementary to the usual and customary care, and a regular medical care group will serve as a control. At this writing, the study is in the pilot stage and training groups are ongoing. To date, the first groups of participants have been regular in attendance, practice the intervention faithfully, and the measurements are well tolerated. In particular, the study is evaluating autonomic tone via 24-hour halter monitoring because of the effect of sympathetic overextension in congestive heart failure.

The first treatment is an adaptation of the mindfulness meditation program developed by Jon Kabat-Zinn at the University of Massachusetts. In this program, participants learn meditation and yoga, are helped to develop a daily stress management practice, and are coached in using the tools in daily life. Clinical research on the mindfulness program has established its effectiveness in the treatment of chronic pain and anxiety (Kabat-Zinn, Lipworth, & Burney, 1985; Kabat-Zinn et al., 1992).

The second treatment will teach the positive emotion enhancement program developed by the Institute of HeartMath. In this program, participants learn how to focus their attention on positive feelings and are taught how to use this focus both to manage their stress and to improve their relationships. The Institute of HeartMath has conducted research that offers suggestive indications (Rein, Atkinson, & McCraty, 1995; Tiller, McCraty, & Atkinson, 1996) that positive emotion can positively affect heart function, while negative emotions such as anger and resentment can jeopardize heart function.

Both programs will be taught over 4 months in a small-group format. Participants are expected to regularly practice the techniques taught, and each program requires a long session of practice as part of the training. In addition, the techniques are adapted so that gentle exercise with a specific psychosocial focus becomes an integral part of the practice. Finally, homework assignments are given so those participants may integrate the practices into their daily life to better manage their disease. This study will measure participants' emotional status, quality of life, symptom intensity, functional capacity, exercise tolerance, and autonomic function.

The second study investigates the effect of phytoestrogen supplementation on postmenopausal women. The phytoestrogens are administered as part of a soy protein supplement. In this study, participants were randomly assigned to either a protein supplement group receiving the phytoestrogens or to a group receiving the protein supplement without the phytoestrogens. The primary purpose of the study is to establish that supplementation with plant-based estrogens can lower cholesterol, in particular LDL, in postmenopausal women. Secondary interests are in quality-of-life and psychosocial improvement.

The study involves 180 women and requires 5 months of regular participation. To participate, the women in this study cannot be taking hormone replacement therapy. The participants agree to be weighed every 2 weeks to guard against unwanted weight gain. Consultation with professional nutritionists also is provided.

This study design emerged from a successful, unpublished pilot study where all participants were given the phytoestrogen supplementation. In this pilot study, the soy protein supplementation was helpful in reducing LDL cholesterol. The pilot was based on population-based research and some laboratory work that suggested soy-based estrogen had a salutary effect on lowering cholesterol.

The two highlighted CAMPS studies were picked to be representative of the range of work taking place at CAMPS. Research conducted at CAMPS is designed to critically evaluate the effect of complementary, primarily lifestyle-modification practices, on the health of elderly men and women with the goal to provide tools to facilitate and enhance successful aging.

FREDERIC LUSKIN

CENTER FOR THE STUDY OF COMPLEMENTARY AND ALTERNATIVE THERAPIES TO REDUCE PAIN AND SUFFERING

The Center for the Study of Complementary and Alternative Therapies at the University of Virginia, one of 10 Centers for Complementary and Alternative Medicine (CAM) Research, was created in October 1995 with funding from the National Institute for Dental Research and the Office of Alternative Medicine, National Institutes of Health. While the infrastructure of the Center was created with this federal award, the majority of the funds needed to conduct specific research projects are sought from private foundations, industry, and appropriate institutes within the National Institutes of Health. The Center, like the nine other funded Centers, is viewed as a first step in expanding the national infrastructure for investigation of complementary therapies.

A major first-year activity involved a review of the literature to determine the state-of-the-art use of complementary therapies in pain management and to establish a database in the area of pain management and the topic of psychosocial individual differences. Using the bibliographic database software Reference Manager, the staff developed an electronic tagging mechanism to document the availability of articles in the Center's files, as well as other characteristics of the articles. The Center has nearly 10,000 citations that include the key word "pain."

The Center identifies and evaluates through rigorous research promising complementary therapies related to the relief or reduction of pain and related symptoms. The Center's core investigators have developed a prioritized list of multidisciplinary research projects that include modalities from four of the broad program areas identified by the National Center for Complementary and Alternative Medicine: manipulative and body-based systems (e.g., chiropractic and massage therapy), biofield (e.g., energy healing, intentional effects on living systems such as therapeutic touch), bioelectromagnetics (e.g., therapeutic application of pulsed electromagnetic fields and static magnetic fields), and mind-body therapies (e.g., music with and without binaural beats).

The Center's researchers and their collaborators have studies under way to test the efficacy of complementary therapies

categorized in the above four program areas. Adult populations being studied include the following: postoperative patients; persons diagnosed with fibromyalgia, chronic low back pain, migraine headaches, temporomandibular disorders, stump pain, or phantom limb pain; patients experiencing anxiety; and patients with wounds that have not healed adequately.

A major focus of the Center is exploration of individual differences and other psychosocial factors that are likely to influence why people choose to use complementary therapies, the extent to which they have used these modalities in the past, and their beliefs and expectations about the use of the therapies. The investigators collect these data on all populations studied, believing that individual psychosocial differences are likely to contribute to "nonspecific" (placebo) treatment effects of the modality being tested.

To implement its goals the Center facilitates collaborations of conventional scientists, clinicians, and individuals who can conduct research related to the Center's research agenda. The Center's researchers and their collaborators publish the results of the studies in the scientific literature and disseminate the findings to the public through presentations and articles.

Administratively based in the School of Nursing at the University of Virginia, the Center is able to connect with multidisciplinary researchers and clinicians to conduct the basic laboratory, preclinical, clinical, and epidemiological research related to its agenda. The university provides the necessary culture of inquiry and research tools, such as outstanding library facilities, well-equipped laboratories, expert statistical support services, state-of-the-art computer facilities, and the interface with other research environments. In addition, resources are readily available for the training of students and other future scientists. Doctoral students interested in complementary therapies connect with the Center to conduct their dissertation research, while master's candidates and undergraduate students conduct research projects and gain research skills through course-related activities in the Center.

The Center is exemplary of the National Center for Complementary and Alternative Medicine's use of the center concept to provide a mechanism to study the potential efficacy, effectiveness, safety, and validity of complementary therapies and to provide scientific and technical assistance to investigators who can develop research projects.

Because researchers have not studied complementary therapies to reduce pain and suffering as much as pharmacological and physical therapies, there is much need to study an array of therapies that have the potential to be integrated into conventional pain management. While there is sufficient data to support the use of selected therapies such as relaxation techniques in promoting comfort and pain reduction for some individuals, there is not yet sufficient evidence to state that one therapy is better for a particular condition than another. To reduce pain and suffering as we enter the 21st century, the Center's challenge is to investigate modalities to determine which of the complementary therapies can be integrated into conventional care, thus providing a full spectrum of modalities to promote comfort to those who suffer from painful conditions.

ANN GILL TAYLOR

Acknowledgment: This manuscript was prepared with partial support from grant award 5 U24 DE11924 funded by the National Institute of Dental Research and the Office of Alternative Medicine, National Institutes of Health

See
Chiropractic: Definition, History, and Theory (IV)
Electromagnetic Heating for Cancer Treatment (IV)
Music Therapy (IV)
Therapeutic Touch: Definition, History, and Theory (IV)

Section 4

Legal, Legislative, and Health Policy Issues

LEGAL RULES AFFECTING COMPLEMENTARY PRACTICE: MALPRACTICE AND VICARIOUS LIABILITY*

Individual as well as institutional health care providers must address concerns about malpractice liability when reaching beyond the bounds of conventional medicine to provide complementary health care. Providers can be categorized into physician, nonphysician, and institutional providers.

Malpractice is unskillful practice that falls below the standard of care in the profession and results in injury to the patient. Most complementary treatments (such as chelation therapy, ozone therapy, homeopathy, and nutritional and herbal treatments) at present are not commonly taught in medical schools or used in U.S. hospitals. Thus, physicians integrating these treatments into conventional care depart from biomedical norms of practice. They face the risk that courts may view a lack of general medical acceptance of specific procedures or a lack of government approval as failure to follow the standard of care, giving an injured patient a viable malpractice claim.

Physicians integrating complementary health practices may find a number of existing legal defenses advantageous. First is the "respectable minority" doctrine. It provides that a physician who undertakes a mode of treatment that a respectable minority within the profession would undertake under similar circumstances does not incur liability for malpractice. However,

courts differ as to what constitutes a respectable minority. Some courts permit the respectable minority defense where there is only one physician in the community following a particular approach, whereas other courts require that the minority's view be adopted by a certain number of physicians. Still others require that the minority view be "reasonable and prudent." The rather fluid and imprecise contours of the defense may be further exaggerated given the controversial nature of complementary approaches, methodological challenges raised, and shifting levels of acceptance within the health care community.

A second possible defense is assumption of risk. As applied to complementary practice, this doctrine provides that a physician may have a defense to malpractice when an individual has expressly accepted complementary care in lieu of conventional treatment and agreed to assume any ensuing risks. Courts may be inclined to honor agreements between provider and patient regarding treatment, so long as the provider has not acted in a manner that is grossly negligent or reckless.

Generally, a practitioner of complementary techniques is held to a standard of care appropriate to the profession. A chiropractor is held to a chiropractic standard of care, a naturopath to the standard of care of the naturopathic profession, an acupuncturist to the same standard as other acupuncturists.

Standards of care are more fluid for complementary practitioners because treatments involve widely varying schools of thought and techniques and highly individualized or nonstandardized methods. Many treatments, such as massage therapy, draw on the provider's intuitive or subjective faculties as much as on uniform, profes-

---

*Note. Portions of this article are excerpted or adapted from *Complementary and Alternative Medicine: Legal Boundaries and Regulating Perspectives* by M. H. Cohen, 1998, Baltimore: Johns Hopkins University Press. Copyright 1998 by Michael H. Cohen. Adapted with permission.

sionally prescribed practices. Despite the less formalized agreement around standards of care, however, some professions have established guidelines for practice that could serve as the basis for standards of care in malpractice actions (for example, clean needle technique in the practice of acupuncture).

In addition, a complementary provider may be held to medical standards of care when professional practice overlaps with biomedicine (for example, performing a physical examination). Further, complementary providers may have a duty to refer clients to medical professionals when such care is necessary and appropriate.

A final area of potential malpractice liability for complementary providers involves misrepresentation. Providers should be cautious in making claims as to the potential healing benefits of complementary care, since courts may view these claims as fraudulent, deceptive, or misleading. Generally, it is sound practice as well as legally advisable to ensure that individuals receive conventional health care treatment alongside complementary treatment, and that the complementary provider does not assume total responsibility for physical recovery from medically defined pathology.

Institutional providers of health care, such as hospitals, nursing homes, clinics, and managed-care organizations, face at least two kinds of malpractice exposure when utilizing health care professionals who provide complementary treatments: direct liability (for an act or omission of the institution, also known as corporate negligence) and vicarious liability (for an act or omission of the individual provider).

Under the doctrine of corporate negligence, courts have imposed direct liability on health care institutions for negligently failing to properly supervise health care professionals. In a groundbreaking case, *Darling v. Charleston Community Memorial Hospital* (1996), the plaintiff broke his leg in a college football game. Negligent care by the medical and nursing staff resulted in amputation of the leg. The Supreme Court of Illinois held the hospital directly liable for failure to take due care in supervising the treatment offered by its medical staff.

Institutions can mitigate such liability by ensuring that complementary providers associated with the institution are properly licensed, certified, or registered and have achieved the highest level of professional certification available. Ideally, complementary providers will have levels of training, skill, and professionalism commensurate with that of medical peers.

Health care institutions should keep accurate records of the selection and review process for such providers and should investigate whether the selected provider has a history of being sanctioned or liable for negligent practice. Institutions also can attempt to meet their duty to nonnegligently retain and supervise individual providers through periodic review and monitoring of complementary providers, and internal risk-management programs.

Finally, the institutions must ensure that providers are delivering services within their legally authorized scope of practice. For instance, massage therapists should not be engaged in spinal manipulation, and chiropractors (absent specific legislative authorization) should not be recommending homeopathic remedies. Institutions need to develop recognized protocols for collaborative practice between providers and clarify providers' specific roles within collaborative or integrated health care.

Even if health care institutions manage to avoid direct liability, they must address the risk of vicarious liability for the negligent acts of complementary providers within their domain. The doctrine of vicarious liability (or *respondeat superior*) considers individual providers to be agents of the health care institution rather than independent contractors. In vicarious liability, negligent acts of the agent are attributable to, and considered to be acts of, the principal. Courts frequently support the imposition of vicarious liability by finding "ostensible agency" or "apparent authority," in which the organization's structure gives the appearance that the provider is an agent of the institution.

Courts tend to find apparent authority lacking when: (1) the individual directly contracts with the health care provider for a specific treatment; (2) the provider arranges for admission to a particular hospital if hospitalization is necessary; (3) the provider is responsible for his or her own income tax, patient billing, and medical equipment; and (4) the provider makes independent clinical judgments, without submitting such judgments to institutional supervisors.

On the other hand, courts tend to find apparent authority when the institution: (1) exercises control over providers through rules relating to staff privileges; (2) requires providers to meet institutional quality of care standards; (3) requires consultation with appropriate staff physicians where appropriate; (4) has exclusive control of billing and fees; and (5) provides clerical and health care support personnel, as well as instruments and supplies, to providers at no cost.

If a health care institution loosens its supervisory control over its providers to reduce the risk of vicarious liability, the organization also increases the risk of direct liability for the negligent acts of its providers. Institutions must balance the risks of direct and vicarious liability. Institutions probably will err on the side of greater control, supervision, and standards, as the legal rules governing malpractice liability for complementary providers and treatments unfold.

MICHAEL H. COHEN

See
Chiropractic: Definition, History, and Theory (IV)
Herbal Therapies (IV)
Homeopathy: Molecular Basis (IV)

FEDERAL REGULATION OF COMPLEMENTARY PRACTICE THROUGH HEALTH AND INSURANCE FRAUD LEGISLATION*

Health care providers generally are subject to numerous federal antifraud statutes and regulations. These include the False Claims Act, the federal mail fraud statute, the federal wire fraud statute, and statutes prohibiting a variety of forms of fraud and abuse, including false or fraudulent statements or representations in billing claims involving Medicare and Medicaid.

Such legal rules and regulations may be enforced by such disparate federal agencies

Note. Portions of this article are excerpted or adapted from chapter 8 of *Complementary and Alternative Medicine: Legal Boundaries and Regulatory Perspectives*, by M. H. Cohen, 1998, Baltimore: Johns Hopkins University Press. Copyright 1998 by Michael H. Cohen. Adapted with permission.

as the Federal Trade Commission, the U.S. Postal Service, and the U.S. Department of Justice. Complementary providers are particularly vulnerable to such enforcement of antifraud regulation because coding complementary and alternative treatments under existing billing systems can equate complementary practice with fraudulent treatment.

A recent statute, the Health Insurance Portability and Accountability Act, exacerbates this issue. The statute authorizes coordinated enforcement efforts by federal entities to prosecute a broadly defined area of health care and insurance fraud. Among other things, the act criminalizes the submission of Medicare or Medicaid claims for "a pattern of medical or other items or services that a person knows or should know are not medically necessary." This language could allow federal prosecutors to find complementary treatment "medically unnecessary," and submission of claims fraudulent.

In response to intervention by complementary providers, legislators have reaffirmed that the practice of "complementary, alternative, innovative, experimental, or investigational medical or health care itself would not constitute fraud," and stated that the "conferees intend that this proposal not be interpreted as a prohibition of the practice of these types of medical or health care."

Nonetheless, the broad enforcement tools created by the act and existing under other federal antifraud statutes, continue to give complementary providers reason to control and monitor their billing and health care practices carefully.

One effort to prevent regulators from treating complementary and alternative treatments as fraudulent is the dedication of federal resources to scientific investigation and research of complementary practice through the National Center for Complementary and Alternative Medicine (NCCAM) at the National Institutes of Health (NIH). Congress created NCCAM in 1992 to facilitate the evaluation of complementary treatment modalities, including acupuncture and Chinese medicine, homeopathic medicine, and physical manipulation therapies. The center, among other things, provides guidance on quantitative studies, including clinical trials, outcomes research, and systematic literature reviews.

The center's existence, mandate, program, and funding have been controversial. Opponents claim that the federal government is wasting taxpayer money on areas of research that lack a scientific basis. Supporters of the NCCAM point to the vast area of unexplored professional healing, which NCCAM is charged with investigating. NCCAM's budget has risen to $50 million, as compared with the more than $12 billion annually allocated to the 24 institutes, centers, and divisions at the NIH.

Other federal institutions beyond NCCAM from time to time engage in research or information gathering and dissemination relating to therapies such as acupuncture, chiropractic, biofeedback, and herbal medicine. Such research, together with the existence of an NIH center for federally sponsored complementary research, suggests the possibility of positive, future expansion for complementary-based healing professions.

MICHAEL H. COHEN

See

Acupuncture and Chinese Medicine (IV)

Biofeedback (IV)

Chiropractic: Definition, History,
    and Theory (IV)
Herbal Therapies (IV)
Homeopathy: Molecular Basis (IV)

THE FEDERAL ROLE IN REGULATING ACCESS TO COMPLEMENTARY PRACTICE*

Although most of the political and legal battles surrounding complementary practice have been fought at the state level, the federal role has centered on three important areas: (1) federal regulation of access to treatments through food and drug law; (2) federal regulation of insurance and health care fraud; and (3) federal sponsorship of scientific investigation and evaluation of complementary practice through institutions such as the National Center for Complementary and Alternative Medicine (NCCAM) at the National Institutes of Health.

Each area has challenged regulators' views of disease, health, medicine, and the appropriate role of the federal government in health promotion and consumer protection. This article addresses the impact of federal food and drug regulation on access to complementary treatments.

New Drugs

The first arena of federal oversight involves regulation of products considered to be new drugs. The federal Food, Drug, and Cosmetic Act provides that no new drug may be distributed in interstate commerce without approval of the U.S. Food and Drug Administration (FDA). Such approval requires proof that a drug is "safe and effective" for its intended use. Satisfactory proof may require a decade or more of research, cost hundreds of millions of dollars, and consume over 100,000 pages of supporting documentation.

Manufacturers and scientists developing unusual, unconventional, or complementary treatments to diseases such as cancer and AIDS—which often strike rapidly, are deadly, and have no approved, satisfactory treatment—have objected to the regulatory requirements as burdensome and inefficient. Similarly, for consumers, the increase in such diseases has made the regulatory approval process seem arcane, unwieldy, and indefensible.

The FDA has responded by providing some mechanisms for expedited approval of and expanded access to certain new drugs. Such efforts to relax regulatory controls have left many complementary proponents unsatisfied. FDA critics note that the agency may delay or even deny approval of access to the therapy or may condition approval on compliance with specified guidelines, excluding certain patients or treatments. The FDA also may intrude excessively in treatment by micromanaging the provider's use of the unapproved therapy.

Congressional consideration of FDA reform legislation may further loosen the approval process for new drugs, as well as FDA control over consumer access to unapproved complementary treatments.

Nutritional Therapies

The second arena of federal food and drug regulation involves nutritional therapies. According to federal law, such therapies

*Major areas of regulation by states include licensure, scope of professional practice, professional discipline, malpractice and vicarious liability, and third-party reimbursement.

Note. Portions of this article are excerpted or adapted from chapter 6 of *Complementary and Alternative Medicine: Legal Boundaries and Regulatory Perspectives* by M. H. Cohen, 1998, Baltimore: Johns Hopkins University Press. Copyright 1998 by Michael H. Cohen. Adapted with permission.

are considered to be drugs if they are "intended for use in the diagnosis, cure, mitigation, treatment, or prevention of disease." For example, if a manufacturer intends to market a nutritional therapy to treat disease (e.g., saw palmetto to treat benign prostatic hypertrophy, or St. John's wort to cure depression), the product is deemed a drug and requires FDA approval.

Because nutritional therapies such as saw palmetto or St. John's wort cannot be patented, companies do not invest in the FDA approval process for such products. In addition, companies may not make unapproved health claims for these products, and they may not market the products as intended to diagnose, cure, mitigate, treat, or prevent disease.

Licensed health care professionals (such as physicians and chiropractors) risk FDA enforcement action when they recommend or prescribe an independently manufactured nutritional product to individuals to diagnose, cure, mitigate, treat, or prevent disease. The FDA has been known to read its jurisdiction broadly in cases against complementary providers using nutritional products for disease care. The best-known example is the 1992 FDA raid on the office of Jonathan Wright, M.D., in which FDA agents seized files and injectable vitamins at gunpoint.

Even if the FDA does not proceed with any enforcement action or criminal penalties, FDA investigation and information sharing with other prosecutorial agents can trigger disciplinary action by the state medical board, as well as civil malpractice litigation by the consumer.

Dietary Supplements

The third arena of federal food and drug regulation involves dietary supplements, products that contain vitamins, minerals, herbs, or other botanicals, amino acids, or other products to supplement the diet by increasing total dietary intake. In 1994, Congress enacted the Dietary Supplement Health and Education Act (DSHEA) in recognition of the use by millions of Americans of dietary supplements for health promotion and disease prevention.

The most important contribution DSHEA makes to complementary practice is classifying dietary supplements as foods. The statute thus exempts dietary supplements from new drug approval.

DSHEA also expands the possibility of consumer education about nutrition by authorizing retail stores to provide literature in connection with the sale of dietary supplements. Among other requirements, the statute requires that the literature be not false or misleading, not promote a particular manufacturer or brand of dietary supplement, present a balanced view of the available scientific information, and be displayed separate and apart from the dietary supplements.

DSHEA further allows manufacturers to include a statement of a supplement's nutritional value under specifically designated circumstances. The manufacturer, though, may not claim that the product will diagnose, mitigate, treat, cure, or prevent a specific disease or class of diseases. Such a claim would bring the product into the realm of drugs, requiring FDA approval.

Expanding Access

Frustrated with FDA control of complementary practice through food and drug regulation, complementary proponents have brought litigation, asserting constitutional challenges to regulatory restrictions on access. Such challenges, by and large, have been unsuccessful. Most federal courts have rejected consumer claim to a right to select their treatment of choice based on the constitutional right to privacy.

The seminal case is *United States v. Rutherford*, in which the U.S. Supreme Court rejected efforts of individuals diagnosed with terminal cancer to obtain laetrile and concluded that Congress reasonably could have intended to protect consumers from ineffective or unsafe drugs such as laetrile. On remand from the Supreme Court, the U.S. Court of Appeals for the Tenth Circuit held that while an individual has a constitutionally protected right to decide whether or not to undergo treatment, the "selection of a particular treatment, or at least a medication, is within the area of governmental interest in protecting public health" and is not encompassed by the constitutional right to privacy. The *Rutherford* decisions have enjoyed support in subsequent cases.

Although unsuccessful in judicial challenges to restrictions on access to complementary treatment, proponents have sought legislative change to broaden access. One such effort is the Access to Medical Treatment Act. This piece of federal legislation gives an individual "the right to be treated by a health care practitioner with any treatment (including one that is not approved, certified, or licensed by the Secretary of Health and Human Services) that such individual desires or the legal representative of such individual desires," if the practitioner personally examines and agrees to treat the individual and the administration of the treatment is within the provider's authorized scope of practice, the treatment is nondangerous, and other conditions are met. Whatever the fate of this particular bill, its

introduction signals expanding congressional recognition of American's desire to utilize complementary treatments.

MICHAEL H. COHEN

STATE LEGISLATION

Popular and professional interest in complementary forms of treatment has increased dramatically in the United States in the final decade of the 20th century. Among the many types of activities associated with complementary care during this period, developments occurring in the legislative arena have been of primary importance in securing for the public a legal right of access to therapies that depart from prevailing medical practices and, for complementary providers, the related right to practice these modalities with less fear of adverse governmental action.

Owing to the primary jurisdiction of the states over matters pertaining to the practice of health occupations, legislative developments concerning complementary practice occur principally at the state level. State statutes in this field generally may be grouped into three categories of enactments: (1) provider practice acts that formally regulate a specific complementary modality through licensure, certification, or registration; (2) isolated references to miscellaneous complementary therapies, usually in the context of a statute defining the scope of practice for, or an exemption from, a more systematically regulated unconventional or conventional form of treatment; and (3) provisions in medical practice acts that conditionally authorize physicians to employ complementary modalities. Statutes that confer full licensure upon a particular therapy generally represent the most formal and extensive authorization of practice rights for a health profession and typically delimit the scope of practice for the modality, qualifications for licensure, authority of the administrative unit exercising regulatory power over the profession, grounds for discipline against providers, and penalties for violation of the licensing act. In some states, however, certification and registration schemes may not differ substantially in content from licensure statutes in other jurisdictions for the same profession.

Provider Practice Acts

Apart from the professions of osteopathy and chiropractic, which have been largely absorbed into the mainstream of American health care and whose practitioners enjoy legislative recognition in all states, the most numerous provider practice acts for complementary practitioners may be found in the fields of acupuncture, massage, and naturopathy. By mid-1997, acupuncture practice statutes had been adopted in some 32 states, massage legislation in 25 states, and naturopathy statutes in 12 states. While little uniformity exists among these laws even within the same profession, the proliferation of enactments for the three modalities since 1990 reflects strong national interest in these professions and in complementary health care generally. Although less numerous, provider practice acts also exist in some states for homeopathy, naprapathy, Chinese medicine, and reflexology.

Miscellaneous Therapies

A variety of less well known complementary therapies are referenced by many state statutes as either within or without the scope of practice for fully regulated forms of treatment. For example, legislative enactments may recognize practice rights for acupressure within the scope of acupuncture; for biofeedback within the practice of psychology, physical therapy, or naturopathy; and for hypnotherapy as part of psychology practice. In Maine, the state massage practice act specifically excludes from its application such modalities as rolfing, Trager, reflexology, shiatsu, Reiki, and polarity therapy, while the Alabama massage act excludes from its purview Native American healers who use traditional healing practices. The very existence of statutory references to the latter group of modalities, even by way of exclusion, is a very recent development and indicates that the practice and access interests of a wide variety of complementary providers and their clients are beginning to form part of the legislative and regulatory agenda in a number of states.

State statutes also contain numerous provisions permitting the use of spiritual healing practices. Many of these laws are in the form of exemptions from licensure requirements under a state medical practice act and serve the dual function of accommodating the guaranty of the free exercise of religion under the First Amendment to the U.S. Constitution and of protecting the spiritual healer from the charge of unauthorized medical practice under sweeping definitions of the practice of medicine common to most state codes. The nature of the accommodation for spiritual healing varies widely throughout the states and may be restricted to healing methods associated with the practices or tenets of a specified church (i.e., Christian Science) or a church of an unspecified denomination, or predicated on the use of an officially approved form of healing (e.g., prayer) or the absence of the use of disfavored procedures (e.g., faith cure, mind healing, or the laying on of hands). More broadly, however, a number of states authorize persons to engage in healing practices through the use of either prayer or mental or spiritual means. In many states, including those whose statutes are generally permissive concerning the use of spiritual healing practices, additional conditions may apply to ensure that spiritual healers avoid the use of medical titles, comply with public health and sanitation requirements, and do not perform surgery or prescribe drugs or other medications.

Medical Practice Act Amendments

Another significant legislative development to occur in the 1990s in this subject area is the adoption of amendments to state medical practice acts to allow physicians to utilize complementary therapies in treating their patients. The amending statute is often popularly referred to as a medical or health freedom law. By mid-1997, eight states had enacted amendatory legislation of this type. These laws are intended to lessen the risk of disciplinary action by the state medical board against a physician who uses these forms of care and simultaneously to enhance public access to therapies that do not correspond to mainstream medical practice. The wording of the statutes and the conditions under which the accommodation is allowed for complementary treatments vary considerably among the enacting jurisdictions. Thus, practice and access rights may largely depend on whether the consumer is demonstrably physically harmed (Alaska) or actually injured or subject to an unreasonable risk of harm (Washington). There is a

safety risk greater than that of the prevailing mode of care or whether the treatment is generally not effective (North Carolina), or is in fact effective (New York), or, without further qualification, is experimental or nontraditional (Oklahoma). Some jurisdictions authorize the use of a complementary modality if there is a reasonable potential for a therapeutic gain that is not outweighed by the associated risk (Colorado), or if the treatment does not pose an unreasonable and significant risk of danger (Georgia). More narrowly, one state (South Dakota) limits the benefit of the accommodation only to physicians who use chelation therapy.

Recent state enactments in the form of practice acts for complementary providers, statutory references to a variety of miscellaneous complementary modalities, and legislative accommodations for physicians to use complementary therapies have functioned synergistically with developments in the nonlegal sphere to promote the progressive development of a more holistic paradigm of health care in the United States. With the continuing reluctance of the courts to recognize a constitutional right for a person to choose any form of health care treatment against a rationally based restriction imposed by the government, as distinguished from the right to refuse treatment altogether, the primacy of the state legislative arena as a forum for securing practice and access rights for unconventional therapies seems strongly indicated for the foreseeable future.

DAVID M. SALE

See

Acupuncture and Chinese Medicine (IV)
Biofeedback (IV)

Homeopathy: Molecular Basis (IV)
Hypnotherapy (IV)
Native American Medicine (IV)
Naturopathy (IV)
Reiki (IV)
Rolfing: Structural Integration (IV)
Shiatsu (IV)
Trager Approach (IV)

NATIONAL CENTER FOR COMPLEMENTARY AND ALTERNATIVE MEDICINE

The National Institutes of Health (NIH) was authorized in 1992 to develop an Office of Alternative Medicine (OAM), which became the National Center for Complementary and Alternative Medicine (NCCAM) in 1998. This center was organized under the Associate Director for Disease Prevention within the office of the director of NIH. The purpose of the center is to serve as a facilitator and coordinator of biomedical research rather than to serve as a referral agency for various alternative medical treatments or individual practitioners. The NCCAM supports and conducts research and research training on unconventional health practices and disseminates information on this research.

In the fall of 1996, the NCCAM established a clearinghouse to serve as a site where complementary and alternative health care information is collected, developed, and distributed to the public. The public can obtain fact sheets, information packages, and publications from the clearinghouse. The clearinghouse is located in Silver Springs, Maryland and will respond to calls, fax, or mail. The NCCAM also publishes a quarterly newsletter that can be obtained and duplicated as needed.

The NCCAM research data base consists of more than 60,000 non-duplicative bibliographic citations from 1966 to 1996. These citations can be obtained from the National Library of Medicine's Medline database. The NCCAM works closely with the NIH library to obtain hard copies of selected research articles. They are mainly interested in those articles reporting clinical trials, either randomized or controlled, on any alternative health practice.

A seven-category classification system has been developed and now contains more than 340 terms representing the major alternative health care practices. This classification system is updated periodically.

In 1996, through efforts of the NCCAM, five new MeSH terms were added for alternative practice and include: acupressure, health food, imagery, medication, and therapeutic touch. Currently there are 22 MeSH headings in Medline under the term alternative medicine. These include: acupuncture, anthroposophy, biofeedback, chiropractic, color therapy, diet fads, eclecticism, electrical stimulation therapy, homeopathy, applied kinesiology, massage, traditional medicine, mental healing, moxibustion, music therapy, naturopathy, organotherapy, radiesthesis, reflexology, relaxation techniques, therapeutic touch, and tissue therapy (National Center for Complementary and Alternative Medicine, 1997). This classification helps to identify the type of research that has been conducted on a specific alternative medicine practice, modality, or system.

The NCCAM has developed evaluation methods for research articles on alternative health care. Studies listed include randomized controlled trials, case-controlled trials, in-vitro study, and case studies. The NCCAM evaluation process is systematic and explicit and provides critical appraisal and/or synthesis of the scientific literature on alternative health practices. The purpose is to determine the quality of individual studies, the amount of evidence available, and the appropriateness of specific practices, including the safety, efficacy, and effectiveness of the specific health practice.

The NCCAM provides research grants in the area of complementary practices. This source of funding has greatly enhanced the research data base for alternative health practices. The NCCAM has been involved with both intramural and extramural research in complementary alternative therapies. Intramural research is conducted by employees of the NIH and FDA. Extramural research are projects conducted by investigators outside the government. These include scientists at universities, hospitals, and other research institutions.

Staff of the NCCAM have worked on collaborating with the international Cochrane Collaboration's (CC) efforts to identify clinical trials on alternative medicine topics internationally. Information about the NCCAM can be obtained from the Internet.

MARY E. HAZZARD

THE EFFECTS OF COMPLEMENTARY THERAPIES ON NATIONAL HEALTH POLICY

During the 1990s, complementary approaches ceased to be an underground consumer movement and began to be integrated into mainstream health care in the United States. This trend was driven by a confluence of forces, including consumers'

seeking alternatives to invasive procedures and potentially toxic drugs; the desire of some physicians to provide their patients with a broader range of treatment options, and the willingness of elected officials and health policymakers alike to evaluate new information and respond to changing attitudes on the part of the public. Perhaps the first clear indication that such a transformation was taking place came in 1993, when the *New England Journal of Medicine* published a study indicating that one third of Americans regularly used some kind of complementary therapy even though they were forced to pay for it themselves. This evidence, coupled with the fact that the great majority of those using complementary approaches did not share this information with their primary care physicians, attracted widespread attention.

In 1992, Congress created a federal Office of Alternative Medicine (OAM) under the auspices of the National Institutes of Health. The leader of the effort to establish the Office, Senator Tom Harkin (D-Iowa), wanted the government to study the therapeutic approaches associated with complementary approaches and reach conclusions about their validity if possible. In a decision that caught some people by surprise, the Food and Drug Administration (FDA) reclassified the acupuncture needle from an experimental to a therapeutic device based on research that established acupuncture's value in providing relief to those suffering from chronic pain and asthma.

So many Americans suffer from acute low back pain that another federal agency, the Agency for Health Care Policy Research (AHCPR), decided to study the problem. It eventually concluded that spinal manipulation techniques associated with chiropractic were more effective in treating this condition than drugs or corrective surgery. On a symbolic level, this decision provides the best illustration of the more cooperative, less confrontational attitude that the government has adopted in its approach toward complementary therapies and its practitioners. Just 50 years ago, chiropractors were often arrested for practicing medicine without a license. All complementary approaches were frequently lumped together when the government investigated medical fraud.

Today, policymakers, physicians, and the public face a very different kind of problem. With so many different units of the federal government involved in medical research and development activities, it is becoming increasingly difficult to grasp the larger picture. Senator Arlen Specter (R-Pennsylvania) requested a government-wide survey of such activities in an effort to provide a clear, comprehensive picture of federal initiatives in this area.

Looking to the future, there are unresolved issues relating to complementary approaches that could help shape federal health policy in the United States for years to come. The first issue is a financial one. Federal entities such as OAM and AHCPR are severely limited by the small budgets they have been accorded. For example, OAM's current budget is just $12 million, while the research budget for the NIH as a whole is $12 billion. While AHCPR enjoys a significantly larger budget of $160 million, that is still far too small to carry out the bulk of outcomes based research that needs to be done. At the current levels of support, it may take years to determine which complementary medical approaches have true therapeutic benefits to offer. Spending the significant sums necessary to support a comprehensive program of outcome-based clinical trials may be one of the most prudent long-term investments that we as a society could make.

MARC MICOZZI

Section 5

Historical
Perspectives

WELLNESS PROMOTION: HISTORICAL ASPECTS

A universal feature of systems of complementary health care, whatever their individual therapies and rationales, is an emphasis on proper lifestyle as the basis for health. It is not health in the common understanding of freedom from patent disease that is intended, but a state of exuberant vitality that in recent decades has come to be identified as wellness. So forceful is this emphasis on wellness, in fact, that one is given to suppose it must represent a modern breakthrough in outlook, a dawning new age awareness of the possibilities of human vigor.

In fact, wellness has been an element of health philosophy for centuries. It can be traced to Hippocrates (ca. 460–370 B.C.), whose writings repeatedly stressed the importance of proper diet, regular exercise, and adequate sleep for the maintenance of health and the enjoyment of life. It was the Greco-Roman physician Galen (129–ca. 210), though, who organized these ideas into a distinct code of hygiene. Derived from Hygeia, the Greek goddess of health, "hygiene" historically has referred to all the components of lifestyle conducive to health, not simply bodily cleanliness, the meaning usually attached to it today.

Galen's code, embracing diet, exercise, sleep, bodily evacuations, air, and emotions, served as the basis for health education for more than 1,500 years, through the 18th century. But while a number of books were written before the 1800s to educate the public in the rules of right living, their impact was minimal. To begin, they were accessible only to the small minority who could read and were specifically directed at the upper classes, those who had the

time and means to look after their health. Even more important, these guides to hygiene were perfused by the religious pessimism that dominated pre-Enlightenment European culture, the conviction that recurrent sickness and early death were the natural order of things, punishments deserved by the whole human race for the original sin of Adam and Eve. The practice of good hygiene might bring health for a time, but ultimately all was in God's hands, and life-long health was highly unlikely.

By 1800, the liberalization of religious thought effected by Enlightenment rationalism had led to a prevailing view of God as a loving father who rewarded those children who were obedient rather than inevitably punishing them. One of the rewards for obedience to the rules of hygiene was health. In the religious context, health became not merely a possibility but an obligation, a duty owed to the Creator of the body that functioned according to divinely instituted laws of physiology. As health came to be regarded as a certainty available to all who fulfilled their moral duty, the production of hygiene literature multiplied accordingly. Demand was increased as well by spreading literacy and by the widely held fear that the new environment—the industrial city—posed unprecedented challenges to physical well-being.

From the turn of the 19th century to the present, there has been a flood of health promotion literature, from books to pamphlets to newspaper columns, assuring the public that higher levels of wellness are freely available to those who make the effort and offering specific recommendations for diet, exercise, maintenance of emotional equilibrium, and other components of daily living. The specific advice offered varies considerably from author to author, with the content divisible into two categories. Much of the hygiene literature of the last two centuries—what might be regarded as the mainstream tradition—was written by physicians, biological scientists, and lay writers promoting the rule of temperance, the avoidance of excess in any activity. Although the details of advice have been continually revised to reflect advancing knowledge in physiology, biochemistry, and epidemiology, the overall philosophy has been that any of the common indulgences of daily living are harmless in moderation. Not until tobacco came to be incriminated in so many health problems—and that quite recently—did this tradition condemn a common activity as dangerous in any amount.

There has been a second stream of literature, though, some of it also written by physicians or scientists, but most of it by lay health reformers, that has seen wellness as attainable only by the complete elimination of one or another indulgence, by abstinence instead of temperance. Typical of this tradition has been the conflation of physiology with morality, the assumption that whatever is morally wrong must of necessity be physically wrong as well. One sees this in the 19th- and early 20th-century movement to prohibit alcohol and more lastingly in the promotion of vegetarianism. Purely a moral crusade prior to the 19th century, vegetarianism was transformed in the 1830s to a physical health movement under the influence of New Englanders William Alcott (1798–1859) and Sylvester Graham (1794–1851), creator of the Graham cracker. At the turn of this century, the vegetarian health rationale was thoroughly updated by John Harvey Kellogg (1852–1943), founder of the modern breakfast cereal industry, but he too supposed meatless diet to be more healthful because it was more virtuous. Subsequent epidemiological studies have in fact confirmed the health benefits of vegetarianism regardless of moral considerations (Whorton, 1982).

The late 19th century also witnessed the emergence of an energetic campaign to promote health through exercise. Under the leadership of Bernarr Macfadden (1868–1955), this "physical culture" movement encouraged esthetic (body building) as well as hygienic improvements, and brought such figures as Charles Atlas (1892–1972) into the limelight. Even the present-day icon of strength and energy Jack LaLanne (1914–) can be linked directly with the physical culture efforts of Macfadden (Green, 1986; Grover, 1989).

The individual's pursuit of wellness continues today along lines laid down in the 1800s, but the activity has become enormously more complicated in the present century. The luxuriant growth of nutrition and exercise physiology as sciences, as well as so many additional areas of expansion of understanding of the human body, has presented the health-minded with a bewildering array of options of foods and activities to adopt or avoid. The confusion has been compounded, furthermore, by the commercialization of hygiene as health assumed greater cultural importance during this century. Dietary supplements, barbells, running shoes—there is no end to the products marketed as health aids, each category bursting with individual brands aggressively competing through seductive advertising for the health conscious consumer's pocketbook. Yet in the end, however much the wellness lifestyle of the modern holistic era is extolled as a veritable revolution in thought and activity (see, for example, Harvey and Marilyn Diamond, *Living Health*), the fundamental things one must do to build health have not changed since Galen's codification of hygiene in the 2nd century (Weil, 1995).

JAMES C. WHORTON

SELF-CARE IN AMERICAN HISTORY

Self-care has always occupied a prominent place in American medical culture. During the colonial period, geographical isolation and a shortage of trained physicians forced people to be medically self-sufficient. Ailments were commonly treated within the family, more often than not by the wife and mother, employing remedies acquired from midwives (often the only medical practitioners in rural areas), folk tradition, or the practices of Native Americans. Lay health care knowledge was codified, furthermore, in any number of books, although until the latter 1700s such works were compendia of general information in which directions for the preparation of medicinals was jumbled up with recipes for jams and pickles, agricultural advice, and other tips for household management (Risse, 1977).

In 1769, a new type of medical guide appeared, with the publication of Scottish physician William Buchan's *Domestic Medicine*. Authored by a medical professional and devoted entirely to the prevention and treatment of disease, *Domestic Medicine* established a model for instruction on home treatment of illness that would continue on to the 20th century. This and the many similar domestic guides that followed reflected the 18th-century Enlightenment faith in the ability of people to manage and improve their lives when given adequate education, a faith that presages the medical "empowerment" movement of recent years.

Though issued in Edinburgh, *Domestic Medicine* quickly became the standard home medical reference throughout America, being outsold only by the Bible. Nevertheless, the work did have to compete with the productions of American physicians, whose volumes were tailored to the diseases and climate distinctive to the United States.

Gradually, by 1840, Buchan's place was usurped by native authors, especially John Gunn, a Tennessee practitioner whose own *Domestic Medicine*, first published in 1830, went through 100 reprintings (with some revision) in its first 40 years. Subtitled *Poor Man's Friend*, Gunn's book was intended to help the many who simply could not afford professional assistance. He was also inspired by philosophical, not just practical, concerns. Writing during a period of burgeoning democratic self-consciousness, Gunn expressed a widespread popular distrust of professional elites, a suspicion that physicians in particular strove to keep the public economically dependent by keeping them medically ignorant. Gunn's position was that commoners could in fact understand all they needed to know to protect themselves from illness if medicine were stripped of its Latin obfuscations and other bewildering scientific language—"demystified," in today's terminology. So confident was he and other domestic medicine authors of the layperson's medical competence that instructions were offered for treating even the most serious ailments (cholera, for example) at home. In at least one home medical guide of the era, precise directions were given for amputation of the limbs of injured family members or neighbors with butcher knife, mitre saw, and other everyday household implements.

Confidence in the ability of people to treat themselves as successfully as any doctor could, rapidly waned during the last quarter of the 19th century. The germ theory gave medicine, for the first time, a scientifically demonstrable explanation of the cause of disease and fostered remarkable advances in treatment. Surgery was revolutionized by aseptic technique in the 1870s and 1880s (performing amputations on the kitchen table simply would not do any more), then drug therapy was transformed by the development of sulfa drugs and antibiotics. The latter did not occur until the 1930s and 1940s, but as early as the 1920s the American public was in awe of "scientific medicine," the phrase cultivated by the medical profession to dramatize its newly acquired power. Popular ambition for self-care shrank to the level of treating the common cold and upset stomach, patching abrasions and bandaging sprains. Typified by the 1935 *Modern Home Medical Adviser*, edited by Morris Fishbein (also long-time editor of the *Journal of the American Medical Association*), this modern genre of domestic manual as dictionary and encyclopedia was intended not to encourage self-treatment but to present basic medical ideas and procedures in lay language so that the public could better understand and cooperate with the treatments prescribed by their physicians. The goal was compliance rather than self-reliance.

Over the last three decades, self-care has made a comeback. The suppression of infectious disease cleared the way for the chronic diseases of aging to assume much more prominence; these are complaints that are difficult to cure through medication or surgery but that can often be monitored and alleviated somewhat by the individual sufferer. As medical costs and physicians' incomes rose dramatically, the public looked for ways to manage illness more economically and, as in the mid-1800s, grew increasingly distrustful of the medical profession. Discomfort with physicians has been intensified as well by the alienating effects of medical specialization and doctors' reliance on the hospital and intimidating technology. These dissatisfactions, coupled with the consumerism and the demand for respect for individual rights (civil, gender, sexual) that have so agitated American culture since the 1960s, have fostered the holistic health movement, with individual responsibility for self-care as one of its major tenets. Self-care literature and lay-organized self-care groups have grown remarkably in number over the past quarter century, yet they might be seen as a return to the Victorian era in their emphasis on the ability of people to take care of themselves (Berkeley, 1978; Weil, 1995).

Contemporary lay medical manuals often recommend complementary health practices for self-care, but that too can be seen as a return. Complementary health care first appeared in America at the beginning of the 19th century, and the earliest actually made self-care its cardinal principle. Thomsonianism, a program of herbal healing created by the farmer Samuel Thomson, made "Every Man His Own Physician" its motto, and sold "Family Right Certificates," conferring the legal privilege of using Thomson's botanicals to individual households. By 1840, more than 100,000 certificates had been sold nationwide. And though Thomsonianism was in steep decline by 1850, other alternative systems stepped in to promote self-treatment (such approaches to healing would not be thought of as "complementary" instead of "alternative" until the late 20th century). Homeopaths sold "domestic kits" of their most useful remedies, along with instruction booklets on their use. Hydropaths, who employed cold water baths (and occasionally warm ones) to purify and stimulate the body, published numerous manuals on water cure in the home. Both hydropaths and Thomsonians, incidentally, demonstrated a particular concern for women's health, striving to educate them to deal with their distinctive health problems and not rely on physicians for gynecological and obstetrical care. Indeed, except for the systems of musculoskeletal manipulation (osteopathy, chiropractic), which could not be taught without practical demonstration, all alternative and complementary systems have attempted to inform people how to treat themselves by the system's methods and have urged them to assume as much responsibility as possible for their health. Throughout the history of alternative and complementary care, self-care has been a central component of philosophy.

JAMES C. WHORTON

See

Midwifery (IV)
Native American Medicine (IV)

THE HISTORY OF HOMEOPATHY IN THE UNITED STATES

Homeopathy was initially developed and systematized by the German physician Samuel Hahnemann (1755–1843). Al-though he never visited the United States, his ideas profoundly affected and divided American medicine.

By the early 20th century, the United States had become the world's leading center for homeopathy, with 66 general and 74 specialized homeopathic hospitals (Nichols, 1988). There were 22 homeopathic schools of medicine, including Boston University, the University of Michigan, Hahnemann Medical College (in Philadelphia), New York Homeopathic Medical College (later called New York Medical College), the University of Minnesota, and the University of Iowa (Coulter, 1975).

Approximately 15% of American physicians considered themselves homeopaths, but even more significant was the fact that many leading citizens considered themselves to be advocates of this new school of medicine. They included Mark Twain, William James, Louisa May Alcott, Harriet Beecher Stowe, Henry Wadsworth Longfellow, Henry David Thoreau, Nathaniel Hawthorne, William Cullen Bryant, William Lloyd Garrison, Susan B. Anthony, and Mary Baker Eddy (Ullman, 1991). Even several U.S. presidents were supporters of homeopathy, including Abraham Lincoln, James Garfield, and William McKinley.

Paul Starr noted in his Pulitzer Prize–winning book, *The Social Transformation of American Medicine*, that there were good reasons for America's educated elite to seek out homeopathy: "Because homeopathy was simultaneously philosophical and experimental, it seemed to many people to be more rather than less scientific than orthodox medicine" (Starr, 1982, p. 97).

Shortly after homeopathy was first introduced in the United States by Danish physician Hans Gram in 1825, its popularity increased rapidly. The American Institute of Homeopathy, founded in 1844, became the first national medical society in the United States. Two years later, a rival medical association was formed. That organization, which became the American Medical Association (AMA), asserted that one of its goals was to slow the growth of homeopathy.

Because homeopaths were trained physicians themselves, they were particularly threatening to orthodox, or allopathic, doctors. The AMA actively sought to attack and marginalize homeopaths. The consultation clause in the AMA ethics code strongly reprimanded any orthodox physician for even consulting with a homeopath. At a time when the AMA did not enforce even egregious ethical violations, it did actively enforce the consultation clause. One physician lost his license for consulting with a homeopath, his wife (Coulter, 1975). In 1882 the New York Medical Society voted to abolish the consultation clause; because of this, the entire state medical society was expelled from the AMA (Starr, 1982).

In the early 20th century the AMA realized that the restrictive consultation clause was not working and decided to repeal it in 1903. Homeopaths were even allowed to become members of the organization. Some historians have asserted that homeopathy began to decline once the AMA stopped being antagonistic to it (Starr, 1982). However, these historians neglected to point out that the homeopaths who were admitted to the AMA were required to stop calling themselves homeopaths and to stop using homeopathic medicines. This suggests that antagonism toward homeopathy was still very evident.

A more accurate explanation for the repeal of the consultation clause is that it was not working and the AMA chose a different, and ultimately more effective, route of attack. Shortly after its repeal, AMA leaders sought to collaborate with Abraham Flexner, who, through the Carnegie Commission, was charged with evaluating medical education in the United States (Brown, 1979).

The Flexner Report of 1910 sought to standardize American medical education and used the Johns Hopkins School of Medicine as the standard. Medical schools that employed full-time teachers and researchers who focused on the pathological and physiochemical analysis of the body received high rankings. Because homeopathic schools preferred to employ teachers who also were clinicians and because they taught homeopathy, they received low rankings. The Flexner Report greatly influenced public and private funding as well as the general prestige of medical schools. In 1900 there were 22 homeopathic medical schools; by 1923 only 2 remained.

Homeopathy continued to decline until the 1970s, when the holistic health movement emerged. Although interest in homeopathy in the 1970s was not significant, it did signal a trend. In the 1980s homeopathy began to grow more substantially. Two leading homeopathic companies from France and one from Germany set up manufacturing plants in the United States. Their increased marketing and educational efforts helped the movement grow. Also, new clinical and laboratory studies were beginning to be published in conventional scientific journals, sowing the seeds for further development of the field.

From 1990 to 1997 the number of schools and training programs in homeopathy grew from 4 to approximately 25. There also were considerably more and larger companies; even some conventional drug companies were manufacturing and marketing homeopathic products. Research showed the efficacy of homeopathic medicines, though not enough to convince hardened skeptics (Bellavite & Signorni, 1995; Ullman, 1996).

Historians have described homeopathy as a medical heresy that rose because conventional medicine was so dangerous, and that fell because it was not found to be effective and because conventional medicine was found to be better (Kaufman, 1971). This analysis is inadequate, because homeopathy's decline started at a time when conventional medicine was being recognized as ineffective, even dangerous. There are, in fact, no conventional medical treatments of that day that have survived. It has been said that history is written by the victors. Considering the present shift in medical paradigms, it appears that history soon may be rewritten.

DANA ULLMAN

See

Homeopathy: Molecular Basis (IV)
Homeopathy: Use in Family Practice Medicine (IV)

THE HISTORY OF THE HYDROPATHIC MOVEMENT IN THE UNITED STATES

The legacy of the 19th-century water-cure movement in the United States is found in hydrotherapy, which consists of exercises performed in water, hot and cold packings, steam baths, and the use of jacuzzis, spas, and other recreational water facilities (Ko-pelman & Moskop, 1981). Recently, hot spring resorts that cater to stress-weary Americans have become popular tourist destinations, further emphasizing the growing interest in hydrotherapy and the curative effects of water.

Hydrotherapy's predecessor, hydropathy, or cold water cure, was introduced into the United States in the 1840s. It was modeled after a system pioneered by Vincent Priessnitz (born 1799) of Austrian Silesia who earned fame as a curer with water. His establishment, called Grafenberg, served as the model for its American counterpart. In the United States, hydropathy followed in the path cleared by earlier sects, such as botanics, Thomsonianism, and phrenology. Yet while hydropathy benefited from the acceptance already accorded these sects, hydropathic living represented a high point in its comprehensive worldview and its emphasis on self-sufficiency. It also provided a scathing critique of allopathic medicine, which utilized evacuative therapeutics and dramatic interventions. Hydropaths believed these therapeutics caused greater illness and death, weakened the patient's constitution, and fostered the patient's passivity and reliance on the omnipotent doctor.

The hydropathic philosophy, conversely, demanded active involvement by the patient in bettering his or her own health. To that end, vegetarianism, physical exercise, abstention from tobacco and alcohol, and "moderation in all habits" were advocated and exacted; water was the sole curative agent.

Water-cure therapeutics were applied according to the condition or ailment. Direct applications of water at a temperature suitable to the patient's "reactive power" were prescribed. Water was credited with the ability to cleanse, purify, give renewed life, soothe, cool, relax, and stimulate. Thus douches (showers) of varying heights and durations were prescribed by water-cure practitioners. Similarly, soaks, wet bandage wraps, and the drinking of large quantities of fresh (not stagnant) water were prescribed. The goal of hydropathic treatment was to rid the body of its "putrid matter," which carried illness. The putrid matter was extracted from the body and replaced by healthy matter transmitted through the clean, fresh water. Both organic and inorganic ailments were treated; fevers and neuromuscular disorders, in particular, were treated with great success.

At the heart of the hydropathic philosophy was the belief that one ought to cooperate with nature through preventive care, rather than reactive counterattacks upon disease through episodic crisis interventionism. Because they believed this, hydropaths and their followers scorned vigorous drug and/or depletion therapeutics.

Hydropaths also greatly critiqued and reconceptualized the allopathic doctor-patient relationship that emerged in the 1840s. Instead of patient passivity and physicians' exclusive hold on knowledge, hydropaths argued for mutual responsibility and ultimate self-determination by consumers. Individuals were encouraged to become their own doctors; hydropaths were merely guides.

This philosophy offered a unique and positive role for American middle-class women of European descent. At the time their physiology was considered frail and was being used as a rationale for their limited social role. Hydropaths rejected this notion and urged women to assume responsibility for their own and their families' health. Through healthful food preparation,

unrestrictive dress, exercise, and applications of water therapies, women could lead their families to better health.

Hydropathic colleges and one-on-one mentoring relationships actively recruited women to become practitioners. Larger water-cure establishments had at least one female physician on staff who specialized in women's diseases and appealed to its female clientele. Hydropathic female followers experienced a communal mission to improve their own and their families' health, while pursuing autonomy and self-determination.

America of the 1840s was hospitable ground for the hydropathic philosophy and its emphasis on self-care. Joel Shew and R. T. Trall were two of the founders of the movement. By the 1860s there were 212 live-in cures offering hydropathy. Patients' stays at the "cures," as these sites were called, lasted from a few weeks to several months. Costs varied, although several cures had "clergy fees" that allowed poorer clients to stay while paying a reduced fee. Weekly rates ranged from $5.00 to $16.00 in the early years. This included all therapies, meals, and accommodations. The cures were mostly situated in pastoral areas, which were themselves thought to be curative.

Hydropathic advocates published prolifically, producing self-help books for home use, disease-specific treatments, and philosophical tracts, as well as the monthly *Water-Cure Journal*, which was published from 1843 until 1913. (The journal's subscription list reached a circulation of 100,000 in the 1850s.) Hydropathic leaders also shared a reformist zeal on many pressing social issues beyond women's appropriate social role: antislavery, dress reform, temperance, vegetarianism, and female suffrage.

The austere and spartan life demanded of water-cure patients became less appealing to late-19th-century middle-class Americans faced with greater opportunities for consumption, leisure, conspicuous display of wealth, and personal indulgence. Other causes for the demise of the movement included the inability of hydropathic leaders to incorporate "larger truths" (e.g., many opposed vaccination), the utilization of a hodgepodge of electrochemical gadgetry, a dwindling patient population for practitioners, and the leadership's refusal to firmly declare allegiance to the cause of antislavery.

At its height (from 1840s to the 1860s, although variations of the movement continued into the 1950s) hydropathy offered unprecedented opportunities for self-care, an emphasis on preventive health practices, a positive view of women's physiology and social role, and a hub for reform-oriented activism.

SUSAN E. CAYLEFF

Part II

Conditions

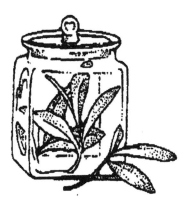

ABUSE

Child abuse is strongly associated with parenting stress and anger expression. Rodriguez and Green (1997) were able to predict child abuse potential by using measures of parenting stress and anger expression.

Childhood physical or sexual abuse is associated with adult health problems, including physical symptoms, psychological problems, HIV risk behaviors, and substance abuse (Briere et al., 1997; Thompson, Potter, Sanderson, & Maibach, 1997). For many variables, this association is as strong as for individuals experiencing current abuse (McCauley et al., 1997). Social isolation and experiencing the death of a mother were significant predictors for abuse before age 12, while the predictors of childhood sexual abuse (CSA) after age 12 were physical abuse and a mentally ill mother. For abuse perpetrated by a family member, the significant predictors of CSA were physical abuse, having no one to confide in, having no caring female adult, and having an alcoholic father. For girls abused by someone outside the family, the significant predictors of CSA were physical abuse, social isolation, the mother's death, and having an alcoholic mother (Fleming, Mullen, & Bammer, 1997).

In one study, women with unexplained chronic pelvic pain with pelvic venous congestion reported more childhood sexual abuse than the noncongested group (Fry, Beard, Crips, & McGuigan, 1997). Bodily shame has been shown to play a mediating role between early abuse and both depression (Moyer, DiPietro, Berkowitz, & Stunkard, 1997) and bulimia (Andrews, 1997). Parenting stress and anger expression predict child abuse potential (Rodriguez & Green, 1997). Adverse childhood experiences are powerful risk factors for adult homelessness. Effectively reducing child abuse and neglect may ultimately prevent social problems, including homelessness (Herman, Susser, Struening, & Link, 1997). Posttraumatic stress disorder (PTSD) has been linked with childhood sexual and physical abuse (Briggs & Joyce, 1997; Rodriguez, Ryan, Vande Kemp, & Foy, 1997). The women who reported multiple abusive episodes that involved sexual intercourse had increased symptoms of PTSD (Briggs & Joyce, 1997).

In a study of 122,824 public school students in grades 6, 9, and 12, physical and sexual abuse were associated with an increased likelihood of the use of alcohol, marijuana, and almost all other drugs for both males and females. Abuse victims also reported initiating substance use earlier than their nonabused peers and gave more reasons for using, including use to cope with painful emotions and to escape from problems (Harrison, Fulkerson, & Beebe, 1997).

Biofeedback

Infant crying can produce intense parental stress and can precede physical child abuse or neglect. Tyson (1996) assigned 15 female participants to either EEG biofeedback pretraining without stress, or pretraining or no pretraining while listening to infant crying. Biofeedback training significantly shifted participant response to infant crying. Stress management training may help ameliorate aversive responses to infant crying and could prevent child abuse.

Drawing

Projective drawings can facilitate awareness and understanding of boundary problems in abused children (Glaister, 1994).

Home Visiting

Logan (1997) reported the use of home visiting to reduce the rates of childhood injuries and abuse.

Licensing Parents

The misuse of parental power in child abuse and the abdication of parental responsibilities in child neglect has led to an increased role for the government in family life. Westman (1997) proposes a parent license to validate parental rights, establish parental responsibility, and provide a basis for the societal support of parenting in the form of financial benefits, parent education and training, and protective services for children when necessary. By increasing competent parenting, the need for governmental interventions in families could be reduced.

Short-term Group Therapy

Short-term group therapy for children with physical and/ or sexual abuse backgrounds has proven useful (Morris, 1994).

Storytelling

Therapeutic storytelling has been used as an intervention for victims of child abuse (Hinds, 1997).

Support Networks

Mulroy (1997) provided the results of an organizational analysis of one interorganizational collaboration to create, implement, and institutionalize a community-based service network of informal and formal family support programs to prevent child abuse and neglect.

CAROLYN CHAMBERS CLARK

See
Anger (II)
Depression (II)
Pain (II)
Stress (II)

See also
Art Therapy (IV)
Biofeedback (IV)
Fibromyalgia (II)
Nutrition (IV)

AGING

Aging is a normal process, but evidence is accumulating that specific behaviors can enhance performance despite age. For example, although brain cells may shrink by 10% between the ages of 20 and 70, response time may be reduced, but not significantly. The power to think is the same even though it may take a little longer to remember things or solve complex problems. Challenging the brain at any age helps sprout dendrites that enhance communication between cells. Although it is believed sensory perception diminishes with age, after 6 years of volunteers smelling lemons and some 40 other scents, including natural gas and bubble gum, Dr. Marc Heft (Daughtry, 1997) determined that aging has little effect on smell, taste, or touch. Using the Pennsylvania Smell Identification Test, in which participants scratched and sniffed cards with different scents on them ranging from licorice to paint thinner, the researchers found that women have better senses of smell than men and were able to identify different scents more easily. There were no differences between gender for the other senses. Heft recommended regular exercise, activities that stretch the mind (such as reading), and staying out of the sun (hurries aging and indirectly affects the skin's senses) as ways to enhance sensory perception.

Animal-Assisted Therapy

Fick (1993) conducted a study to determine the effect of the presence and absence of a dog on the frequency and types of social interactions among nursing home residents during a socialization group. Point sampling was used to evaluate the behavior of 36 male residents at a Veterans Administration medical center. A significant difference in verbal interactions occurred among residents with the dog present, providing additional support for the value of animal-assisted therapy for increasing socialization among residents in long-term care facilities.

Exercise

Resistance-training intervention studies have demonstrated important health benefits in older adults. Most have used exercise performed at specific intensities on expensive equipment. Rooks, Kiel, Parsons, and Hayes (1997) tested two self-paced less expensive exercise protocols with community-dwelling adults 65 to 95 years of age. One hundred and thirty-one individuals were randomly assigned to a novel resistance training program, walking, or a control group. Muscle strength, balance, reaction time, stair-climbing speed, and a timed pen pickup task were measured before and after the intervention period. Significant improvements in tandem stance and single-legged stance with eyes open and stair-climbing speed occurred in both exercise groups. Resistance trainers also improved

their muscle strength and ability to pick up an object from the floor and reduced the number of missteps taken during tandem walking. Walkers also reduced tandem walking time. Controls showed no significant improvement in any variable.

Walking or cycling more than 1/2 hour a day was associated with reduced risk of vertebral deformity in women (as measured by interviewer-administered questionnaire and lateral thoracolumbar radiographs). The same study found that heavy levels of activity in early and middle adult life were associated with increased risk for vertebral deformity in men (Silman et al., 1997).

Only walking improved at least one measure of all major outcomes (strength, gait, endurance, balance, and health status) in a single-blind, randomized trial of 106 sedentary adults age 68 to 85 with at least mild deficits in balance (Buchner et al., 1997). Seals, Silverman, Reiling, and Davy (1997) demonstrated that regular aerobic exercise can produce clinically important reductions in resting blood pressure (without any change in maximal aerobic capacity, body weight, or dietary intake) in Caucasian postmenopausal women with mild to moderately elevated initial levels.

Moderate-intensity exercise programs can improve self-reported sleep in healthy older adults (age 50 to 76), according to a study by King and colleagues (1997). Forty-three adults participated in the research. Exercise group participants had four sessions of exercise per week, two sessions at the local YMCA lasting 1 hour and two sessions at home lasting 40 minutes, for 16 weeks. Controls continued their usual activities. Exercise participants had significant improvement on the self-report Pittsburgh Sleep Quality Index for sleep duration, quality, and onset.

Falls are the leading cause of death for persons 75 years and older. Exercise can have important benefits on balance and flexibility, thus protecting older adults from falls. In one study, 20 individuals 65 years of age participated in an 8-week low-intensity aerobic exercise program, including stretching and strengthening exercises, mostly performed from a seated position. Twenty-seven individuals in a comparison group maintained their usual level of exercise. Significant differences between groups were found for flexibility of the ankles and right knee following the treatment program. Individuals in the treatment group also improved their balance by 22% (Mills, 1994).

Food and Supplements

Selhub and colleagues (1995) found that high concentrations of homocysteine and low concentrations of folate and vitamin B6 (through their role in homocysteine metabolism) are associated with an increased risk of extracranial carotid-artery stenosis in individuals age 67 to 96.

Perrig, Perrig, and Stahelin (1997) examined the relationship between antioxidants and memory performance in the old and very old. Noting that aging processes, specifically brain aging, are believed to be associated with free radical action, they hypothesized that plasma antioxidant vitamin levels would correlate with cognitive performance in healthy older adults. In a total of 442 participants, the researchers found that free recall, recognition, and vocabulary were correlated significantly with vitamin C and beta-carotene. The two antioxidants remained significant predictors, especially of semantic memory, after controlling for possible confounding variables including age, education, and gender.

Lindenbaum and others (1994) found that vitamin B12 deficiency was extremely common in apparently healthy older people. None showed signs of pernicious anemia, the classic cause of B12 deficiency. A more likely cause identified by the lead researcher is that a sizable group of the elderly population doesn't secrete enough acid and pepsin to liberate B12 from food. Part of the problem could be corrected, he added, because people who secrete too little stomach acid can still absorb the crystalline B12 in supplements. Because B12 deficiency is dangerous and can lead to irreversible damage to the nervous system, Lindenbaum advised that anyone with an unexplained neuropsychiatric problem should be tested for B12 deficiency. If the result is less than 258, not the usual 149 cutoff, there is a definite suspicion of B12 deficiency.

Snowdon, Gross, and Butler (1996) investigated the relationship between plasma antioxidants and reduced functional capacity in the elderly, specifically dependence in self-care, in a cross-sectional study of 88 Catholic nuns who lived and ate together. This was the first study to report an association between lycopene (found in tomatoes) and self-care, including assistance with bathing, walking, dressing, standing, toileting, and feeding.

Researchers at the Bilboa Medical Unit in London examined age-related chromium levels in 51,665 hair, sweat, and serum samples obtained from 40,871 individuals referred by their physicians. Males were found to have significantly lower mean chromium levels than females, and there was good correlation between chromium levels in the collected samples, using graphite furnace atomic absorption spectrophotometry. The researchers pointed out the role that decreases in chromium levels and the use of refined carbohydrates play in the development of compromised chromium status and the increased risk of age-related impaired glucose metabolism, disordered lipid metabolism, coronary heart disease, arteriosclerosis, and type II diabetes mellitus (Davies, McLaren, Hunnisett, & Howard, 1997).

A group of Massachusetts researchers using a double-blind, placebo-controlled intervention, found that consuming 200 mg of vitamin E (more than the recommended daily dietary allowance) enhances immune responses (including an increase in antibody titer to tetanus vaccine) in older individuals without resulting in any adverse effects (Meydani et al., 1997).

Dance

Twenty-six individuals were selected at random from the psychogeriatric population at the Psychiatric Hospital in Havana, Cuba. During a year of participation in psychoballet (elemental ballet techniques as therapy), there was an improvement in interpersonal relationships and a decrease in the need for psychopharmaceuticals (Acadna Roque, Gonzales Valente, & Fialio Sanza, 1990).

Herbs

Drabaek and others (1996) tested the effects of *Ginkgo biloba* extract versus a placebo in a randomized-double-blind crossover study. Questionnaires based on visual analogue scales were used to quantify the severity of leg pain, impairment of concentration, and inability to remember. The researchers did not find any significant changes in peripheral blood pressures, walking distances, or the severity of leg pain. Systemic blood pressure was reduced both by placebo and by the gingko. The impairment of concentration and the inability to remember were both reduced when comparing results during active treatment (gingko) to placebo. Short-term memory did not change significantly, but the researchers concluded that treatment with the gingko extract did improve some cognitive functions in older individuals with moderate arterial insufficiency.

Stimulation of collagen synthesis prevents the aging process. Metori, Furutsu, and Takahashi (1997) found a formula ratio of ginseng to u-Zhong leaf of 1:3 was the most effective for stimulation of collagen synthesis and the prevention of decreased protein metabolism in aging.

Two types of herbals, Toki-Shakuyaku-San and Boui-Jiou-Tou, were studied using the Senescence-Accelerated Mouse, thought to be a useful model of human aging. Median survival time tended to be longer and acquisition time for learning tasks shorter in the treated group than in the control group. A Chinese herb known as NaO Li Su was used in a double-blind, placebo-controlled crossover trial with 100 elderly Danish volunteers who complained of deteriorating memory. After 3 months of treatment, a battery of psychological and biochemical tests were completed. No desirable effects on memory functions were achieved by the active treatment, but increases in the number of red blood cells and in the serum creatinine levels were seen. In the subgroup initially showing a number of red blood cells below the median, a significant positive correlation was found between changes in the number of red blood cells and changes in the Wechsler Memory Scale (Iversen et al., 1997).

Socializing

Friendships and support groups prevent stress-inducing isolation, build confidence, and keep the mind engaged. Activities like classes and volunteer work enhance social lives and mental dexterity (Crowley,1996).

Tai Chi Chuan (TCC)

In a case-control study of a TCC group and a group of sedentary controls in a hospital-based exercise physiology laboratory, 76 community-dwelling senior persons (mean age 69.3 years) were used to evaluate the health-related fitness of Tai Chi Chuan. In the peak exercise, men in the TCC group showed 19% higher peak oxygen uptake compared with the sedentary group: they also were more flexible and had a lower percentage of body fat (Lan, Lai, Wong, & Yu, 1996).

Wolfson et al. (1996) also studied the beneficial effects of Tai Chi Chuan. They found significant gains in balance and strength after participation in T'ai Chi training, with gains persisting after 6 months.

Yoga

Bowman and colleagues (1997) examined the effect of aerobic exercise training and yoga. They found the heart rate decreased and the alpha High Frequency (reflecting parasympathetic activity and fluctuations in heart rate and blood pressure) increased following yoga, but not aerobic training.

CAROLYN CHAMBERS CLARK

See
Animal-Assisted Therapy (IV)
Dance/Movement Therapy (IV)
Exercise (IV)
Lifestyle Change (IV)
Nutrition (IV)
T'ai Chi (IV)
Yoga (IV)

See also
Alzheimer's Disease (II)
Antioxidants and Free Radicals (III)
Chromium (III)
Diabetes (II)
Heart and Blood Vessel Conditions (II)
High Blood Pressure (II)
Lung Disorders (II)
Memory Problems (II)
Stress (II)
Gingko (III)
Vitamin E (III)

AIDS/HIV

Acquired immunodeficiency syndrome (AIDS) is a progressive condition characterized by suppression of the immune system. There is an increased risk of developing Kaposi's sarcoma, a rare type of cancer. Wolffers and de Moree (1994) analyzed alternative/complementary questionnaires of 206 respondents with human immunodeficiency virus (HIV)/AIDS: 30.6% used alternative/complementary treatments, half of the participants used alternative/complementary therapies on the instigation and with the support of their family physician, 37% felt better using alternative/complementary therapies, and 34% were satisfied because the therapies gave them the feeling they were actively increasing their own resistance capacity.

Food and Supplements

Many people infected with the HIV virus remain AIDS-free for over 20 years, according to a study of 111 men with hemophilia who also had HIV. Nutritional factors may play a role in staying well. Studies have found evidence that HIV depletes selenium in infected cells. Look and colleagues (1997) found that stages I through III of HIV disease are characterized by significant impairments of antioxidative defenses provided by selenium, glutathione (GSH, GSH-Px), and plasma thiol (SH-groups). One theory suggests that the HIV virus needs selenium, which preserves the elasticity of body tissue and slows the aging process to trigger its growth. Once the virus uses up all the selenium in one cell, it breaks out in search of more, spreading the infection to new cells.

Researchers at the University of Georgia suggest that the latency period may be attributed to the period of time it takes to deplete the body of selenium storage (Cheung, 1995). Micronutrients (zinc, copper, selenium, vitamins A and E, and carotenoids) are essential for the integrity of host defenses. Periquet and colleagues (1995) found that children at the Paediatric Haematology and Oncology Unit of Toulouse Hospital, France, who were infected with human immunodeficiency virus type 1 (HIV-1) had statistically significant deficiencies in these important micronutrients at the non-AIDS stage and were confirmed at the AIDS stage: P less than .05 for lycopene, retinol, tocopherol and P < .001 for transthyretin and serum albumin. Levels of copper and long-chain polyunsaturated fatty acids were higher in the non-AIDS group than in the controls. Thus biological impairing of the micronutrient levels was observed in the non-AIDS stage without clinical signs. This information could be useful in delineating nutritional intervention strategies to improve clinical status of HIV-1-infected children with the hope of altering the disease course.

Due to its antiviral effects and its importance for all immunological functions, Schrauzer and Sacher (1995) urged the administration of selenium as a supportive measure in early and advanced stages of HIV-induced disease. Tang and colleagues (1993) examined the intake of micronutrients associated with the progression of HIV-1 infection to AIDS. A total of 281 HIV-1 seropositive homosexual/bisexual men were seen at the Baltimore/Washington, D.C., site of the Multicenter AIDS Cohort Study. Participants completed a self-administered semiquantitative food frequency questionnaire at baseline. The highest levels of total intake from food and supplements of vitamins C and B1 and niacin were associated with a significantly decreased progression rate to AIDS. Those reporting the lowest and highest intake of vitamin A did most poorly, whereas the middle two quartiles were significantly associated with slower progression to AIDS. Increased intake of zinc was significantly associated with an increased risk of progression to AIDS. The risk of developing AIDS was 40% to 50% lower in those who consumed, either from food or supplements, more than 61 mg of niacin, between 9,000 IU and 20,000 IU of vitamin A, and more than 715 mg of vitamin C a day. Risk started to climb in the men who consumed more than 15 mg of zinc a day.

Liang and colleagues (1996) reviewed the interactions between vitamins and the immune system in human AIDS and animal models of AIDS. They found that vitamins A, E, and B12 deficiency accelerated the development of AIDS with low T cells, whereas their normalization retarded the development of immune dysfunction. Other supplements of importance for preventing progression toward AIDS include oral glycyrrhizin and licorice extract (Pierson, 1994). Licorice root is of special interest because it is one of the best nontoxic substances in the food supply that has anti-HIV activity.

Cryptococcal meningitis, an opportunistic infection in people with AIDS, has been treated effectively with intravenous garlic (Davis et al., 1994). In a recent Chinese study reported by Weil (1995), garlic worked better than the antibiotic amphotericin B and caused no toxicity at any dose.

Herbs

Preliminary and anecdotal studies indicate aloe vera juice may offer some "tonic" and antiulcer effects on the gastrointestinal tract (McDaniel, Combs, & McDaniel, 1990). The polysaccharide component of aloe vera, acemannan, has significant immune-enhancing and antiviral activity that could prove useful as an adjunct to current AIDS therapy.

In a preliminary study, St. John's wort (hypericin) was shown to interfere with viral infection. The researchers (Meruelo, Lavie, & Lavie, 1988) suggested that hypericin could become a therapeutic tool against retroviral-induced diseases such as AIDS.

See, Broumand, Sahl, and Tilles (1997) reported the in vitro effects of echinacea and ginseng on natural killer and antibody-dependent cell cytotoxicity in healthy subjects with chronic fatigue syndrome or AIDS. They found both *Echinacea purpurea* and *Panax ginseng* enhance the cellular immune function of peripheral blood mononuclear cells both from normal individuals and from those with depressed cellular immunity.

Yao, Wainberg, and Parniak (1992) found that the herb *Prunella vulgaris* antagonizes HIV-1 infection of susceptible cells by preventing viral attachment to the CD4 receptor.

Massage

Massage has been used successfully to facilitate weight gain in neonates born to HIV-seropositive women, to improve neonatal performance, and to reduce stress behaviors in babies born to HIV women (Field, 1993). In another study 42 people with HIV and moderately immunocompromised were randomly assigned to one of four groups: massage only; massage and two 45-minute aerobic exercise sessions; massage, aerobic exercise, and a 1-hour per week stress management session; and a control group, with members receiving the usual medical treatment. The massage and stress management group missed work less often than the other groups, but this did not reach statistical significance. For use of medical care, the massage and stress management group was significantly better than massage alone. For symptoms of distress, the massage group was better or had fewer feelings of distress but was not significantly different from the other three groups. The researchers concluded that 40 minutes of massage a week does not significantly increase the function of the immune system, as measured by CD4 and natural killer cell counts in moderately compromised persons with HIV. When massage is combined with stress management, significantly less use of medical care occurs.

Stress and AIDS

Stress can accelerate the progression of the early stages of HIV disease, as reported by researchers from the University of Florida and the University of North Carolina at

Chapel Hill. Researchers studied 93 homosexual men, age 18 to 51, who tested positive for HIV but showed no symptoms when they entered the trial. Subjects were recruited from rural and urban areas of North Carolina through state health departments, though advertisements in gay publications and gay organizations, and by word of mouth. Participants were asked about more than 100 possible stresses at 6-month intervals, including death of a mate, arrest, trouble with a boss, chronic financial difficulties, and breakup of a love relationship. The results showed that only severe stress had any influence on the course of illness (Petitto, 1997).

CAROLYN CHAMBERS CLARK

See
   Esalen Massage (IV)
   Exercise (IV)
   Nutrition (IV)

See also
   Aloe (III)
   Echinacea (III)
   Ginseng (III)
   Infection (II)
   Selenium (III)
   Vitamin A (III)
   Vitamin C (III)
   Vitamin E (III)
   Ulcers (II)

ALCOHOLISM

Alcoholism is a leading form of drug abuse in the United States, affecting millions of people. The ingestion of alcohol contributes to countless arrests and thousands of suicides and traffic fatalities every year. Alcoholism costs billions of dollars annu-

ally in lives, health care, time lost from work, and property damage.

Ayurveda

Chronic ethanol ingestion in rats shows metabolic and physiological changes similar to alterations reported in human alcoholism. Administration of SKV, an Ayurvedic formula produced by fermentation of cane sugar with raisins and 12 herbal ingredients, brought down voluntary ethanol ingestion in rats and increased food intake. ECG and EEG evidence of cardiac depression, augmentation of frequency and amplitude of alpha, delta, and theta waves, and weakness in beta waves were reversed during SKV-induced voluntary alcohol restriction. SKV appeared to have no adverse reactions with ethanol and may be a promising way to combat alcoholism (Shanmugasundaram & Shanmugasundaram, 1986).

Exercise

A group of participants being treated for alcoholism were assigned to a physical fitness program as an adjunct to the usual program. Participants in the exercise group showed significantly less craving for alcohol than members in the standard treatment group. The group who participated in exercise also saw themselves as having more internal locus of control and being less controlled by powerful others (Ermalinski et al., 1997).

Guided Imagery

Relapsed alcoholic individuals often report that negative emotions trigger their return to drinking. Cooney and colleagues (1997) provided a negative guided imagery to 50 men with alcoholism to induce negative emotions before exposing them to their favorite alcoholic beverage or spring water. Both alcoholic beverage presentation and negative imagery increased participants' reports of a desire to drink, which predicted time to relapse after inpatient discharge.

CAROLYN CHAMBERS CLARK

See
Imagery (IV)

ALLERGIES

An allergy is an abnormal reaction by the immune system to a usually safe substance. A generally weakened immune system provides a fertile environment for allergens. In a heightened state of alert, the body considers itself vulnerable to attack and prepares to launch a defense against a perceived invader.

A complementary approach to allergies is based on the theory that there is an underlying process that leads to symptoms and a communication link between brain biochemistry and psychoneuroimmunology. These pathways provide an understanding of the links between nutritional intake and central nervous system, immune function, and psychological health (Miller, 1996). The complementary approach seeks not only to reduce symptoms but also to deal with the underlying processes that lead to symptoms.

Allergies range from mildly bothersome to life threatening. An allergic reaction occurs when the immune system releases histamine to attack harmless substances as if they were threats. Symptoms of allergy include sneezing, wheezing, nasal congestion, and coughing (drug or respiratory allergies); itchy eyes, mouth, and throat (respiratory allergies); stomachache, frequent indigestion, and heartburn (food sensitivities); stiffness, pain, and swelling of joints (food or drug allergies); fatigue, difficulty concentrating, emotional upset or irritability, and insomnia (food or seasonal allergies); and irritated itchy, reddening, or swelling skin (drug, food, and insect-sting allergies).

Complementary approaches to allergies include reducing allergic threshold through dietary and lifestyle changes (eliminating/rotating offending foods, increasing certain foods and supplements, and taking environmental actions) and implementing procedures that either reduce symptoms or tackle processes underlying allergic responses. Primary approaches involve reducing airborne and food allergens.

Other complementary approaches that have been used successfully with allergies include acupressure, affirmations, aromatherapy, Ayurveda, Chinese medicine, color therapy, herbs, homeopathy, hydrotherapy, reflexology, and yoga.

Lifestyle and Dietary Procedures

Environmental Actions

A high-efficiency particulate air cleaner (HEPA filter) removes pollen and mold spores that can prompt allergic responses. Turning on the air conditioner in the car and at home and cleaning damp areas with bleach or a citrus cleaner may help. Avoiding household pets and/or giving them frequent baths can reduce noxious dander. Using a vacuum cleaner with a HEPA filter can eliminate many airborne allergens.

A "sick building syndrome" occurs in structures with increased insulation and sealed windows. Wall-to-wall carpeting invites roaches and their detritus. Symptoms of the syndrome include eye, nose, throat, and skin irritation, headache, lethargy, and respiratory problems. Chronic colds and/or dull headaches have also been identified as symptoms of sick building syndrome. Symptoms can be relieved if new buildings are aired for several months before being used and air circulation system filters, drip pans, and humidifiers are changed regularly.

Carbonless paper, toners (from laser printers and copy machines), adhesive floor coverings, and smoking can increase symptoms and are common causes of sick building syndrome. Permanent-press clothes (containing formaldehyde) have been associated with allergies. A clue is the concentration of a rash in clothing-covered areas and/or areas where clothing fits tightly. To avoid allergic responses, wear natural fiber clothes. Bird antigens linger in a house for as long as 18 months. The best action for people who develop lung irritations (hypersensitivity pneumonitis) as a result is to avoid the room in which the bird was kept.

Other actions include making the bedroom allergy-proof by encasing the mattress in allergen-proof plastic; washing sheets, blankets, pillowcases, and mattress pads every week in water that is at least 140° F; and using hypoallergenic bedding materials.

Food Diary/Eliminating Offending Foods

A food diary is used to record all foods, beverages, medications/drugs, and supplements, along with the time of day, mood, and symptoms, for 6 hours after ingestion. Any of the following could suggest a food allergy: warmth, itchiness, stuffiness, headache, fatigue, gastrointestinal symptoms (stomach upset, canker sores, chronic diarrhea, gas, ulcers), genitourinary symptoms (bladder infections, bedwetting, kidney disease), immune system symptoms (chronic infections, frequent ear infections), brain symptoms (anxiety, depression, insomnia, irritability, mental confusion), musculoskeletal problems (joint pain, low back pain), respiratory problems (asthma, chronic bronchitis, wheezing), skin symptoms (acne, hives, rashes, itching), and other miscellaneous symptoms (sinusitis, edema, fainting, fatigue, headache, hypoglycemia, itchy nose or throat, migraines, sinusitis). In young children, bedwetting, sleep disorders, excessive coughing, bad breath, growing pains, abdominal pains, constant runny nose, nausea, recurring middle ear infections, ringing in the ears, or hyperactivity could mean a food allergy. Food additives such as yellow dye no. 5 (tetrazine) and benzoates can increase the production of mast cells, elevating the propensity to allergies. The following may produce allergies and/or asthma: azo dyes or colorings, salicylates, aspartame, benzoates, nitrites, sorbic acid, hydroxytoluene, sulfites, gallates, polysorbates, and vegetable gums (Murray, 1994).

Fatty acids are important mediators of inflammation because of their ability to form prostaglandins. Animal foods (meat and dairy products) contain saturated fats and arachidonic acid, both of which can increase the inflammatory process. Decreasing the intake of animal foods and increasing the intake of omega-3 oils found in flaxseed oil and cold-water fish such as mackerel, herring, sardines, and salmon can reduce the inflammatory/allergic response (Murray, 1994).

Food Rotation

By rotating offending foods, allergic reactions can be reduced. Dairy products, yeast, wheat, rye, corn, soybeans, eggs, oranges, white potatoes, peanuts, chocolate, various spices, beef, coffee, tomato, malt, and pork are among the most common food allergens. By not eating offending foods more often than once every 5 days, allergic symptoms can often be controlled.

Foods and Supplements

Caffeinated and decaffeinated beverages and sugar can overstimulate the immune system and aggravate allergies. Vitamin C and bioflavonoids in citrus fruits or supplements are natural antihistamines. Vitamins A and B-complex can reduce respiratory allergic symptoms. Capsicum (cayenne or chilies) boost the immune system and circulation, clean the blood, and thin secretions. Onions build the immune system, provide quercetin, and heal lung tissue. In one supporting study, children who ate an Indian diet (more vegetables, less meat, and fewer additives and packaged and processed foods) had fewer symptoms of allergy and asthma than Indian youngsters eating a primarily Western diet (Carey, Cookson, Britton, & Tattersfield, 1996). Excluding meat, fish, eggs, and dairy products; maintaining a vegetarian diet; drinking nonchlorinated tap water; avoiding coffee, ordinary tea, chocolate, sugar, green peas, soybeans, and salt; and limiting or excluding potatoes, grains, apples, and citrus fruits have all been shown to be helpful. Eliminating common food allergens and eating berries and onions, two foods that have been shown to produce antiasthmatic effects in controlled studies, can help in the treatment of many chronic allergic or inflammatory diseases (Murray, 1994).

A case-control study nested in a cross-sectional study of a random sample of adults (Soutar, Seaton, & Brown, 1997) concluded that diet may have a modulatory effect on bronchial reactivity. They found an increased risk of symptoms associated with low intakes of zinc and magnesium. The lowest intakes of vitamin C and manganese were associated with a fivefold increased risk of bronchial reactivity. A prospective case-control study provided 279 infants with high atopic risk for allergic symptoms with dietary interventions (prolonged milk feeding, primarily breastfeeding, followed by hypoantigenic weaning diet and avoidance of parental smoking in the presence of the infants for the first 2 years of life). The control group (80 infants) received no intervention. The preventive measures (exclusive breastfeeding and/or hydrolyzed milk feedings, delayed and selective introduction of solid foods, and environmental advice), were effective at the third year of follow-up, greatly reducing allergic manifestations in the high-risk babies in the intervention group (Marini, Agosti, Motta, & Mosca, 1996).

Herbal Therapies

Some of the herbs that have been used as infusions for their anti-inflammatory, immune system–building, respiratory-soothing, and antimucus effects include cubeb berry, stinging nettle, fenugreek seed, rose hips, saw palmetto berry, chamomile, elder flower, eyebright, garlic, yarrow, and pau d'arco bark (Landis & Khalsa, 1997). Ginger tea has been used to reduce sinus inflammation. The steam from grated ginger simmering in water is breathed in (for

5 to 7 minutes, 2 or 3 times a day) until symptoms subside. It is believed that herbs can strengthen the immune system. Once it has been strengthened, offending foods can often be gradually reintroduced with no allergic response. Immune system tonic herbs include astragalus, licorice, pau d'arco, ginseng, ginger, and garlic (Landis & Khalsa, 1997).

Homeopathy

In a randomized, double-blind, controlled trial, Reilly and colleagues (1994) in Glasgow, Scotland, used homeopathically prepared dilutions of grass pollens or dust mites in the treatment of nasal allergies. The results provided evidence that individuals treated with homeopathically prepared allergens improved considerably more than those treated with a placebo. Runny noses, itchy throats, and sneezes may be helped by homeopathic remedies *Arsenicum album* or sabadilla. Remedies for temporary relief of allergies include monkshood, windflower, eyebright, red onion, trioxide of arsenic, phosphate of iron, iodide of potassium, quicksilver, and poison-nut. Since most allergies are long-term problems, they require consultation with a trained homeopathic practitioner.

CAROLYN CHAMBERS CLARK

See
Affirmations (IV)
Aromatherapy (IV)
Ayurveda (IV)
Color Therapy (IV)
Homeopathy (IV)
Psychoneuroimmunology (IV)
Reflexology (IV)
Yoga (IV)

See also
Anxiety/Panic (II)
Asthma (II)
Back Pain (II)
Capsaicin (III)
Caffeine (III)
Chronic Fatigue Syndrome (II)
Cold Symptoms (II)
Depression (II)
Diarrhea (II)
Echinacea (III)
Fatty Acids, Essential (III)
Flavonoids (III)
Garlic (III)
Ginseng (III)
Headache (II)
Insomnia (II)
Licorice (III)
Saw Palmetto (III)
Skin Disorders (II)

ALZHEIMER'S DISEASE

Alzheimer's disease (AD) is a neurodegenerative disorder characterized by loss of memory and other cognitive abilities. Crawford (1996) reviewed the literature and found a link between reduced cerebral blood flow in Alzheimer's. Neurofibrillary tangles, senile plaques, cell loss, and impaired synaptic function characterize the problem. Cholinergic, noradrenergic, and dopaminergic neurons are lost. Oxidative stress and the accumulation of free radicals lead to neuronal degeneration and excessive lipid peroxidation in the brain. A number of complementary approaches have been found helpful.

Foods and Supplements

Sugar has been identified as a potential risk factor in AD because it is linked to reduced cerebral blood flow (Crawford, 1997). Some other foods and supplements have proved helpful.

A double-blind, placebo-controlled, randomized, multicenter trial was conducted with individuals with Alzheimer's of moderate severity. In the study, 341 participants received either 10 mg of the monoamine oxidase inhibitor selegiline, 2,000 I.U. of vitamin E, or a placebo. Both selegiline and vitamin E slowed the progression of Alzheimer's (Sano et al., 1997).

A study at the University of Basel, Switzerland by geriatric professor Hannes Staehelin (1997) on Swiss men and women age 65 to 94 years for 20 years found those who had high levels of vitamin C and beta-carotene in their blood performed better in memory tests. Vitamin C and beta-carotene were significant predictors of ability in tests of vocabulary and beta-carotene in tests of recognition. The study had a 20-year follow-up period. The research showed that memory functions could be linked to increased oxidative stress with aging. Neurons in brain cells are challenged by free radicals and antioxidants, which protect the neurons from damage. Dr. Shaehelin suggested that antioxidants are ideally obtained from natural sources such as fruits and vegetables, but supplements might be necessary.

Pettegrew and colleagues (1995) used a double-blind placebo study to test the effect of acetyl-L-carnitine (an amino acid–like substance) with 7 probable AD individuals, who were then compared over the course of a year by clinical and 31P magnetic resonance spectroscopic measures with 5 placebo-treated probable AD individuals and 21 age-matched healthy controls. Compared to AD individuals on placebo, acetyl-L-carnitine-treated partici-pants showed significantly less deterioration in their Mini-Mental Status and Alzheimer's Disease Assessment Scale test scores.

Also, the decrease in phosphomonoester levels observed in both the acetyl-L-carnitine and placebo AD groups at entry was normalized, as were high-energy phosphate levels, but only in the treatment group. This was the first direct in vivo demonstration of the beneficial effect of L-carnitine on both clinical and central nervous system (CNS) neurochemical parameters in AD. Thal and colleagues (1996) also studied the effect of L-carnitine, using an acetyl-L-carnitine hydrochloride (ALCAR) formulation. Their 1-year, double-blind, placebo-controlled, randomized, parallel-group study compared the efficacy and safety of ALCAR with placebo in individuals with mild to moderate probable AD, age 50 or older. The participants were given 3 g per day of ALCAR or placebo (1 g tid) for 12 months. Of those who entered the study (4,311), 83% completed 1 year of treatment. Early onset AD individuals (age 65 or younger at study entry) on ALCAR declined more slowly than those on placebo and tolerated the supplement well.

Herbs

Itil and Martorano (1995) reported findings from a pilot bioequivalency study. Findings indicated significant quantitative CNS effects in Ginkgold similar to other psychoactive compounds classified as cognitive activators. Recent studies in which EGb (*Ginkgo biloba*) 761 demonstrated therapeutic effects in the treatment of dementia and have earned EGb the approval of the German Bundesgesundheits Amt used in the treatment of dementia. Kanowski and colleagues (1996) used a prospective, randomized, double-blind, placebo-controlled, multicenter study using *Ginkgo biloba* special extract EGb 761 (240 mg) or placebo with 216 individuals diagnosed with presenile or senile primary degenerative dementia of the Alzheimer type. Those taking gingko showed a significant positive difference from the placebo group on the Clinical Global Impressions test, the Syndrom-Kurz test for attention and memory, and the Nurnberger Alters-Beobachtungs-skala test for behavioral assessment of activities of daily life.

Haase, Halama, and Horr (1996) had similar results with short-term intervenous infusion therapy for those with moderate dementia. Results included an improvement in cognitive performance and increased ability to cope with the demands of daily living.

LeBars and colleagues (1997) at the New York Institute for Medical Research reported that an extract of *Ginkgo biloba* (EGb 761) may be as effective as any drug, hormone (primarily estrogen), or vitamin (E) currently used to treat Alzheimer's. In the study, 27% of participants ($n = 309$, with a one-third dropout rate) who took 120 mg a day of the herb for 6 months or longer showed improvement in mental functioning (reasoning, memory, and ability to learn), compared to those who took a placebo (14%). Although these results are encouraging, the researchers suggested that a larger trial should be undertaken.

Mirror Use

Tabak, Bergman, and Alpert (1996) reported the use of the mirror as a therapeutic tool for patients with dementia. The sample was comprised of 100 people suffering from dementia, 67 women and 33 men between the ages of 67 and 95. The findings showed that most responses to looking in the mirror were positive and raised awareness regarding self-care. In a few participants, looking into the mirror aroused feelings of anger or despair, but this was followed by relief and calmness. The use of mirrors allowed caregivers to communicate more clearly with participants. Staff reported that the use of mirrors was an inexpensive and efficient therapeutic tool for improving care.

Music

Dinner music can help nursing home residents eat more calmly, feed themselves more than usual, show decreased restlessness (Ragneskog, Kihlgren, Karlsson, & Norberg, 1996), and appear less depressed, irritable, and fearful (Ragneskog, Brane, Karlsson, & Kihlgren, 1996). Significant reductions were observed in the cumulative incidence of total agitated behaviors, physically nonaggressive behaviors, and verbally agitated behaviors (Goddaer & Abraham, 1994).

Support and Counseling

In a randomized controlled intervention study of 206 spouse-caregivers of individuals with Alzheimer's, members of the treatment group were provided with 6 sessions of individual and family counseling and were required to join support groups. Counselors were also available for further counseling as needed. The program substantially increased the time spouse-caregivers were able to care for their spouses at home, especially in the early to middle stages of dementia (Mittelman et al., 1997).

CAROLYN CHAMBERS CLARK

See
  Music Therapy (IV)
  Imagery (IV)

See also
  Aging (II)
  Anger (II)
  Antioxidants and Free Radicals (III)
  Depression (II)
  Memory Problems (II)
  Vitamin C (III)
  Vitamin E (III)

ANEMIA

In anemia, body tissues are deprived of oxygen due to a reduction in the number of circulating red blood cells. There are more than 400 forms of anemia. Symptoms include weakness, fatigue, and a general feeling of malaise (mild anemia); burning tongue (vitamin B12 anemia); weakness, tiredness, shortness of breath, and faintness or dizziness (severe anemia); pasty or yellowish skin and bluish lips, pale gums, nail beds, eyelid linings, or palm creases (strong signs of anemia); and movement or balance problems, slick tongue, confusion, depression, memory loss, and tingling in extremities (pernicious anemia). Other possible symptoms include headache, insomnia, decreased appetite, poor concentration, and irregular heartbeat. Iron overload can occur from taking iron supplements. Symptoms include vomiting, bloody diarrhea, fever, jaundice, lethargy, and seizures.

Chinese Medicine

Anemia, or deficient blood, is treated with acupuncture and herbal therapies. Asian ginseng is used as a general tonic for fatigue. Dong quai (dang gui) has been used alone for thousands of years as a blood tonic. It may be combined with Chinese foxglove root or astragalus.

Zhou and Zhou (1990) reported a study treating anemia using the principle of bu-shen yi-qi. In their study, 60 people with orthostatic dysregulation were randomly divided into a treatment group (received Chinese herbs under the principle of bu-shen yi-qi) and a control group (received oryzanol and vitamins B1 and B6). Herbs selected were rich in trace elements, including iron (enhances red blood cell action) and zinc. After 1 month, results showed that 16 members of the treatment group and 4 members of the control group had significantly improved. Of the total group, 43, or 71%, also clinically expressed mild anemia. Blood was drawn before and after treatment. Blood values for red blood cells, hemoglobin, and hyperchromia in 20 participants in the treatment group were significantly improved; 17 of the controls remained unchanged.

Zee-Cheng (1992) reported the use of Shi-quan-da-bu-tang (10 significant tonic decoction, or SQT), a combination traditionally used for anemia, anorexia, extreme exhaustion, fatigue, kidney and spleen insufficiency, and general weakness. In the study, the combination was used to restore immunity in people diagnosed with cancer, potentiate the therapeutic effect, and ameliorate the adverse toxicity of anticancer agents. Zee-Cheng reported the results of 8 years of animal and human studies showing that SQT ameliorates anemia, among other conditions, by "toning the blood and strengthening Q (vital energy)."

Su, He, and Chen (1993) reported on a study of an herbal preparation, Man-Shen Ling, which consists of medicinal herbs such as astragalus and rehmannia. The combination was markedly effective for anemia and showed no adverse effects on liver, kidney, heart, or gastrointestinal tract functions.

Zhang, Shi, and Fan (1995) reported the use of Chinese medicinal herbs and vitamin C for 43 children with aplastic anemia treated with fetal blood transfusion. The treatment group receiving Chinese medicinal herbs and blood transfusion improved by 88.9% (chronic aplastic anemia) and 62.5% (acute aplastic anemia), as compared to 46% for the blood transfusion–alone group.

Foods and Supplements

Caffeinated or decaffeinated tea, coffee, or cola should be avoided with meals because caffeine and the tannin in black tea inhibit iron absorption. Instead, citrus juices rich in vitamin C are recommended to enhance iron absorption. The chronic use of alcoholic beverages should also be avoided. These can interfere with the ability to absorb folic acid.

Iron-rich foods include parsley (also contains vitamin C, which promotes iron absorption), broccoli, tomatoes, dried beans, blackstrap molasses, dried fruits, almonds, liver, poultry, and red meat. Vitamin C and copper also promote iron absorption.

To enhance red blood cell production, the following foods should be eaten fresh or minimally cooked to preserve their folic acid content: dark green vegetables, milk, wheat germ, brewer's yeast, pumpkin, liver, and eggs. Salmon and mackerel are good sources of vitamin B12, and black-eyed peas, beans, and lentils provide folate.

Vegetarians are at risk for vitamin B12 anemia because the vitamin is found only in animal products and fermented foods. Vegetarians need to include dairy products, eggs, and fermented foods, such as miso, tofu, and tempeh, in their diet. Iron supplements and/or some vitamin supplements can provide excess iron that can be harmful.

CAROLYN CHAMBERS CLARK

See
Acupuncture and Chinese Medicine (IV)

See also
AIDS/HIV (II)
Caffeine (III)
Dang Gui (Dong Quai) (III)
Depression (II)
Diarrhea (II)
Headache (II)
Heart and Blood Vessel Conditions (II)
Insomnia (II)
Memory Problems (II)
Tea (III)
Vitamin C (III)

ANGER

Anger is a strong feeling or condition of displeasure and antagonism that can depress the immune system and induce abnormal electrical activity in the heart (Wenneberg et al., 1997). Common sources of anger are illness and the health care experience (Whyte & Smith, 1997).

Some other sources of anger include: attacks from others (including other health care workers), lack of assistance and support, and differential treatment based on unchangeable characteristics (age, gender, ethnicity, etc.).

Work-related anger can result in severed relationships, feelings of guilt, powerlessness, isolation, humiliation, and incompetence (Brooks, Thomas, & Droppleman, 1996), or problem-focused coping (Manderino & Berkey, 1997; Thomas & Droppleman, 1997). A result of unresolved anger can be depression (Rosal et al., 1997). Robbins and Tanck (1997) asked 77 undergraduate students to complete the Beck Depression Inventory and keep a psychological diary for 10 consecutive days, answering questions dealing with felt anger and expressed anger and several measures of depressed affect. The tendency to attribute the cause of angry feelings to their own actions was positively related to depressed affect, and the tendency to inhibit expression of anger was positively related to the measure of depression.

Changes in health care management can lead to grief in the health care professional. Change involves loss and grief (including denial, anger, bargaining, depression, and acceptance) and are expected responses (Daugird & Spencer, 1996). Although medical providers may recognize anger in clients, they may not have been educated to deal with it effectively, according to Doblin and Klamen (1997).

Research shows that anger can affect blood pressure negatively and can bring on asthma symptoms and angina attacks. Even recalling angry events from the past can trigger abnormal electrical activity and heartbeats in individuals with heart disease (Siegman & Snow, 1997), and high levels of expressed anger may be a risk factor for coronary heart disease, at least for older men (Kawachi et al., 1996). Learning to forgive, staying submissive, reducing negative attitudes, taking on a confidant, taking care of a pet, and avoiding overstimulation are key solutions (Gabay et al., 1996; Shapiro, Goldstein, & Jamner, 1996; Spicer & Chamberlain, 1996; Whiteman, Deary, Lee, & Fowkes, 1997).

A study by Wenneberg and colleagues (1997) found that modes of anger expression may be associated with increased platelet aggregation. Raikkonen and colleagues (1996) linked anger with insulin resistance syndrome.

Anger Management Training

Larkin and Zayfert (1996) provided anger management training for 13 people with essential hypertension. The program included 6 weeks of relaxation training, self-statement modification, and role-play assertiveness training. Participants in the program exhibited significantly lower diastolic blood pressures, significantly more assertive skills, and lesser diastolic blood pressure reactivity after training than did controls.

Breathing Therapy

Appels and colleagues (1997) reported the use of breathing therapy to reduce anger and the risk of new cardiac events after a percutaneous coronary angioplasty. Thirty postangioplasty participants and 65 controls comprised the sample that was studied for an average period of 16 and 18 months, respectively. Breathing therapy resulted in a significant decrease of the mean exhaustion scores and reduced the risk of a new coronary event (cardiac death, coronary artery bypass grafting, myocardial infarction, angioplasty, and restenosis) by 50%. The results indicated that breathing therapy can reduce vital exhaustion and hostility, thereby reducing the risk of a new cardiac event.

Cognitive-Behavioral Treatment

Employing a randomized group design, Chemtob, Novaco, Hamada, and Gross (1997) used a 12-session anger treatment with severely angry Vietnam War veterans with combat-related posttraumatic stress disorder. Controlling for pretreatment scores, the researchers found significant effects on anger reaction and anger control measures even at 18-month follow-up.

Linehan, Tutek, Heard, and Armstrong (1994) used a l-year clinical trial with 26 chronically suicidal female individuals assigned to either a dialectical behavior therapy or a usual treatment. The cognitive-behavioral treatment group had significantly better scores on measures of anger, interviewer-rated global social adjustment, and the Global Assessment Scale and tended to rate themselves better on overall social adjustment than treatment-as-usual subjects.

Exercise

Petajan and colleagues (1996) randomly assigned 54 people diagnosed with multiple sclerosis to exercise or nonexercise groups. Anger scores were significantly reduced.

Jette and colleagues (1996) reported a videotaped, home-based strength training program (Strong-for-Life) with older adults age 66 to 87. Participants were iden-

tified from the Medicare beneficiary list and randomized to exercise or no exercise. Older males achieved significant differences in perceived anger, tension, and overall social functioning.

Forgiveness

According to Hargrave and Sells (1997) forgiveness and anger are mutually exclusive concepts. Once forgiveness occurs, anger leaves. The researchers reported the development of a forgiveness scale and presented data to support the validity and reliability of the instrument.

Laughter

Keltner and Bonanno (1997) investigated the use of laughter to reduce distress and anger. To test their hypothesis that laughter facilitates an adaptive response by increasing the psychological distance from stress and enhancing social relations, they created measures of bereaved adults' laughter and smiling. Duchenne laughter, which involves orbicularis oculi muscle action, related to self-reports of reduced anger and increased enjoyment, dissociation of distress, better social relations, and positive responses from strangers.

Mirrors

Tabak, Bergman, and Alpert (1996) reported a novel response to anger. They examined changes in the behavior of 67 women and 33 men between the ages of 67 and 85. Looking in the mirror at first aroused feelings of anger or despair, followed by relief and calmness.

Social Support

Brownley, Light, and Anderson (1996) examined the effects of anger and social support on clinic, work, and blood pressure in 129 black and white healthy adults. Angry black men with high tangible support tended to exhibit lower blood pressure than other black men. For white women, high belonging support was associated with lower blood pressure and low tangible support; high anger was also related to higher clinic blood pressure. Regardless of ethnicity or gender, high appraisal support was associated with lower overall blood pressure. The researchers' findings suggest that the adverse effects of anger on blood pressure can be reduced by social support.

CAROLYN CHAMBERS CLARK

See
Cognitive-Behavioral Therapy (IV)
Diet and Mood (IV)

See also
Anxiety/Panic (II)
Asthma (II)
Depression (II)
Heart and Blood Vessel Conditions (II)
Syndrome X (II)

ANXIETY/PANIC

Anxiety is a state of unexplained discomfort that is frequently coupled with guilt, doubt, fears, and obsessions. It is apt to occur in interpersonal situations that threaten prestige and dignity. A little anxiety is helpful to the learning process, but as it escalates, selective inattention to details occurs, until a state of disorganizing behavior called panic is reached. At that point, the heart races, and a feeling of impending doom takes over. Physiological symptoms of sweating, weakness, nausea, numbness,

and dizziness, along with feelings of unreality and "going crazy," are common.

At some point in their lives, 24 million Americans suffer from anxiety so intense that it interferes with their ability to function in everyday situations. Complementary therapies have been shown to be effective treatments for moderate and intense anxiety. Some treatments for which there is clinical, but not research support, include avoiding drinking more than 4 cups of coffee, tea, or cola drinks a day; pressing acupressure calming points; using Bach flower remedies; breathing from the abdominal area; keeping a panic diary of each attach, what triggers it, and the individual coping responses to the attack; using homeopathic remedies such as *Aurum* met. and ignatia; and taking antistress vitamins (B-complex, or B-complex and C).

Autogenic Training

Sakai (1996) reported the use of the second autogenic training exercise for panic disorder with 34 individuals treated by the researcher. Fifteen participants had no further symptoms, 9 were much improved, 5 improved, and 5 remained unchanged.

Combined Treatments to Reduce Anxiety

Field and colleagues (1997) reported a study testing the immediate effects of brief massage therapy, muscle relaxation with visual imagery, and muscle relaxation and social support group session for job stress among health care workers. All groups reported decreases in anxiety, depression, fatigue, and confusion, as well as increased vigor, which suggests that all therapies were equally effective.

Gagne and Tove (1994) found that both relaxation (treatment) and therapeutic touch (placebo, control group) produced significant reductions in reported anxiety in 31 individuals in a Veterans Administration psychiatric facility. Rest, music therapy, and music-video therapy were equally helpful in producing a relaxation response in a study of individuals undergoing heart surgery (Barnason, Zimmerman, & Nieveen, 1995).

Cognitive Therapy

Brown and colleagues (1997) found that both focused and standard cognitive therapy worked well for panic disorder. Both groups (20/group) reported significant decreases in panic, and over 84% in both groups were free from panic attacks a year later.

Dance

Leste and Rust (1984) studied the effects of modern dance on anxiety. State anxiety was assessed before and after a 3-month education program, using the Spielberger State-Trait Anxiety Inventory. The class in modern dance was compared with a physical education group, a music group, and a mathematics control group. Dance training significantly reduced anxiety, but no control activities did.

Noreau, Martineau, Roy, and Belzile (1995) investigated the use of aerobic dance–based exercise for 19 people with rheumatoid arthritis who participated in a 12-week biweekly program. Ten people served as controls. Besides improvement in movement and decrease in pain, the treatment group showed positive changes in anxiety and other negative feelings.

Desensitization Through Reexposure

Swinson and colleagues (1992) found that people who experienced panic attacks often headed for the emergency room of the hospital, fearing they were having a heart attack. In a study of 33 people who came to the emergency room of one hospital, half were given reassurance and half were advised to reexpose themselves to the situation as soon as possible and to wait there until their anxiety decreased. During the next 6 months, people who had been reassured experienced an increase in panic-related behaviors. Those who had been given exposure (desensitization) directions showed a significant decrease in panic behavior.

Distraction

Distraction may be a better coping device for upsetting situations than discussion of what happened. Sharing thoughts about the day's woes can worsen mood, according to a study of 79 men who tracked their biggest upset of the day, how they coped with it, and what their moods were that day. As a reliability check, their wives also kept notes on what their husbands' moods were. The most effective coping strategies, in terms of lifting mood, were distraction (e.g., cleaning house, quietly meditating, or pumping iron in the gym), relaxation, and acceptance of the ill-fated day. Distraction allows the mental screen to clear and allows the mind to focus on less aggravating things (Stone, 1996).

Exercise

Positive changes in anxiety and tension were observed after a 12-week exercise program for individuals with arthritis (Noreau et al., 1995). Exercise was also found useful in significantly decreasing anxiety in women during radiation therapy treatment for breast cancer (Mock et al., 1997).

Kugler and colleagues (1994) completed a meta-analysis of 15 studies on the psychological effects of exercise programs on people diagnosed with coronary heart conditions. They found a positive effect size both for anxiety and depression.

Pierce and Pate (1994) examined the effects of a single bout of physical activity among older participants. Sixteen trained women completed an abbreviated Profile of Mood States prior to and immediately following a 75-minute session of aerobic line dancing. A series of one-way analysis of variance with repeated measures from pre- to posttest scores showed significant decreases in scores on tension.

O'Connor, Bryant, Veltri, and Gebhardt (1993) reported the effect of resistance exercise in females on state anxiety and ambulatory blood pressure. Young women undergoing high-intensity exercise reported significantly less stress than participants in the less intense exercise groups. However, the relationship between stress and anxiety/depression/ hostility weakened at the end of the training period, but strengthened in the less intense exercise groups. The study provided evidence to support the hypothesis that, in an adolescent population, aerobic exercise has positive effects on well-being.

Raglin, Turner, and Eksten (1993) also provided evidence for the use of exercise as an anxiety reducer. Eleven female and 25 male collegiate varsity athletes completed 30-minute sessions of leg cycle ergometry or weight training in a randomized order on separate days. State anxiety and systolic (SBP) and diastolic (DBP) blood pressure were measured at baseline prior to exercise and 20 and 60 minutes postexercise. State anxiety increased significantly following weight training, but decreased significantly below baseline 50 minutes following ergometry. SBP (but not DBP) was reduced by 6.5 mm/Hg below baseline at 60 minutes following ergometry.

Rejeski, Thompson, Brubaker, and Miller (1992) evaluated the experimental hypothesis that aerobic exercise buffers psychosocial stress responses in low to moderately physically fit women. Forty-eight (24 white, 24 black) 25- to 40-year-old women participated in either an attention control group or a 40-minute bout of aerobic exercise at 70% heart rate reserve. Both groups were followed by 30 minutes of quiet rest, exposure to mental and interpersonal threat, and 5 minutes of recovery. Aerobic exercise reduced both the frequency and the intensity of anxiety-related thoughts after the interpersonal threat as compared to the placebo group.

Homeopathy

Individually selected homeopathic remedies were used on an outpatient basis to treat 12 adults who had social phobia, panic disorder, or major depression. Overall response rates were 58% according to the clinical global improvement scale and 50% on the SCL-90 and the Brief Social Phobia Scale.

Meditation

Miller, Fletcher, and Kabat-Zinn (1995) found that an intensive, time-limited group stress reduction based on mindfulness meditation significantly reduced anxiety and panic for 22 individuals with *DSM-III-R*–defined anxiety disorders.

Music

A convenience sample of 97 adults receiving chemotherapy for the first time was assigned to either an experimental group offered taped music and a message from their physician ($n = 47$), or a "no intervention" control group ($n = 50$). After the fourth chemotherapy treatment, Sabo and Michael (1996) found significant results on the Spielberger State Anxiety Inventory (as compared to initial evaluation) for the taped music group, but not for the control group. These preliminary findings indicate that this simple and cost-effective intervention can decrease anxiety when receiving chemotherapy.

Relaxation

Using a conceptual framework of holism Weber (1996) investigated the effects of relaxation exercises on anxiety levels in an inpatient general psychiatric unit. The researcher used a convenience sample of 39 participants. Anxiety levels were measured prior to and after the relaxation exercises using the state portion of the State-Trait Anxiety Inventory. Treatment included progressive muscle relaxation, meditative breathing, guided imagery, and soft music. There was a significant reduction in anxiety level on the posttest.

Self-Hypnosis

Ashton and colleagues (1997) hypothesized that self-hypnosis relaxation techniques would have a positive effect on individuals' mental and physical condition following coronary artery bypass surgery. The researchers used a prospective, randomized trial ($n = 32$) and followed participants from 1 day prior to surgery until the time of discharge. The treatment group was taught self-hypnosis relaxation techniques preoperatively, whereas the control group received the usual care. Individuals who were taught self-hypnosis were significantly more relaxed postoperatively compared to the control group. Pain medication requirements were also significantly lower for the treatment group.

Therapeutic Touch

Simington and Laing (1993) studied the effect of therapeutic touch versus a backrub on anxiety level in 105 institutionalized elderly. A double-blind, three-group experimental design was used. State anxiety was measured using the Spielberger State-Trait Anxiety Inventory. The anxiety level of subjects who received therapeutic touch was significantly lower than for those who received a back rub without therapeutic touch. The researchers suggested that therapeutic touch has some potential for enhancing the quality of life for this population.

CAROLYN CHAMBERS CLARK

See
Autogenic Training (IV)
Bach Flower Remedies (IV)
Cognitive-Behavioral Therapy (IV)
Dance/Movement Therapy (IV)
Esalen Massage (IV)
Exercise (IV)
Homeopathy (IV)
Hypnotic Preparation for Surgery (IV)
Imagery (IV)
Music Therapy (IV)
Therapeutic Touch (IV)

ARTHRITIS

There are more than 37 million diagnosed cases of arthritis in the United States. By age 40 most people have experienced an arthritic attack, if only a flare-up of an old sports injury or stiffness upon rising. Arthritis, or inflammation of the joint, is not a single entity. The two major types are osteoarthritis and rheumatoid arthritis, but there are more than 100 variations. Obesity is an important risk factor for osteoarthritis of the knee (McAlindon et al., 1996).

Chinese Medicine

Chen and Zuoxu (1994) reported treating osteoarthritis of the knee joint using traditional Chinese medicine. In traditional Chinese medicine, the condition falls into the Bi syndrome (rheumatic pain) and is considered to be due to a deficiency of yin of the kidney and liver; stagnation of qi, causing blood stasis; and a superimposed invasion of wind, cold, and dampness. The principle of treatment is to reinforce the liver and kidney, thus activating the blood and resolving stasis, promote smooth circulation of blood and vital energy to relax muscles and tendons, and disperse blockage of channels to relieve pain. In the Chen and Zuoxu study, the basic prescription was oral administration of the Radix Angelicae Pubescentis and Ramulus Loranthi decoction. For individuals who could not take the decoction orally, Radix et Rhizoma Rhei, frankincense, and Pericarpium Zanthoxyli were used in a hot fomentation placed directly over or under the knee twice a day for 10 days. Gentle manipulations were also done, including tapping the following points with fingertips: Xuehai (Sp 10), Xiyan (Extra 32), Yanglingquan (GB 34), Yinlingquan (Sp 9), Fengshi (GB 31), Ganshu (UB 18), Shenshu (UB 23), and Weizhong. Additional treatment involved kneading and rolling of the quadriceps muscle, knee joint, and patella. Of the 28 cases treated, 7 were "cured," 13 showed marked effect, 6 were improved, and 2 had no effect. The overall effective rate was 93%. The shortest duration of treatment was 3 weeks; the longest, 3 months.

Cognitive-Behavioral Pain Management

Walco and colleagues (1992) reported a cognitive-behavioral self-regulatory program in the management of juvenile rheumatoid arthritis. Self-regulatory techniques were taught to 13 children ranging in age from 4.5 to 16.9 years. Baseline data included an initial comprehensive assessment of pain, disease activity, and level of functional disability, as well as pain intensity ratings gathered over a 4-week period. Participants were seen for eight individual sessions and taught progressive muscle relaxation, guided imagery, and meditative breathing. Parents were seen for two sessions, during which key aspects of behavioral pain management techniques were reviewed. These techniques led to a substantial reduction of pain intensity, which generalized to outside the clinic setting. Six- and 12-month follow-up data showed consistent decreases in pain and improved adaptive functioning.

Dance

Three research studies have shown the benefits of using dance for rheumatoid arthritis symptoms. Van Deusen and Harlowe (1987) showed how dance enhanced the upper extremity range of motion. Perlman and colleagues (1990) provided evidence that dance has positive effects on lower extremity function and quality of life. Noreau and colleagues (1995) showed the effect of dance on depression, anxiety, fatigue, and tension.

Exercise/Rest

Keeping mobile is a major goal for those with arthritis. Joint movement nourishes the cartilage, and the resulting pressure forces synovial fluid out of the cartilage. Pressure is relieved when the joint relaxes and the fluid flows back into the cartilage, carrying with it nutrients and oxygen to keep the cartilage healthy. Stretching exercises can reduce stiffness and enhance circulation, as can laughter and other types of exercise. Suggestions for safe exercising include the following: (1) incorporate warm-up and cool-down periods of stretching and slower-paced activity before and after exercise to prevent injury, (2) take naps, and (3) add regular stretch breaks from work to help avoid fatigue and overexertion.

In one study, low-load resistive muscle training worked well with individuals diagnosed with functional class 2 rheumatoid arthritis. Participants reported increased functional capacity. Screening for dormant coronary artery disease was recommended by the researchers (Komatireddy et al., 1997).

Food and Supplements

Hansen and colleagues (1996) used a prospective, single-blind study of 6 months' duration with 109 active rheumatoid arthritis participants, who were randomly assigned to either treatment with or without a specialized diet. A daily food diary was completed by each individual and the total intake of 47 different food elements was calculated. Although 28 participants dropped out, of the remaining 81, the ones who followed the special diet (adjusted energy intake, fish meal, and antioxidants) demonstrated a significant improvement in morning stiffness, number of swollen joints, pain status, and reduced cost of medicine.

A significant improvement can also occur with a vegetarian regime. Kjeldsen-Kragh, Haugen, Borchgrevink, and Forre (1994) found the following variables were significantly different for those who responded to a diet change to vegetarianism than for those who didn't: pain score, duration of morning stiffness, Stanford Health Assessment Questionnaire index, and number of tender and swollen joints.

Other studies have indicated that the inflammatory process can be reduced by switching to a vegetarian diet because it significantly alters the intake of fatty acids. Haugen and colleagues (1994) examined the relationship between fatty acids and a vegan diet. Although a clinical enhancement occurred, the fatty acid profiles could not explain the improvement.

The effect of fish oils was evaluated in a multicenter, randomized, double-blind study. Fifty-one participants were allocated 12 weeks of treatment with either six *n*-3 polyunsaturated fatty acid (PUFA) capsules (3.6 g) or six capsules with a fat composition averaging the Danish diet. Small but significant improvements in morning stiffness, joint tenderness, and C-reactive protein were observed. A study of women (Shapiro et al., 1996) examined the relationship between ingestion of fish and arthritis. Consumption of broiled or baked fish, but not of other methods of preparing fish, was associated with a decreased risk of rheumatoid arthritis in the 324 incident rheumatoid arthritis cases (as opposed to the controls). Their results support the hypothesis that omega-3 fatty acids may help prevent rheumatoid arthritis.

Flynn, Irvin, and Krause (1994) examined the effect of cobalamin-folate supplements in 26 participants diagnosed for an average of 5.7 years with idiopathic osteoarthritis of the hands who had been medicated with prescribed nonsteroidal and anti-inflammatory drugs (NSAID). After a 10-day washout period from use of all antiarthritis drugs, vitamins, and minerals, participants were randomly assigned to 6,400 mcg folate or 6,400 mcg folate plus 20 mcg cobalamin (vitamin B12) or lactose placebo each for 2 months within self-selected diets. Pain was medicated by acetaminophen as needed. When participants were assessed, mean right- and left-hand grip values were higher with combined vitamin B12–folate ingestion than with other "vitamin" supplements and were equivalent to NSAID use. Number of tender hand joints was greater with use of NSAID than with use of cobalamin-folate. There were many side effects with NSAID, whereas there were no side effects with the vitamin combination and the cost was lower.

Kremer and Bigaouette (1996) found that people diagnosed with rheumatoid arthritis tended to ingest too much total fat and too little polyunsaturated fat, and their diets are deficient in zinc, magnesium, pyridoxine, copper, and folate. The researchers collected information from a detailed dietary history and analyzed it for nutrient intake. They suggested that routine dietary supplementation with multivitamins and trace elements is appropriate for this population.

Leventhal and colleagues (1993) used a randomized, double-blind, placebo-controlled, 24-week trial. Thirty-seven individuals attending a rheumatology clinic of a university hospital were randomly assigned to treatment with 1.4 g/d gammalinolenic acid in borage seed oil or cottonseed oil (placebo). Treatment resulted in clinically important reductions in the number of tender and swollen joints compared to the control group. Leventhal, Boyce, and Zurier (1994b) used blackcurrant seed oil (BCSO) in a randomized, double-blind, placebo-controlled, 24-week trial. The oil is rich in gammalinolenic acid as well as alphalinolenic acid. Both are known to suppress inflammation and joint tissue injury in animal models. The treatment group in this study showed a significant reduction in disease activity, but many participants withdrew because both BCSO and its placebo had to be administered in 15 large capsules daily.

Selenium may be an essential factor in many of the biochemical pathways associated with rheumatoid arthritis because it is involved in the production of prostaglandins and leukotrienes, which regulate the inflammation process. Glutathione peroxidase is a selenium-dependent antioxidant enzyme that modulates the effect of free radicals, which promote inflammation and degrade collagen and cartilage in joints. Low selenium levels have been found in individuals with inflammatory rheumatic disorders. In study, symptoms improved in 40% of participants after selenium supplementation. Some drugs used to treat arthritis may lower available selenium; in these cases, selenium supplementation may be of value (Peretz, Neve, & Famaey, 1991).

Evidence suggests that pathophysiologic processes in bone are important in the development of osteoarthritis of the knee. Low intake and low serum levels of vitamin D may compromise usual protective responses and predispose individuals to progression of the condition (McAlindon et al., 1996). People taking middling to high doses of vitamin C (in food or supplements) had a threefold reduction in risk for osteoarthritis and knee pain. A reduction in the risk of progression also occurred, possibly due to beta-carotene and vitamin E, but only in men (McAlindon, 1997).

Relaxation Therapy/Cognitive-Behavioral Treatment

Although the cause of arthritis is unknown, it is believed to be a disturbance of the immune system. The effects of stress on the immune system have been well documented, so it seems logical to assume that reducing stress can reduce arthritic symptoms. O'Leary, Shoor, Kate, and Holman (1988) examined the effect of a program in self-relaxation, cognitive pain management, and goal setting. The control group members received an arthritis helpbook containing information on arthritis self-management. The treated group experienced reductions in depression and stress, coped more effectively with their arthritis, and slept longer and better.

Yoga

Yoga and relaxation techniques traditionally have been used by nonmedical practitioners. A study by Garfinkle and associates (1994) at the University of Pennsylvania School of Medicine examined the effect of yoga on the hands of patients with osteoarthritis. Participants were randomly assigned to either yoga or no therapy. The yoga-treated group improved significantly more than the controls in terms of pain during activity, tenderness, and finger range of motion.

CAROLYN CHAMBERS CLARK

See
   Acupuncture and Chinese Medicine (IV)
   Cognitive-Behavioral Therapy (IV)
   Dance/Movement Therapy (IV)
   Imagery (IV)
   Vegetarianism (IV)
   Yoga (IV)

See also
   Antioxidants and Free Radicals (III)
   Anxiety/Pain (II)
   Chronic Fatigue Syndrome (II)
   Depression (II)
   Fatty Acids, Essential (III)
   Heart and Blood Vessel Conditions (II)
   Pain (II)
   Stress (II)
   Vitamin C (III)
   Vitamin E (III)

ASTHMA

Asthma is an allergic overreaction to airborne particulates, such as pollen and dust, in which a flood of antibodies can lead to lung inflammation, airway restriction, and a life-threatening shortness of breath. Most authorities recognize an emotional component of asthma and allergies, often associated with stress.

Adult-onset asthma has been linked to estrogen use. In an analysis of more than 23,000 postmenopausal women participating in the ongoing Nurses' Health Study (Trois, Speizer, et al., 1995), past or current users of hormone replacement therapy had a 60% higher risk of being afflicted with asthma than women who had never taken estrogen. The risk for women who had been on the hormone therapy for 10 years or more was double that of nonusers.

Breathing Exercises

Breathing exercises have been used, especially with children, to help individuals ward off asthma attacks. Fluge and colleagues (1994) examined the effects of breathing exercises and yoga on the course of bronchial asthma in 36 people with mild symptoms. Participants were randomly divided into 3 groups: 3 weeks of breathing training, 3 weeks of yoga training, and no additional treatment (control group). Both breathing and yoga created a significant amelioration of mental state, but only the breathing exercises induced a significant improvement in lung function parameters compared to the individual baseline values on the forced expiratory volume in 1 second (FEV1) test.

Chinese Medicine

In Chinese medicine, the lungs are associated with grief. It is notable that chest prob-lems often follow a loss, and that chest infections are apt to strike when individuals feel depressed, perhaps as a result of unhappiness at work or home. The breath is associated with qi (vital energy) and controls its flow. Respiratory conditions are viewed as damaging to the vital energy and as a sign of qi weakness and imbalance.

Dietary Approaches

In a complementary approach to asthma, the diet consists primarily of fresh fruits and vegetables, nuts and seeds, oatmeal, brown rice, and whole grains. Processed foods are avoided because they often contain allergy-producing preservatives such as BHA and BHT. Dairy products are avoided because they generate additional mucus.

Vitamin E may have a modest protective effect for asthma (Troisi, Willett, et al., 1995). In a study comparing wheeze, atrophy, and bronchial hyperreactivity in Asian and white children, researchers found that Indian children living in England whose diet consisted largely of foods from their native country were less likely to have symptoms of asthma and allergy than Indian youngsters who kept to a primarily Western diet. Indian diets tend to include more vegetables, less meat, and fewer additives and processed and packaged foods than the typical Western diet. Findings were similar for children following vegetarian and nonvegetarian diets. The study provides additional evidence that adoption of an affluent, Western, urban lifestyle may increase the risk of asthma and allergic disease (Carey, Locke, & Cookson, 1996).

According to the National Health and Nutrition (NHANES II) survey, the diets of many Americans are below the recommended daily allowances for zinc, calcium, magnesium, B vitamins, vitamin C, and other nutrients (Yong et al., 1997). People with asthma have an even greater need for good nutrition, especially if they are taking medications that may decrease the absorption of important nutrients from the body. Salt has been implicated as an asthma aggravator, at least in men. In one study (Carey, Locke, & Cookson, 1993), 22 men with mild to moderate asthma were placed on a low-sodium diet (80 mmol a day). Half received a tablet containing 200 mmol of sodium (the amount many Americans ingest daily), and the other half were given a placebo. After 5 weeks, the men receiving the extra sodium switched to the placebo and vice versa. Those on the low-sodium regime were found to use bronchodilators less often, were able to exhale more air, and had fewer symptoms, such as wheezing. Another study found that selenium supplementation increases glutathione peroxidase activity, thus improving cellular oxidative defense, which might counteract the inflammation and disordered respiration associated with asthma (Hasselmark et al., 1993).

Vitamin C

Preliminary results by E. Neil Schachter, M.D., of Yale University, provide evidence that vitamin C may help with exercise-induced asthma. Taken orally 1 1/2 hours before exercise, 500 mg of vitamin C reduced bronchospasm in 12 participants with exercise-induced asthma.

Imagery

Imagery exercises are used to picture the lungs and breathing apparatus working calmly and efficiently. A recent study (Halper, 1997) examined the use of guided imagery via a controlled, randomized study. Participants were recruited from the Lenox Hill Hospital, in New York City, by referral in response to a letter and by advertisements in community newspapers and stores. Inclusionary criteria were appropriate medical history, decreased FEV1, diminished mid-expiratory flow rate (MEFR), and bronchodilator reversibility. All participants were matched with respect to illness severity, medication use, and age, then randomly assigned to a mental imagery group or a control group. Sixty-eight participants were accepted in the study; 17 completed the experimental protocol, and 16 were in the control group. All participants received an asthma diary and peak flow meters with instructions on their use. Pulmonary function was assessed by spirometery every 4 weeks during this 16-week study. Data examined were drawn from pulmonary function tests, including FEV1 and the MEFR-forced vital capacity test; the Beck Depression Scale; the Spielberger Anxiety Scale; and the Asthma Quality of Life Scale. Also studied were asthma symptoms and medication use. The study found that significantly more participants in the mental imagery group than in the control group discontinued their use of medication. They also had lower Beck Depression scores and Spielberger Anxiety scales than those who remained on their medications. The researchers concluded that mental imagery had a major impact on medication use (Halper, 1997).

Music versus Breathing Exercises

In another study, 96 individuals suffering from bronchial asthma were given music or breathing exercises. Anxiety level and bronchial resistance were reported in the treatment group, but not in the control group, who used the traditional breathing kinesytherapy (Janiszewski, Kronenberger, & Drozd, 1996).

Relaxation Therapy

Relaxation therapy has been used, including desensitization procedures, to learn how to keep the body calm while in a stressful situation. Kohen and Wynne (1997) reported the use of relaxation, imagery, hypnosis, and storytelling in a preschool program for children and parents. Physician visits for asthma were significantly reduced, as were symptom severity scores.

Yoga

A common trigger for asthma is stress. Yoga can help relieve asthma suffering by teaching deep breathing and relaxation, two antidotes to stress. In one study (Jain & Talukdar, 1993), 46 people suffering from bronchial asthma were compared for exercise capacity, pulmonary function, and blood gases. Exercise capacity was measured by three tests: a 12-minute walk test; the physical fitness index, modified by the Harvard step test; and the Exercise-Liability Index. The yoga therapy program resulted in a significant increase in pulmonary function and exercise tolerance. A 1-year follow-up study showed a good to fair response with reduced symptoms scores and drug requirements in participants. The researchers concluded that yoga therapy was beneficial for bronchial asthma.

CAROLYN CHAMBERS CLARK

See
Acupuncture and Chinese Medicine (IV)

Interactive Guided Imagery (IV)
Music and Imagery in Healing (IV)
Vegetarianism (IV)
Yoga (IV)

See also
Allergies (II)
Calcium (III)
Depression (II)
Vitamin C (III)
Vitamin E (III)

ATTENTION DEFICIT HYPERACTIVE DISORDER

Approximately 3% to 10% of school-age children in the United States are diagnosed with attention deficit hyperactive disorder (ADHD). The primary treatment is the use of stimulant drugs. Twenty-five percent of these children do not respond to this therapy, however, some complementary therapies show promise.

Acupuncture

Sonenklar (1997) investigated the efficacy of using single-point acupuncture (ear) treatment for children with ADHD. Seven children completed the study; 3 showed improvement during the treatment phase; 1 showed improvement during the placebo phase; 2 showed worsening throughout. The researcher suggested that acupuncture, a simple procedure with minimal risk, might be effective for some children.

Food and Supplements

In a double-blind, placebo-controlled food challenge with 16 children, Boris and Mandel (1994) demonstrated a significant improvement on placebo days compared to open challenge days, when children reacted to many foods, dyes, and/or preservatives. The study demonstrated the beneficial effect of eliminating reactive foods and artificial colors in children with ADHD. The researchers concluded that dietary factors may play a significant role in the cause of ADHD.

Carter and colleagues (1993) studied 78 children referred to a diet clinic because of hyperactive behavior. Participants were all placed on a few foods elimination diet. Fifty-nine improved their behavior during this open trial. For 19 of the participants, it was possible to disguise foods or additives by mixing them with other tolerated foods and testing their effect in a double-blind, placebo-controlled challenge. The results of the challenge showed a significant effect for the provoking foods to worsen behavior ratings and impair psychological test performance.

In a 21-day double-blind, placebo-controlled, repeated-measures study of 200 children, Rowe and Rowe (1994) showed that behavioral changes in irritability, restlessness, and sleep disturbance were associated with the intake of tartrazine, a synthetic food coloring, in 24 children.

Lifestyle Factors

A study by Milberger and colleagues (1996) investigated the role of maternal smoking during pregnancy in the etiology ADHD in 140 boys ages 6 to 17 and a normal comparison group ($n = 120$). Twenty-two percent of the ADHD children had a maternal history of smoking during pregnancy, compared with 8% of the non-ADHD children. This positive association remained significant after adjustment for socioeconomic status, parental IQ, and parental ADHD status. Significant differences in IQ were found between those children whose mothers smoked during pregnancy and those whose mothers did not smoke.

Symmetric Tonic Neck Reflex Exercises

Dr. Miriam L. Bender and her students' research (1971, 1973; O'Dell, 1973) and clinical writings (O'Dell & Cook, 1997) indicated that many children experience behavioral and academic difficulties, including ADHD, due to an immature symmetric tonic neck reflex (STNR).

During normal growth and development, the STNR governs head position until 2 years of age. Retention of this reflex past that age is abnormal and can lead to muscular tension in the child's arms and legs in relation to head movements. Involuntary movements occur that interfere with the child's gaining control of the body. When this happens, the body controls the child.

Children with immature STNR can be diagnosed as hyperactive or as having attention deficit disorder because they have difficulty sitting still, may get up and sit down to relieve the tension caused by the reflex, or may have poor penmanship because they cannot hold a pen or pencil comfortably. Copying from the board to their paper may be especially difficult and inefficient because of the positional changes effected by the reflex in their arms and neck.

Any of the following difficulties may be due to immature STNR: sitting "inappropriately," squirming, daydreaming, writing poorly, writing laboriously, moving awkwardly or clumsily, reversing letters or numbers, avoiding athletics, or developing poor athletic skills.

If for any reason a baby does not crawl long enough or in the proper manner, the STNR will continue, keeping the top half of the body straight when the bottom half bends and vice versa. Bender and her students have developed exercises that can be used with anyone over the age of 5 (O'Dell & Cook, 1997).

CAROLYN CHAMBERS CLARK

See
Diet and Mood (IV)

BACK PAIN

In the United States alone, it is estimated that $24 billion is spent annually on the treatment of back pain. A large percentage is spent on surgery, such as fusion of the lower (lumbar) spine, which is frequently unsuccessful. Magnetic resonance imaging (MRI) can reveal what looks like a trouble spot in the lumbar spine, but abnormal-looking disks are almost as likely to show up in people with no back pain as with those in pain, and some people with severe back pain have normal-looking MRIs. This suggests that other factors are involved in lower back pain.

Surgery benefits only about 1 in 100 people with acute lower back problems and may only be appropriate when there is severe, disabling, and persistent sciatica. Lifestyle changes and exercise are still the most effective means to treat back pain. The following treatments are *not* supported by scientific evidence: extended bed rest (more than 4 days); use of oral steroids, colchicine, antidepressants, and phenylbutazones (potential side effects range from gastrointestinal irritation to bone marrow suppression); and injections of local anesthetics, corticosteroids, or other substances into the back (can have serious side effects, such as nerve damage and hemorrhage). Other treatments for which the federal Agency for Health Care Policy and Research (1994) could find no evidence of effectiveness include heat/diathermy, massage, ultrasound, spinal traction, transcutaneous electrical nerve stimulation, acupuncture, lumbar corsets (except when used preventively for persons who do frequent lifting), support belts, back machines, and cutaneous laser treatment and other forms of electrical stimulation.

There is relatively weak agreement between the results of physical examination and the subjective reporting of pain and disability (Michel, Kohlmann, & Raspe, 1997). With chronic pain, more psychosocial, demographic, and occupational aspects come into play (Valat, Goupile, & Vedere, 1997).

Chiropractic/Spinal Manipulation

Some studies have shown short-term benefits of chiropractic care for acute low back pain, and the Agency for Health Care Policy and Research (1994) suggests it can be helpful in relieving pain, especially within the first 4 weeks of injury.

Ergonomics

Ergonomics involves the design and arrangement of things people use to maximize safety and efficiency, particularly in the workplace. Back pain can result if the environment is not ergonomically sound (Scheer & Mital, 1997).

A study of 1,216 nurses in hospitals in Belgium and the Netherlands found that ergonomic interventions alone were not sufficient to control musculoskeletal problems. Lifetime prevalence rates for musculoskeletal problems and low back pain were significantly lower in the Dutch hospitals (where heavy workload was prevalent in a higher proportion of nurses) than in the Belgian hospitals. The Dutch nurses were significantly less depressed and more positive about pain, work, and activity (Burton et al., 1997).

Exercise

A majority of people seeking advice for back problems have a weak back due to sedentary lifestyle and poor body mechanics. Strengthening the leg muscles as well as including regular sit-ups and arm/leg raises from a lying, face-down position can strengthen back muscles.

Harreby, Hesselsoe, Kjer, and Neergaard (1997) studied a cohort of 38-year-old men and women for leisure time physical exercise in relation to low back pain. Those who were physically active for at least 3 hours per week reported a reduced risk of lower back pain. Gymnastics and swimming reduced lower back pain significantly.

Bentsen, Lindgarde, and Manthorpe (1997) reported a prospective, randomized investigation of two back pain programs for 57-year-old women. Seventy-four women participated in the study. Both training groups (a dynamic supervised strength muscle training program and a home training program) showed significant improvement at the 3- and 12-month follow-ups. There was a significant reduction in the number of women on sick leave and in use of health care services after 1 year, but not after 3 years. The home training program was as effective as the supervised. The adherence rate was better when the training was supervised.

Ljunggren, Weber, Kogstad, Thom, and Kirkesola (1997) used an open, randomized, multicenter parallel-group study with an observation period of 12 months. Four Norwegian physiotherapy institutes took part. After ordinary physiotherapy treatment for low back problems, participants were randomly allocated either to a conventional training program designed by physiotherapists or to a training program using a new training apparatus called the TerapiMaster. Both exercise programs reduced work absenteeism significantly. No differences in the effects of the two programs were discernible. Regular follow-up and variation in the training programs were important in motivating individuals to adhere to regular exercise programs.

Ferrell, Josephson, Pollan, Loy, and Ferrell (1997) conducted a pilot study to evaluate a practical exercise program for elderly people with chronic musculoskeletal pain. Thirty-three participants were randomly assigned to one of the groups: a 6-week supervised program of walking; a pain education program, which included the demonstration of the use of heat and cold, massage, relaxation, and distraction; or usual care. Pain, self-reported health, and functional status were evaluated at baseline and at 2 and 8 weeks (end of study). Attendance was 100% for the education sessions and 93% for walking sessions. Both intervention groups demonstrated significant improvements in pain and functional status. The researchers concluded that both education and walking can improve pain management.

Lifestyle Interventions

Inactivity can weaken needed muscles. Nine out of ten people with acute back pain who resume normal activity after a brief rest period of a day or two can expect to recover on their own within a month. Practitioners who use the following protocol are usually the most successful: (1) Tell the client that his or her low back pain is amenable to self-care, that it usually goes away in a reasonable time, and that it is manageable; (2) teach the client specific ways to deal with his or her own back problems through exercise and lifestyle changes, and (3) prescribe drugs less frequently or not at all.

Women who are overweight or with a large waist have a significantly increased likelihood of low back pain (Han, Schouter, Lean, & Seidell, 1997). Therefore, losing weight can be a significant intervention for lower back pain in overweight women.

High-heeled shoes (3 inches or higher) increase pressure on the balls of the feet by 76% and can lead to lower back pain (American Academy of Orthopaedic Surgeons, 1995). Women who wear high heels should consider wearing flat shoes or shoes with heels lower than 3 inches.

Tobacco use and other behavioral factors are associated with chronic back pain. McPartland and Mitchell (1997) found that people with chronic back pain consumed over twice as much caffeine as those without such pain, although there were possible confounding variables that were not explained by their research.

Psychosocial Aspects of Pain

Papageorgiou and colleagues (1997) found that people dissatisfied with work were more likely to report low back pain, for which they did not consult a physician.

Bendix, Bendix, Lund, Kirkbak, and Ostenfeld (1997) tested the theory that a multifaceted pain management program was more economical and beneficial than a less intensive program. Using a randomized, blinded study, they compared an (1) intensive 3-week multidisciplinary program, (2) an active physical training and back school, and (3) a psychological pain management program with active physical training. There was no significant difference between programs 2 and 3 in most parameters except for sick leave and leg pain.

Trigger Point Therapy

The efficacy of trigger point injection therapy in the treatment of lower back strain was evaluated in a prospective, randomized, double-blind study. Sixty-three individuals with a diagnosis of nonradiating lower back pain participated. They were treated conservatively for 4 weeks before entering the study. Injection therapy was of four different types: lidocaine, lidocaine combined with a steroid, acupuncture, and vapocoolant spray with acupressure. Results indicated that therapy without injected medication (63% improvement rate) was at least as effective as therapy with drug injection (42% improvement rate). The researchers concluded that trigger point therapy is a useful treatment for lower back strain. The injected substance apparently is not the critical factor. Direct mechanical stimulus to the trigger point gave equal or better symptomatic relief to the injected medication.

Kovacs and colleagues (1997) also examined the use of trigger point therapy for treating chronic lower back pain. They used a randomized, double-blind, controlled, multicenter trial. Thirty-seven participants were assigned to a control group and received a sham trigger point therapy;

41 participants were assigned to the treatment group and received a real trigger point treatment. Those in the treatment group showed immediate and significant lessening of pain compared to the control group.

CAROLYN CHAMBERS CLARK

See also
Pain (II)
Pregnancy (II)
Repetitive Strain Injuries (II)

BALANCE DISORDERS

Balance is a term used to describe the ability to maintain or move within a weight-bearing posture without falling. It has three aspects: steadiness, symmetry, and dynamic stability. Steadiness refers to the ability to maintain a given posture without swaying. Symmetry is the equal weight distribution between the weight-bearing components, either the feet in a standing position or the buttocks in a seated position. Dynamic stability is the ability to move without falling.

There is a substantial population of people with balance disorders who are at risk for injury from falls. Traditional physical therapy may not prove effective, but biofeedback and *t'ai chi* may.

Biofeedback

Recent advances in technology have resulted in the availability of force platform systems for retraining the balance function, especially for people who have suffered strokes. These systems provide visual or auditory biofeedback about the center of force or center of pressure, as well as training protocols that enhance stance symmetry, steadiness, and dynamic stability (Nichols, 1997).

T'ai Chi

A study by Wolf, Barnhart, Ellison, and Coogler (1997) explored whether two exercise programs affected the ability to minimize postural sway for 72 relatively inactive, older participants. All were evaluated under four postural conditions, then randomly assigned to one of the following 15-week interventions: (1) a computerized balance training group ($n = 24$), (2) a *t'ai chi* group ($n = 24$), or (3) an educational group serving as a control for exercise ($n = 24$). All participants were evaluated on the four postural conditions immediately after the program and 4 months later. Platform balance measures showed greater stability after training in the balance training group but not in the other two groups. Participants in the *t'ai chi* group were less afraid of falling after training compared with the other two groups. The major benefit of *t'ai chi* is that it promotes confidence without reducing sway, rather than primarily focusing on a reduction in sway-based measures.

Jacobson, Chen, Cashel, and Guerrero (1997) assessed the effect of *t'ai chi* training on lateral stability, kinesthetic sense, and strength of voluntary knee extension with 12 naive volunteer men and 12 naive volunteer women, age 20 to 45 years. Pre- and 12-week posttests examined lateral body stability, kinesthetic sense in the glenohumeral joint (for 30, 45, and 60 degrees), and strength of knee extension. One half of the participants performed *t'ai chi* three times per week for 12 weeks, while a control group continued with their usual activities. An analysis of variance showed significant group differences in lateral body stability, kinesthetic sense at 60 degrees (but not at 30 and 45 degrees, angles used less frequently in *t'ai chi* training, according to film analysis). The researchers concluded that *t'ai chi* provided a low-stress method to enhance stability, selected kinesthetic sense, and knee extension strength.

Hain (1995) examined the effect of *t'ai chi* on the balance of persons with balance disorders by comparing functional tests of balance and self-reports of balance and falls prior to and following 8 weeks of daily *t'ai chi* practice. Another evaluation was performed 3 months after the beginning of exercise sessions. Measures used included the Romberg, Duncan Reach test, Moving platform Posturography, Duke Mobility Skill inventory (MOS), Jacobson dizziness disability inventory (DHI), Mini-Mental status questionnaire, and Falls self-report. Highly significant improvements in posturography (average score changed from 59.5 to 64.3), the tandem Romberg, and Mos and DHI tests were found. The Duncan Reach test scores were not significantly changed, but improvement on the other measures was found in all age groups. The researcher concluded that *t'ai chi* can provide significant improvement in balance.

CAROLYN CHAMBERS CLARK

See
T'ai Chi (IV)

See also
Aging (II)

BLADDER PROBLEMS

Almost 40 million American women develop cystitis each year, the second most common condition (after the common cold). Men and children can develop cystitis, but an overwhelming number of sufferers are women. The two main types of cystitis are bacterial and interstitial. Symptoms can be triggered by environmental and food allergies and by general infections in the body. Available complementary research exists for cranberry juice, reflexology, and some lifestyle behaviors.

Cranberry Juice

Cranberry juice is a simple, nonpharmacologic means to reduce or treat urinary tract infections. A study by Fleet (1994) indicated that bacterial infections (bacteriuria) and associated influx of white blood cells into the urine (pyuria) can be reduced by nearly 50% in elderly women who drank 300 ml of cranberry juice cocktail each day over the course of 6 months. Avorn and colleagues (1994) replicated these findings with a sample of 153 elderly women volunteers. The researchers assigned the women to drink 10 oz of cranberry juice or an identical-tasting red placebo beverage. Those on cranberry juice were about 4 times more likely than the placebo group to have white blood cells and bacteria cleared from their urine. The researchers explained that cranberry juice may contain an as-yet unidentified substance that keeps bacteria from attaching to the lining of the bladder.

Lifestyle Interventions

Foxman, Geiger, Palin, Gillespie, and Koopman (1995) studied the relation between sexual and health behaviors of women and first-time urinary tract infection (UTI). The population included unmarried women using a university health service who had no history of UTI and who had engaged in sexual activity at least once. Having a sex partner for less than 1 year versus 1 year or more was associated with about twice the risk of UTI. Drinking carbonated soft drinks and using deodorant sanitary napkins or tampons was also associated with increased risk. Lifestyle interventions include not wearing pantyhose or tight jeans, drinking 8 to 10 glasses of water a day, and avoiding foods that may trigger infection or irritation (citrus fruits and juices; red wine; aged proteins such as yogurt, pickled herring, cheese; aspartame; bananas; avocados; and foods containing tyrosine and phenylalanine).

Reflexology

Kesselring (1994) reported a small pilot study using reflexology postoperatively on gynecological patients. The intervention group showed a lesser need for medication to enhance bladder tonus than did the control group. The literature describes foot reflexology as enhancing urination.

CAROLYN CHAMBERS CLARK

BURNS

Oxidative stress may contribute to secondary tissue damage and impaired immune function after burn injury. Rock and associates (1997) examined the plasma antioxidant micronutrients in 26 adults admitted with extensive burn injuries. They also administered beta-carotene in a prospective randomized design in which people with burns received either a placebo or 30 mg/day of beta-carotene in an enteral feeding. They found vitamin C tocopherol and retinol concentrations were low at baseline but increased significantly over the 21-day study period in both groups. Plasma beta-carotene concentration increased only when this carotenoid was provided in the oral feeding.

Chai and colleagues (1995) examined the protective function of vitamin E. Half of the 22 participants with severe burns were given vitamin E; the control group did not receive vitamin E. The results showed a significant elevation and impairment of neutrophil phagocytic (immune) function in the control group, as opposed to healthy normals and the group who received vitamin E. The results suggested that, for severely burned people, the free radical scavenger and antioxidant vitamin E could protect the neurophil function.

Simon and colleagues (1994) reported the use of vitamin E for skin burns with animals. Laser radiation on the skin of Yorkshire pigs was treated with topical or intramuscular vitamin E. Healing time was significantly decreased for wounds that were pretreated with vitamin E.

Haberal and colleagues (1988) reported both animal and human studies using vitamin E to show its positive effect on immune regulation. In the animal study, vitamin E was given intramuscularly to the treatment group. In the groups that received vitamin E, the spleen weight and complement fixation test increased significantly while the acid phosphatase in serum decreased. In the clinical study, 17 people who had been burned over 20% were compared with eight healthy persons. Half of the people who had been burned received vitamin E on 3 consecutive days. On the fourth day, blood was taken. An analysis showed that the number of T cells decreased significantly in the controls, but increased significantly in the participants who had received vitamin E. The researchers concluded that vitamin E stimulated both cellular and humoral immunity, and they recommended it for all burn victims.

Bekyarova, Yankova, and Galunska (1996) evaluated the effect of a topical application of vitamin E and FC-43 perfluorocarbon emulsion, alone and in combination. The best results were from combining the two. Immediately after thermal skin injury, the emulsion was applied. By the third hour after injury, there were increases in plasma antioxidant capacity, decreases in free radical mediated damage of erythrocytes, and suppression of their aggregation.

In another animal study, LaLonde, Nayak, Hennigan, and Demling (1997) studied the effect of an oral administration of a water-soluble antioxidant solution containing ascorbic acid, glutathione, and a precursor for glutathione synthesis, N-Acetyl-L-cysteine, on liver antioxidant activity, liver cell energetics, and mortality in rats in response to a 20% third-degree burn injury. They found that the oral administration of the antioxidants prevented death. They concluded that a 20% burn produced a modest decrease in liver energy charge potential and antioxidant defense without producing death. Antioxidants given after burns restored antioxidant defenses, attenuated the altered cell energetics, and prevented death, indicating oxidants were the cause of death.

Zhang and colleagues (1992) studied the contents of serum lipid peroxides and vitamin E in 35 severely burned people. Eighteen individuals were given vitamin E. A comparative survey showed that the serum vitamin E decreased significantly from days 6 to 8 postburn in both groups of burned people, while serum lipid peroxides increased significantly, reaching a peak. In the control group, serum vitamin E levels were lower and lipid peroxides higher than those of a comparison group of 113 healthy people from days 20 to 22 postburn. At that time, serum vitamin E levels increased and lipid peroxides decreased to the level of the health comparison group in the participants who had received vitamin E. The researchers suggested that supplementation with vitamin E for people with burns is necessary.

Gao (1991) observed the influence of various doses of vitamin A on the serum and liver levels of vitamin A, and the effect of prevention and treatment on the injured spleen, liver, thymus, and small intestine mucosa. The researcher studied third-degree burns in rats. In the control group that had suffered burns, the spleen was swollen and the hepatocytes were decreased significantly. The small intestine villi were atrophic and the muscosa thinned. In order to obtain prevention and adequate treatment of postburn lesions, the investigator had to use a dose 4 times the normal requirement.

CAROLYN CHAMBERS CLARK

See also
Vitamin A (III)
Vitamin C (III)
Vitamin E (III)

CANCER

Cancer mortality in the United States has been relatively stable over the past 25 years. Some cancers, such as lung and prostate, have experienced increased mortality; others, such as colorectal, have shown a decline. One-third of all cancer deaths are related to tobacco and one-third to diet. The data show modest improvement in the eating habits of adults over the past decade in dietary fat intake (Healthy People Progress Report, 1994), but white women, especially, are eating fewer dark green leafy vegetables (Nebeling et al., 1997).

Of great concern is the increase in childhood cancer. A 2-day conference sponsored by the U.S. Environmental Protection Agency (EPA) (Allen, 1997) attempted to develop a national strategy to combat childhood cancer. The EPA has started an Office of Children's Health Protections to coordinate work on setting health and safety standards to protect children, who face higher exposures to pesticides and other environmental toxins through diet and play.

Two processes may have a role in limiting tumor growth: necrosis and apoptosis. Necrosis occurs due to an adverse environment. Apoptosis is believed to be programmed at birth and later triggered when cell death benefits the host. Cancer may occur due to a failed effort of apoptosis to remove cells with damaged DNA (Schwartzman & Cidlowski, 1993).

Cancer risk may be increased by some chemicals (e.g., phenophthalein, an ingredient found in a common laxative, and chlorinated drinking water), chlorine, alcohol consumption (raises levels of estrogen, a physiologic variable most closely linked to breast cancer), and exposure to electromagnetic fields (Fackelmann, 1992; Guenel et al., 1993; Lindbohm et al., 1992; Loomis & Savitz, 1995; Loomis et al., 1994; Swanson et al., 1997).

Behavioral Interventions

Gruber and others (1993) examined the effect of relaxation, guided imagery, and biofeedback training on 13 lymph node negative individuals who had recovered from a modified radical mastectomy. The women were randomly assigned to either immediate or delayed treatment. Significant effects were found in natural killer cell (NK) activity, mixed lymphocyte responsiveness, and the number of peripheral blood lymphocytes. These results provided additional evidence to those of an earlier pilot study from the researchers' center that behavioral interventions correlate with immune system measures.

Chalmers, Thomson, and Degner (1996) found that information, support, and communication were important for the adaptation to the risk of breast cancer for women. Despite their importance, the 55 women studied had difficulty meeting these needs. Communication patterns within the family and with health professionals were generally not helpful.

Haase (1997) found that teenagers diagnosed with cancer and other chronic illnesses coped most successfully when they were optimistic, hopeful, and had a spiritual perspective. Family protective factors included family support and resources. Social protective factors included the nature and availability of health resources and connectedness with peers and others with the same or a similar condition.

Chinese Medicine

According to traditional Chinese medicine, cancer can develop from any of the three primary causes of disease and one of four broad categories of patterns can be diagnosed: phlegm, toxins, qi and blood, vacuity and qi, and blood stagnation (Boik, 1996).

Zee-Cheng (1992) screened and evaluated 15 compounds to restore immunity in people diagnosed with cancer, potentiate the therapeutic effect, and ameliorate adverse toxicity of anticancer agents. *Shi-quan-da-bu-tang* was selected as the most effective biological response modifier. It contains 10 significant herbs, including *Rehmannia glutinosa*, *Paeonia lactiflora*, *Liquisticum*, *wallichii*, *Angelica sinesis*, *Glycyrrhiza uralensis*, *Poria cocos*, *Atractylodes macrocephala*, and *Panax ginseng*. Eight years of studies provided evidence of its (1) extremely low toxicity; (2) immunomodulatory, immunopotentiating, and chemotherapy-potentiating effects; (3) inhibitory effect on malignancy; (4) ability to prolong survival; and (5) ability to ameliorate and/or prevent anorexia, nausea, vomiting, hematotoxicty, immunosuppression, leukopenia, anemia, and liver damage of many anticancer drugs. The author explained the therapeutic action tones the blood and strengthens Qi.

Environmental Risks

Bra Use

A 1990 study by Ashizawa, Sugane, and Gunji (1990) showed that breasts swelled under the influence of wearing a bra. Singer and Grismaijer (1995) put forth the novel hypothesis that this edema may be do to the buildup of lymph in constricted tissue. They used a questionnaire to interview women in five major cities in the United States. Four hundred women in each city who had been diagnosed with breast cancer were interviewed. In each city 500 women without breast cancer were also interviewed. In this study of 2,674 women, the researchers found that women who do not wear bras had a 20-fold lower incidence of breast cancer than did women who wore bras. They noted that this finding has about the same statistical significance as a comparison of the health risk of non-smokers with smokers. Conversely, women who slept with bras or breast-supporting garments were 6 times more likely to be diagnosed with breast cancer. Ninety-nine percent of the women who developed breast cancer wore bras more than 12 hours a day. The researchers' theory was that bras constricted breast tissue, restraining the normal lymphatic drainage that cleans the breasts of toxins and repairs damage. Over the years, this chronic constriction of breast tissue takes its toll. Overburdened, the immune system is worn down, and this may serve as a trigger for some breast cells to become malignant.

Method of Food Preparation

Yo (1997) reported a case-control study of cooking methods associated with increased or decreased risk of stomach cancer. For meat or fish, pan frying was associated with decreased risk, while stewing or broiling was associated with increased risk.

Perineal Powdering

Chang and Risch (1997) pointed out the dangers of using powder on the genitals. Clinical and epidemiologic studies have already indicated an association between ovarian carcinoma and talcum powder use. Talc particles have been detected in histologic sections of ovarian carcinomas. Inert particles travel from the perineum to the ovaries. Chang and Risch identified 450 respondents with borderline and invasive ovarian carcinoma and 564 population controls in metropolitan Toronto. Participants were interviewed about their reproductive and menstrual histories and their use of dusting powders. Exposure to talc, via sanitary napkins, direct application to the perineum, or both, was significantly associated with risk of ovarian carcinoma.

Radiation

No single factor probably "causes" cancer. Radiation, even in small exposures, may be one link in the chain of events leading to cancer (Trosko, 1996). Some sources of radiation mentioned in the literature include sunlight, large power lines, unnecessary dental and medical x-rays, faulty wiring, electric blankets, waterbed heaters, electric clocks, and baby monitors placed too close to nightstands or baby cribs, electric shavers, daily use of hair dryers/curlers or curling irons, beds placed too close to major appliances, and TV screens too close to viewers. In the workplace, sources of radiation listed include electrical heating units or other field generators, printers, facsimile machines and copiers, computer monitors, and fluorescent lights (Barnes, 1995; Darius & Leverett, 1995). Milham (1996) found that cumulative magnetic field exposure may explain cancer incidence in a cohort of 410 office workers exposed to strong magnetic fields by three 12 kV transformers located beneath their first-floor office.

Dolk and colleagues (1997) found a significant decline in risk for adult leukemia with distance from radio and television transmitters in Great Britain. A significant decline in risk with distance was also found for skin and bladder cancer.

Sakagami and colleagues (1997) found that vitamin E protected the cell membranes from UV irradiation. However, the protective effect only occurs when the vitamin E is available to cells prior to irradiation.

Tobacco Use and Lung-Colorectal Cancers

Although tobacco is well known as a cause of lung cancer, Potter (1996) found that tobacco smoking was also a clear and consistent risk factor for colorectal cancer.

Exercise

Potter (1996) found that physical activity had the most consistent inverse (protective activity) association with colorectal cancer. Martinez and colleagues (1997) found a significant inverse association between leisure-time physical activity and incidence of colon cancer in women, consistent with what has been found in men. The researchers recommended increased physical activity and maintenance of lean body weight as part of a feasible approach to the prevention of colon cancer. Exercise can affect estrogen production and menstrual cycle patterns, thereby reducing the risk for breast cancer. Bernstein and colleagues (1994) showed that women who exercised an average of 3.8 hours per week had an odds ratio of breast cancer of 0.28 for women who had full-term pregnancies and 0.73 for those who did not. The results provide evidence that regular physical exercise is a critical component in breast cancer prevention. Rosengren and Wilhelmsen

(1997) found similar results for men. They found that leisure-time physical activity has a protective effect against cancer death.

Thune, Brenn, and Lund (1997) found that the risk of breast cancer was reduced by 72% in lean, regular-exercising pre-menopausal women. Exercise may also be beneficial in reducing symptoms caused by radiation treatment in women diagnosed with breast cancer. Using an experimental, two-group pretest, posttest design, Mock and associates (1997) tested the hypothesis that women participating in a walking exercise program during radiation therapy treatment for breast cancer would show lower symptom intensity and higher levels of physical functioning than women who did not participate. Forty-six women beginning a 6-week program of radiation therapy for early-stage breast cancer comprised the sample. The exercise group scored significantly higher than the usual care group on physical functioning ($p = 0.003$) and symptom intensity, particularly in terms of fatigue, anxiety, and difficulty sleeping.

Fiber Protects

Le Marchand and colleagues (1997) conducted a population-based case-control study among different ethnic groups in Hawaii using personal interviews with 698 males and 494 females diagnosed during 1987–1991 with adenocarcinoma of the colon or rectum as compared to 1,192 population controls matched by age, sex, and ethnicity. They found a protective association in both sexes with fiber intake from vegetable sources (but not from fruits, except bananas, and cereals). Intakes of carotenoids, light green and yellow-orange vegetables, broccoli, corn, carrots, garlic, and legumes (including soy products) reduced risk, even after adjustment for vegetable fiber. The data supported a protective role of fiber from vegetables against colorectal cancer independent of its water solubility property and the effects of other phytochemicals.

Food and Supplements

Animal Fat

Giovannuci and colleagues (1993) found dietary fat to be a risk factor for prostate cancer. Red meat represented the food group with the strongest positive association with advanced cancer. Fat from dairy products, with the exception of butter, and fish were unrelated to risk. High intake of foods from animal sources (meat, eggs, cheese) was slightly, but not statistically, related to elevated risk for endometrial cancer. The only significant dose-response relation observed was for processed fish and meat (Zheng et al., 1995b).

Risch and associates (1994) found that eating 10 g per day of saturated fat may raise a woman's risk of ovarian cancer by 20%. They compared the eating habits of 450 women age 35 to 79 years with newly diagnosed ovarian cancer to those of 540 demographically similar healthy women in Ontario, Canada. Participants were surveyed about their number of pregnancies, history of oral contraceptive use, and diet. For every 10 g of saturated fat consumed daily, the risk of ovarian cancer rose 20%. Women who lowered their saturated fat consumption by 10 g per day experienced a 20% drop in risk. Nonsaturated fat had no effect on ovarian cancer risk. Women who added 10 g of vegetable fiber to their diet lowered their risk of ovarian cancer by 37%. Full-term pregnancy lowered risk by 20%, and each year of oral contraceptive use lowered it another 5% to 10%.

Potter (1996) found that meat consumption was associated with increased risk for colorectal cancer but was not fully explained by its fat content. Yo (1997) reported a case-control study finding an increased risk of stomach cancer for people who frequently consumed broiled meats and fish.

Peters and others (1994) found a persistent significant association for childhood leukemia and children's intake of hot dogs and fathers' intake of hot dogs with no evidence that fruit intake provided protection. Their results are consistent with experimental animal research and the hypothesis that human N-nitrosos compound intake is associated with leukemia risk.

Citrus Pectin/Citrus Oils

Prostate cancer is the most prevalent type of cancer diagnosed in men in the United States and remains incurable once it metastasizes to other parts of the body. Many stages of the metastatic cascade involve cellular interactions mediated by cell surface components, such as carbohydrate-binding proteins, including galectins and galactoside-binding lectins. One soluble component of plant fiber derived from the white portion of citrus fruit, modified citrus pectin, has been shown to interfere with cell-cell interactions mediated by cell surface carbohydrate-binding galectin-3 molecules. Pienta and colleagues (1995) examined the ability of citrus pectin to inhibit spontaneous metastasis of prostate cancer cells in rats. Compared with 16 control rats that had lung metastases on day 30 of the study, 7 of 14 rats in the 0.1% and 9 of

16 rats in the 1.0% modified citrus pectin group had statistically significant reductions in lung metastases. Studies showing the ability of modified citrus pectin to inhibit human prostate metastasis are needed. Citrus fruit oils and d-limonene, the major constituent of citrus fruit oils, have cancer inhibitory effects (Ren & Lien, 1997).

Coenzyme Q10

CoQ10 is necessary for normal human physiology. A deficiency can lead to ill health and disease. Low blood levels of CoQ10 have been found in American and Swedish women diagnosed with breast cancer, and clinical success with small populations has been reported (Ren & Lien, 1997).

DHEA and Cancer Prevention

DHEA and its sulfate ester (DHEAS) are major secretions of the human adrenal gland. Epidemiologic studies have shown subnormal plasma levels of DHEA and DHEAS in people with breast cancer, as compared to controls; additionally, DHEA has been shown in animal studies to be broadly cancer chemopreventive. There are significant adverse effects that can be overcome through the use of synthetic analogs of DHEA (Ren & Lien, 1997).

Essential Oils of Vegetables

Celery seed oil, parsley leaf oil, dillweed oil, and caraway oil are essential oils present in *Umbelliferae* plants. All have shown promise in cancer chemoprevention (Ren & Lien, 1997).

Olive Oil

Increased olive oil consumption (more than once a day vs. once a day) was associated with significantly reduced breast cancer risk, whereas margarine consumption was associated with a significant risk increase, in a large study of Greek women (Trichopoulou et al., 1995). This study duplicates findings of the protective effect of olive oil in a study of American women (Martin-Moreno et al., 1994).

Protective Plant Foods and Supplements

Knekt and colleagues (1997) studied the relation between the intake of antioxidant flavonoids and subsequent risk of cancer among 9,959 Finnish men and women age 15 to 99 and initially cancer free. Food consumption was estimated by the dietary history method. During a 25-year follow-up there was an inverse association between intake of flavonoids and incidence of all sites of cancer combined. The association between flavonoid intake and lung cancer incidence was not due to the intake of antioxidant vitamins or other potentially confounding factors because adjustment for factors such as smoking, energy intakes, vitamin E, vitamin C, and beta-carotene did not significantly alter results. The association between flavonoids and protection from lung cancer was strongest in persons under 50 years of age and in nonsmokers. The consumption of apples showed an inverse association with lung cancer incidence. These results support the hypothesis that flavonoid intake may be involved in the cancer process, resulting in lowered risks.

Slattery and associates (1997) used a population-based case-control study with 1,993 people in Northern California, Utah, Minneapolis, and St. Paul and 2,410 controls. Higher intakes of vegetables were associated inversely with cancer risk, as was dietary fiber. Other nutrients plant foods contributed that were associated with lower risk were vitamin B6, thiamin, and niacin (women only).

Pool-Zobel and colleagues (1997) completed a human intervention study with vegetable products with 23 healthy, non smoking males, age 27 to 40. Participants consumed their normal diets but abstained from vegetables high in carotenoids throughout the study period. After a 2-week depletion period, they received 330 ml of tomato juice daily with 40 mg of lycopene (weeks 3 and 4), 330 ml of carrot juice with 22.3 mg of beta-carotene and 15.7 mg of alpha-carotene (weeks 5 and 6), and 10 g of dried spinach powder (in water or milk) with 11.3 mg of lutein (weeks 7 and 8). Blood was collected and DNA damage was detected. Supplementation with tomato, carrot, or spinach products resulted in a significant decrease in endogenous levels of strand breaks in lymphocyte DNA. Oxidative base damage was significantly reduced during the carrot juice intervention. Their findings support the hypothesis that carotenoid-containing plant products are cancer-protective by decreasing oxidative and other damage to DNA.

Although the evidence to date is primarily in vitro and in vivo only in rats, broccoli has shown inhibitory effects on mammary tumor formation in females. Isolation studies from broccoli show sulforaphane is the principal component that blocks tumor cell formation (Ren & Lien, 1997).

Epidemiologic evidence indicates that diets high in fruits and vegetables are associated with a reduced risk of several cancers, including cancers of the stomach and esophagus. One explanation is that vegetables, especially green ones, contain chlorophyll, a green plant pigment, which limits carcinogen bioavailability by interfering with cytocohrome P450–mediated activation of chemical carcinogens.

Dashwood and Guo (1995) conducted a number of studies providing evidence that chlorophylls operate as interceptor molecules. This may be the process that limits bioavailability.

Blot and colleagues (1993) sought to discover whether dietary supplementation could lower mortality from incidence of cancer and other conditions. Individuals age 40 to 69 were recruited from four Linxian communes, an area with one of the world's highest rates of esophageal/gastric cardia cancer and low intakes of several micronutrients. The study randomly assigned 29,584 adults to intervention groups: retinol and zinc; riboflavin and niacin; vitamin C and molybdenum; and beta carotene, vitamin E, and selenium in doses 1 to 2 times the U.S. recommended daily allowance. Lower mortality, especially due to lower stomach cancer rates, occurred among those receiving supplementation with beta-carotene, vitamin E, and selenium.

Using data from the Iowa Women's Health Study, Zheng and colleagues (1995a) reported on the association of retinol and antioxidant vitamins (carotene and vitamins C and E) and cancers of the upper digestive tract. After adjusting for age, smoking, and total energy intake, intakes of carotene and vitamins C and E were related to lower risks of both gastric and oral/pharyngeal/esophageal cancers. Retinol was associated with a lower risk of gastric cancer only. This study provided evidence that high intake of antioxidant vitamins may be important in preventing cancers of the upper digestive tract. Zheng

and associates (1995b) assessed the relationship between eating plant and animal foods and cancer. Stratified analyses of a mailed questionnaire to 23,000 postmenopausal Iowa women suggested that intake of energy from plant foods (vegetables, fruits, etc.) may be inversely associated with endometrial cancer risk. In another study, frequent consumption of vegetables, fruits, and grains was associated with decreased polyp prevalence (Witte et al., 1996). After adjusting for potentially anticarcinogenic constituents of foods, high carotenoid vegetables, cruciferous vegetables, garlic, and tofu (or soybeans) remained inversely associated with polyps (Zheng et al, 1995b).

Potter (1996) reviewed the epidemiologic evidence on the relation between nutrition and colorectal cancer. Vegetables were associated with lower risk, unless they were pickled (Yo, 1997), as were folate and calcium.

Freudenheim and colleagues (1996) found only intake of vegetables had a strong inverse relationship to premenopausal breast cancer risk, while in the Iowa Women's Health Study, Kushi and colleagues (1996) found that vitamins A, C, and E may play a protective role in preventing and reversing postmenopausal breast cancer.

Gerster (1997) found a remarkable inverse relationship between lycopene (found almost exclusively in tomatoes and tomato products) and cancers of the prostate, pancreas, and, to a certain extent, stomach.

Key and associates (1997) found statistically significant associations between vitamin B6, garlic, baked beans, and garden peas and prostate cancer. Giovannucci and colleagues (1995) found that four foods were inversely associated with risk of prostate cancer: tomatoes, tomato sauce, tomato juice, and pizza. All contain lycopene. Franceschi and colleagues (1994) found that tomatoes provided a significant protection against all digestive tract cancers.

Lignans and isoflavonoids are diphenolic compounds found in plant foods, particularly whole grains and legumes. They have anticarcinogenic properties in animal and human cells and have been associated with reduced cancer risk in epidemiological studies (Kurzer, Lampe, Martini, & Adlercreutz, 1995; Ziegler, 1994).

Yong and associates (1997) examined the relationship between the dietary intake of vitamins E, C, and A (estimated by a 24-hour recall) and lung cancer incidence in the First National Health and Nutrition Examination Survey Epidemiologic Followup Study. In the study, 3,968 men and 6,100 women age 25 to 74 comprised the sample. When vitamins E and C and carotenoid intakes were studied in combination, a strong protective effect was observed. While smoking is the most important risk behavior to reduce, a daily consumption of a variety of vegetables and fruits provided the best dietary protection against cancer of the lung.

Helicobacter pylori (HP) infection is involved in the development of stomach cancer. Antitumor stomach defense is weakened by the decrease in the stomach of ascorbic acid (vitamin C), carotene, and tocopherol (vitamin E) resulting from HP-infection.

Gastric cancer is the major type of cancer in the developing world and one of the top two worldwide. The incidence of stomach cancer is lower in individuals and populations with *Allium* vegetable intakes.

Allium vegetables, particularly garlic, have antibiotic activity.

Sivam and colleagues (1997) investigated garlic's antimicrobial activity against *H. pylori*, the bacterium implicated in the etiology of stomach cancer. In a laboratory test, *H. pylori* was inhibited by garlic. The researchers suggest the use of garlic as a low-cost intervention, with few side effects, in populations at high risk for stomach cancer, particularly where antibiotic resistance and the risk of reinfection are high. Riggs, DeHaven, and Lamm (1997) also found evidence that garlic may provide a new and effective form of therapy for transitional cell carcinoma of the bladder.

Sigounas and colleagues (1997) concluded from their study that aged garlic extract was an effective antiproliferative agent against erythroleukemia cells that induce cell death by apoptosis. Pinto and colleagues (1997) found that garlic may modulate tumor growth in human prostate carcinoma cells in culture.

The milk thistle family of plants (including artichokes) may provide protection against skin cancer (Katiyar et al., 1997). Unlike sunblock, the therapeutic effects work just as well when applied after sun exposure. A compound called silymarin acts as an antioxidant and prevents swelling associated with free radical damage. Although only tested on mice, when used before and after exposure to UV rays, the tumor rate was 25% in treated mice and 100% in unprotected ones. It is not clear if eating artichokes or taking silymarin supplements will reduce skin cancer risks, but clinical testing is warranted.

Comparative international epidemiological data indicate that the difference between the highest and lowest colon cancer incidence is approximately 10-fold, suggesting a causal role for environmental, rather than genetic, sources, with the dominant environmental cause being the typical low-fiber diet of Western industrialized nations. In a study of tumors in rats that consumed high-fat, Western-style diets, the researchers found a synergistic protective effect of wheat bran and soluble fiber psyllium, while the combination of wheat bran with beta-carotene showed only an additive effect (Alabaster, Tang, & Shivapurkar, 1997). Vitamin E and beta-carotene inhibited progression of preneoplastic foci to colon cancer, while wheat bran and folic acid had a weak cancer-preventive potential at a late stage of carcinogenesis.

Trichopoulou and colleagues (1995), at the Athens School of Public Health, analyzed data from a comprehensive, semiquantitative food-frequency questionnaire administered to 820 women with breast cancer and 1,548 control women. They found evidence that vegetables and fruits are inversely and significantly associated with breast cancer risk. Another study found that flaxseed contains omega-3 fatty acids, which may inhibit cancer growth and metastasis, especially in mammary tumorigenesis (Serraine & Thompson, 1992).

Dietary supplements that have a reported positive effect on cancer (Boik, 1996) are DMSO (may perform as a free radical scavenger), bovine and shark cartilage (may be useful as antiangiogenic agents in treating solid tumors, stimulating the immune system, or inhibiting collagenase), multienzyme formulas and bromelain (may stimulate the immune system, enhance globulin degradation, and inhibit inflammation and platelet aggregation), and urea (may affect the fibrin matrix of tumors and inhibit angiogenesis).

Vitamin D, a nutrient made by the skin when exposed to sunlight, may be an important breast cancer protective. Ren and Lien (1997) reviewed the literature on natural products and their derivatives as cancer chemopreventive agents. Based on examples in many different malignant cells, they suggested that vitamin D appears to be antiproliferative and promotes cellular maturation. The vitamin must be viewed as an important cellular modulator of growth and differentiation, as well as a regulator of calcium homeostasis and its analogs, may prove useful in cancer prevention. Evidence includes the fact that women who live in the southern states below Kansas tend to get significantly less breast cancer than those who live in states north of Kansas. Southern women get more exposure to year-round sunlight. In laboratory studies, vitamin D–related compounds inhibited cancer cell growth (Rozen, Yang, Huynh, & Pollak, 1997). John (1997) presented findings from a study comparing the health habits of 133 women with breast cancer and women who did not have cancer. Exposure to sunlight significantly reduced the risk of breast cancer. Besides exposure to sunlight, which is a risk factor for skin cancer, vitamin D is available in fish oil, fatty fish, egg yolks, and liver. Fortified foods, including milk and some breads and cereals, also contain vitamin D.

Malvy and colleagues (1997) investigated the serum antioxidant levels of vitamin A (retinol), E (alpha-tocopherol), beta-carotene, zinc, and selenium for 170 children with newly diagnosed malignancies. Measurements were taken at diagnosis and 6 months after initiation of conventional treatment. A total of 170 children age 1 to 16 years and 632 cancer-free controls participated in the study. At diagnosis, serum concentrations of retinol, beta-carotene, zinc, and alpha-tocopherol were significantly inversely associated with cancer. The only significant decreases in mean values at 6 months were the alpha-tocopherol-to-cholesterol ratio in children with bone tumors, and serum zinc in bone tumors and central nervous system malignancies. Retinol and selenium increased in children with leukemia during the period of treatment. These findings provide evidence about the micronutrient requirement for children diagnosed with cancer.

Polyunsaturated Fatty Acids

Polyunsaturated fatty acids of the omega-6 class, as found in corn and safflower oils, can act as precursors for the growth of mammary tumors, but polyunsaturated fatty acids of the omega-3 class, as found in fish oil, can inhibit these effects. Bagga and colleagues (1997) found that by feeding women with breast cancer a low-fat diet and a fish oil supplement, they could alter breast tissue, significantly reducing the total omega-6 polyunsaturated fatty acids in their plasma. (It should be noted that the 25 women in the study also consumed a diet heavy in soy products, green leafy vegetables, broccoli, brussels sprouts, cauliflower, and carrots.)

Processed Foods and Sugar

Monosaccharides, or simple sugars, inhibit T cells, part of the immune system, by reacting as aldehydes (Rhodes, Zheng, & Lifely, 1992). Moerman (1993) examined 111 case studies of biliary tract cancer and compared them to 480 controls for dietary factors. She found a more than double risk for biliary tract cancer associated with the intake of sugars independent of any other

energy source. The researcher suggested that sugars may be a risk due to their relationship with blood lipids and gallstone formation.

Slattery and associates (1997a) also found a connection between dietary sugars, especially a diet high in simple carbohydrates relative to complex carbohydrates and increased risk of colon cancer. Wu, Yu, and Mack (1997) found a risk of small intestinal adenocarcinoma in men and women associated with adding sugar regularly in coffee or tea and daily intake of nondiet carbonated soft drinks.

Franceschi and colleagues (1995) conducted a study involving 2,569 women with incident breast cancer (median age: 55 years) and 2,588 control women hospitalized with nonacute neoplastic diseases. The participants were interviewed in six different regions of Italy. The researchers found significant trends increasing breast cancer risk with increasing intake of the following foods, many of which are highly processed and/or contain sugar: bread and cereal dishes, pork and processed meats, sugar, and candies. High intake of milk, poultry, fish, raw vegetables, potatoes, coffee, and tea exerted a protection against the development of breast cancer. Soups, eggs, other meats, cheese, cooked vegetables, citrus and other fruits, cake, and desserts were not significantly related to breast cancer risk. The variety of vegetable types consumed weekly had a beneficial effect beyond high vegetable intake.

Retinol and Squamous Cell Skin Cancers

Moon and others (1997) reported the results of two chemoprevention randomized clinical trials to evaluate retinoids in the prevention of skin cancers. People with moderate risk with a history of at least 10 actinic keratoses and at most two prior skin cancers were randomly assigned to either 25,000 IU retinol or a placebo daily for 5 years. People with high risk (at least four prior skin cancers) received either 25,000 IU retinol, 5 to 10 mg isotretinoin, or placebo daily for 3 years. Daily retinol was effective in preventing squamous cell cancers in people with moderate risk, but the retinols had no significant benefit for the high risk group.

Sesame Oil

Frequent consumption of sesame oil was found to decrease risk of stomach cancer in a case-control study (Yo, 1997).

Soybeans and Peanuts

Seeds of many plants belonging to the legume family, especially soybeans and peanuts, are rich sources of protease inhibitors. There is epidemiologic evidence that the consumption of legumes is associated with a decrease in prostate, colon, breast, oral, pharyngeal, pancreas, and stomach cancers (Ren & Lien, 1997).

A great deal of evidence suggests that compounds present in soybeans can prevent cancer in many different organ systems (Knight & Eden, 1996; Stoll, 1997). Isoflavones, protease inhibitors, saponins, and genistein are all compounds present in soybeans that may suppress carcinogenesis (Barnes et al., 1996; Clawson, 1996). There is also evidence suggesting that diets containing large amounts of soybean products (tofu, tempeh, soy milk, etc.) are associated with overall low cancer mortality rates, particularly for colon, breast, endometrial, and prostate cancer (Goodman et al., 1997; Wu et al., 1996; Zava et al., 1997). It is believed that supplementation of diets with soybeans and soybean products could markedly reduce cancer mortality rates (Kennedy, 1995).

Herbs and Spices That Protect

Although individualized combinations of herbs are used to treat cancer using the traditional Chinese medicine method, the ones showing the most promise, based on clinical studies, include indirubin, rhein, emodin, psoralen, matrine, and oxymatrine (Boik, 1996).

Turmeric, a spice from the root of the plant *Curcuma longa*, has long been used in foods. It is a major phenolic antioxidant and has been used as a naturally occurring medicine for the treatment of inflammatory diseases. The spice also has strong anticarcinogenic effects in several tissues, including skin, stomach, colon, small intestine, breast, and tongue. It may be that curcumin induces apoptosis in malignant cancer cell lines by blocking the cellular signal transduction (Ren & Lien, 1997).

Nishino and others (1986) demonstrated the skin tumor–suppressing effect of berberine sulfate, an alkaloid isolated from *Hydrastis canadensis*, or goldenseal.

Luettig and colleagues (1989) showed that *Echinacea purpurea* was effective in activating macrophages to cytotoxicity against tumor cells. This finding may be important in the defense against tumors.

Yo (1997) reported that case-control and cohort studies have provided evidence that ginseng intake decreased the risk of gastric cancer.

Green Tea

The effect of drinking green tea in reducing human cancer risk is unclear, although a protective effect has been reported in some animal and epidemiological studies. Ji and others (1997) examined the hypothesis that green tea consumption reduces the risk of cancers of the colon, rectum, and pancreas in a large population-based case-control study in Shanghai, China. In the study, 1,552 controls were matched by gender and age to newly diagnosed cancer cases (931 colon, 884 rectum, and 451 pancreas). Adjustments were made for age, income, education, and cigarette smoking. Dietary intake and body size were found to have minimal impact. An inverse association with each cancer was observed with increasing amount of green tea consumed, with the strongest trends for pancreatic and rectal cancer.

Other Promising Herbs

Other herbs reported to show promise for the treatment of cancer include horse chestnut, aloe vera gel, dang gui, and astragalus.

Guided Imagery

Kolcaba (1995, 1997) tested the hypothesis that guided imagery tapes would increase comfort for women receiving radiation for breast cancer. The tapes contained messages that personalized the radiation equipment as "a powerful friend," radiation as "healing ray," and experiences with therapy and therapists as positive and health-providing. Participants listened to the tapes every day at their convenience and answered the comfort questionnaire three times during the 10-week study period. An equal number of participants in the control group did not receive tapes but answered the same questionnaires all three times. Differences in comfort increased over time among individuals who received the inter-

vention compared to the control group. At the end of the study, both groups were given tape players and other audiotapes designed for enhancing wellness.

Imagery/Hypnosis and Quality of Life

Rapkin, Straubing, and Holroyd (1991) used imagery-hypnosis preoperatively with a sample of 15 individuals scheduled for head and neck cancer surgery and compared them with 21 others who received usual care and were followed through their hospital charts. Within the hypnotic intervention group, hypnotizability was negatively correlated with surgical complications, and there was a trend toward negative correlation between hypnotizability and surgical blood loss. The findings suggested that imagery-hypnosis may reduce the probability of postoperative complications, thereby keeping hospital stay within the expected range. Controlled, randomized, clinical trials with a larger sample are needed to provide statistical analysis with appropriate power.

Justice (1997) reported randomly assigning 47 women to imagery (practice with audiotapes providing training in relaxation, imaging ability, and basic breathing), 1-hour group support (nonstructured, support-oriented, and aimed at decreasing stress, minimizing feelings of isolation, and enhancing self-esteem), or standard care after treatment for breast cancer. Groups did not differ in natural killer activity or immune changes, but the imagery and support groups both showed a (not statistically significant) lowering of opioid stress hormones than the standard treatment group. The imagery group showed improvement over the support group in decreased stress, increased vigor, and improved quality of life.

Lactobacillus Acidophilus

Lactobacillus acidophilus, an ingredient in many yogurt products, has been shown to exhibit antitumor qualities by stimulating the production of immunologic factors (Rangavajhyala et al., 1997).

Massage and Aromatherapy

Kirshbaum (1996) reported using massage and aromatherapy to reduce pain and discomfort of lymphoedema of the arm, a complication of treatment for breast cancer.

Weight Gain

Huang and colleagues (1997) examined the body mass index at the age of 18 years and at midlife and adult weight change in relation to breast cancer incidence and mortality for 95,256 U.S. female nurses age 30 to 55 years. The population was followed for 16 years. Weight gain after the age of 18 years was unrelated to breast cancer incidence before menopause but was positively associated with incidence after menopause. Weight gain alone in women accounted for approximately 16% of postmenopausal breast cancer; hormone replacement therapy alone accounted for 5%. When taken together, these two variables accounted for about one third of postmenopausal breast cancers.

Support Groups Enhance

Gregoire, Kalogeropoulos, and Coreos (1997) investigated the effectiveness of support groups for men with prostate cancer. A total of 54 men and some family members participated in seven separate groups. They met for a series of 10, 90-minute weekly sessions. The meetings were led by a nurse and a psychologist. The researchers provided information on the medical aspects of treatment, focused on the emotional reactions of participants to their diagnosis, and encouraged participants to adopt more active, health-promoting actions. Participants were surveyed anonymously by questionnaire at the end of the last session. The participants described having a better understanding of their illness and being more involved in treatment and more positive in their outlook as a result of the group experience. The researchers concluded that support groups were useful in facilitating perceptions of enhanced coping in men diagnosed with prostate cancer.

Davison and Degner (1997) explored the hypothesis that assisting men with prostate cancer to obtain information would enable them to assume a more active role in treatment and decrease their anxiety and depression. Using a sample recruited from one community urology clinic, 60 men newly diagnosed with prostate cancer were randomly assigned to receive either a written information package with discussion, a list of questions they could ask their physician and an audiotape of medical consultation, or a written information package alone. Results showed that men in the intervention group assumed a significantly more active role in treatment decision-making and had lower state anxiety levels at 6 weeks. Levels of depression were similar for both groups at 6 weeks.

CAROLYN CHAMBERS CLARK

See
Exercise (IV)

CARPAL TUNNEL SYNDROME

Carpal tunnel syndrome (CTS) is a painful condition of the flexor retinaculum. The carpal tunnel is in the wrist and is composed of the flexor retinaculum, which extends across the carpal bones and attaches to the hook of harnate and pisiform bones and extends across the carpal bones to the trapezium tubercle and scaphoid tubercle. Going through this tunnel are arteries, veins, lymphatic vessels, nine tendons and their synovial sheaths, and the radial nerve.

CTS has been categorized under a variety of physiological classifications, including repetitive stress injuries (RSIs), cumulative trauma disorders (CTDs), and repetitive use injuries (RUIs). Although representing slightly different viewpoints, each of these classifications refers to the same physiological condition.

The Merck Manual of Diagnosis and Therapy (1985) defines CTS as "a deposition of mucinious ground substance in the wrist." The ground substance, or amorphous ground substances, are a gel-like matrix produced by the same cells that generate the fibrocomponents of connective tissue. It contains a variety of combinations of fats, proteins, and sugars. This matrix is the major component of soft tissue content and part of the lymphatic system. Its unique characteristics are contributing factors to the carpal tunnel condition.

The ground substance's characteristics are affected by temperature change, water content, and colloidal content. Normally this ground substance oozes through the connective tissue at a very sluggish rate that is dependent on muscle function; that is, its movement through the soft tissues is dependent on muscles pumping it through.

In addition to being dependent on muscles for movement, the combination of muscle contractions and variables in viscosity affect the material's ability to flow through the pores of the tissues. This sets the condition for a natural buildup of hydraulic pressure in the tissues, which in turn creates a situation for the breakdown of tissue structures. When this occurs, the alarm bell goes off and a sensation of pain is perceived. At a molecular level, when this occurs it is called "micro-tearing" of the tissues; that is, at a molecular level there are tiny tears in the fabric of the tissues to relieve the built-up pressures. When that occurs, the pressurized ground substance oozes out through the tear, thus relieving the internal pressures. The pain then goes away and in the normal course of events, the components of the ground substance then glaze over the micro-tear and inside the compartment fibroblasts begin to lay down a collagen fiber mat in repair of the tear.

When a micro-tear occurs in the carpal tunnel area, the compactness of the tissues in the area and the normal healing process of micro-tearing combine to make a unique condition for supporting adhesions between moving tissues of the tendons and their sheaths. Thus, with the normal functioning of the hand and independent movement of the fingers, these micro-tears will go through a continuous process of healing over and adhering to adjacent tissues, then being torn open again as the adjacent tissues move through normal hand function. This action lays the foundation for cumulative trauma and RUIs. This normal interaction with the connective tissue and lymphatic system can occur not only in the carpal tunnel but also in other parts of the arm and body.

CTS Indicators

Some of the indicators of the physiological changes in the soft tissue content pressure are pain, tingling, and/or numbness in the hands and fingers; burning and/or pain in the wrist area; difficulty buttoning, grasping, opening jars, and/or writing; pain in the elbow area; pain from hand to shoulder; pain in the shoulder when sleeping; swelling of the hand, wrist, elbow, or arm; weakness in the morning. Symptoms often are worse at night.

Common tests to confirm a diagnosis of CTS include Tinel's Sign, where a tap on the inside of the wrist causes tingling or pain in the hand; Phalen's Sign, where tingling or pain occurs if the wrist is bent to 90 degrees and held for 3 minutes; and a nerve conduction test, which is administered and interpreted by a physician.

Prevention

Although CTS and related conditions are considered to be related to keyboarding and computer usage, people in virtually any profession or trade can be affected. Many hobbies, including carpentry, needlework, and playing musical instruments, can also be conducive to CTS. The most effective methods of prevention are good posture and ergonomically correct work environment, planned periodic breaks from repetitive motions, rest, proper food regimen, exercise, and a regular program of self-massage.

Intervention After Onset

Because the onset and progression are lifestyle-based, CTS is insidious with a variable rate of progression. Application of the factors mentioned under "Prevention" will help to limit the progress of the condition. Treatments can be noninvasive or invasive.

The least invasive method of treatment is a professionally administered program of massage combined with a complete evaluation of the patient's work and hobby environments, resulting in improved ergonomics, appropriate rest, proper food regimen, and exercise. A 1992 test conducted on the effectiveness of Specific Lymphatic Massage, a technique created by this author for the treatment of CTS and related conditions, was found to be 95% effective 2 years post-treatment. Patients who learn and self-apply Specific Lymphatic Massage while continuing the ergonomic and lifestyle improvements can maintain a CTS-free state and avoid recurrence of the condition.

Braces and other orthotic devices can bring some relief to certain patients. These devices include splints with aluminum or plastic inserts to keep the hand at a specific angle, thus alleviating the pressure on the carpal tunnel. Some patients cannot accomplish necessary daily tasks efficiently with splint-type braces. For these people, nonsplint devices, such as fingerless gloves made of stretch-type fabric, allow more natural use of the hand. Usually these patients wear the splint-type devices at night.

The most invasive and expensive alternative is surgery, which is employed in extreme cases where the patient has lost most of the use of either or both hands due to CTS. Surgery is controversial and cannot be guaranteed to work in every case. Furthermore, unless the patient employs preventive measure, the condition may return.

STEPHEN E. CHAGNON

See
Aromatherapy (IV)
Biofeedback (IV)

CATARACTS

Defined as a partial or complete clouding of the lens of the eye, cataracts are the leading cause of blindness and visual impairment. Cataracts have been linked to aging, radiation or infrared light, certain medications (including steroids), and various injuries and conditions.

Preventive treatments include diet and supplementation. Vitamins with antioxidants may affect cataract development by protecting against free radical damage. Seddon and colleagues (1994) found that men who took multivitamin supplements tended to experience a decreased risk of cataract. The Linxian Cataract Studies suggested that vitamin/mineral supplements may decrease the risk of nuclear cataracts (Sperduto et al., 1993).

Mares-Perlman (1995) found that taking vitamin supplements lowered the risk of cataracts by 40%. Study participants who ate more fiber in breads and cereals also had less severe cataracts.

Jacques and Chylack (1991) studied the relationship between antioxidant nutrient status and senile cataracts in 77 people with cataracts and 35 controls with clear lenses. Participants who consumed fewer than 3.5 servings of fruit or vegetables a day had an increased risk of both cortical and posterior subcapsular cataracts.

A 1993 study by Vitale and colleagues (1993) found that higher levels of plasma alpha-tocopherol (vitamin E) was associated with a reduced risk of cataracts in 660 people enrolled in the Baltimore Longitudinal Study on Aging.

Birlouez-Aragon and colleagues (1993) conducted a study to evaluate the relationships between milk and yogurt consumption, galactose metabolism, and cataract risk. Yogurt intake had a protective effect on cataract formation for the whole population, while milk ingestion was dose-related with cataract risk in lactose digesters (particularly diabetics, but not in lactose maldigesters).

Jacques and associates (1988) found that people age 40 to 70 ($n = 112$) with a cataract in at least one lens had low levels of vitamin C and higher levels of vitamin B6 and selenium. Risk was reduced for individuals in the highest quintile of vitamin D and total carotenoids.

Jacques and Taylor (1997) found that taking vitamin C supplements for 10 years or more may lower the risk of developing cataracts in women by 77% for loss of transparency in a small area of lens and by 83% for the risk of moderate opacities. Their findings support some earlier studies finding that vitamin C use may help reduce age-related cataract development and suggest it is the antioxidant properties of the vitamin that are protective.

CAROLYN CHAMBERS CLARK

See
Nutrition (IV)

See also
Antioxidants and Free Radicals (III)
Diabetes (II)
Vitamin C (III)
Vitamin E (III)

CAVITIES

Dennison (1997) reviewed the cause of cavities in infants. Nursing bottle cavities has long been recognized as a consequence of feeding juices in bottles to babies and using the bottle as a pacifier.

Pierson (1994) found that licorice inhibited the bacteria that cause dental decay. Osawa (1996) reported that an ethanol extract of the dried leaves of eucalyptus has an appreciable antibacterial action on typical bacteria associated with both dental caries and periodontal disease.

CAROLYN CHAMBERS CLARK

See also
Dental Problems (II)

CHRONIC FATIGUE SYNDROME

Chronic fatigue syndrome is diagnosed (Hickie, 1995) when four or more of the following symptoms occur concurrently:

- impairment of short-term memory or concentration;
- sore throat;
- tender cervical or axillary lymph nodes;
- muscle or multi-joint pain;
- headaches;
- unrefreshing sleep;
- post-exertional malaise

Herbs and exercise have been tested for their use in treating chronic fatigue. Evidence for the usefulness of both has been provided in the research literature.

Herbs

Herbs that have been used successfully in treating fatigue are licorice root, echinacea, and *Panax schinseng*. See, Broumand, Sahl, and Tilles (1997) reported the use of both echinacea and ginseng with individuals exhibiting chronic fatigue syndrome. Both significantly enhanced natural killer function.

Licorice root soothes the digestive system and the lungs and may provide support to the adrenal glands. Baschetti (1995) found that licorice may be useful for people complaining of fatigue who have mild adrenal insufficiency.

Exercise

White and Fulcher (1997) found that walking, swimming, and other forms of mild to moderate aerobic exercises tailored to specific needs can help people with chronic fatigue syndrome. Fifty-five percent of participants in a regular, graded aerobic exercise program reported feeling "much better" or "very much better" after 3 months, as compared to 26% of individuals introduced to flexibility and relaxation exercises only.

CAROLYN CHAMBERS CLARK

See
Fibromyalgia (II)

See also
Licorice (III)

COLD SYMPTOMS

Symptoms of the common cold include: cough; headache; hoarseness; muscle ache; nasal drainage; scratchy throat; nasal congestion; sore throat; sneezing; or oral temperature over 37°C (Ricchini, 1997).

Rhinoviruses are probably the world's leading cause of respiratory illness and are spread chiefly by aerosol, rather than by fomites or personal contact. Rhinovirus transmission can be completely interrupted by careful use of virucidal facial tissues, which smother aerosols generated by coughing, sneezing, and nose blowing (Jennings & Dick, 1987).

Susceptibility to colds may decrease with increased diversity of social network (Cohen et al., 1997). The researchers found that increased diversity was a more significant predictor of cold symptoms than the number of members of a network, intake of more than 85 mg of vitamin C daily, exercising more than two times a week, or not smoking.

Research has provided evidence of the effectiveness for echinacea, garlic, and ginseng as immune enhancers. Zinc gluconate has shown promise for reducing cold symptoms, and onions and garlic have antibiotic properties. Intake of vitamin C may have a physiological effect on susceptibility to common cold infections, especially for those with low dietary vitamin C intake (Hemila, 1997) and people who do heavy exercise or have frequent upper respiratory infections (Hemila, 1996). However, taking between 1 and 6 g/day may decrease the duration of cold episodes for all populations by between 21% (Hemila & Herman, 1995) and 23% (Hemila, 1994).

Echinacea

Several researchers have shown that the herb echinacea provides a defense against infectious conditions (Bauer, 1996; Luettig et al., 1989; See, Broumand, Sahl, & Tilles, 1997).

Garlic

Garlic has been shown to exhibit broad-spectrum antimicrobial activity (Naganawa et al., 1996), including inhibiting gram-positive bacteria (e.g., *Bacillus cereus*, *Bacillus subtilis*, *Mycobacterium smegmatis*, *Streptomyces griseus*, *Staphyloccus aureus*, and *Lactobacillus plantarum*) and gram-negative bacteria (*Escherichia coli*, *Klebsiella pneumoniae*, and *Xanthomonas maltophilia*).

Ginseng

Ginseng has been shown to enhance killer cell activity in both normal individuals and those with either chronic fatigue syndrome or acquired immune deficiency syndrome (See et al., 1997).

Onions and Garlic

Onion and garlic contain sulfur active substances mainly in the form of cysteine derivatives with antibiotic properties (Augusti, 1996).

Zinc

Using a randomized, double-blind, placebo-controlled study, Mossad, Macknin, Medendorp, and Mason (1996) studied the effectiveness of zinc gluconate lozenges as a treatment for reducing the duration of cold symptoms with 100 employees of a Cleveland medical clinic. Participants had all developed cold symptoms in the prior 24 hours. They were divided into a zinc group (who were given 13.3 mg of zinc gluconate for as long as they had a cold) and a placebo group (who were given lozenges containing 5% calcium lactate pentahydrate).

The zinc group recovered quicker (a median of 4.4 days compared to 7.6 days for the placebo group), had fewer days with cough (2 days compared to 4 days), headache (2 days compared to 3 days), hoarseness (2 days compared to 3 days), nasal congestion (4 days compared to 6 days), nasal drainage (4 days compared to 7 days), and sore throat (1 day compared to 3 days). No significant difference was noted between the two groups in the resolution of fever, muscle ache, scratchy throat, or sneezing. The zinc group reported more nausea (20% compared to 4%) and greater bad taste reactions (80% compared to 30%).

CAROLYN CHAMBERS CLARK

See also
AIDS/HIV (II)
Allergies (II)
Chronic Fatigue Syndrome (II)
Echinacea (III)

Garlic (III)
Ginseng (III)
Vitamin C (III)

CONSTIPATION

Lifestyle factors play a large role in constipation. Increasing fiber in the diet, exercising (to stimulate peristaltic movement), and taking in sufficient fluids all contribute.

Beverley and Travis (1992) found that a mixture of prune juice blended with raisins, currants, prunes, figs, and dates was as effective as drugs, enemas, and suppositories for older adults. Participants found the mixture palatable and drank it willingly.

Biofeedback can also be an effective treatment for constipation. Patankar and colleagues (1997) reported its use in a multicenter statewide study. One hundred and sixteen people with chronic constipation had a mean of eight weekly biofeedback sessions. Eighty-four percent had a significant improvement in their constipation with biofeedback treatment. The mean number of weekly unassisted bowel movements increased from 0.8 to 6.5.

CAROLYN CHAMBERS CLARK

See
Exercise (IV)

CYSTIC FIBROSIS

Cystic fibrosis (CF) is a chronic multisystem disease affecting nearly 30,000 Americans. In CF, a chronic lung infection occurs with progressive pulmonary insufficiency. *Pseudomonas aeruginosa* is the prominent organism found in individuals with this disease.

Song and colleagues (1997) used a rat model of chronic *P. aeruginosa* pneumonia mimicking that found in people with CF. They studied whether the inflammation and antibody responses could be changed by using ginseng. An extract of ginseng was injected subcutaneously in study participants, and saline and cortisone were used as controls. Two weeks later, the ginseng treatment group showed a significantly improved bacterial clearance from the lungs, less severe lung pathology, lower lung abscess incidence, and fewer lung mast cells. Findings indicate that ginseng may have potential as a treatment for people with CF.

Individuals with CF may be more susceptible to oxidative-cell injury due to impaired absorption of dietary antioxidants. Brown, McBurney, Lunec, and Kelly (1995) collected the first morning void of urine for 13 children with CF, and 10 same-aged controls, in an attempt to correlate its excretion with clinical status. They found a significant positive correlation between urinary oh8dG concentration and plasma alpha-tocopherol (vitamin E) concentration. Their results confirmed that individuals with CF are susceptible to oxidative-induced DNA damage.

Goodill (1995) studied the effectiveness of a short-term dance/movement therapy for hospitalized adults with CF. Forty-one adults were randomly assigned to either the treatment or the control group. Twenty-four adults ranging in age from 18 to 67 comprised the treatment group, and 17 adults ranging in age from 18 to 67 comprised the control group. Both groups were pretested, then posttested at discharge and 1 month later using the Profile of Mood States and the Draw-a-Person test.

Neither group received physical therapy. The treatment group participated in sessions that included guided stretching and mobilization, verbal and movement interaction regarding their condition and its effects on their body posture, guided imagery focused on breathing, and deep muscle relaxation work.

There were statistically significant differences between pre- and posttest for participants on the Total Mood Disturbance, with mood state improving. On Vigor and Fatigue, two subscales, significant changes also occurred from pre- to posttest.

CAROLYN CHAMBERS CLARK

See
Dance/Movement Therapy (IV)
Deep Tissue Therapy (IV)

See also
Antioxidants and Free Radicals (III)
Ginseng (III)
Lung Disorders (II)
Vitamin E (III)

DENTAL PROBLEMS

Peridontal disease has recently been shown to be a risk factor for diabetes, coronary heart disease, and preterm low birth weight. Use of xylitol-containing chewing gum reduced *Streptococcus mutans* counts in plaque and saliva. At the same time, it fostered remineralization of early cavities (Toors, 1992).

CAROLYN CHAMBERS CLARK

See also
Cavities (II)

DEPRESSION

The American Psychiatric Associations' *Diagnostic and Statistical Manual of Mental Disorders* (DSM-IV, 1994) identifies numerous features of unipolar depression, including the psychological (lowering of mood over several weeks or months; low self-esteem; lack of motivation; irritability; feelings of worthlessness, hopelessness, or inappropriate guilt; suicidal ideation; forgetfulness; distractibility; indecisiveness) and the somatic (fatigue, weakness, insomnia, and/or change in appetite or body weight). Bipolar depression includes both manic and depressive phases.

Depression is a major condition that is approximately twice as common in women as in men. This gender difference may be due to social pressures on women to be "feminine" (Oakley, 1994), or to the "chronic overload" that women face, including spending significantly more time doing housework than men and caring for children and sick and elderly relatives. Distressing thoughts can contribute to depletion of the immune system, indirect disruption of sleep, and depressive symptoms (Azar, 1996).

Depression has been linked to anger (Robbins & Tanck, 1997). The researchers asked 77 undergraduate students to complete the Beck Depression Inventory and keep a diary for 10 consecutive days, answering questions about felt and expressed anger and depressed affect. They found a tendency to attribute the cause of angry feelings to one's own action. This tendency was positively related to depressed affect. Inhibiting expression of anger was positively related to the measure of depression.

Depression is one of the 10 most frequently reported medical problems and may be linked with pain (Ross, 1996). Pharmacological interventions fail to provide lasting relief, but a number of complementary procedures offer promise.

Acupuncture

Allen and Schnyer (1994) reported the use of acupuncture for unipolar depression for 33 women age 18 to 45. The treatment group received acupuncture designed to treat depressive symptoms. The nonspecific group first received acupuncture for symptoms not related to depression, and later acupuncture for depressive symptoms. The waiting list group received no treatment for 8 weeks, followed by specific acupuncture treatment. Sixty-four percent of the women who received treatment specifically designed for depression experienced full remission, indicating sufficient promise to warrant a larger clinical trial.

Yang, Liu, Luo, and Jiu (1994) compared the use of acupuncture ($n = 20$) with amitriptyline ($n = 21$) for depression. Using the Hamilton Rating Scale for Depression, researchers determined the factor of anxiety somatization decreased significantly in the acupuncture group (as compared to the antidepressant group). After 6 weeks, slow wave delta decreased in the treatment group and fast wave alpha increased significantly.

Assertiveness Training

Sanchez et al. (1980) reported assigning 32 depressed individuals to either group assertion training or traditional group psychotherapy. Assertion training was more effective than traditional psychotherapy in increasing self-reported assertiveness and in alleviating depression.

Bibliotherapy

Bibliotherapy is the therapeutic use of books and reading as treatment for depression. Smith, Floyd, Scogin, and Jamison (1997) examined the durability of cognitive bibliotherapy for mild to moderately depressed persons in a 3-year follow-up of participants from a previous study. The Hamilton Rating Scale for Depression, the Beck Depression Inventory, and questions related to participants' perceptions of the program were used to measure effects. Treatment gains were maintained over the 3-year follow-up period. The results support the usefulness of cognitive bibliotherapy as an adjunct to traditional treatment for depression.

Biofeedback

Rosenfeld, Cha, Blair, and Gotlib (1995) reported the use of biofeedback to teach depressed undergraduates to control left-right frontal (brain) alpha power differences. The researchers suggested that biofeedback has potential for treating depression.

Cognitive Behavioral Therapy

Thirty-one unmedicated people with depression were given 16 weekly sessions of cognitive therapy and compared to 45 who received placebo treatment. Right-ear accuracy (as measured by dichotic syllable and complex tone tests) for syllables was the best predictor of response to cognitive therapy for depression (Bruder et al., 1997).

Cognitive behavioral treatment has also been found helpful for depression for some people after their hospitalization for stroke (Lincoln, Flannaghan, Sutcliffe, & Rother,

1997). Conclusions were based on visual inspection, and comparison during baseline and treatment phases and proportion of scores below lowest baseline on the Hospital Anxiety and Depression Scale and the Beck Depression Inventory. The sample was small, so further evaluation of this treatment for depression with this population is warranted.

Abraham, Neundorfer, and Currie (1992) compared the effects of cognitive-behavioral group therapy, focused visual imagery group therapy, and education-discussion groups on cognition, depression, hopelessness, and dissatisfaction with life among depressed nursing home residents. Seventy-six men and women with mild to moderate cognitive decline participated in nurse-led 24-week protocols. Data were collected 4 weeks before the treatments and 8 and 20 weeks after treatment. Participants in the cognitive-behavioral and focused imagery groups showed a significant improvement on cognitive scores beginning 8 weeks after treatment initiation. The researchers suggested that both of these kinds of groups may reduce cognitive impairment in depressed nursing home residents with mild to moderate cognitive decline.

Dance

Noreau, Martineau, Roy, and Belzile (1995) examined the use of a dance-based exercise program in a group of 19 persons with arthritis (mean age: 49.3) in a 12-week, twice weekly format. Positive changes occurred in ratings for depression, anxiety, fatigue, and tension.

Exercise

Singh, Clements, and Fiatarone (1997) tested the use of a progressive resistance training (PRT) program, hypothesizing it would reduce depression while improving physiologic capacity, quality of life, morale, function, and self-efficacy without adverse events in an older, significantly depressed population. Volunteers, age 60 and older, were randomly assigned to a 10-week exercise program or an attention-control group. PRT significantly reduced all depression measures (Beck Depression Inventory and Hamilton Rating Scale for Depression) and improved quality of life, social functioning, role emotion (morale), and strength.

Testing a group ($n = 58$) of ethnically diverse pregnant adolescents, Koniak-Griffin (1994) found that aerobic exercise significantly decreased depressive symptoms and increased total self-esteem. Thayer, Newman, and McClain (1994) completed four studies evaluating the success of behaviors and strategies used to self-regulate bad moods, raise energy, and reduce tension. The four studies (open-ended questionnaire, fixed-response surveys, and therapist and self-rating measures) confirmed previous findings that exercise is the most effective mood-regulating behavior and that the best general strategy to change a bad mood is a combination of relaxation, stress management, cognitive, and exercise techniques.

Guided Imagery and Music Therapy

McKinney and colleagues (1997) found that healthy adults who participated in 13 weeks of the Bonny Method of Guided Imagery and Music (a depth approach to music psychotherapy) sessions reported significant decreases between pre- and postsession depression, fatigue, and total mood disturbance (on the Profile of Mood States) as opposed to a waiting-list control group. According to the results of blood tests, participants also exhibited a reduced level of cortisol, which may have health implications for chronically stressed people.

Herbs

The ability of *Ginkgo biloba* extract (GBE) to improve the general mood in people suffering from cerebral vascular insufficiency led researchers to investigate the antidepressive effects of the herb. Forty depressed participants (ranging in age from 51 to 78 years) who had not benefited fully from standard antidepressant drugs were given either 80 mg of GBE three times daily or a placebo. By the end of the fourth week of treatment, the total score on the Hamilton Depression Scale was reduced from an average of 14 to 7. After 8 weeks of treatment, the total score in the GBE group dropped to 4.5. In comparison, the placebo group dropped from 14 to 13. The researchers concluded that GBE offers a significant benefit as an antidepressant on its own or in combination with standard drug therapy (Schubert & Halama, 1993).

Two meta-analyses of 23 (Linde et al., 1996), and 25 (Nordfors & Hartvig, 1997) randomized trials showed extracts of *Hypericum perforatum* (Saint-John's-wort) were more effective than placebo in the treatment of depression, and as effective as standard antidepressive treatment. Saint-John's-wort also had fewer side effects than the standard antidepressant drugs.

Lifestyle Behaviors

Koenig and colleagues (1997) examined models of relationships between religious activities, physical health, social support, and depressive symptoms for a sample of

4,000 people age 65 and older. Frequency of church attendance was positive related to physical health and negatively related to depression but unrelated to social support. Frequent churchgoers were about half as likely to be depressed. Private prayer/Bible reading was negatively associated with physical health and positively associated with social support but unrelated to depression. Religious TV/radio listening was unrelated to social support, negatively associated with good physical health, and positively associated with depression.

Light Therapy

Seasonal affective disorder (SAD) represents a subgroup of depression that includes hypersomnia, anergia (lack of energy), increased appetite, weight gain, and carbohydrate craving. The symptoms occur in autumn and winter in northern climates and are in full remission in spring and summer.

Light therapy, or phototherapy, continues to be under study as a treatment for depressive symptoms. In treating SAD, individuals are exposed to a full light screen 2 hours early in the morning, between 6:00 and 9:00 a.m. The most common side effects are headache, eyestrain, and muscle pain. It is not used with tricyclic antidepressants, neuroleptics, and other medication containing a tricyclic, heterocyclic, or porphyrin ring system because of the potential negative reaction (Sartori & Poirrier, 1996). Beauchemin and Hays (1997) randomly assigned depressed inpatients to high and low levels of artificial light. Both unipolar and bipolar depression responded when phototherapy was used as an adjunct to pharmacotherapy. Mood improvement was significantly related to intensity of illumination.

Massage and Relaxation Therapy

Field and colleagues (1996) examined the effects of relaxation and massage therapy on depression and anxiety in depressed teen mothers who recently gave birth and were recruited from an inner-city hospital maternity ward. All mothers showed elevated scores on the Beck Depression Inventory but were not being treated for depression or taking medications. They were randomly assigned to either a relaxation therapy (RT) group or a massage therapy (MT) group for 30 minutes a day for 2 successive days for 5 successive weeks. The MT group reported less anxiety, anxiety behaviors, depression, and stress than the RT group. Participants perceived the RT as "too much work," so results may have been biased, suggesting further research is needed to avoid this bias.

Meditation

Smith, Compton, and West (1995) reported the use of meditation to enhance Fordyce's Personal Happiness Enhancement Program (PHEP) to reduce depression and anxiety. A control group received no instruction. The Happiness Measure, Psychap Inventory, Beck Depression Inventory and State-Trait Anxiety Scale were dependent measures. The meditation plus PHEP group significantly improved on all dependent measures, including depression, over both the PHEP-only group and the control group.

Social Support

Home-visit programs can bring positive results for depressed mothers. Gelfand, Teti,

Seiner, and Jameson (1996) examined a home-visit intervention program for depressed mothers with infants age 3 to 13 months. Public health nurses made 29 visits to homes ($n = 37$) at 2-week intervals. The nurses modeled positive interactions with infants, taught new parenting skills, and reinforced maternal competencies. They also suggested resources and positive coping responses for mothers. The interventions successfully reduced maternal depression, increased new mothers' perception of social support, and decreased levels of perceived daily hassles.

Patten and colleagues (1997) found that depressive symptoms in adolescents were associated with a perceived lack of support from parents who are present, not with family structure.

Yoga

Berger and Owen (1992) found that both yoga and swimming participants reported greater decreases in scores on anger, confusion, tension, and depression than did the control group. Among male participants, the acute decreases in tension, fatigue, and anger after yoga were significantly greater than those after swimming. The researchers concluded that aerobic exercise was not necessary to reduce depression.

CAROLYN CHAMBERS CLARK

See
Acupuncture and Chinese Medicine (IV)
Biofeedback (IV)
Cognitive-Behavioral Therapy (IV)
Dance/Movement Therapy (IV)
Exercise (IV)
Herbal Therapies (IV)

Imagery (IV)
Lifestyle Change (IV)
Yoga (IV)

See also
Anger (II)
Cancer (II)
Gingko (III)
Heart and Blood Vessel Conditions (II)
Pain (II)
Premenstrual Syndrome (PMS) (II)

DIABETES

Diabetes is characterized by an elevated concentration of glucose in the bloodstream and/or a deficiency of insulin leading to long-term complications involving the eyes, kidneys, nerves, and blood vessels. Syndrome X (insulin resistance) has also been linked to diabetes as well as to cardiovascular conditions and obesity (Cichoke, 1997).

At least 13 million Americans are believed to be diabetic, but up to half of them do not know it. A simple glucose test can reveal the condition. Low magnesium levels may predict diabetes (Brancati & Kao, 1997).

Autogenic Training

In one study (Gohr, Ropcke, Pistor, & Eggers, 1997), a group of 21 youngsters age 9 to 14 years with diabetes mellitus type I attended an 11-week course in autogenic training. After training, five scales and one second-rank factor on the Multidimensional Questionnaire for Children showed significant changes. Significant reduction was observed in "need for aggressive forms of dominance behavior," "feeling of submission with respect to others," "emotional lability," and "tendency for dependence on adults." A significant increase occurred in the scale measuring "self-confidence regarding one's own meaning, decisions and planning ability." In subjective ratings of training, most of the course members and their parents described fewer problems with attention, less test anxiety, and less aggression and nervousness.

Biofeedback

McGrady (1996) randomized 10 males and 8 females with diabetes (type I) to either 12 sessions of biofeedback and relaxation therapy or their usual regimen. All participants were asked to record their blood glucose levels and insulin dosages daily and remained under the care of their physician. They all had blood drawn for biologic indicators of blood glucose and completed psychological inventories measuring anxiety, hassles, and depression. All participants were retested 4 weeks and 3 months after baseline treatment or control. Biofeedback-assisted relaxation was associated with a decrease in blood glucose, as indicated by self-report and biologic assay, for more than half of the participants. The researcher concluded that persons exhibiting depression are less likely to benefit from biofeedback-assisted relaxation and that lengthy, complicated treatment protocols have a negative effect on participant performance.

Exercise

Manson and colleagues (1992) found evidence that men who exercised at least once a week reduced their risk of developing non-insulin-dependent diabetes mellitus (NIDDM). Risk decreased with frequency of exercise. The inverse relation of exercise to risk of NIDDM was especially pronounced in overweight men. Their research suggests that increased physical activity may be a promising approach to primary prevention of NIDDM because it reduces excess weight and body fat and helps the body handle sugars more normally. Laboratory research indicates that exercise also makes body cells more sensitive to insulin.

Exercise and Dietary Fish

Dunstan and colleagues (1997) studied the effect of moderate aerobic exercise and the incorporation of fish into a low-fat diet on serum lipids and glycemic control in people with dyslipidemic NIDDM. They found that a reduced fat diet incorporating one daily fish meal reduces serum triglycerides and increases HDL2 cholesterol in this population. Associated deterioration in glycemic control (as measured by self-monitoring of blood glucose) was prevented by a concomitant program of moderate exercise.

Food and Supplements

According to Barnard and colleagues (1994), diabetes can be controlled without insulin or any medication by following a low-fat, low-cholesterol, high-complex-carbohydrate, high-fiber diet combined with daily aerobic exercise. In the study, 652 men and women, all diagnosed with type II diabetes, attended the Pritikin Longevity Center's 26-day live-in program. Seventy-six percent of the participants reduced their blood glucose levels to the normal range within 3 weeks. The second part of the study involved 197 people who were taking oral hypoglycemic agents. Seventy percent were able to discontinue their medication, and their glucose levels decreased to the normal range within 3 weeks.

The third group in the study consisted of 212 participants taking insulin injections. After 26 days, 39% were able to discontinue insulin injections. Additionally, participants in all three groups reduced their cholesterol levels by more than 20% over the 26 days. The researchers stated the diet and exercise approach not only controls diabetes but also significantly reduces the risk factors associated with cardiovascular disease. On the average, people with diabetes die 10 years earlier than those without the condition due to premature cardiovascular disease, especially heart attack and stroke.

Compared with more buoyant low-density lipoprotein (LDL), dense LDL (D-LDL) is more susceptible to oxidation and less readily protected from oxidation by antioxidant enrichment. Diets enriched with monounsaturated fatty acids (MUFAs) were particularly effective in protecting D-LDL from oxidation. Individuals with non-insulin-independent diabetes mellitus (NIIDM) frequently have increased amounts of D-LDL. Garg and colleagues (1988) compared a high-carbohydrate diet with a monounsaturated fat diet (MUFD) for people with NIIDM. Participants were randomly assigned to receive first one diet, then the other, each for 28 days, while on a metabolic ward. The MUFD lunch included a main dish of chicken breast sautéed in olive oil with seasonings and a small serving of rice, lettuce salad with olive oil and lemon juice dressing, bread, peaches, and iced tea.

The most pronounced difference in results between the two diets was the effect on total triglycerides (25% lower on the MUFD). The MUFD also excelled in raising good cholesterol (HDL) 13% and in lowering blood sugar levels and daily insulin requirements for most participants. Total cholesterol and bad LDL cholesterol did not differ significantly. The results suggest that partial replacement of complex carbohydrates with a diet higher in fat is beneficial and more palatable.

Salmeron and colleagues (1997) found that people, especially women, who eat high-glycemic-index foods like white bread, white rice, and potatoes and do not also include whole or less refined grains are at risk for non-insulin-dependent diabetes mellitus. The researchers' findings support the hypothesis that there is an increased risk of NIDDM associated with a high glycemic load and low cereal-fiber content diet.

Bitter Melon

Two ounces of bitter melon juice from the bitter melon (balscem pear), long used in folk medicine as a remedy for diabetes, has been shown in clinical trials to improve glucose tolerance (Srivastava et al., 1993; Welihinda et al., 1982).

Chromium

Anderson and colleagues (1997) reported on the effect of chromium picolinate taken two times per day. The researchers divided 180 men and women diagnosed with type II diabetes in three groups: a placebo group, a 100-mcg chromium picolinate group, and a 500-mcg chromium picolinate group. The two chromium picolinate groups showed lower values on tests of fasting glucose, 2-hour insulin, and plasma total cholesterol.

The data provided evidence that supplemental chromium had significant beneficial effects on glucose, insulin, and cholesterol variables in men and women with type II diabetes.

Fenugreek

Fenugreek seeds show significant antidiabetic effects in clinical and experimental studies. Defatted fenugreek seed powder given twice daily at a 50-g dose to people with insulin-dependent diabetes resulted in significant reduction in fasting blood sugar and improved results on the glucose tolerance test (Sharma, Raghuram, & Rao, 1990). These results suggest that fenugreek seeds or defatted fenugreek powder should be considered as part of the diet for those with diabetes.

Onions and Garlic

Onions and garlic have demonstrated the ability to help lower blood sugar levels. Experimental and clinical evidence supports the theory that allyl proply disulphide lowers glucose levels by competing with insulin for insulin-inactivating sites in the liver. The results are similar in both raw and boiled onion extracts (Augusti, 1996; Sharma, 1977; Sheela & Augusti, 1992). The cardiovascular effects (lowering blood pressure and cholesterol) provide further support for the liberal use of onions and garlic by people with diabetes (Murray, 1994).

Vitamins A and E

Reaven, Grasse, and Barnett (1996) evaluated the effect of supplementation with vitamin E (1,600 IU/day) or probucol alone and in combination with a monosaturated fatty acid diet with 12 NIIDM participants.

In both the vitamin E and probucol-supplemented groups, the benefit of adding MU-FAs was greatest for D-LDL.

People with diabetes face an increased risk of atherosclerosis, or hardening of the arteries, which can be curbed with high doses of vitamin E (1,200 IU/day). In a placebo-controlled, randomized study conducted by Fuller and colleagues (1996), the supplemented group (including people with both type I and type II diabetes) had significant reductions in LDL oxidation. In the study, 52 healthy volunteers were given somatostatin, a drug that stops natural insulin secretion. Blood sugar levels were measured while insulin and glucose were being administered. Participant dietary surveys revealed that the more vitamin A reported, the more effective insulin was in controlling blood sugar (Facchini, 1996). This suggests that vitamin A may help control blood sugar.

Vitamin C

Ting and colleagues (1996) found that vitamin C improves vascular reactivity in NIDDM. Their findings support the hypothesis that nitric oxide inactivation by oxygen-derived free radicals contributes to abnormal vascular reactivity in diabetes.

Herbs

Bearberry, Goldenseal, Mistletoe, and Tarragon

Bearberry, goldenseal, mistletoe, and tarragon counter diabetic symptoms hyperphagia and polydipsia (Swanston-Flatt, Day, Bailey, & Flatt, 1989).

Cayenne

Tandan and colleagues (1992) used a topical cream containing capsaicin for 22 individuals with chronic severe painful diabetic neuropathy who were unresponsive or intolerant of drug therapies. Controls were rubbed with a vehicle cream. The treatment group showed a statistically significant improvement.

Evening Primrose Oil

Evening primrose oil was used by Tulloch, Smellie, and Buck (1994) to test its effectiveness in reducing urine calcium excretion in animal-induced diabetes. The researchers found that urine calcium excretion was significantly less in the primrose oil–fed rats during both the prediabetic phase and the diabetic phase compared with the rats on the normal diet. These results indicate that evening primrose oil, a rich source of gamma-linolenic acid, helps to reduce urine calcium excretion in diabetic rats. The researchers suggest that dietary modifications with long-chain omega-6 and omega-3 fatty acids might be a useful adjunct in the treatment of idiopathic hypercalciuric urolithiasis.

Ginseng

Ginseng is an adaptogen that can help the body fight fatigue and stress. Sotaniemi and colleagues (1995) conducted a study of 36 volunteers with newly diagnosed type II diabetes mellitus. Participants were given 100 to 200 mg per day of ginseng or a placebo for 8 weeks. The herb produced no side effects and was associated with improved psychophysical performance, elevated mood, lowered fasting blood glucose levels, and lower body weight when compared with typical levels of these indicators in the control group. The study found that 200 mg of ginseng enhanced physical activity.

Licorice

Basso and colleagues (1994) found that licorice extract ameliorated postural hypotension (quick drop in blood pressure when moving from a prone to sitting and/or standing position) caused by diabetic autonomic neuropathy.

Yoga

Changes in blood glucose and glucose tolerance were investigated by Jain, Uppal, Bhatnagar, and Talukdar (1993). They used an oral glucose tolerance test (OGTT) after 40 days of yoga therapy in 149 non-insulin-dependent diabetics. The response to yoga was categorized according to a severity scale index based on area index total under OGTT curve. One hundred and four participants showed a fair to good response. There was a significant reduction in hyperglycemia and oral hypoglycemia.

CAROLYN CHAMBERS CLARK

See
Autogenic Training (IV)
Biofeedback (IV)
Exercise (IV)
Herbal Therapies (IV)

See also
Heart and Blood Vessel Conditions (II)
Syndrome X (II)

DIABETIC RETINOPATHY

Lanthony and Cosson (1988) investigated the use of *Ginkgo biloba* extract in a 6-month double-blind trial with 29 individuals suffering from diabetic retinopathy. Individuals treated with gingko showed a significant improvement compared to the control group. These findings corroborate the expected pharmacological actions of gingko on diabetic retinopathy.

CAROLYN CHAMBERS CLARK

See also
   Diabetes (II)
   Gingko (III)

DIARRHEA

Nonspecific chronic diarrhea, or "toddler's diarrhea," has been associated with fruit juice consumption, especially juices high in fructose and sorbitol. In the United States, 11% of healthy preschoolers consume 12 oz or more per day of fruit juice, which is excessive (Dennison, 1997).

CAROLYN CHAMBERS CLARK

DIARRHEA, ACUTE CHILDHOOD

In the developing world, there are an estimated 5 million deaths annually attributed to diarrhea in children under the age of 5. Dehydration from acute diarrhea is a significant factor in childhood morbidity and mortality in the United States as well. It is estimated that 17 million children under the age of 5 experience up to 37 million cases of diarrhea resulting in nearly 4 million physician visits annually. It accounts for the hospitalization of 220,000 children under 5 and 400 deaths annually. It is also estimated that diarrhea is responsible for 10% of preventable postnatal deaths, especially among disadvantaged families (Reis, Goepp, Katz, & Santosham, 1994; Cohen et al., 1995). In Springfield, MA, dehydration was the leading cause of death in infants in 1992.

Oral Rehydration Therapy

In light of this world-wide problem, the World Health Organization (WHO) (1984) developed recommendations for the treatment of acute diarrhea which included oral rehydration therapy (ORT). ORT combines the use of a balanced oral solution of electrolytes and carbohydrates with early refeeding. ORT is noninvasive, inexpensive, can be readily taught to the child-caregiver and performed in the home. Prompt and appropriate therapy prevents the progression to severe dehydration and has been credited with dramatically reducing the death rate from infectious diarrhea in developing countries.

In response, the American Academy of Pediatrics (1985) published recommendations for the use of oral rehydration solutions (ORS) to treat mild (< 5%) and moderate (6 to 9%) dehydration. Despite numerous studies done in this country supporting the efficacy of ORT (Cohen et al., 1995), physicians in the United States have not universally accepted its use. In 1991 (Snyder) fewer than 30% of surveyed physicians advised the use of ORS and fewer than 50% advised prompt refeeding (Bezerra, Stathos, Duncan, & Gaines, 1992). A 1994 survey of pediatricians by Reis, Goepp, Katz, and Santosham, found that 97% used ORS for mild dehydration only. Moderate dehydration and vomiting were identified by one third of the pediatricians as contraindications to ORS, and less than 50% of the pediatricians adhere to the AAP recommendations for prompt refeeding. In addition, only 3% recommended direct use of a spoon or syringe for specific measurements of fluid to be given, as is recommended by AAP guidelines.

The AAP recommendations (1985) included the use of ORS with sodium concentrations ranging from 75 to 90 MEg/L for rehydration, and a separate solution with sodium concentrations ranging from 40-60 MEg/L for maintenance hydration. Cohen and colleagues (1995) studied the efficacy of using a single solution by comparing results obtained from two commonly used solutions in the rehydration of infants with mild to moderate dehydration caused by acute diarrhea in the United States. Pedialyte and Infalyte were the solutions used for both the rehydration and maintenance phase. Both of these solutions fall below the AAP recommendations for sodium concentrations; each containing 50 and 75 MMoL, respectively. Cohen and colleagues found that infants in each of the study groups (pedialyte and infalyte) were successfully rehydrated using ORS without the use of intravenous fluids. No significant differences were detected between the two ORS groups in time to rehydration or percentage of weight gain after rehydration.

Each infant's fluid deficit was estimated by multiplying the admission weight by the estimated percent dehydration and a randomly assigned solution was offered in a volume twice as great as the estimated fluid deficit over the next 8 hours. Rehydration was judged clinically by the presence of tears, return of skin turgor, moist mucus membranes, weight gain, increased urine output, decreased urine specific gravity, correction of acidosis and/or other electrolyte abnormalities and lowering of blood urea nitrogen. After rehydration was achieved, early refeeding was begun.

During the maintenance phase breast milk or a soy-based formula in a volume of 120 ml/kg/day was offered. In addition, children over 1 year were given their routine solid diet with the exception of lactose-containing food. After each diarrhea stool, a volume of oral rehydration solution equal to the volume of stool was offered. The mean time to rehydration was 15–16 hours in this study—prolonged compared to the AAP's recommendation of 4–6 hours. They believe their rehydration evaluation may have been prolonged due to the reliance of blood tests obtained at 12 hours and weights obtained at 16 hours before assessing "rehydration." They also identified the labor-intensive effort required by ORT from parents and the fact that most of the rehydration periods began in the evening into the night when both parent and child were interested in resting as well as rehydrating.

Homeopathy

Jacobs, Jiménez, Gloyd, Gale, and Cruthers (1994) performed a study in Nicaragua to determine whether homeopathy is useful in the treatment of acute diarrhea. They acknowledged that ORT can prevent death from dehydration, but it does not reduce the duration of individual episodes.

Infants and children with mild to moderate signs of dehydration were included in this study. Children with severe dehydration were transferred to the hospital for intravenous therapy and were not included in this study.

An experienced homeopathic practitioner from the United States interviewed and examined each child. Information about the nature of the stools, abdominal pain and/or vomiting, the mood and temperament of the child, degree of thirst and appetite, presence of a fever, abdominal bloating, sleep disturbance, amount of perspiration, and other signs or symptoms were collected and entered into a computerized homeopathic expert system (RADAR, Archimed, Inc., Namur, Belgium). The results were used to prescribe an individualized homeopathic medicine for each child. Only one remedy was prescribed for each child for the duration of the study.

Eighteen different homeopathic medicines were prescribed to children in the study. Podophyllum, Chamomilla, and Arsenicum album were the three most commonly prescribed remedies in nearly 60% of the cases.

Jacobs, Jiménez, Gloyd, Gate, and Cruthers found that the treatment group had a statistically significant ($p < .05$) decrease in duration of diarrhea, defined as the number of days until there were less than 3 unformed stools daily for 2 consecutive days. There was also a significant difference ($p < .05$) in the number of stools per day between the two groups after 72 hours of treatment. They conclude that children treated with homeopathic remedies as an adjunct to ORT had a 15% decrease in duration of the episode of diarrhea. This may have clinical significance by decreasing dehydration, post-diarrheal malnutrition, and reduce the burden to the mother or caregiver.

In each one of the previously discussed studies, etiology of the diarrhea was *not* a significant variable, except in Cohen and colleagues' study. Children with cholera and related disorders, requiring high sodium content and an additional source of fresh water, were excluded in his study.

ORT has been shown to be an effective therapy for the treatment of acute diarrhea in children. Research studies show that Pedialyte and Infalyte are effective oral rehydration solutions for both the rehydration and maintenance phase in noncholera diarrhea. When individually prescribed homeopathic remedies were given as an adjunct to ORT to Nicaraguan children, there was a 15% decrease in duration of the episode of diarrhea. Jacobs, Jiménez, Gloyd, Gate, and Cruthers' study was designed to see *if* homeopathic treatments had an effect on acute childhood diarrhea, not how they worked. This is one of the first research reports to appear in a medical journal that scientifically demonstrates the effect of combined application of allopathic and homeopathic knowledge.

MARGO A. DROHAN

DIVERTICULAR DISEASE

Aldoori and colleagues (1994) studied a cohort of 47,888 American men. Total dietary fiber intake was inversely related to the risk of diverticular disease after adjustment for age, energy-adjusted total fat intake, and physical activity. The inverse relationship was primarily due to fruit and vegetable fiber. The prospective data supported the hypothesis that a diet low in total dietary fiber increases the incidence of symptomatic diverticular disease. The study also provided evidence that the combination of high intake of total fat or red meat and a diet low in total dietary fiber especially augments risk.

CAROLYN CHAMBERS CLARK

See also
Fiber (III)

EATING DISORDERS

Eating disorders have existed since ancient times. They vary in frequency, manifestations, and possible motivation. Sociocultural factors may influence the frequency and type of disorder (Bemporad, 1996).

Anorexia nervosa, or self-induced starvation, is believed to result from eating-related family conflict (Robin, Siegel, & Moye, 1995), sexual abuse, and parental care. Troop and Treasure (1997) found a higher rate of childhood helplessness and a lower rate of childhood mastery in women with eating disorders. There may also be an association between eating disorders and running in women. In one study, Estok and Rudy (1996) found that 25% of the women who ran 30 or more miles per week had Eating Attitude Test scores indicating a high risk for anorexia.

The condition afflicts 0.5% to 1.0% of female adolescents in the United States. The course is chronic in 50% of cases, leading to substantial bone loss with osteoporotic fractures after a few years of amenorrhea (Maugars et al., 1996), and to insulin resistance and overt diabetes mellitus for others (Koffler & Kisch, 1996).

Because individuals with eating disorders are often of normal weight, they can sometimes hide their conditions. Studies generally report decreased concentrations of phosphorus for both bulimia and anorexia nervosa. Elevated serum phosphorus levels may serve as an additional objective marker for the presence of bulimia (Bonne, Gur, & Berry, 1995), as may total body potassium. Powers, Tyson, Stevens, and Heal (1995) found that even when serum potassium was normal in anorectic individuals, total body potassium may be low, which can lead to heart arrhythmias and other physiological abnormalities.

Cognitive-Related Treatments

A cognitive-behavioral program for the treatment of anorexia is based on the assumptions that anorexia, including food phobias, develops as a way of coping with life stresses. Such a program is aimed at confronting fears and avoidance behavior; identifying deficient problem-solving skills, especially in the interpersonal arena; and cultivating new problem-solving skills (Kleifield, Wagner, & Halmi, 1996).

Treasure and colleagues (1995) compared the use of cognitive analytical therapy program with an educational-behavioral therapy program. Thirty participants were randomly assigned to one or the other program. Both programs led to an improvement in nutritional outcome in two thirds of the cases.

Cooper, Coker, and Fleming (1996) tested the use of a supervised, highly structured self-help manual with 82 bulimic individuals. For the 67 individuals who completed the self-help course, the frequency of bulimic episodes and self-induced vomiting decreased by 80% and 79%, respectively. Those who had a poor outcome or dropped out of treatment were more than twice as likely to have had anorexia nervosa in the past and were somewhat more likely to have a personality disorder. Clinical gains were well maintained a year later: Almost two thirds still did not induce vomiting nor have bulimic episodes.

Connors, Johnson, and Stuckey (1984) reported significant improvements in psychological functioning, including self-esteem, depression, assertiveness, and pathological attitudes about eating. The researchers used two groups of 10 normal-weight bulimic women who received short-term structured group treatment beginning 3 weeks apart. The researchers' multiple baseline design used a multifaceted treatment approach incorporating education, self-monitoring, goal setting, assertion training, relaxation, and cognitive restructuring. Women in the treatment group showed an overall reduction of 70% in binge/purge episodes.

Schneider and Agras (1985) used a cognitive-behavioral approach with 13 bulimic women, with a self-reported average of 24 self-induced vomiting episodes per week. Participants were treated in two groups that met for 16 weeks each. The primary outcome was the number of self-reported vomiting episodes. Vomiting frequency decreased to an average of 2.2 times per week (91% improvement), with seven women abstinent by the end of treatment. Significant pre- to posttreatment changes were also demonstrated on measures of depression, eating attitudes, and assertiveness. At 6-month follow-up, 11 women indicated a mean vomiting frequency of 3.8 per week.

Feldenkrais Method

Laumer, Bauer, Fichter, and Milz (1997) studied the therapeutic effect of a 9-hour Feldenkrais method "Awareness through Movement" course with 15 eating disordered individuals. Results were compared to a control group without eating disorders who did not participate in the course. The treatment group showed increased contentment with the problematic zones of their body and health, decreased feelings of helplessness, and a decreased wish to return to the security of early childhood. The

researchers suggested that these findings indicated the development of a felt sense of self, self-confidence, and a general process of maturation of the personality.

Videotape Feedback

Rushford and Ostermeyer (1997) used a videofeedback session with 18 individuals diagnosed with anorexia and 18 normal controls. Body-image distortion was evaluated before and after videofeedback. Sensation of fatness and size compared with other young women decreased significantly with videotape feedback for the treatment group.

Television and Eating Disorders

The media, especially television, play a significant social and cultural role in behavior. Verri and associates (1997) examined the influence of television on body image. Twenty-four female adolescents with eating disorders showed a psychological dependence on television (spent more time watching TV, and buying attitudes were more influenced by TV advertising than a comparable group of controls without eating disorders). The researchers concluded that, to reduce the prevalence and incidence of eating disorders among adolescents, it is appropriate to control the myths, propagated by media, TV in particular.

Dietary Intervention

Rock and Vasantharajan (1995) claim that vitamin abnormalities in individuals with eating disorders may contribute to altered neuropsychological status and the development of sequelae such as cognitive dysfunction. They examined the relationship between vitamin status and clinical indices in 13 hospitalized low-weight individuals with eating disorders. Thirty-one percent initially had riboflavin and vitamin B6 deficiencies; 23% had elevated plasma cholesterol concentrations. At discharge, thiamin, riboflavin, and vitamin B6 status indicators were normal in all cases. Suboptimal vitamin status is common in individuals with eating disorders, but can be normalized with dietary intervention.

CAROLYN CHAMBERS CLARK

See
Feldenkrais (IV)

See also
Osteoporosis (II)
Syndrome X (II)

ECTOPIC PREGNANCY

Researchers (Kendrick et al., 1997) studied the effect of douching on ectopic pregnancy in a case-control study of black women with ectopic pregnancy conducted at a major public hospital in Atlanta. The researchers found an odds ratio of ectopic pregnancy associated with douching to be 3.8. No douching behavior was found to be without risk, even among occasional users of douches. The researchers concluded that as many as 65% of the ectopic pregnancies among black women in the United States may be associated with douching.

The reasons for douching aren't completely understood but probably are related to viewing douching as a harmless activity that promotes hygiene. Less invasive means of vaginal cleansing, such as vaginal washing, is recommended. Also, women should be taught that clear, odorless vaginal secretions are normal.

CAROLYN CHAMBERS CLARK

EPILEPSY

In the United States, it's estimated that 2 million children have epilepsy. Most have seizures easily controlled by medication; however, the side effects including hyperactivity, clumsiness, aggression toward other children, upset stomach, headaches, and severe tremors, can be difficult to tolerate. Each year, up to 7,000 new cases of so-called intractable seizures, those that are difficult to control, develop in children, according to the Epilepsy Foundation of America. For these reasons, complementary treatments are often sought.

Biofeedback

Kotchoubey and colleagues (1996) carried out 20 sessions of biofeedback training with 12 drug-resistant individuals with focal epilepsy who learned to produce either negative or positive shifts of their slow cortical potentials. In the study, the mean severity of seizures, estimated as the frequency of seizures as weighted by their subjected strength, decreased significantly after training as compared to the pretraining phase. The data suggest that individuals can learn to achieve a state of cortical disfacilitation and, with progressive learning, show less fear and less motivation to produce negative shifts associated with early signs of seizure.

Environmental Interventions

Flashing lights can trigger seizures in people with epilepsy who are photosensitive (about 2% to 3% of the total epileptic population). Video games have been linked to seizures in youngsters. Television, disco strobe lights, even sunlight seen flashing through leaves while riding in a car can touch off a seizure in susceptible individuals. For that reason, photosensitive persons with epilepsy should avoid flickering lights.

Food

Ballaban-Gil and colleagues (1996) reported the use of a ketogenic (high-fat) diet with adults. In their study, heavy whipping cream was used as the base of a creamy shake. This beverage was given at each meal, and other foods consumed were carefully measured, with complex carbohydrates and simple sugars eliminated. This kind of diet is most commonly used to treat children with refractory epilepsy and was thought to be ineffective with adults. However, Ballaban-Gil and colleagues treated four adults age 22 to 29 years using this diet. All participants had generalized epilepsy or multifocal disorder and were mildly or severely cognitively impaired. All experienced fewer seizures; one experienced a 75% decrease in seizure frequency, and another dropped from one convulsion every 2 to 3 days to fewer than four a month.

Yoga

Panjawani and colleagues (1996) reported the effect of sahaja yoga meditation on seizure control and electroencephalographic alterations in 32 individuals diagnosed with idiopathic epilepsy. Participants were randomly assigned to practicing sahaja yoga for 6 months ($n = 10$), practicing exercises mimicking sahaja yoga for 6 months ($n = 10$), or a control group. Individuals in the treatment group reported a 62% decrease in seizure frequency at 3 months and a further decrease of 86% at the end of 6 months. Power spectral analysis of EEG showed a shift in frequency from 0–8 Hz to 8–20 Hz. The ratios of EEG powers in delta, theta alpha, and beta bands were increased. The percent of delta power decreased, and the percent of alpha power increased. No significant changes in any of the parameters were found in the mimic or control groups, indicating that sahaja yoga practice may bring about seizure reduction and EEG changes.

CAROLYN CHAMBERS CLARK

FAILURE TO THRIVE

Excess fruit juice consumption has been reported as a contributing factor for some children for nonorganic failure to thrive and in some children with decreased stature (Dennison, 1997).

Zinc is important in reducing infant morbidity and mortality. It helps ensure optimal birth weight (Friel et al., 1993).

CAROLYN CHAMBERS CLARK

See also
Zinc (III)

FATIGUE

A condition of being very tired as a result of physical or mental exertion. There is a loss of energy, lessened activity, and decreased response to stimulation.

CAROLYN CHAMBERS CLARK

See also
Chronic Fatigue Syndrome (II)

FIBROMYALGIA

Fibromyalgia syndrome (FMS) is characterized by a history of diffuse, widespread neuromuscular pain, fatigue, and a high incidence of multiple nonrheumatic symptoms. In 1990, the American College of Rheumatology (ACR) established a diagnostic definition for fibromyalgia with two primary criteria. According to ACR criteria, a person diagnosed with fibromyalgia must have a "history of widespread pain of at least 3 months duration," and pain in at least 11 of 18 paired tender points evidenced by digital palpation and present in all four body quadrants at time of examination (Wolfe et al., 1990). Pain usually is associated with the fibrous connective tissue areas of muscles, tendons, and ligaments. Although no definitive evidence of muscle disease has been found, ultrastructural evaluations of quadricep muscle biopsy has demonstrated pathologic degenerative changes.

Multiple nonrheumatic symptoms, often synchronous in patients with FMS, fall into the four general categories of neurological, smooth muscle dysmotility, increased skeletal muscle tone, and inflammatory symptomology. Specific symptoms include rhinitis, cystitis, tension and migraine headache, irritable bowel syndrome, chest pain, fatigue, affective disorder such as depression, esophageal dysmotility, dysmenorrhea, cognitive dysfunction, peripheral neuropathy, hypersensitivity to cold, Raynaud's disease, sleep disturbance, and parethesias. Mitral valve prolapse has been found in 75% of patients with FMS (Pellegrino et al., 1989).

There is indication that fibromyalgia occurs at higher frequencies in familial groups and that there may be a genetic tendency toward its development. Two classifications of FMS are commonly recognized: primary and secondary. Secondary FMS occurs after a triggering event such as an emotional or physical trauma or after a viral illness. With primary FMS, no specific triggering event or associated illness can be identified.

Differential diagnoses include rheumatoid arthritis, polymyalgia rheumatica, polymyositis/dermatomyositis, systemic lupus erythematosus, hypothyroidism, hypo- and hyper-parathyroidism, viral hepatitis, human immunodeficiency virus infection, parasitic infections, metastatic carcinoma, multiple sclerosis, myasthenia gravis, amyotrophic lateral sclerosis, myofascial pain syndrome, yeast infections, alcohol myopathy, and, most difficult of all, muscle pain of psychogenic origin. Chronic fatigue syndrome and fibromyalgia are, at this time, considered as possible variations of the same disorder.

Differential Diagnosis by Etiology

Neurologic—Multiple sclerosis, myesthenia gravis, amyotrophic lateral sclerosis, myofascial pain syndrome, alcohol myopathy.

Infectious—Viral hepatitis, human immunodeficiency virus infection, parasitis infections, yeast infections.

Cardiovascular—Chest pain of undetermined origin.

Endocrinologic—Hypothyroidism, hypoparathyroidism, hyperthyroidism.

Rheumatologic—Rheumatoid arthritis, polymyalgia rheumatica, polymyositis, dermatositis, systemic lupus erythematosus.

Metabolic—Vitamin and mineral disorders.

Psychological—Psychogenic muscle pain, cognitive processing disorder.

It is widely reported that there are no specific biochemical tests for diagnosing FMS; however, in 1996 Samborski and colleagues were able to confirm the diagnosis of FMS in 60 patients by findings of significantly decreased levels of serotonin, somatomedin C, calcitonin, and prostaglandin E 2, and significantly increased levels of prolactin when compared with healthy controls. Electroencephalographic findings indicate that people with FMS experience about 60% alphawave intrusion into slower stage IV deltawave sleep, compared with 25% alphawave intrusion rate into control subjects (Boissevian & McCain, 1991).

History

Muscle aches and pains have been noted since earliest times. One of the earliest recorded references to musculoskeletal aches and pains was made by the great Greek physician Hippocrates about 400 B.C. Hippocrates used the word *rheumatismos* to describe generalized aches and pains that occur throughout the body. Over the years since Hippocrates, the condition of bodily aches and pains has been given many names, often depending on the description of the disease process that is occurring ("muscle gelling"), the etiology of the condition ("occupational myalgia"), or the location of the condition ("soft tissue rheumatism"). Physician and author Paul Davidson identified 64 different names for the aches and pains we now call fibromyalgia (Davidson, 1991). The term "fibrositis," the most immediate and most commonly recognized predecessor of the term "fibro-myalgia," was suggested by William Gowers in an article in *The British Medical Journal* in 1904. Believing that there was inflammation present in the muscles that would explain the aches reported by patients, Gowers proposed that the condition was the result of an "inflammation of the fibrous tissue" that had not yet been discovered or identified (Davidson, 1991).

Since Gowers there has been a great deal of debate as to what to name the condition of diffuse muscular aches and pains. In 1936, Hench introduced the term "fibromyalgia," meaning pain in fibrous tissue, to replace the term "fibrositis." This change of terminology removes the concept of inflammation from the name of the condition. In 1976, Drs. Hugh A. Smythe and Harvey Moldofsky proposed that fibromyalgia was the occurrence of exaggerated muscle tenderness in specific locations that were caused or exacerbated by sleep disturbances.

Studies of morbidity conducted around the world have found that the diagnosis of fibrositis or fibromyalgia occur in from 5% to 33% of individuals, depending upon from where the study is reported. In the United States, it is estimated that from 3 million to 6 million people have symptoms of FMS. The age range for diagnosis of FMS is 34 to 53 years.

LESLIE ELLIS

FRACTURES

Dawson-Hughes and colleagues (1997) showed that nutrients can stave off osteoporosis in men and reduce fractures. Inexpensive daily supplements of calcium and vitamin D can significantly cut the risk of fractures. In one study, scientists at the Jean Mayer USDA Human Nutrition Research Center on Aging at Tufts University tracked the results of moderate supplementation with the two nutrients in a group of 389 healthy men and women age 65 and older over a 3-year period. Half the participants received daily supplements of 500 mg of calcium and 700 IU of vitamin D; the other half took placebos.

Those receiving the supplements fared better when measured for bone loss that commonly occurs with age and leads to osteoporosis. They did much better when it came to broken bones. Over the course of the study, nearly 13% of the placebo group suffered fractures, compared to less than 6% of the group receiving supplements.

Participants in the study had been getting slightly more than 700 mg of calcium per day from their diets alone. With the added supplements, those who showed beneficial results obtained about 1,200 mg of calcium per day, an amount that matches the National Institute of Medicine's new recommended intake of calcium for persons over 50 years of age.

CAROLYN CHAMBERS CLARK

See also
   Aging (II)
   Hip Fractures (II)
   Osteoporosis (II)

HEADACHE

Headaches are the most commonly treated medical complaint. There are many different types of headaches, and they don't always fit into neat clinical diagnoses. Chronic daily headache (CDH) accounts for 40% of the complaints seen in headache clinics (Matthew, 1993). CDH includes chronic tension headache, migraine with interparoxysmal headache, transformed migraine, evolutive migraine, mixed headache syndrome, and tension-vascular headache. Headache pain relief requires a multifaceted approach, and there are numerous such approaches available.

Biofeedback and Cognitive-Behavioral Therapy

Kropp and colleagues (1997) studied the use of biofeedback and cognitive-behavioral therapy with 28 people diagnosed with migraine headache. Half received biofeedback followed by cognitive-behavioral therapy; the other half received cognitive-behavioral therapy followed by biofeedback. In the study, the effects of receiving biofeedback first were significantly better than the reverse order. The researchers concluded that the application of biofeedback helps the migraine sufferer recognize the influence of thoughts and emotions on bodily reactions, preparing the way for successful cognitive treatment.

Biofeedback and Relaxation Therapy

Arena, Bruno, Hannah, and Meador (1995) studied the use of a 12-session trapezius EMG biofeedback training regimen ($n = 10$) and compared its effects with a standard 12-session frontal EMG biofeedback training regimen ($n = 8$), and a standard 7-session progressive muscle relaxation therapy regimen ($n = 8$). After 3 months, posttreatment assessment showed clinically significant decreases in overall headache activity (50% or greater) in 50% of the participants in frontal biofeedback,

100% in the trapezius biofeedback group, and 37.5% in the relaxation therapy group. Chi-squared analyses revealed that the trapezius biofeedback group showed more effective significant clinical improvement than the other two groups.

Chiropractic

In a prospective randomized controlled trial with a blinded observer, 53 individuals suffering from frequent headaches who fulfilled the International Headache Society's criteria for cervicogenic headache (excluding radiological criteria) were recruited from 450 headache sufferers who responded to newspaper advertisements (Nilsson, Christensen, & Hartvigsen, 1997). After randomization, 28 participants received high-velocity, low-amplitude cervical manipulation twice a week for 3 weeks. The remaining 25 participants received low-level laser in the upper cervical region and deep friction massage (including trigger points) in the lower cervical/upper thoracic region twice a week for 3 weeks. The use of analgesics decreased by 36% (statistically significant) in the manipulation group but not in the laser group. Headache intensity decreased by 36% (statistically significant) per incident in the manipulation group, compared to 17% in the soft-tissue group.

Estrogen

Women who take estrogen after menopause or extended oral contraceptive use are more likely to have headaches and temporomandibular disorder (TMD). In a study examining the group health plan records of 1982–1992, 1,291 postmenopausal women over age 40 referred for TMD were compared with 5,164 age-matched women not referred for TMD treatment. The results were significant. Twenty-eight percent of the TMD sufferers had filled a prescription for estrogen in the 9 months before referral compared to 19% of the controls. Those who had used estrogen replacement were 77% more likely than nonusers to be referred for TMD treatment. When 1,400 35- to 45-year-old women with TMD were matched with 5,600 controls, those who used oral contraceptives had a 20% greater chance of suffering from TMD than those who did not (DeAngelis, 1994).

Food and Supplements

Detection and removal of allergic/intolerant foods can reduce headache symptoms. The most common allergens are milk, wheat, chocolate, food additives (MSG by itself or in foods like bouillon cubes, some canned foods/soups, and soy sauces), artificial sweeteners, tomatoes, and fish (Murray, 1994). Chocolate, aged cheese (e.g., cheddar or blue), beer, scotch, champagne, red wine, and aspartame can precipitate a headache because they contain compounds known as vasoactive amines, which cause blood vessels to expand. Too much caffeine (coffee, tea, colas) can also cause a rebound headache as blood vessels dilate (Murray, 1994).

Magnesium may be a useful supplement to prevent and treat headaches. One of the key functions of magnesium is to maintain the tone of blood vessels. Low magnesium levels have been implicated in chronic daily headaches (Gallai et al., 1994; Ramadan et al., 1989; Swanson, 1988). Low brain tissue magnesium concentrations have been found in people with migraines, indicating a need for supplementation.

Aloisi, Marrelli, and Porto (1997) treated children suffering from migraine with and without aura in a headache-free period. A 20-day treatment with oral magnesium picolate normalized the magnesium balance in 90% of the children. After treatment, a reduced P100 amplitude in visual-evoked potential confirmed the inverse correlation with serum magnesium level. The study suggested that higher visual-evoked potential amplitude and low brain magnesium level can both be an expression of neuronal hyperexcitability of the visual pathways and the lowered threshold for migraine attacks.

Magnesium deficiency has also been linked to mitral (heart) valve prolapse, which in turn is linked to migraines because it leads to a change in blood platelets, causing them to release vasoactive substances. Eighty-five percent of people with mitral valve prolapse have a chronic magnesium deficiency that can be improved with supplementation (Galland, Baker, & McLellan, 1986).

McCarty (1996) theorized that magnesium taurate and fish oil could prove useful in preventing headaches. Clinical investigations and known drug activity suggest that neuronal hyperexcitation, cortical spreading depression, vasospasm, platelet activation, and sympathetic hyperactivity often play a role in the development of migraine. Taurine and magnesium could dampen hyperexcitation, counteract vasospasm, increase tolerance to focal hypoxia, stabilize platelets, and lessen sympathetic outflow. Fish oil, too, has promising qualities, especially platelet stabilization and antivasospastic action. McCarty suggested that these two nutritional measures have particular merit because of their versatility, safety, lack of side effects, and long-term impact on vascular health.

Guided Imagery

Ilacqua (1994) compared guided imagery to biofeedback in the treatment of migraine headache. Forty men and women with migraine headache diagnosis at Sunnybrook Health Sciences Centre in Toronto comprised the sample. They were randomly assigned to six sessions of training in guided imagery or biofeedback or a control group. The results did not reveal significant reduction in migraine activity in either treatment group, but subjective reports favored guided imagery for its positive influence on the perception of migraine pain.

Headache Medication Use

The overuse of headache medication can lead to analgesic-rebound headache. In one study (Isler, 1982) sufferers of migraine headaches who took more than 30 analgesic tablets per month had twice as many headache days per month as those who took fewer than 30 tablets. In another study, 70 people with daily headaches who were consuming 14 or more analgesic tablets per week were told to discontinue their use (Rapoport et al., 1985). Sixty-six percent improved after a month and 81% improved after 2 months.

Analgesic-rebound headache should be suspected in anyone with daily predictable headaches who is taking large quantities of analgesics. Analgesic medications typically contain substances in addition to the analgesic, such as caffeine or a sedative like butalbital, both of which can lead to withdrawal headaches and other symptoms including nausea, abdominal cramps, diarrhea, restlessness, sleeplessness, and anxiety. Regular use of ergotamine is also associated with an increase in headache intensity upon cessation of the medication (Murray, 1994).

Herbs

Murphy, Hepinstall, and Mitchell (1988) assessed the use of feverfew (*Tanacetum parthenium*) in a randomized, double-blind, placebo-controlled crossover study. After a 1-month single-blind placebo trial, 72 volunteers were randomly assigned for 4 months to either one capsule of dried feverfew leaves a day or a placebo capsule, then transferred to the other treatment for another 4 months. Diary cards were used to chart frequency and severity of migraine attacks and were issued every 2 months. Efficacy of each treatment was assessed by visual analog scores. Feverfew was associated with a reduction in the mean number and severity of migraines, degree of vomiting, and a significant improvement in visual analog scores.

Lifestyle Factors

Pharmacological treatment of headache overlooks the underlying precipitating factors, including food allergies, low magnesium levels, emotional changes (especially letdown after stress) and anger, hormonal changes, too little or too much sleep, exhaustion, poor posture, muscle tension, eyestrain, withdrawal from caffeine or other drugs that constrict blood vessels, and continuous use of headphones or plastic hearing aids.

Muscle Tension

In one study, 112 young female headache sufferers were tested and compared with 31 headache-free controls when all were free from headache (Lipchik & LeResche, 1994). Subjects with headaches reported greater muscle tenderness than controls. Those with chronic tension headaches experienced the most tenderness, followed by those with migraines (without aura), those with episodic tension headaches, and those with migraines with aura. All the participants with chronic tension headaches had muscle tenderness in at least one muscle, compared to 52% of the controls.

Reflexology

Although samples were small, Kesselring (1994) reported the findings from several reflexology studies that showed the method was as effective as medication for headache. The advantage of reflexology was that users had fewer side effects.

Smoking

Smoking has been associated with some types of headache. Hannerz (1997) compared 27 women with episodic cluster headache with 27 age-matched women with migraine headache. The extent of smoking was significantly greater in the cluster headache group than in the migraine group, both as to the number of cigarettes smoked per day and the years of smoking.

CAROLYN CHAMBERS CLARK

See also
   Allergies (II)
   Caffeine (III)

HEAD INJURY

Damage to the head and brain can occur due to internal or external events. Both music and apitherapy in treatment situations have been reported in the research literature.

Music

Eslinger (1995) reported the effect of music on 15 pairs of adults diagnosed with chronic brain damage from traumatic brain injury or stroke. Measures of self-perception, empathy, emotion processing, and depression were used to track this effect over a 3-month period; a stratified randomized procedure was used to assign participants to either treatment or control group. All participants were given psychological testing prior to entering the study. The treatment group received a 10-week music therapy–based intervention, and the control group received casual and nonorganized socialization. Music therapy was structured to address psychosocial adjustment and group process. All participants were tested after 10 weeks, then 15 weeks later. Measures included the Competency Rating Scale; Emotional Empathy measure; Hogan's Cognitive Empathy Inventory; Profile of Nonverbal Sensitivity (PONS); Beck Depression Inventory; Emotional Expression through Videotaping; and clinician ratings on the Music, Cognition, and Social Behavior scale. The neuropsychological measures showed a statistically significant improvement in emotional empathy measures in the treatment group. The depression measure showed a positive change, but it was not significant. The Music, Cognition, and Social Behavior scale showed statistically significant improvement for each individual in the music group. The social support group also showed improvements in emotional empathy, but not in depression.

Apitherapy

Ludianskii (1990) reported studying 856 people with brain trauma. Three syn-dromes of dissociated hypotension of the cerebrospinal fluid (CSF) were described: (1) at the level of the Magendi-Luschka openings, (2) at the level of the aquduct of Sylvius, and (3) at the level of the third ventricle. The parameters of the progressive course and early identification made it possible to begin rehabilitation. Special attention was given to apitherapy, phytococktails, and instillations of special cocktails for controlling the dissociation between CSF hypotension and hydrocephaly. Rehabilitation made it possible to significantly reduce the incidence of crises indicative of the decompensation of brain injury.

CAROLYN CHAMBERS CLARK

See
Apitherapy (IV)

See also
Phytochemicals (III)
Stroke (II)

HEART AND BLOOD VESSEL CONDITIONS

The human heart beats millions of times during a lifetime. Heart problems vary widely in their nature and severity. Many types of conditions are closely linked to diet and lifestyle. The metaphysical basis for heart problems includes serious emotional problems of a long-standing nature, lack of joy, rejection of life, and belief in strain and pressure. Research has recently provided support that mental stress affects heart conditions. Gullette and colleagues (1997) investigated whether high levels of generalized emotional arousal trigger an obstruction of the inflow of arterial blood (ischemia) in persons with coronary artery disease (CAD). One hundred and thirty two participants underwent electrocardiographic (ECG) monitoring and kept diaries of positive and negative emotions. Findings included: mental stressors such as tension, frustration, and sadness are common triggers of myocardial ischemia in persons with stable CAD.

Everson and colleagues (1996) found that high hopelessness predicted incidence of myocardial infarction (heart attack) in a population-based sample of middle-aged men. Participants were 2,428 men, age 42 to 60, from the Kuopio Ischemic Heart Disease study, an ongoing longitudinal study of unestablished psychosocial risk factors for heart disease and other outcomes.

Biofeedback

Forty individuals with advanced heart failure were randomly assigned to either biofeedback-relaxation or a control group. Both groups had comparable clinical profiles at baseline. Those undergoing biofeedback-relaxation showed an increase in skin temperature of 3.1 ± 2.8 degrees Fahrenheit in the finger and 1.5 ± 5.2 degrees Fahrenheit in the foot, as well as an increase in cardiac output of 0.30 ± 0.33 L/minute, a decrease in systemic vascular resistance, and a decrease in respiratory rate of 4.5 ± 3.2 breaths/minute. No changes in any of these parameters were observed in the control group. The treatment group exhibited no changes in catecholamine levels or oxygen consumption.

Breathing

There is some evidence that unilateral forced nostril breathing (UFNB) can positively affect heart function. The rapid rate of respiration yogic breathing technique called "breath of fire," or *kapalabhatti*, employs a very shallow but rapid breath in which the abdominal region acts like a bellows. UFNB can increase end diastolic volume (Shannahoff-Khalsa & Kennedy, 1993).

Chinese Medicine

In the Chinese medicine system, the heart is associated with the nervous system and the spirit. It is believed that when the heart system is strong, the mind is clear, the emotions are positive and calm, and the spirit is strong. Joy is the main emotion associated with the heart, and the experience of joy is thought to have a beneficial effect on the heart. A lack of love and guidance during the formative years, traumatic experiences or illness, or a lack of joy can promote heart and vascular disease like arteriosclerosis. Just as there can be too little joy, there can be too much. Mania can damage the adrenal and nervous systems as well as the heart. Traditional Chinese medicine recognizes that certain flavors will stimulate the function of various organs. In this system, bitter foods are used to stimulate the heart.

Dance and Meditation

De Lone (1996) reported the use of dance and meditation for 13 women in a 10-week cardiac risk reduction program. All behavioral risk factors contributing to cardiac disease were affected. Not only was weight loss significant, but other health factors changed. By the end of the study, the group, who fit into the moderate risk profile for cardiac disease, dropped a whole standing, to average risk. Ten of 13 participants decreased their total cholesterol an average of 26.1 mg/dl. Blood pressure dropped for 11 of 13 individuals.

Exercise

Risk of stroke may be reduced by regular physical activity in women and men (Gillum et al., 1996), and exercise training is recommended by the American College of Sports Medicine (1994) for individuals with coronary heart disease. There is some evidence that high triglycerides can increase risk of heart attack (Hodis et al., 1997).

One way to lower triglycerides is to do aerobic exercise at least three times per week. Water exercise can improve cardiovascular endurance and decrease body fat when done properly, including maximizing traveling (leg) movements, wearing shoes for better traction, and monitoring heart rate (Frangolias & Rhodes, 1995; Michaud et al., 1995).

Rest may not be best for those diagnosed with chronic heart failure (Ross, 1996). Moderate exercise may help counteract the harmful effects of high hormone levels that cause the failing heart to work too hard. These hormones—angiotension II, aldosterone, and vasopressin—are hallmarks of heart failure. When these hormones continue to be released in high levels, individuals retain excessive water, increase the work of the failing heart, and are associated with poor long-term prognosis and overall survival. After 4 months of walking on a treadmill at 50% to 70% of peak heart rate 3 days per week, half of the participants (mean age: 61 years) had a 30% reduction in these hormones. The other group, who did not exercise, did not (Ross, 1996).

Hardin and colleagues (1997) studied the effect of diet and exercise on Syndrome X (coronary artery disease, hypertension, hyperinsulinemia, and hyperlipidemia) in children. They recruited 36 obese children known to have high fasting cholesterol levels. Each participated in a 6-week protocol in one of three groups: control, diet, or exercise. There was a significant decline in triglyceride levels and fasting insulin levels in both the diet and exercise groups. Due to the large noncompliance in the diet group, the researchers suggested that exercise is the best treatment for improvement in Syndrome X in children.

The National Institutes of Health (1995) Concensus Statement encourages the use of cardiac rehabilitation programs that combine physical activity with reduction in other risk factors for those with known cardiovascular disease. Rosengren and Wilhelmsen (1997) set out to examine the long-term effect of work-related and leisure-time physical activity on risk of death from coronary heart disease and other causes. They prospectively studied 7,142 men age 47 to 55 years with symptoms of coronary heart disease. They assessed activity via questionnaires. After 20 years, men with physically demanding work had a slightly higher death rate from all causes but not from heart disease. This association disappeared after controlling for smoking, occupational class, and alcohol abuse. Men who were physically active during leisure time had a lower risk of death from coronary heart disease and all causes.

Food and Supplements

Nutritional factors play an important role in the prevention and treatment of heart and blood vessel conditions. Kendler (1997) reviewed the literature on the use of nutrition with heart conditions. Favorable effects have been reported with the use of unsaturated fatty acids, vegetarian and semivegetarian food regimes, dietary fiber, plant sterols, vitamins (niacin, E, C, B6, B12, folate), minerals (potassium, calcium, magnesium, selenium), other supplements (coenzyme Q10, L-carnitine, taurine), and botanical agents (garlic, hawthorn, guguli-pid). Nutritional substances associated with undesirable heart and blood vessel effects include transfatty acids, homocys-teine, carbohydrate intolerance, and exces-sive sodium and iron intake.

Coffee and Its Negative Effects

Nygard and colleagues (1997) reported that there was an association between coffee consumption and the concentration of total homocysteine in plasma, a risk factor for cardiovascular disease and for adverse pregnancy outcome. The researchers stud-ied 7,589 men and 8,585 women age 40 to 67 with no history of hypertension, dia-betes, ischemic heart disease, or cerebro-vascular disease. Although coffee drinking was associated with smoking and lower intake of vitamin supplements and fruit and vegetables, the coffee-homocysteine asso-ciation was only moderately reduced after these variables were adjusted for. Guttorm-sen and associates (1996) also found a rela-tionship between lower plasma folate and cobalamin levels, as well as lower intake of vitamin supplements, coffee consumption, and smoking. Folic acid, a B vitamin found in leafy green vegetables and other pro-duce, could provide a deterrent.

Magnesium Protects

Magnesium deficiency increases the risk of cardiovascular damage, including hy-pertension, cerebrovascular and coronary constriction and occlusion, arrhythmias,

and sudden cardiac death. High intakes of fat and/or calcium can intensify magne-sium inadequacy, especially under condi-tions of stress (Seelig, 1994).

Magnesium intake may be important in preventing heart attack. Singh and col-leagues (1996) studied the relationship be-tween dietary and serum levels of magne-sium in a case-control study of primary and secondary care for acute myocardial infarction. They found that for individuals with ventricular arrhythmias, magnesium intake was relatively low compared to the control group.

Brodsky and colleagues (1994) con-ducted a double-blind, placebo-controlled study of magnesium supplementation and its effect on atrial fibrillation. Eighteen par-ticipants with less than 7 days' duration of atrial fibrillation received either digoxin plus a placebo or digoxin plus intravenous magnesium (20% of a 10 g magnesium sulfate solution in 500 ml of 5% dextrose in water).

The benefit of magnesium was obvious in the first 15 minutes, as heart rate de-creased immediately from an average of 130 to 120. After 24 hours, the group re-ceiving magnesium had an average heart rate of approximately 80, whereas the group receiving only digoxin had an aver-age heart rate of 105. The results provide evidence that magnesium either greatly im-proves the efficacy of digoxin or exerts significant effects on its own.

Murray (1994) pointed out the benefits of magnesium over drugs. Magnesium has no side effects and is more effective. Also, over a 24-hour period, 6 g of esmolol (cost-ing $400) or 300 mg of diltiazem (costing $200) are used for an individual with new-onset atrial fibrillation. These prices are much higher than the cost of 10 g of magnesium sulfate ($1) or 2 mg of digoxin ($2), or their combination.

Protective Effect of Fish and Fish Oil

The risk of death from coronary disease is lower among people who eat fish. However, frequent consumers of fish do not appear to have lower coronary risks than those who eat it once or twice per week (National Institutes of Health, 1995).

Studies have consistently demonstrated that fish oils may prevent cardiac arrhythmias (Kang & Leaf, 1996) and lower total cholesterol, triglycerides, and lipoprotein levels (Pauletto et al., 1996).

Garlic and Fish Oil

Adler and Holub (1997) found the coadministration of garlic with fish oil was well tolerated by people with moderately high cholesterol levels and had a beneficial effect on serum lipid and lipoprotein concentrations by lowering total cholesterol and triglycerol concentrations as well as the ratios of total cholesterol to HDL-C and LDL-C to HDL-C.

Morcos (1997) had similar results with a fish oil and garlic combination. Forty consecutive people with lipid profile abnormalities were enrolled in a single-blind, placebo-controlled crossover study. Supplementation for 1 month resulted in an 11% decrease in cholesterol, a 34% decrease in triglycerides, and a 10% decrease in low-density lipoprotein (LDL) levels, as well as a 19% decrease in cholesterol/high-density lipoprotein (HDL) risk. There was no significant placebo effect. The cholesterol lowering and lipid improvement in risk ratios suggests a combination of fish oil (1,800 mg of eicosapentanoic acid and 1,200 mg of docosahexanoic acid) with garlic powder (1,200 mg) capsules daily may have antiatherosclerotic properties and may protect against coronary artery disease. Rimm and colleagues (1996) examined the relationship between dietary fiber, specifically vegetable, fruit, and cereal sources, and risk of coronary heart disease in men. They found that increasing dietary fiber was an important dietary component for the prevention of coronary heart disease.

Folic Acid and Vitamin B6

A number of studies have shown the protective effect of folic acid (Chasan-Taber et al., 1996; Tucker, Selhub, Wilson, & Rosenberg, 1996) on the heart. Eating more green leafy vegetables (brussels sprouts, spinach, lettuce) and fruits (apples, oranges, etc.) or including folic acid supplements could protect against heart attacks and strokes. Other researchers (Dalery et al., 1995) found that low folic acid and vitamin B6 blood levels were associated with high homocysteine levels (a heart risk factor). Vitamin B6 is plentiful in whole grains, legumes (e.g., peanuts and dry beans), and fish.

Coenzyme Q10 (CoQ10)

CoQ10 supplementation has been used successfully to enhance heart action, stabilize blood pressure, reduce shortness of breath and palpitations, and lessen heart muscle thickness (Lampertico, 1993; Mortensen, 1993). As the safety of prescription cholesterol-lowering medications is increasingly questioned, natural, nutritious alternatives are being used to prevent clogged arteries and lower the risk of heart attack.

Citrus Pectin Lowers Cholesterol

Studies of more than 200 individuals have shown that the equivalent of the pectin in two whole grapefruit can lower the LDL (bad) cholesterol between 25% and 30% in just 4 weeks (Cerda, 1996).

Nuts Protect the Heart

Nuts have shown to be heart protective in several studies. In one, walnuts decreased serum levels of total cholesterol and favorably modified the lipoprotein profile in healthy men (Sabate et al., 1993). In another, researchers examined the eating habits of 25,000 Seventh Day Adventists, looking for a relationship between 65 different foods and good health. People who ate nuts five or more times per week were half as likely to suffer a heart attack or die of heart disease than those who rarely or never ate nuts. The benefit held constant despite age, weight, or activity level.

Another study found that women who ate nuts more than two times per week reduced their heart disease risk by 60% (Fraser, Lindsted, & Beeson, 1995). Even though nuts contain a high percentage of fat, volunteers who ate 3.5 oz of almonds per day (590 calories) did not gain a pound. Nuts also contain mono- and polyunsaturated fats, fiber, and vitamin E, all of which protect the heart. Walnuts also contain omega-3 fatty acids (found in fish oils) and the amino acid arginine, which inhibits blood clotting and protects arteries.

Oats and Buckwheat Are Helpful

Oats and buckwheat intake has been associated with lower body mass index, lowering blood pressure and total cholesterol, and increase the ratio of HDL (good) cholesterol to total cholesterol (He et al., 1995).

L-Arginine May Increase Exercise Capacity

Ceremuzynski, Chamiec, and Herbaczynski-Cedre (1997) studied the effect of supplemental oral L-arginine on exercise capacity in individuals with stable angina pectoris (heart pain). A randomized, double-blind, placebo-controlled study showed that 6 g per day for 3 days of L-arginine increased exercise capacity (tested on a Marquette case 12 treadmill according to the modified Bruce protocol).

Importance of Reducing Saturated Fat and Sugar

The best way to lower triglycerides, now linked with the risk of heart attack (Stampfer et al., 1997), is to cut down on saturated (animal-source) fats, candies, and fruit juice (rich in simple sugars). Vitamin E offered the strongest protection against heart attack and angina in a study conducted by Meyer (1994).

Vitamin E Decreases Risk of Death

Vitamin E supplementation lowered the risk of death from ischemic heart disease in a 5-year study that tracked 2,226 men, 45 to 76 years old. The study controlled for high blood pressure, high cholesterol, and heart disease risk factors.

A study by Martin, Foxall, Blumberg, and Meydani (1997) may explain why vitamin E is helpful in decreasing heart disease risk factors. They found that vitamin E has an inhibitory effect on LDL-induced production of adhesion molecules and adhesion of monocytes to human aortic endothelial cells, one of the early events in the development of atherogenesis.

The Cholesterol Lowering Atherosclerosis Study (CLAS) found less carotid wall thickness for a group of 29 subjects who took 250 IU per day of supplementary vitamin E versus 22 who took 100 IU or less per day. The researchers (Azen et al., 1996) concluded that supplementary vitamin E was effective in reducing the progression of atherosclerosis in subjects not treated with lipid-lowering drugs.

Vitamin C Protects

Vitamin C may exert a protective function by lowering atherogenic risk (Hallfrish et al., 1994). The researchers compared plasma lipids and vitamin C levels for 316 women and 511 men age 19 to 95. After adjusting for age, sex, obesity, and smoking and excluding participants with diagnosed diseases that might affect lipids, the association persisted.

Combined Antioxidants Lower Risk

Losonczy, Harris, and Haulik (1996) examined vitamins E and C supplement use in relation to mortality risk in 11,178 persons age 67 to 105. Simultaneous use of the two vitamins was associated with a lower risk of total mortality and coronary mortality, adjusted for alcohol use, smoking history, aspirin use, and medical conditions.

Stephens and colleagues (1996) used a double-blind, placebo-controlled, randomized trial of vitamin E in individuals with coronary disease in the Cambridge Heart Antioxidant Study. Of 1,035 individuals, 546 were assigned capsules containing 800 IU vitamin E daily. The rest were given 400 IU daily. Both treatment groups showed a significantly reduced risk of nonfatal heart attacks, and the effects were apparent even after 1 year of treatment.

Singh, Niaz, Rastogi, and Rastogi (1996) combined antioxidant vitamins A, C, E, and beta-carotene in the treatment group and compared the results with the control group. They found that the vitamin combination protected against cardiac necrosis and oxidative stress and suggested it could be beneficial in preventing complications and cardiac event rate.

Kushi and colleagues (1996) studied the role of vitamins A, E, and C from food sources in women ($S = 34,486$ postmenopausal women). There was little evidence that the intake of vitamin E from supplements was associated with a decreased risk of death from heart disease, but the effects of high-dose supplementation and the duration of supplement use were not addressed. The researchers concluded that the intake of vitamin E from food sources could lower the risk of death from heart disease in women.

Selenium Lowers Risk

Low levels of selenium are associated with a significantly higher risk for developing ischemic heart disease (Stratment & Lardy, 1992), and selenium and other antioxidant supplementation (at least for men) improves the cardiac risk profile and reduces the risk of cardiovascular disease (Salonen et al., 1991; Suadicani, Hein, & Gyntelberg, 1992).

Soy Protein Lowers Cholesterol

Eating 31 to 47 g/day of soy protein (rather than animal protein) lowers serum levels of total cholesterol, LDL, and triglycerides. The effect is greatest for individuals with high serum cholesterol levels (Anderson, Johnstone, & Cook-Newell, 1995). Sources of soy protein include soy milk, tofu, tempeh, and soy burgers.

Benefits of Vegetarianism

In a study of vegetarians who ate milk and eggs, Krajcovicova-Kudlackova and colleagues (1996) found the participants had a favorable atherosclerosis (hardening of the arteries) profile, including significantly reduced fatty acids in plasma, and higher levels of vitamin C, beta-carotene, and vitamin E/cholesterol ratio—all demonstrating a reduced risk for lipoperoxidation, a factor involved in heart and cancer conditions.

Manson and colleagues (1994) examined the incidence of stroke in 87,245 U.S. female nurses using a food frequency questionnaire. After adjustments for age and smoking, the strongest associations for reduced risk of stroke were for carrots and spinach.

Herbs

Hawthorn, garlic, and motherwort are three of the most effective herbs used for preventing and treating heart conditions.

Curcumin, the yellow pigment of turmeric, is one of the most powerful anti-inflammatory agents in nature and can lower cholesterol levels and inhibit platelet aggregation. Huang, Jan, and Yeh (1992) demonstrated the effect of curcumin on the smooth muscle and discussed how it may become a remedy for the prevention of pathological cardiovascular changes such as atherosclerosis and may be used by those

recovering from coronary artery bypass surgery or angioplasty. Curry leaf and mustard seeds have also been shown to reduce total serum cholesterol (Khan, Abraham, & Leelamma, 1996).

Gingko was shown to be significantly superior to placebo for enhancing pain-free walking for 79 individuals suffering from peripheral arteriopathy (Bauer, 1984). Cayenne protects against blood clot formation by increasing fibrinolytic or clot-dissolving activity in the red blood cells. An association has been established between high income of capsicum and extremely low blood-clotting activity (Visudhiphan et al., 1982).

Massage

Studies have shown that underwater massage is an effective method of conditioning in the outpatient setting. Its positive action on the cardiovascular system improved clinical condition in 70% of those treated. Episodes of angina pectoris disappeared or became less frequent, the pains lessened, and exercise tolerance was enhanced. Nearly 67% of those treated retained the effects for 6 months, 53.3% for 12 months (Davydova et al., 1994).

Meditation

Twenty-one individuals with documented coronary artery disease were tested at baseline and assigned to either stress reduction using the transcendental meditation (TM) program or a waiting-list control. After 8 months, the TM group had almost a 15% increase in exercise tolerance, an 11.7% increase in maximal workload, and significant reductions in rate-pressure product at 3 and 6 minutes and at maximal exercise compared with the control group (Zamarra et al., 1996).

Music

A study conducted by Byers and Smythe (1997) supported the idea that music intervention with cardiac surgery patients during the first postoperative day decreased noise annoyance, heart rate, and systolic blood pressure, regardless of individual sensitivity to noise.

Other Lifestyle Factors

Researchers at the University of Florida (Ross, 1997) found that the severity of heart disease could depend on how well people handle anger, hostility, or mental stress. They found that different types of ischemia (or insufficient supply of blood to an area) are associated with different types of psychological factors. Daily-life ischemia occurs without symptoms in people with lower levels of hostility and anger. This suggests they are suppressing or internalizing these feelings. Individuals who had angina (or chest pain) were more anxious and more aware of physical symptoms, like muscle tension.

Gould and colleagues (1995) provided 5-year follow-up evidence that changing lifestyle, as opposed to usual care by physician of antianginal therapy (control group), was more effective in reducing heart perfusion abnormalities as measured by positron emission tomography. The treatment group was randomized to a low-fat vegetarian diet, mild to moderate exercise, stress management, and group support.

Watching television may become the latest risk factor for cardiovascular disease. A study of 4,280 adults age 23 to 35 who watched television an average of 2.5 hours per day linked hours of viewing to elevated triglyceride levels, obesity, tobacco and alcohol use, anger or anxiety, and junk food consumption (Sidney, 1996).

Kawachi and colleagues (1995) studied female nurses. They found that those who worked 6 or more years on rotating shifts increased their risk of coronary heart disease.

Mark (1994) found that optimism is a powerful predictor of who will live and who will die after the diagnosis of heart disease. Giving up and feeling as if one will not survive seems to be a self-fulfilling prophecy. Pessimism appeared to be even more damaging than depression (which has also been shown to be detrimental for those with heart conditions). Other factors that had an effect on heart disease survival were feeling hostile, being unmarried, and having no one at home to talk to.

Relaxation and Guided Imagery

Collins and Rice (1997) reported on the effects of relaxation and guided imagery on psychological and physiologic outcomes in adults with cardiovascular disease who participated in a phase 2 cardiac rehabilitation program. They used a prospective, quasi-experimental design with random group assignment. No statistical differences were found in state anxiety scores or reported symptoms, but there were reductions in depression and interpersonal sensitivity in the relaxation group. Control group participants had a greater number of dose increases in cardiac medications and fewer dose reductions than did those in the treatment group. The researchers wondered whether more instruction sessions on the relaxation method may have resulted in more positive outcomes.

CAROLYN CHAMBERS CLARK

See also
   Anger (II)
   Caffeine (III)
   Depression (II)
   Garlic (III)
   Gingko (III)
   Lung Disorders (II)
   Syndrome X (II)

HEPATITIS

There are several varieties of hepatitis, or inflammation of the liver. Hepatitis A is infectious or viral and is transmitted by urine, saliva, semen, or, most commonly, fecal contamination of food or liquid. Poor food in handling restaurants is often the cause.

Hepatitis B, or serum hepatitis, is transmitted mainly via contaminated needles. The virus is not always destroyed by putting the needle in boiling water. Instead, steam sterilizing, pressure cooking, or passing the needle through a flame may be required. Hepatitis C (virus-RNA positive) occurs in chronic liver disease.

Kents and Mavrodii (1995) evaluated the effectiveness of magnet therapy, inductothermy, UNF electric field, and electromagnetic waves of a decimetric wave band (460 MHz) on the liver, adrenals, and thyroid gland in controlled trials. Eight hundred and thirty-five individuals with viral hepatitis (types A, B, and associated forms) comprised the sample. Sixty-nine percent of the sample benefited from the treatment.

Arase and others (1997) undertook a retrospective study to evaluate the long-term preventive effect of glyzyrrhizin (licorice extract) on hepatocellular carcinoma. Of the 453 individuals diagnosed with chronic hepatitis C, the glyzyrrhizin group exhibited the greatest effectiveness in preventing liver carcinogenesis.

Yamashiki, Nishimura, Suzuki, Sakaguchi, & Kosaka (1997) tested the effects of the Japanese herbal medicine Sho-saiko-to (TJ-9) on cells of patients with chronic hepatitis C. Sho-saiko-to is widely prescribed for chronic viral liver disease. TJ-9 is known to suppress liver cancer and may have macrobiotic effects. The addition of TJ-9 to cell cultures strongly induced IL-10 (interleukin-10). This induction was mainly attributable to the effects of scutellaria and glycyrrhiza roots.

CAROLYN CHAMBERS CLARK

See
   Magnet Therapy (IV)

HIGH BLOOD PRESSURE (HYPERTENSION)

It is estimated that 40 million Americans have hypertension, or high blood pressure, with the risk notably among people over the age of 50. Hypertension puts people at risk for cardiovascular disease, stroke, and kidney disease. Lifestyle factors such as obesity, drinking habits, diet, and physical-inactivity are well-established determinants of high blood pressure. Hostile individuals display significantly greater blood pressure reactivity compared with individuals rated low in hostility (Christensen & Smith, 1993; Spicer & Chamberlain, 1996). Work stress can affect blood pressure, depending on whether coping skills are adaptive or maladaptive (Lindquist, Beilin, & Knulman, 1997).

Acupressure

Yu and colleagues (1991) treated 291 cases of essential hypertension with acupressure (auriculoacupressure) and compared the results with 51 similar cases treated with Fufang Jiangya (composite hypotensive) tablets. Efficacy was higher in the acupressure group, and the level of blood lipids significantly dropped. Regulatory effects on sinus arrthymia also were demonstrated.

Autogenic Training

A study by Watanabe and colleagues (1996) used autogenic training to lower blood pressure and heart rate of ten individuals diagnosed with hypertension. Participants practiced autogenics three times a day and were monitored at 30-minute intervals for 7 days before training and again for 7 days at 1- or 2-month intervals after training. The overall group reduction was 8 mm Hg (3 to 17 mm Hg). In five participants, reductions were between 7 and 17 mm Hg, a statistically significant amount.

Biofeedback

Hunyor and colleagues (1997) found that among mildly hypertensive individuals, almost half could lower systolic blood pressure at will for short periods. This capability was independent of the real or placebo nature of the feedback signal, as shown by a randomized double-blind study of active or placebo biofeedback groups.

Nakao and associates (1997) randomized 30 participants to either biofeedback or self-monitoring of blood pressure. In the biofeedback group, blood pressure remained unchanged during the control period and was later decreased during the biofeedback treatment phase. The researchers concluded that people whose blood pressure increases with stress may be suited to biofeedback intervention.

Chinese Medicine

The Chinese herbal drug *Evodia rutaecarpa* is used to lower blood pressure. It has been shown to have a vascular muscle relaxant effect (Chiou et al., 1997).

Zhou and Zhou (1990) used a combination of traditional Chinese herbs (under the principle of Bu-Shen Yi-Qi) to treat high blood pressure. The treatment group was comprised of 30 men and women suffering from hypertension. The control group, also comprised of 30 individuals, received oryzanol, vitamin B1, and B6. All 60 suffered from orthostatic dysregulation. The cure rate in the treatment group was significantly better than in the control group. The researchers theorized that the selected herbs were rich in trace elements, including iron and zinc, both of which could have increased the chronotropic effect of blood vessels.

Exercise

Almost 25% of people in industrialized societies are believed to have high blood pressure. They are 2 to 3 times more likely than people with normal blood pressure to have a heart attack or stroke or to develop heart failure. There is now evidence that regular physical activity, including jogging, walking, cycling, and aerobics, reduces blood pressure (Hagberg et al., 1996).

Food and Supplements

Intakes of vitamin C and carotene were found to be inversely related to blood pressure in 1,802 men ages 40 to 56 using the generalized Estimating Equation method for longitudinal analysis (Stamler et al., 1994). In a systematic review of epidemiological studies of vitamin C and blood pressure, Ness and colleagues (1997) found a consistent cross-sectional association between higher vitamin C intake or status and lower blood pressure.

Calcium supplementation has been shown to have a protective effect on blood pressure in inner-city children (Gillman et al., 1994), men (Gillman, Belanger, D' Agostino, Ellison, & Posner, 1994), and pregnant women (Bucher et al., 1996). Potassium, too, has been shown to lower blood pressure, even in people with normal blood pressure. Whelton and colleagues (1997) combined results from nearly three dozen experiments involving more than 2,000 participants to show that taking potassium supplements can help reduce blood pressure. Potassium was found to be even more helpful for people with severe high blood pressure, with high salt intake, and slight more helpful for African-Americans who are particularly susceptible to hypertension. Potassium-rich foods may also be helpful: bananas, cantaloupes, orange juice, baked potatoes, and low-fat yogurt.

Appel and associates (1997) studied the relationship between diet and blood pressure. They found that a healthy diet high in fruits, vegetables, and low-fat milk can help lower blood pressure.

He and colleagues (1995) found that a higher intake of total protein (39 g) was associated with a lower systolic and diastolic blood pressure. High fiber intake (19 g) was significantly associated with both a lower diastolic and systolic pressure.

Epidemiologic studies from divergent geographic locations have consistently shown an inverse correlation between potassium intake and hypertension. Potassium depletion is associated with an increase in blood pressure (Krishna, 1994).

Smith, Klotman, and Svetkey (1992) found that potassium chloride can lower blood pressure in older people with hypertension. In their study, 22 people 60 years of age or older were admitted to a Clinical Research Unit for 8 days after a 2-week period free of antihypertensive medication. They were placed on an isocaloric diet containing 200 mmol/day of sodium, 70 mmol/day of potassium, and 500 mg/day of calcium. Participants were randomized to receive potassium chloride (120 mmol/day) or placebo. After 4 days, participants were switched to the alternate treatment. Systolic blood pressure decreased 8.6 mm Hg and diastolic blood pressure decreased 4.0 mm Hg during potassium chloride supplementation, but there were no significant changes during placebo treatment.

Fotherby and Potter (1997) also used a randomized cross-over study using a potassium supplement versus placebo and checked its effect on blood pressure in eight hypertensive people. They found a significant fall in mean 24-hour systolic blood pressure between 4 months of potassium supplementation and placebo treatment. They concluded that a modest increase in dietary potassium intake could have significant effect on lowering blood pressure in the large proportion of older adults with hypertension.

Magnetotherapy

Miasnikov (1992) studied 147 participants who underwent magnet therapy, with the unit "Magniter-AMT-01" applied to the cervical area. The treatment group included 102 people; 45 participants served as control. The greatest effect on cerebrovascular disorders in hypertension was with the use of the Magniter-AMT-01.

Ivanov and colleagues (1990) reported the use of MKM2-1 magnets on individuals suffering from essential hypertension. Continuous action of the magnetic field was noted to decrease arterial pressure without any side effects and simultaneously reduce the need for drugs.

Massage

The only recent study found concerning massage and blood pressure used an animal model. Massage-like stroking of the abdomen of anesthetized rats lowered their blood pressure (Kurosawa, Lundeberg, Agren, Lund, & Uvnas-Moberg, 1995).

Transcendental Meditation

Wenneberg and colleagues (1997) evaluated the effects of transcendental meditation or a cognitive-based stress education control group on ambulatory blood pressure. Regularly practicing TM demonstrated a significant reduction of 9 mm Hg in average ambulatory diastolic blood pressure compared to controls.

CAROLYN CHAMBERS CLARK

See
Acupuncture and Chinese Medicine (IV)
Auriculotherapy (IV)
Autogenic Training (IV)
Biofeedback (IV)
Exercise (IV)
Nutrition (IV)
Transcendental Meditation (IV)

See also
Calcium (III)
Heart and Blood Vessel Conditions (II)
Vitamin C (III)

HIGH CHOLESTEROL

Lopez and colleagues (1996) assessed the effect of a high monounsaturated fatty acids (MFA) diet on serum lipids for 30 healthy adults volunteers and 37 adults with mild hypercholesterolemia (15 of them with associated type II diabetes mellitus). In the healthy adults, there was a 16% decrease in serum total cholesterol level following the high MFA diet, while it rose after the control diet (MFA 34 g, saturated/unsaturated ratio 0.7). In hypercholesterolemic participants, a significant decrease in serum total cholesterol, LDL-cholesterol, and triglycerides and an increase of HDL-cholesterol levels occurred with the avocado diet, while no significant changes were noted with the control diet.

CAROLYN CHAMBERS CLARK

See also
Garlic (III)
Heart and Blood Vessel Conditions (II)

HIP FRACTURES

The two main causes of hip fracture are bone loss leading to femoral fragility and falls. Vitamin D and calcium deficiencies are common in older adults.

The risk of hip fracture over the remaining life of a 50-year-old Caucasian woman currently is 17%. The increase in life expectancy is expected to cause a threefold rise in worldwide fracture incidence over the next 60 years, for both men and women, and the cost of hip fracture is expected to increase dramatically.

Dirschel, Henderson, and Oakley (1995) examined 97 older adults with acute fractures of the proximal femur sustained as a result of minimal trauma. They found a preferential loss of bone mineral from the femoral neck in younger individuals with hip fractures. Mean daily calcium intake was well below the recommended levels, and calcium intake less than 500 mg per day was associated with lower lumbar spine bone mineral density scores. The researchers suggested that calcium supplementation may play a role in decreasing the incidence of hip fracture.

Meunier (1996) reported a 3-year controlled prospective study of daily supplementation of 1.2 g of calcium and 800 IU of vitamin D3 for 3,270 older women living in nursing homes. The treatment reduced hip fractures and other nonvertebral fractures by 23%. After 18 months of treatment, the bone density (total proximal femoral bone) in the vitamin D3–calcium group increased (significantly) by 2.7% but decreased by 4.6% in the placebo group.

Bonjour, Schurch, and Rizzoli (1996) found that a deficiency in vitamin K may also contribute to bone fragility. In their study, reduced protein intake was also associated with lower femoral neck bone mineral density and poor physical performance. The clinical outcome after hip fracture was significantly improved by daily oral nutritional supplements normalizing the protein intake. The supplementation also resulted in a reduction in complication rate and length of hospital stay.

Meyer and colleagues (1996) used a matched case-control study in Oslo to assess risk factors for hip fracture in older adults. Two hundred forty-six individuals with hip fractures admitted to two hospitals in the course of 1 year comprised the sample. The researchers found increased risk of hip fracture in the following people: the lean, those who had reported weight loss because of poor appetite, and people who had low food intake. No relationship was found between calcium intake and hip fracture, but higher risk was suggested in people with low vitamin D intake, low physical activity, low hand grip strength, smoking, low level of education and frequent admissions to the hospital prior to the study.

Meyer, Pedersen, Loken, and Tverdal (1997) used dietary data from a prospective study to relate factors influencing calcium balance to the incidence of hip fracture. In their study, 19,752 women and 20,035 men filled in and returned a semiquantitative dietary questionnaire. The sample was followed for an average of 11.5 years. At follow-up, 213 hip fractures were found. Fractures associated with high-energy trauma and metastatic bone disease were excluded. There was no clear association between calcium intake or nondairy animal protein intake and hip fracture, but there was an elevated risk of fracture for women with a high intake of protein from nondairy animal sources in the presence of low calcium intake. Women who drank nine or more cups of coffee per day also had an increased risk of fracture. Other studies show that seniors can improve their balance and prevent falls by learning martial arts.

CAROLYN CHAMBERS CLARK

See
T'ai Chi (IV)

HUNTINGTON'S DISEASE

Beal and Matthews (1997) studied the effect of coenzyme Q10 on the central nervous system and its potential use in the treatment of neurodegenerative disease. Coenzyme Q10 is an antioxidant as well as an essential cofactor in the electron transport chain. The researchers found the enzyme effect in both animal and human studies. They fed rats a dose of 200 mg/kg for 1 to 2 months. There were significant liver concentration increases but no significant increase in brain concentrations of either reduced or total coenzyme Q10 levels. There was a reduction in malonate-induced increases in 2,5-dihydroxybenzoic acid to salicylate, consistent with an antioxidant effect.

The oral administration of coenzyme Q10 significantly reduced increased concentration of lactate in the occipital cortex of people diagnosed with Huntington's disease. Taken together, these findings suggest that coenzyme Q10 might be useful in treating neurodegenerative disease.

CAROLYN CHAMBERS CLARK

INCONTINENCE

Urinary incontinence, the loss of bladder control, affects an estimated 10 million Americans, according to the National Institutes of Health. Most of them are women. More than 8 million people affected by incontinence are age 60 or older. In a telephone survey of 1,140 randomly selected men and women over age 65, Branch and colleagues (1994) found that the majority of respondents believed that involuntary loss of urine was a normal result of aging and that surgery was the best treatment.

Incontinence can be treated without medication or surgery. In fact, some drugs can cause incontinence (Branch et al., 1994), and surgery may only help in a certain percentage of people with urinary incontinence (Weinberger & Ostergard, 1996).

Actions found to be helpful include voiding by the clock (making frequent trips to the bathroom, then gradually increasing the time between trips), performing pelvic muscle exercises (Davilla, 1994), and using guided imagery/hypnosis (picturing how much the bladder will hold, then giving a self-suggestion to wake up when the bladder is full; Ack, Norman, & Schmitt, 1984).

Behavioral Management Reduces Urinary Incontinence

Bear and colleagues (1997) used a home-based program for treating urinary incontinence in older rural adults. Women 55 years old and older who had episodes of urinary incontinence two or more times per week comprised the sample. Participants were taught self-monitoring, scheduling regimens, and pelvic muscle exercise with biofeedback. Urine loss was determined by weighing incontinence pads. The behavioral management resulted in a significant decrease in urinary incontinence, but there was a marked lack of response to the project by frail elders and their caregivers.

Gerard (1997) also reported a behavioral management program for 85 women between the ages of 40 and 78 years of various ethnic backgrounds. Participants attended a 2-hour class that covered anatomy and physiology, the causes of incontinence, possible treatment/management alternatives (behavioral methods and dietary changes), and specific exercises to identify pelvic muscles. Following training at 3 and 6 months' follow-up, there was a significant reduction in the number of absorbency products used, especially during the day, and in the need to urinate for women with urge incontinence.

Biofeedback Reduces Fecal Incontinence

Patankar and colleagues (1997) conducted a multicenter study of 72 individuals with fecal incontinence. All participants attended an average of seven weekly biofeedback sessions. Compliance and satisfaction were high. Incontinence decreased significantly from to 11.8 weekly gross incontinent episodes to 2.0.

Rieger and associates (1997) reported on a biofeedback pelvic floor retraining program for fecal incontinence. Participants included 28 women and 2 men, with an age range of 29 to 85 years. In the study, 20 had improved incontinence scores that persisted for 6 weeks.

Kegels for Urinary Incontinence Equal to Surgery Results

Bo and Talseth (1996) compared the long- and short-term effects of a structured, intensive pelvic floor muscle exercise pro-

gram. They followed 23 30- to 70-year-old women with stress incontinence for 5 years. Women who performed pelvic floor muscle exercises three or more times per week had significantly less leakage by pad test than those who performed the exercises less often. Differences by age were not significant. The researchers found that the eventual effect of continuing pelvic floor muscle exercises was equal to surgical intervention.

CAROLYN CHAMBERS CLARK

INFECTION

Onion and garlic exhibit many antibiotic actions (Augusti, 1996). In one study (Ramanoelina, Terrrom, Bianchini, & Coulanges, 1987), essential oils from Madagascar plants, including *Thymus vulgaris*, *Ocimum gratissimum*, and *Eugenia caryophyllata*, showed antimicrobial activity. The essential oil of *Melaleuca viridiflora* also had a high inhibitory effect on gram-positive bacteria.

Peters, Goetzsche, Grobbelaar, and Noakes (1993) found that vitamin C supplementation (600 mg) reduced the incidence of upper respiratory tract infection (URT) in ultramarathon runners. The researchers matched ultramarathon runners with controls of similar ages and randomly divided them into placebo and experimental groups. Symptoms of URT infection were monitored for 14 days after the race. Sixty-eight percent of the runners in the non–vitamin C group, significantly more than in the treatment group, reported symptoms of URT infection after the race. The severity and duration of reported symptoms of URT infections were also significantly less in the nonrunning vitamin C–supplemented group than in the nonrunning non-supplemented group. The study provided evidence that vitamin C supplementation may enhance resistance to postrace upper respiratory tract infections and may reduce the severity of symptoms in nonracers.

CAROLYN CHAMBERS CLARK

INFERTILITY

Infertility is defined as failure by a couple to conceive after 1 year of unprotected intercourse. The condition affects an estimated 20% of couples in the United States (nearly five million). Growing incidence may reflect deferment of marriage and age of first delivery. Major causes include male sperm factors (40%), abnormal tubal function (30%), ovulatory dysfunction (20%), unidentified factors (10%), and cervical factors (Berkow & Fletcher, 1992).

Other factors include eating well (refined foods, sugar and additives may limit the liver's ability to metabolize hormones, and milk consumption may reduce fertility) and keeping body fat at 18% of weight. Falling below this level of body fat may hinder the production of estrogen. Being overweight can cause an excess of estrogen (Weil, 1997).

Taking vitamin C can increase fertility in men and vitamin E may enhance the ability of men's sperm to fertilize an egg. Caffeine can elevate stress levels and should be eliminated. Even moderate alcohol use can reduce fertility, and toxins from cigarettes may kill egg-containing ovary follicles. Marijuana, ulcer medications, and steroids can also reduce fertility (Weil, 1997).

Drugs that dry up cervical fluid should be avoided, including antihistamines, progesterone and Clomid. Men need to avoid exposing their tests to high temperatures from hot tubs, saunas, heated work environments, or the sweat and friction generated while bicycling. Douching can lead to vaginal infections and pelvic inflammatory disease, and can impede sperm survival (Weil, 1997).

Stress may also be a factor by altering the way the hypothalamus regulates estrogen and progesterone. Infertile women have been found to be as anxious and depressed as women diagnosed with cancer, heart disease, or AIDS. A new double blind randomized five-year study funded by the National Institute of Mental Health will study 120 infertile women and assign them to either a mind-body program, a support group, or routine care to see how they compare in terms of pregnancy rate and psychological health (Weil, 1997).

Pilot data revealed the vast majority of women reported feeling significantly better after participating in the program of breathing techniques, progressive muscle relaxation, meditation, cognitive restructuring (avoiding self-punishing thoughts), self-care (taking a warm bath or buying flowers), and guided imagery. Forty-four percent became pregnant after participating in the program (Domar, 1990; Domar & Dreher, 1996).

Salvati and colleagues (1996) reported treating 66 males with *Panax ginseng C.A. Meyer* extract. Thirty were of the oligoastenospermic sine causa (group A) and 16 were of the oligoastenospermic with idiopathic varicocele (group B). Twenty age-matched volunteers were used as control (group C). Use of *Panax ginseng* extract showed an increase in spermatozoa number/ml and progressive motility, an increase in plasma total and free testosterone, DHT, FSH, and LH levels. There was also a decrease in mean PRL. The researchers concluded that ginsenosides may work at different levels of the hypothalamus-pituitary-testis axis.

Buck, Sever, Batt, and Mendola (1997) summarized the epidemiologic evidence of the effect of lifestyle factors on female infertility. Risk factors that affect the risk of primary tubal infertility and were corroborated in two or more studies and included use of intrauterine devices (especially the Dalkon Shield) and cigarette smoking. Extremes in body size were identified as a risk factor for primary ovulatory infertility. Cocaine, marijuana, and alcohol use, exercise, caffeine consumption, and overuse of thyroid medications were possible risk factors for various subtypes of primary infertility.

CAROLYN CHAMBERS CLARK

INSOMNIA

Insomnia is a disturbance or perceived disturbance in the usual sleep pattern that has troublesome consequences, including daytime fatigue and drowsiness, irritability, anxiety, depression, and somatic complaints. It is estimated that 100 million Americans have sleep problems. While sedatives may be indicated for short-term insomnia, such as that caused by stress or jet lag, the long-term use is associated with alteration of sleep stages, daytime residual effects, tolerance, dependence, and rebound insomnia.

Winslow and Jacobson (1997) reported a review of 59 studies conducted from 1974 to 1993 involving 2,102 individuals with problems in sleep-onset, sleep maintenance, or mixed insomnia. Participants kept daily sleep diaries to evaluate the benefits of each procedure.

Stimulus control (go to bed only when sleepy; use the bed only for sleep and sex; get up and go into another room if unable to fall asleep in 10 minutes and return only when sleepy; set the alarm and get up at the same time every morning, no matter the amount of sleep), and sleep restriction (staying in bed only when sleeping) were the most successful strategies. However, relaxation therapy produced important improvements. Paradoxical intention (a cognitive intervention that uses suggestion to tell the person with insomnia to stay awake as long as possible) was also successful for maintenance insomnia in the one study testing its use. Results were maintained for an average of 6 months and were statistically significant when compared to placebo or no treatment.

Pasche and colleagues (1996) reported treating chronic psychophysiological insomnia with low energy emission therapy, an amplitude-modulated electromagnetic field approach. One hundred and six individuals from two different centers participated in their study. Sleep rating forms and polysomnography were used to measure the effect. There was a significant decrease in sleep latency and an increase in total sleep time for the active treatment group and an increase in sleep cycles, compared to the control group.

Buchbauer and colleagues (1991) tested the sedative properties of the essential oil of lavender with laboratory mice. They found a significant decrease in motility in both males and females. After an injection of caffeine, hyperactivity was observed, which was reduced to nearly normal motility after inhalation of lavender oil. The researchers contended that this demonstration of the sedative effects of lavender confirms the use of lavender herbal pillows to bring on sleep.

CAROLYN CHAMBERS CLARK

INSULIN SENSITIVITY

One change associated with aging is a decline in glucose tolerance. Causes reported include increased insulin resistance (from receptor and/or post receptor disturbances) and diminished pancreatic islet B-cell sensitivity to glucose. Insulin resistance may contribute to or even be causal in many chronic disorders associated with aging: noninsulin-dependent diabetes mellitus, obesity, hypertension, lipid abnormalities, and atherosclerosis (Preuss, 1997).

In aging, similar to diabetes, the elevation in circulating glucose (and other sugars secondary to age-induced insulin resistance) can react with proteins and nucleic acids to form products that diminish tissue elasticity and affect bodily functions. These changes in metabolism are associated with enhanced lipid peroxidation secondary to greater free radical formation. Oxygen free radicals are known causes of tissue damage and have been associated with aging conditions including inflammatory diseases, cataracts, diabetes, and heart conditions. Augmented free radical formation and lipid peroxidation are not uncommon in diabetes mellitus.

Ingestion of sugars, fats, and sodium have been linked to decreased insulin sensitivity, while calorie restriction, exercise, ingestion of chromium, vanadium, soluble fibers, magnesium, and antioxidants are associated with greater insulin sensitivity. By manipulating the diet to obtain the substances associated with increased insulin sensitivity, lifespan may be favorably affected and the incidence of chronic disorders associated with aging reduced (Preuss, 1997).

CAROLYN CHAMBERS CLARK

See also
   Aging (II)
   Antioxidants and Free Radicals (III)
   Diabetes (II)
   Heart and Blood Vessel Conditions (II)
   High Blood Pressure (II)
   Syndrome X (II)

IRON OVERLOAD

Iron is a paradoxical nutrient. A minute amount makes life possible. Excessive quantities can be toxic. Iron overload occurs when dietary iron is absorbed by the small intestine and deposited.

Iron overload is related to heart disease, cancer, diabetes, osteoporosis, arthritis, and possibly other conditions. Iron plays a role in oxidative damage. An evaluation of age-related dietary trends and factors involved in iron absorption led Crawford (1995) to the conclusion that a combination of citric acid and ascorbic acid (vitamin C) may lead to iron overload in aging populations.

Not only aging populations are subject to iron overload. Individuals in their thirties may show the characteristic symptoms if they carry the double gene that results in hemochromatosis. Symptoms of this condition include fatigue, bronze or gray skin tone, weight loss, anemia, abdominal pain, joint pain, impotence, menstrual irregularity, early onset of menopause, diabetes, heart attack, heart irregularities and/or failure, non-alcohol-related cirrhosis, liver cancer, headaches, and premature death (Gravess, 1998; Tuomainen et al., 1998).

CAROLYN CHAMBERS CLARK

See also
Aging (II)

IRRITABLE BOWEL SYNDROME

Irritable bowel syndrome is diagnosed when individuals have experienced abdominal discomfort with a change in bowel habits for at least 3 months. The disorder is common, affecting between 10% and 20% of Americans. Common symptoms include bloating, abdominal pain, bouts of diarrhea and constipation (often alternating), and a persistent urge to defecate (Purpura & Henry, 1997).

Van Dulmen, Fennis, and Bleijenberg (1996) investigated the use of cognitive-behavioral group therapy in treating irritable bowel syndrome, charting its effects and long-term follow-up results. Previous studies had used only small samples, and long-term follow-up was lacking. In the first study, the researchers conducted a controlled study with 25 individuals in the group treatment condition and 20 in the waiting-list control condition. Treatment included eight 2-hour group sessions over a period of 3 months. In study 2, all participants were treated and followed for an average of 2.25 years after the completion of

group treatment. Abdominal complaints of participants in the treatment group improved significantly more than the complaints of individuals awaiting treatment. The number of cosuccessful coping strategies was found to increase more and participants' avoidance behavior was found to decrease more in the treatment group than in the waiting-list control group. Positive changes persisted during follow-up.

Other complementary approaches reported to be successful are fiber-rich diet; avoidance of fatty foods, caffeine, and chewing gum or candies that contain sorbitol, manitol, or xylitol (all of which are associated with intestinal problems); and exercise, meditation, yoga, and other forms of stress management (Purpura & Henry, 1997).

CAROLYN CHAMBERS CLARK

KIDNEY DISEASES

Nephritis, or glomerulonephritis, results from immunologic damage to the glomeruli of the kidney. Proteinuria is a marker of renal damage.

Chinese Medicine

A Chinese herbal preparation, Man-Shen Ling (MSL), consisting of herbs including astragalus and rehmannia, was used by Su, He, and Chen (1993) to treat chronic nephritis, a long-term inflammation of the kidneys. Although tested on animals, the laboratory findings and histopathological investigation confirmed that MSL has therapeutic effects on chronic nephritis.

MSL exhibited antiallergy, immunosuppressive, diuretic, hypotensive, anti-inflammatory, and anticoagulatory activity.

It enhanced renal blood flow and glomerular filtration and promoted urea nitrogen excretion, potassium and sodium function, and immunity. Acute and chronic toxicity tests showed no toxic, mutagenic, teratogenic, or carcinogenic effects. The researchers concluded that the MSL herb combination was safe and effective.

Diet Affects Kidney Stone Formation

Parivar, Low, and Stoller (1996) reviewed the research on the influence of diet on the formation of kidney stones. They found that stone formers do not have an adequate fluid intake and consume too much protein, salt, and foods high in oxalates, such as spinach, beets, peanuts, and chocolate.

Individuals with kidney stones are routinely advised to increase their fluid intake to decrease the risk of stone recurrence. There has been little detailed examination of the type of beverage that is most protective. Curhan, Willett, Rimm, Spiegelman, and Stampfer (1996) used a semiquantitative food frequency questionnaire to measure beverage use and type. During 6 years of follow-up of the sample of 242,100 people, 753 incident cases of kidney stones were documented. After adjusting simultaneously for dietary intake of calcium, age, animal protein and potassium, thiazide use, geographic region, and total fluid intake, apple juice and grapefruit juice were the two beverages that significantly increased risk of stone formation.

Hobbs, Rayner, and Hower (1996) found that stroke-prone spontaneously hypertensive rats fed a high salt diet rapidly developed proteinuria. Fish oil inhibited the elevation of blood pressure, prevented the development of proteinuria, and minimized histological lesions. In the rats fed canola oil, hypertension and renal damage were as severe as that found in rats fed olive or safflower oil. The researchers postulated that the prevention of hypertensive renal damage by dietary fish oil may be attributable to the increased incorporation of long-chain omega-3 fatty acids in the kidney.

Rattan, Thind, Jethi, and Nath (1993) examined the contribution of exogenous calcium and oxalate in magnesium deficiency. They found that magnesium deficiency leads to an increased risk of kidney stone formation.

Ankri, Miron, Rabinkov, Wilcheck, and Mirelman (1997) found that allicin, one of the active principles of garlic, inhibits amebic virulence. However, the research was conducted on baby hamster kidney cells, not on humans.

Exercise Enhances Blood Pressure

Boyce and colleagues (1997) examined the effect of exercise on individuals with predialysis renal failure. Only eight individuals completed the study of 4 months of exercise training. Aerobic capacity, muscular strength, and blood pressure improved, but renal failure, as measured by creatinine clearance, continued to deteriorate during the course of the study.

CAROLYN CHAMBERS CLARK

See also
Heart and Blood Vessel Conditions (II)
High Blood Pressure (II)

KIDNEY STONES

Approximately 12% of men and women in the United States develop kidney stones sometime during their lives. After one episode, recurrences are common. Stone formers are urged to increase their fluid intake and reduce their consumption of protein, salt, and foods high in oxalates, including spinach, beets, peanuts, and chocolate (Parivar et al., 1996).

Dietary Factors

Preventive therapy for kidney stones has included recommendations for a low-calcium diet. A study by Curhan, Willett, Speizer, Spiegelman, and Stampfer (1997) cast considerable doubt on that treatment, however. The Curhan sample comprised 91,731 women who were a subset of the Nurses' Health Study. Participants answered a 1992 questionnaire about lifetime history of kidney stones and completed at least one dietary intake questionnaire. Additional information about diet was obtained from a random sample of 100 women who reported taking supplemental calcium in 1994. After controlling for age and dietary intake, a higher risk for kidney stones was associated with supplemental calcium, sucrose, and sodium. A decreased risk for kidney stones was associated with dietary calcium, potassium intake, and fluid intake. The researchers suggested that restriction of dietary calcium in women at risk for kidney stone formation is not warranted and that the possible risk may be reduced by taking supplemental calcium with meals.

CAROLYN CHAMBERS CLARK

See also
Calcium (III)

LUNG DISORDERS

Normal breathing is smooth, relaxed, rhythmic, and quiet. Numerous conditions can interfere with breathing.

Breathing Practice

Joshi, Joshi, and Gokhale (1992) explored the use of short-term Pranayam practice on breathing rate and ventilatory lung functions. Thirty-three normal males and 42 normal females with an average age of 18.5 years took part in a 6-week course in yogic breathing exercise (Pranayam). Ventilatory lung functions were studied before and after practice. All participants improved ventilatory functions, including lowered respiratory rate and increased forced vital capacity, forced expiratory volume, maximum voluntary ventilation, peak expiratory flow rate, and prolongation of breath holding time.

Chinese Herbs

Kong and colleagues (1993) evaluated the use of Chinese herbs Shunag Huang Lian in a randomized, single-blind trial in 96 children with acute bronchiolitis and serological evidence of recent respiratory virus infection. The mean duration of symptoms from the start of treatment was 6.2 days in the groups treated with herbs and with antibiotics and herbs. The mean duration of symptoms for the group treated with antibiotics alone was 8.6 days.

Food and Supplements

Landon and Young (1993) discussed the interaction of magnesium and calcium. The possibility exists that magnesium deficiency contributes to lung complications. Serum magnesium levels are used to detect deficiencies, but cells can be deficient despite normal serum values. The researchers suggested that people being treated for lung conditions should be monitored routinely for magnesium deficiency.

Britton and colleagues (1994) studied a random sample of 2,633 adults age 18 to

70 in the United Kingdom. They tested the hypothesis that high dietary magnesium intake is associated with better lung function and a reduced risk of airway hyperreactivity and wheezing. The researchers measured dietary magnesium intake using a semiquantitative food frequency questionnaire, lung function using 1-second forced expiratory volume (FEV1), and atopy using the mean skin prick test response to three common environmental allergens. Dietary magnesium intake was independently related to lung function and the occurrence of airway hyperreactivity and self-reported wheezing in the general population. Britton and colleagues concluded that low magnesium intake may be involved in the etiology of asthma and chronic obstructive airway disease.

Sempertegui and colleagues (1996) assessed the effect of zinc sulfate supplementation on respiratory tract disease, immunity, and growth in malnourished children at a day care center in Ecuador. Fifty children, age 12 to 59 months, comprised the sample. On a random basis, half received zinc supplementation and half did not. The incidence of fever, cough, and upper respiratory tract secretions was lower in the supplemented group than in the nonsupplemented group at day 60.

Dow and colleagues (1996) investigated whether dietary antioxidant intake in older adults was related to lung function in 178 men and women age 70 to 96. For every extra milligram increase in vitamin E in the daily diet, FEV1 (forced expiratory volume in 1 second) increased by an estimated 42 ml and FVC (forced vital capacity) by an estimated 54 ml. The results suggest that vitamin E may influence lung function in older adults.

Fawzi and associates (1994) examined the relationship between dietary vitamin A intake and cough, diarrhea, and mortality in children. The researchers found that vitamin A intake was especially protective for children who were wasted or stunted or who had cough or diarrhea symptoms. Rahman and colleagues (1996) found that a large proportion of infants remained vitamin A deficient even after large doses of vitamin A supplementation because of frequent respiratory infections, particularly those accompanied by fever.

Humphrey and colleagues (1996) conducted a placebo-controlled trial among 2,067 Indonesian neonates who received either 50,000 IU of orally administered vitamin A or a placebo on the first day of life. Infants were followed for 1 year. During the first 4 months after treatment, 73% and 51% more control infants were brought for treatment for cough and fever, respectively. The researchers concluded that giving neonates vitamin A could reduce the prevalence of severe respiratory infection.

Peters, Goetzsche, Grobbelaar, and Noakes (1993) studied the effect of daily supplementation with 600 mg of vitamin C on the incidence of upper respiratory tract (URT) infections after participation in competitive ultramarathon races. Vitamin C was shown to enhance resistance to URT infections in ultramarathon runners and may reduce the severity of such infections in those who are sedentary.

Guided Imagery

Moody, Fraser, and Yarandi (1993) examined the use of guided imagery and inspiratory muscle training in a group of 10 males and 9 females, age 56 to 75, with moderate bronchitis and emphysema. Guided imagery significantly improved participant-perceived quality of life. Because the inspiratory muscle training could not be tolerated, the effects on dependent variables were precluded.

Yoga

Madanmohna and colleagues (1992) investigated the effect of yoga training on visual and auditory reaction times, maximum expiratory pressure, breath holding time after expiration and inspiration, and hand grip strength. Twenty-seven student volunteers participated in a 12-week yoga training course. The yoga practice resulted in significant reduction in visual and auditory reaction times and significant increase in respiratory pressures, breath holding times, and hand grip strength.

Telles, Narendran, Raghuraj, Nagarathna, and Nagendra (1997) examined the use of yoga for 20 community home girls and 20 age-matched girls from a regular school. One member of the pair was randomly assigned to either yoga or games groups. At the end of 6 months both groups showed a significant decrease in resting heart rate, and the yoga group showed a significant decrease in breath rate. The results suggest that a yoga program, including relaxation, awareness, and graded physical activity, is a useful addition to the routine of community home children.

CAROLYN CHAMBERS CLARK

See
Herbal Therapies (IV)
Imagery (IV)
Yoga (IV)

See also
Asthma (II)
Cold Symptoms (II)
Cystic Fibrosis (II)
Vitamin A (III)
Vitamin C (III)
Vitamin E (III)

MACULAR DEGENERATION

Macular degeneration is the slow deterioration of the center of the retina. It destroys some or all vision in 1 in 20 people in the United States age 70 or older. An estimated 10 million Americans suffer from some visual loss due to the condition.

Although not well understood, macular degeneration may occur due to the failure of blood vessels to properly nourish the tissue beneath the retina of the eye. A diet rich in saturated fat and cholesterol and low in lycopene (tomato products primarily) may increase the risk of macular degeneration by 80% (Mares-Perlman, 1995), whereas a diet rich in vegetables containing carotenoids (especially spinach and collard greens) may decrease the risk of macular degeneration by 43%. Sweet potatoes, cabbage, cauliflower, brussels sprouts, and squash also may be beneficial, whereas supplements of vitamins A, C, E, and retinol (a form of vitamin A) do not decrease the risk (Seddon et al., 1994).

In a multicenter study at eight medical centers, Richer (1996) found that a specific 14-antioxidant capsule (20,000 units of beta-carotene, 200 units of vitamin E, 750 mg of vitamin C, plus zinc, selenium, and other nutrients) twice daily stabilized patients' vision. The researcher concluded that eating green leafy vegetables provides an adequate supply of antioxidants, but high-dose supplements may be needed to stabilize advanced macular degeneration.

West and colleagues (1994) found alpha-tocopherol (vitamin E) exerted a protective effect for age-related macular degeneration. An antioxidant index, composed of plasma ascorbic acid, alpha-tocopherol, and beta-carotene, was also protective.

Mares-Perlman and associates (1996) found a weakly protective effect for zinc in the development of some forms of early age-related maculopathy. Ishihara, Yuzawa, and Tamakoshi (1997) compared serum levels of vitamins A, C, and E and carotenoid, zinc, and selenium in 35 people with age-related macular degeneration with the levels of 66 controls. Serum zinc was significantly lower in the condition group, as compared to the control group. Vitamin E levels also tended to be low. The researchers concluded that subnormal levels of zinc and vitamin E may be associated with development of age-related macular degeneration.

Snodderly (1995) examined the epidemiologic data on other risk factors for macular degeneration. The researcher found that individuals with low plasma concentrations of carotenoids and antioxidant vitamins and those who smoked cigarettes were at increased risk for age-related macular degeneration.

CAROLYN CHAMBERS CLARK

See also

Vitamin A (III)
Vitamin C (III)
Vitamin E (III)
Zinc (III)

MEMORY PROBLEMS

Memory problems are a major concern for many individuals, particularly older adults. Several complementary approaches have been tested for improving memory performance.

Antioxidants

Swiss researchers (Perrig et al., 1997) concluded that two antioxidants, vitamin C and beta-carotene, play an important role in brain aging and memory. Their cross-sectional study evaluated the association between current and long-term plasma levels of these antioxidants, as well as vitamin E, and various memory functions in 6,400 healthy older adults. Vitamin C (ascorbic acid) and beta-carotene were significant predictors of improved free recall, vocabulary, and recognition, even after adjusting for confounding variables.

Affirmations

Chakalis and Lowe (1992) studied the effect of subliminally embedded auditory material on short-term memory recall. Sixty volunteers took a face-name-occupation memory test before and after a 15-minute intervention. Participants were randomly assigned to one of three groups: (1) no sound, (2) supraliminal presentation of relaxing music, or (3) subliminal presentation of memory-improvement affirmations embedded in relaxing music. After intervention, only the subliminal group significantly improved their performance on recall of names.

Cognitive Memory Restructuring

Lachman and colleagues (1992) studied the effect of several different methods of improving memory performance and beliefs about memory ability and control. They assigned participants to one of five treatment groups: cognitive restructuring to promote adaptive beliefs about memory, memory skills training, combined cognitive restructuring and memory skills training, practice on memory tasks, and a no-contract control group.

Beliefs about participant ability and effectiveness in controlling memory, memory performance, including working memory, recall of text materials, categorizing a word list, and identifying names and faces were assessed pre- and posttest. As predicted, those receiving the combined treatment showed the greatest increases in their perceived ability to improve memory and their sense of control. All groups improved equally on memory tasks, but those who received memory training were more likely to report that at the second posttest they had begun using new strategies for remembering.

Herbal Treatment

Several herbs have been associated with enhanced memory. A study by Hong, Qin, and Huang (1994) showed that the aqueous extract of *Astragulus membranaceus* improve memory.

Drabaek and colleagues (1996) tested the effects of *Ginkgo biloba* extract versus a placebo in a randomized double-blind, crossover study. Questionnaires based on visual analog scales were used to quantify the severity of leg pain, impairment of concentration, and inability to remember. The impairment of concentration and the inability to remember were both reduced when comparing results during active treatment (gingko) to placebo. Short-term memory did not change significantly, but the researchers concluded that treatment with the *Ginkgo biloba* extract did improve some cognitive functions in older individuals with moderate arterial insufficiency.

CAROLYN CHAMBERS CLARK

See
Cognitive-Behavioral Therapy (IV)
Herbal Therapies (IV)

See also
Aging (II)
Antioxidants and Free Radicals (III)
Vitamin C (III)
Vitamin E (III)

MENTAL RETARDATION

Liu and colleagues (1994) reported the use of hyoscyamus, self made Retarde Recovery Pill and acupuncture with 80 infants diagnosed with infantile mental retardation due to perinatal brain injury. Fifty other infants comprised the control group. They were treated with Nao An Tai, Nao Fu Kang, etc. After 3 months of treatment, the IQ increased by 15 points in 29 of the treatment group and 3 infants in the control group. After treatment for 6 months, IQ increased in 41 of the treatment group and 5 of the control group. In 59%, speech and motion greatly improved. The researchers stated that combining traditional Chinese and Western medicine proved effective.

CAROLYN CHAMBERS CLARK

MORNING SICKNESS

Nausea and vomiting associated with early pregnancy have been treated effectively with acupressure. Hyde (1989) reported the use of acupressure using a two-group, prospective, random assignment crossover design. Eight women in one group used acupressure wristbands for 5 days, followed by 5 days not wearing the wristbands. The Multiple Affect Adjective Checklist and Sickness Impact Profile were used, and extent of nausea was assessed at baseline and on days 5 and 10. The acupressure wristbands relieved morning sickness in 12 of

16 women, resulting in a statistically significant reduction in anxiety, depression, behavior dysfunction, and nausea.

De Aloysio and Penacchioni (1992) also reported on the antiemetic effect of acupressure at the Neiguan point on the wrist. Sixty women in early pregnancy entered into a randomized, double-blind, crossover, placebo-controlled trial. Use of acupressure resulted in a significantly lower frequency of morning sickness compared with placebo treatment. Changing from unilateral to bilateral pressure on the Neiguan point produced no significant statistical difference.

CAROLYN CHAMBERS CLARK

MULTIPLE SCLEROSIS

Multiple sclerosis (MS) is a progressive, degenerative disorder affecting the white (and occasionally, gray) matter of the central nervous system. The result is abnormal nerve conduction. The cause is not clear, but some research suggests an immune-mediated response to a viral trigger (Frozena, 1997). Prevalence of multiple sclerosis has been increasing (Schwyzer, 1992), and traditional medical therapies offer treatments that are only temporarily effective (Goodkin, Ransohoff, & Rudick, 1992).

Use of Complementary Therapies

Fawcett, Sidney, Riley-Lawless, and Hanson (1996) described complementary therapies used by 16 people diagnosed with MS. Types of symptoms reported included numbness ($n = 16$), weakness ($n = 44$), visual disturbances ($n = 25$), paresis ($n = 19$), sensory changes ($n = 19$), loss of balance ($n = 13$), paralysis ($n = 13$), bladder dysfunction ($n = 13$), fatigue ($n = 6$), tremor ($n = 6$), tingling ($n = 6$), and verbal dysfunction ($n = 6$).

Kinds of complementary therapies included having mercury dental fillings removed (56%), homeopathy (50%), massage (50%), nutrition (44%), acupuncture (44%), physical therapy (32%), psychological counseling (32%), aquatic therapy (19%), shiatsu (13%), biofeedback (13%), chelation (13%), therapeutic touch (6%), and yoga (6%).

All of the respondents reported that the severity of their symptoms decreased as a direct result of the complementary therapy. There was a statistically significant improvement in symptom severity following use of complementary therapies.

Many participants reported using more than one complementary therapy, suggesting they continued to search for the one treatment that will relieve their symptoms and improve their functional status. Whether the relief they experienced represented a real or placebo effect is not known.

Aerobic Training

Petajan and colleagues (1996) reported the use of aerobic training and its effect on fitness and quality of life in multiple sclerosis. Fifty people diagnosed with MS were randomly assigned to exercise or nonexercise groups. Measures of aerobic training, including maximal aerobic capacity, isometric strength, body composition, and blood lipids were measured before and after training. Information about daily activities, mood, fatigue, and disease status were gathered via the Profile of Mood States Sickness Impact Profile, Fatigue Severity Scale, and neurological examination. Training consisted of three 40-minute sessions per week. There was improved bowel and bladder function in the exercise group and significant increases in maximal aerobic capacity, upper and lower extremity strength, skinfolds, triglycerides, very-low-density lipoprotein, depression, anger, and fatigue ratings.

Electromagnetic Therapy

Sandyk (1997) reported the use of weak electromagnetic fields to reduce sleep paralysis in a woman with multiple sclerosis. Sleep paralysis has been reported in people with MS, including frightening vivid hallucinations and dreams, and the sensation of struggling to move. A 40-year-old woman who had complained of episodes of sleep paralysis since the age of 16 was given AC pulsed applications of picotesla intensity electromagnetic fields (EMFs) of 5 Hz frequency extracerebrally one to two times per week. During the course of treatment her vision, mobility, balance, bladder control, fatigue, and short-term memory improved. In addition, her baseline pattern reversal visual evoked potential normalized 3 weeks after the initiation of magnetic therapy and continued normal for more than 2.5 years. Sleep paralysis gradually abated over the next 3 years. The researcher theorizes that AC pulsed EMFs enhanced melatonin, circadian rhythms, and cerebral serotoninergic neurotransmission.

Hypnosis

Recent reports suggest an emotional component to MS. Sutcher (1997) reported the use of hypnosis for individuals with multi-

ple sclerosis. One man had been wheel chair bound for 35 years. The second man had recently been diagnosed and was minimally affected, but had difficulty with balance and walked with the aid of a cane. The third case was a women who reported pain in her right leg. Sutcher reported that all three showed improvement either immediately or within several weeks after the hypnotist suggested improvement or the displacement of symptoms. No attempt was made to deal with the psychodynamics or to suggest alternate symptoms. Symptoms substitution did not occur. A secondary effect of the hypnosis session was that all three people exhibited increased hopefulness.

CAROLYN CHAMBERS CLARK

See
  Acupuncture and Chinese Medicine (IV)
  Apitherapy: Research and Clinical Use (IV)
  Biofeedback (IV)
  Exercise (IV)
  Nutrition (IV)
  Shiatsu (IV)
  Therapeutic Touch: Uses, Research and Standards for Practice (IV)
  Yoga (IV)

NAUSEA AND VOMITING

In addition to the discomfort the symptoms evoke, detrimental effects including dehydration, weight loss, and fluid and electrolyte imbalance must be considered. Some complementary approaches that have been used include music therapy, hypnosis, progressive muscle relaxation, dietary modifications, and acupressure (Keller, 1995).

Acupressure

Nausea is the most common postoperative complication of anesthesia. Ferrara-Love, Sekeres, and Bircher (1996) used acupressure to prevent the problem. Ninety individuals scheduled for surgery were randomly assigned to the treatment group (received bilateral elastic bands designed to exert pressure on the appropriate location on the distal aspect of the wrist during the perioperative period), the placebo group (wore elastic bands incapable of pressure on the acupoint), or the control group (routine health care). The incidence of post-surgery nausea and vomiting was 10% in the treatment group, 20% in the placebo group, and 50% in the control group. The study provided evidence that incidence of nausea can be significantly decreased with placebo and further reduction can be obtained by using acupressure.

Fan and colleagues (1997) studied 200 healthy people undergoing a variety of short surgical procedures in a randomized, double-blind study. The acupressure group included 108 individuals, and the control group, 92. Spherical beads of acupressure bands were placed at the P6 points in the anterior surface of both forearms in the treatment group and inappropriately on the posterior surface for the control group. The acupressure bands were put in place before induction of anesthesia and were removed 6 hours after surgery. All bands were covered with a soft cotton wrapping to conceal them from the blinded observer, who evaluated all participants for the presence of nausea and vomiting and checked the order sheet for any antiemetics prescribed. Age, gender, height, weight, and type and duration of surgical procedures were comparable in both groups. In the treatment group, 23% of the participants had nausea and vomiting. In the control group, 41% did.

Belluomini, Litt, Lee, and Katz (1994) used acupressure to reduce the nausea and vomiting of pregnancy of 60 women. The treatment group used acupressure point PC-6, and a sham control group used a placebo point. Participants were blind to group assignment. For 10 consecutive evenings, participants completed an assessment scale describing the severity and frequency of their symptoms. Data from the first 3 days were used as baseline scores. On the morning of day 4 (through day 7), each woman used acupressure on her assigned point for 10 minutes four times a day. Data from day 4 were discarded to allow a treatment effect to result. There were no differences between groups in attrition, parity, fetal number, gestational age at entry, maternal age, or pretreatment nausea and vomiting scores. Nausea improved significantly in the treatment group compared to the sham control group.

Vitamin B6

Sahakian, Rouse, Sipes, Rose, and Niebyl (1991) used a randomized, double-blind, placebo-controlled study of pyridoxine hydrochloride (vitamin B6) for the treatment of nausea and vomiting associated with pregnancy. Thirty-one women received vitamin B6, 25 mg tablets every 8 hours for 72 hours, whereas the control group of 28 received a placebo following the same regime. Twelve of 31 women in the vitamin B6 group had a pretreatment nausea score greater than 7 (on a scale of 1 to 10), as did 10 of the women in the placebo group. Following therapy, there was a significant difference in the mean difference in nausea score (baseline minus posttherapy nausea) between women with severe nausea receiving vitamin B6 and placebo at the .01 level. Fifteen of 31 women in the treatment group had vomiting before therapy, compared to 10 of 28 in the placebo group (not significant). At the completion of 3 days of therapy, only 8 of 31 women in the vitamin B6 group had any vomiting, compared with 15 of 28 women in the placebo group.

CAROLYN CHAMBERS CLARK

See
  Hypnotherapy (IV)
  Music Therapy (IV)
  Nutrition (IV)

NEURAL TUBE DEFECT

The incidence of neural tube defects (NTDs) in the United States is 1 to a:1000 births. Spina bifida (defective closure of the vertebral column) or anencephaly (absence of the cerebral hemispheres) are inherited as multifactorial disorders.

Willett (1992) reviewed a series of non-randomized and randomized intervention trials and case-control and cohort studies examining the use of supplements to reduce the risk of neural tube defects. Women using multivitamins or folic acid supplements (usually 200-400 mcg per day) during the first 6 weeks of pregnancy experienced a three- to fourfold reduction in neural tube defects in their offspring. The data provided strong evidence that many U.S. women were not receiving sufficient folic acid to minimize their risk of a defective pregnancy.

Folate is widely distributed in foods and is found in especially high levels in dark green leafy vegetables, legumes, some citrus fruits and juices, and organ meats, such as liver. Folic acid has also been added to many ready-to-eat breakfast cereals and appears in multivitamin supplements.

CAROLYN CHAMBERS CLARK

See
  Nutrition (IV)

NOISE, NOXIOUS, EFFECTS OF

Noxious noise levels can interfere with physiological and behavioral balance. Music has been used to induce relaxation states and reduce stress responses. Kaminski and Hall (1996) examined the effect of calming music for newborns in hospital nurseries, theorizing that noxious noise levels in the nursery could interfere with neonatal efforts to achieve a healthy physiological and behavioral balanced state.

Their study used a one-group, pretest, posttest design. A convenience sample of 20 term, Caucasian neonates comprised the sample. The number of high arousal behavioral states and the number of state changes of the newborns was recorded for a control and treatment group. Soothing, lyrical music was played in the baby's bed for the treatment group. A significant difference was observed at the .01 level. Their results suggested that soothing music may help reduce high arousal states and state lability in newborns.

CAROLYN CHAMBERS CLARK

See
  Music Therapy (IV)

See also
  Balance Disorders (II)

OBESITY

Obesity occurs when energy intake chronically exceeds energy expenditure. Obesity contributes to non-insulin-dependent type II diabetes mellitus, cardiovascular (heart and blood vessel) conditions, and all-cause mortality. To date, drugs have not produced and sustained a significant body weight loss. Even those that have produced short-term weight loss can have significant side effects. Given the problems of polypharmacy in older adults and the physiological changes that occur with aging, it is debatable whether obesity should be treated with drug intervention (Dvorak et al., 1997).

In the United States, one out of four children is obese. By the age of 3 many American children have fatty deposits in their aortas. Excess fruit juice consumption (12 fl oz/day) by preschool-aged children is associated with short stature and obesity (Dennison, Rockwell, & Baker, 1997). Obesity is also a problem in the adult population and is increasingly being recognized as a problem for the older adult.

Chromium and Exercise Training

Grant, Chandler, Castle, and Ivy (1997) examined the effects of supplementing obese young women diagnosed with non-insulin-dependent diabetes mellitus with 400 mcg of chromium, with or without exercise training. Chromium picolinate supplementation alone resulted in significant weight gain, whereas exercise training combined with chromium nicotinate supplementation led to significant weight loss and lowered insulin response.

Healthy Lifestyle

The only effective long-term strategy for obesity is the adoption of a healthy lifestyle, including exercise and prudent eating. The needed behavior modification may be supplied by a health care or mental health care practitioner.

Mellin, Croughan-Minihane, and Dickey (1997) used a 2-year program called the Solution Method, a developmental skills training program for adult weight management. The program is an adult application of the Shapedown Program used in the management of pediatric obesity. A questionnaire was used to indicate the extent to which weight was a medical and/or psychosocial risk for potential participants. Twenty-two adults completed the group intervention conducted by a dietitian and a mental health professional. They attended 2-hour weekly sessions for an average of 18 weeks. Participants learned six developmental skills: effective limit-setting, strong nurturing, good health, balanced eating, body pride, and mastery living. Data were collected at the beginning of treatment and at 3-, 6-, 12-, and 24-month intervals and included weight, 7-day exercise recalls, blood pressure, and self-rated depression. Weight decreased gradually throughout the 2-year period of study from a mean weight change of −4.2 kg at 3 months to −7.9 kg at 24 months. Compared to baseline, blood pressure (both systolic and diastolic) showed significant improvement during the study period. Depression did not improve significantly, but most participants reported improvement in a broad range of functioning.

CAROLYN CHAMBERS CLARK

See
Exercise (IV)
Nondieting (IV)
Nutrition (IV)

See also
Chromium (III)
Diabetes (II)

OBSESSIVE-COMPULSIVE SYMPTOMS

People affected with obsessive-compulsive symptoms show recurrent, persistent thoughts, as well as impulses or urges (obsessions), leading to the performance of repetitive rituals (compulsions). Psychotherapy is often not effective, but 70% of individuals are helped by behavior therapies such as exposure therapy. In this treatment, the person is brought into contact with the feared object (e.g., dirty clothes, door locks, or elevators) but not permitted to perform the compulsive behavior.

Cognitive-Behavioral Treatment

Freeston and colleagues (1997) randomly assigned 29 people with obsessive-compulsive disorder who did not have overt rituals to a treatment or waiting list. Those in the treatment condition received cognitive-behavioral therapy, including a detailed explanation of the occurrence and maintenance of obsessive thoughts, exposure to obsessive thoughts, response prevention of neutralizing strategies, cognitive restructuring, and relapse prevention.

Individuals in the treatment group improved significantly on measures of severity of obsessions, current functioning, self-reported obsessive-compulsive symptoms, and anxiety. After waiting-list participants were given the same treatment, the combined group improved on all outcome measures and maintained treatment gains at 6-month follow-up.

Yoga

Shannahoff-Khalsa and Beckett (1996) reported the use of yogic techniques in the treatment of eight adults diagnosed with obsessive-compulsive disorder. For 1 year participants practiced a specific yogic breathing pattern. Although not a controlled study, of the five people who completed the study, all showed a mean improvement of 54% based on the Symptoms Checklist-90-R. Three participants stopped their medication after 7 months or less and two significantly reduced it, one by 25% and the other by 50%.

Imagery

Imagery is also a useful approach. In this treatment, the person imagines the feared situation while performing a relaxation exercise. Riskind, Wheeler, and Picerno (1997) reported a variant of imagery, during which individuals were taught to reduce fears of contamination and avoidance behavior by imagining that the contamination was frozen in place and unable to move. The freeze imagery reduced self-reports of anxiety and worry and indirect assessments of fear and avoidance behavior.

CAROLYN CHAMBERS CLARK

See
Cognitive-Behavioral Therapy (IV)
Imagery (IV)
Yoga (IV)

OSTEOPOROSIS

Osteoporosis is a condition resulting in the loss of bone density. In the United States alone, more than 1.5 million bone fractures occur every year, costing more than $10 billion. The disorder afflicts 25 million Americans, most of them women. As the elderly population continues to increase, the magnitude of the problem will grow. As young children, age 1 to 5 years, are drinking more fruit juice, consumption of milk has declined. At present, only 50% of children in this age group meet the recommended daily allowance for calcium (Dennison, 1997), putting them at risk for osteoporosis. Individuals with eating disorders are also at risk for osteoporotic fracture (Maugars et al., 1996). Many of these risks could be prevented or lessened in severity if proper attention is given to lifestyle factors.

Carbonated Beverages

Wyshak and Frish (1994) surveyed 76 girls and 51 boys, asking them about the frequency with which they drank soft drinks. In females, a distinct relationship was found between cola beverage consumption and bone fractures. High calcium intake provided some protection against the phosphoric acid in colas that causes calcium to leave bones faster, a major risk factor for osteoporosis in postmenopausal women. Mazariego-Ramos and colleagues (1997) carried out a comparison of 57 children with low serum calcium concentrations and 171 controls. The intake of at least 1.5 l/ week of soft drinks containing phosphoric acid was found to be a risk factor for the development of hypocalcemia. As noted above, low calcium levels in childhood are linked to osteoporosis in later adulthood.

Calcium

There is now unequivocal evidence that high intakes of calcium may prevent or stall the development of osteoporosis both early in life and in early adulthood. There is some evidence that high urine flow caused by alcohol or caffeine intake may contribute to body calcium loss year by year (Hernandez-Avila, 1991). Dairy products, green vegetables, canned fish, and tofu provide good sources of calcium as well as magnesium, vitamin D, magnesium, and vitamin C, nutrients needed for effective bone metabolism (Whiting, Wood, & Kim, 1997). For those who cannot obtain the needed amount of calcium in food, supplementation with either calcium citrate, calcium gluconate, or calcium citrate-maleate is more easily absorbed than calcium carbonate (Smith, Heaney, Flora, & Hinders, 1987).

There is no evidence that calcium and magnesium must be ingested together except in populations with impaired renal function or diabetes, gastrointestinal malabsorption syndrome, or alcoholism. In these cases, a calcium supplement of 100 mg of magnesium for each 500 mg of calcium is recommended (Whiting et al., 1997).

Exercise

Cline (1993) studied that effect of deficient calcium intake, decreased bone density, and lack of exercise and their relationship to risk of stress fractures in female U.S. Army recruits undergoing basic training. Forty-four female recruits with medically confirmed stress fractures were compared with 72 soldiers without stress fractures. Both groups were similar in height, weight, and body mass. Calcium intake during adolescence, as measured by a food frequency questionnaire, showed no difference between the two groups. Bone density for both groups was below the age and gender-specific norms, suggesting a possible lower peak bone mass. Leisure activity energy expenditure in kcal/day during adolescence had a protective effect against stress fracture, and sports participation during high school was positively associated with bone density in the hip.

Fifty healthy volunteers between the ages of 62 and 82 who were leading relatively sedentary lifestyles participated in the study. Using a MedX lumbar extension (lower back) machine, participants were guided through a set of exercises consisting of 15 to 20 repetitions once a week. The machine allowed researchers to isolate and exercise the lumbar muscles by stabilizing the pelvis. Bone measurements were taken at the beginning of the study and at its end 6 months later using an x-ray absorptiometer, which measures density by sending low levels of radiation through bone and muscle. Bone mineral density was increased by 14% after 6 months of exercise (Dohn, 1994).

Dohn (1996) reported that almost 100% of the people who undergo heart transplants develop ostenpenia, or weaking of the bones, and one half of these people will develop osteoporosis unless they begin strength-training. Those who participated in a strength-training program were able to restore and maintain bone mineral density to the same level prior to surgery. Bone mineral density measurements were taken at the onset of the study, at 3 months and again at 6 months for a control group who performed only cardiovascular exercises and another group that combined cardio-

vascular exercises with weight training three times a week. In the weight-training program, participants performed one set (10 to 15 repetitions) of exercises using a machine that isolated the lower back where bones demineralize quickly and fracture easily. They also used eight different upper and lower body exercise machines to stimulate the entire skeleton to grow and remineralize. The rehabilitation strength-building program counterbalanced the effects of the prednisone they were given after transplant.

Puntila and colleagues (1997) studied the association between sports participation during adolescence and peri- and postmenopausal bone mineral density, a risk factor for osteoporosis. In the study, 881 women stated that they had taken part in sports during adolescence. Bone mineral density was measured using dual x-ray absoptiometry in lumbar vertebrae and the left femoral neck. After adjusting for age, weight, time from menopause to densitometry, and duration of estrogen replacement therapy, bone mineral density was significantly higher in the spine among women who had taken part in sports during adolescence. This study provides evidence that recreational physical activity in adolescence could play a role in preventing osteoporosis in later life.

Hip Fracture Risk

According to one longitudinal study of 9,516 white women age 65 years or older who had no previous hip fracture, risk factors that increased the chance of hip fracture included long-acting benzodiazepine therapy, high caffeine intake, less than 4 hours per day on feet, weighing less than they had at age 25, and maternal hip fracture (Cummings et al., 1995).

Salt Intake

Matkovic and colleagues (1995) evaluated 381 girls age 8 to 13 years, during early puberty, for urinary calcium levels and bone mineral density. Excess intakes of calcium were excreted in the urine, and the more salt the girls ate, the more calcium they excreted and the lower their bone density levels.

Based on diets and bone changes over 2 years, a similar study of 124 postmenopausal women showed that for sodium levels beyond 2,600 mg/day, as much as 891 mg of calcium was lost. Switching to fresh vegetable condiments (slices of tomato instead of ketchup or salsa) can reduce sodium intake by 175 mg or more.

CAROLYN CHAMBERS CLARK

See

Exercise (IV)
Nutrition (IV)

See also

Aging (II)
Eating Disorders (II)
Fractures (II)
Hip Fractures (II)

PAIN

Pain can be either acute or chronic. In the United States estimated annual costs of chronic pain are $90 billion in direct or indirect health care costs, or loss of productivity due to work absences (Ross, 1996).

In one study (White, LeFort, Amsel, & Jeans, 1997), people with chronic pain reported higher pain intensity, higher anxiety and distress, less certainty that their pain would resolve, longer hospitalization, less independence in ambulation, a diagnosis of trauma, and less need for surgery. Chronic pain is also linked with depression (Ross, 1996).

Acupressure and Postoperative Pain

Felhendler and Lisander (1996) studied the analgesic effect of acupoint pressure on postoperative pain in a controlled, single-blind study. Forty participants undergoing knee arthroscopy in an ambulatory surgery unit were randomized to receive either an active stimulation (AS) or a placebo stimulation (PS) 30 minutes after awakening from anesthesia. Fifteen classical acupoints were stimulated in the AS group on the side opposite surgery, with firm pressure and a gliding movement across the acupoint. In the PS group, 15 nonacupoints were subjected to light pressure in the same areas as the acupoints in the AS group. Pain was assessed using a 100 mm visual analog scale (VAS) before sensory stimulation, at 30 and 60 minutes and after 24 hours. The results (VAS pain scores) indicated that pressure on acupoints decreased postoperative pain.

He, Hsu, Tsai, and Lee (1996) used stimulation of the P-6 (Neiguan) acupoint to relieve nausea and vomiting following administration of epidural morphine for post–cesarean section pain relief. Using a randomized, double-blind, and controlled trial, the researchers sampled 60 women. Participants received either acupressure bands or placebo bands on the P-6 acupoint before administration of spinal anesthesia and were observed over a 48-hour period. The incidence of vomiting and nausea was significantly decreased from 43% and 27% in the control group, to 3% and 0% in the acupressure group.

Acupuncture and Pain

Tavola, Gala, Conte, and Invernizzi (1992) randomly chose 30 people with tension-type headache to undergo a trial of acupuncture and sham acupuncture. Five measures were used to assess symptom severity and treatment response: intensity, duration and frequency of headache pain episodes, headache index, and analgesic intake. Measures were assessed during baseline, and after 4 weeks, 8 weeks, and 1, 6, and 12 months thereafter. Frequency of headache episodes, analgesic consumption, and the headache index (but not the duration or intensity of headache episodes) significantly decreased over time for both acupuncture and placebo treatment.

Sun, Li, and Si (1992) compared the effect of acupuncture and epidural anesthesis in 80 people having appendectomies. There was less respiratory distress, hypotension, and cardiac arrhythmias, as well as less liquid infusion needed, for the acupuncture anesthesia group. Intestinal gas excreted, number of analgesics and antibiotics administered, and rate of wound infection were significantly better for the acupuncture anesthesia group.

Aromatherapy Helps Perineal Discomfort

In a blind, randomized clinical trial involving three groups of mothers, Dale and Cornwell (1994) studied 635 women. Participants were divided into three groups: One group used pure lavender oil for perineal discomfort following childbirth, one used a synthetic lavender oil, and one used an inert substance as a bath additive for 10 days following normal childbirth. No side effects were found. The women using lavender oil as a bath additive recorded lower mean discomfort scores between day 3 and 5, a time when the mother usually finds herself discharged home and perineal discomfort is high.

Exercise and Education Reduce Musculoskeletal Pain

Ferrell and colleagues (1997) reported a pilot study to evaluate an exercise program for older adults with chronic musculoskeletal pain. Thirty-three people with back, knee, or hip pain were randomly assigned to (1) a 6-week supervised program of walking; (2) a pain education instruction program with demonstration of use of heat, cold, massage, relaxation, and distraction; (3) usual care. Outcomes included pain, self-reported health and functional status, and performance-based measures of functional status. All were evaluated at baseline and at 2 and 8 weeks (end of study). Both intervention groups demonstrated significant improvements in pain and performance-based measures of functional status, whereas the control group showed no change.

Hypnosis

Crawford (1995) examined the effect of hypnosis on chronic pain, the most frequent symptom presented by clients to the primary care physician. The researcher studied how hypnotically suggested analgesia affected the electrophysiology of the brain during either electrical stimulation (assessed by somatosensory event-related potentials) or ice cold water (assessed by EEG brain wave activity). Participants included 17 adults with chronic low back pain and 20 without pain. In the study, participants kept daily pain and sleep diaries for 1 week prior to the first session, then for a minimum of 3 subsequent weeks. They were interviewed about their pain and medical histories and participated in a hypnosis assessment. During a training procedure, participants placed their left hand in ice water for five 60-second dips. During three dips, they learned hypnotic techniques of imagery, distraction, redefinition, and dissociation to reduce or eliminate the perception of pain and distress. In session 2, they were given 30 electrical stimulations to the middle finger in conditions of waking and hypnosis. Participants were told to ignore or attend to the pain they felt. Accompanying somatosensory event–related potentials were recorded at 109 scalp sites. During session 3, each participant's EEG at 19 scalp sites was recorded during 60-second cold pressor pain dips in conditions of waking and hypnosis while each was told to ignore the pain using hypnotic analgesia suggestions. The results were the following: During the hypnotic analgesia condition, participants reduced their pain and distress significantly, and successful transfer to home and work occurred for learned laboratory skills. Thirty-five percent reported a decrease or cessation of medications to assist in nighttime sleep. Time to fall asleep also was reduced from 1 hour to less than 30 minutes, and the depression rating was significantly reduced.

Music Therapy Decreases Pain

Henry (1995) reviewed the literature on the use of music therapy and found the procedure can reduce both pain and anxiety in critical care patients. Zimmerman, Nie-

veen, Barnason, and Schmaderer (1996) examined the effects of second- and third-day postoperative music interventions (music or music video) on pain and sleep for 96 individuals having coronary artery bypass graft surgery. The McGill Pain Questionnaire results indicated no difference between rest period control group and music groups, but the music group had significantly lower scores on the evaluative component of pain on postoperative day 2 than did the rest control group.

Schorr (1993) investigated the use of music as a means of altering the perception of chronic pain among women with rheumatoid arthritis. Thirty women responded to the McGill Pain Questionnaire prior to listening to music of their choice, during music, and 1 to 2 hours after completing the treatment. Results were analyzed using the Number of Words Chosen and the Pain Rating Index-Rank of the McGill Questionnaire. Results provided evidence of the use of music for altering the perception of chronic pain.

CAROLYN CHAMBERS CLARK

See
Acupuncture and Chinese Medicine (IV)
Aromatherapy (IV)
Exercise (IV)
Hypnotherapy (IV)
Music Therapy (IV)

PAIN, CHRONIC

Neurochemical Abnormalities and Their Treatment

All persons with chronic pain have some degree of depression; many have severe psychosocial distress and/or depression preceding onset of pain. The following are some of the neurochemical abnormalities found at the Shealy Institute based on thousands of blood tests done through Nichols Lab (Quest Diagnostics):

1. Taurine deficiency is common in 86% of the individuals treated.
2. Other essential amino acid deficiencies (1 to 7 deficient amino acids are common).
3. Magnesium deficiency in 80% to 100% of patients.
4. Vitamin B6 deficiency in 80% of smokers, 35% of nonsmokers.
5. Norepinephrine excess or deficiency 60% of patients.
6. Dopamine excess or deficiency 10% of patients.
7. Serotonin excess or deficiency 80% of patients.
8. B-endorphin deficiency; very small percent of highly agitated patients have excess.
9. Melatonin excess or deficiency 20% of patients.
10. DHEA or low deficient (about 50% of patients are deficient; 25% in lowest quartile and 25% in second lowest quartile; none in upper 2 quartiles, except rare highly agitated or psychotic patients).

These individuals also have striking EEG abnormalities, demonstrated with computerized EEG mapping:

1. Focal excess activity, any frequency. 75% of the time in right frontal lobe; may be any area.
2. Failure to follow photostimulation appropriately; i.e., 10 Hz may elicit 3 Hz or 20 Hz response, but not 10 Hz.
3. Increased EEG asymmetry when an electric clock is placed within 6 inches of the head. This does not occur in healthy individuals.

The following program has been found most effective in relieving depression as well as improving neurochemical balance and EEG symmetry:

1. Magnesium, 2,000 mg, and vitamin B6, 100 mg; 50 cc IV fluid daily for 10 days.
2. Meat broth, prepared with 8 oz of any type flesh flood and 1 qt water, cooked in slow-cooker 12 hours; daily for 1 month.
3. Cranial electrical stimulation (CES) 1 hour each morning for 1 month. This is a special type of TENS that uses 15,000 Hz at 1 to 2 milliamps of current applied transcranially.
4. Vibratory music (music bed with speakers), classical music 1 hour daily for 2 weeks.
5. Photostimulation using the Shealy RelaxMate at 1 to 7.5 Hz, 1 hour daily for 1 month.
6. Videotaped educational lectures, 1 hour per day for 10 days. These cover a wide variety of topics related to physical and psychological health.
7. Videotaped educational lectures, 1 hour per day for 10 days. These cover a wide variety of topics related to physical and psychological health.

Fifty percent of those with depression improved just with CES as measured by the Zung Test for Depression. Using all four modalities, there was an improvement in 85% of patients as measured by the Zung Test for Depression and the MMPI. Using just the music, photostimulation, and educational videotapes, 55% improve. With no further intervention, 80% remain without depression 3 to 6 months after treatment. A longer follow-up is currently under way.

For pain relief, bromelain 1,000 mg, 4 times a day, 30 minutes a.c. and h.s., has been as effective as NSAIDS, without side effects.

C. NORMAN SHEALY

PARKINSON'S DISEASE

Up to two million older Americans are estimated to be affected by Parkinson's disease (PD), a chronic, progressive neurological disorder. Classic symptoms include tremors (intensified by stress or fatigue that disappear during sleep or concentrated effort), muscular stiffness or rigidity, slowing of body motion, and a characteristic shuffle.

Approximately 90% of people diagnosed with PD are labeled cause unknown. A current theory is that PD may be caused by a toxic environmental agent or chemical compound. Reports of greater prevalence in rural areas suggest a possible link to exposure to agricultural chemicals. The herbicide Parquat is a likely culprit (Reis, 1995). Dieldrin and DDT have also been implicated (Fleming et al., 1994).

Antioxidants and Free Radicals

Scheider and colleagues (1997) used a case-control study to examine the possible role of long-term dietary antioxidant intake in PD etiology. Participants include 57 men age 45 to 79 with at least two cardinal signs of PD and age-matched friend controls chosen from lists provided by partici-

pants. Antioxidant intake, except for lycopene (primarily tomatoes and related products), was not associated with reduced PD risk. Intakes of sweet foods, including fruit, were associated with higher PD risk. The researchers theorized that pesticide residues in the fruits and vegetables may have contributed to the development of PD.

Using a much larger sample, de Rijk and colleagues (1997) investigated whether high dietary intake of antioxidants decreased the risk of PD. The community-based Rotterdam Study studied 5,342 individuals living independently without dementia. Participants were between the ages of 55 and 95 years of age. The researchers used a semiquantitative food frequency questionnaire to study the association between dietary intake of antioxidants and PD. Results were adjusted for age, sex, smoking habits, and energy intake. Those with PD who had a Hoehn-Yahr stage of 2.5 or 3.0 were excluded. The data still suggested that a high intake of dietary vitamin E may protect against the occurrence of PD (de Rijk et al., 1997).

Ayurveda

Manyam (1996) examined *Mucuna pruriens*, an herb claimed to be active in treating Parkinson's. Using an animal model, the researcher examined the use of *Mucuna Prurien endocarp* (MPE) and found it effective as a treatment for PD.

Electromagnetic Restoration of Dream Recall

Sleep disorders occur in 74% to 98% of people with Parkinson's disease, adversely affecting their quality of life (Partinen, 1997). Markedly reduced or absent REM sleep with cessation of dream recall and associated right hemispheric dysfunction has been documented in numerous neurological disorders including Parkinson's. Sandyk (1997) reported treatment of a 69-year-old man who had experienced complete cessation of dreaming since the onset of motor disability and treatment with levodopa and dopamine. Dreaming was restored after six treatments of AC pulsed picotesla range electromagnetic fields (EMFs) applied extracranially over three successive days (three sessions) followed 6 months later with three additional sessions. After treatment, hypnagogic imagery prior to the onset of sleep and vivid dreams with intense colored visual imagery were reported, indicating improvement in visual memory known to be subserved by the right temporal lobe.

CAROLYN CHAMBERS CLARK

See
Ayurveda (IV)
Magnet Therapy (IV)

See also
Antioxidants and Free Radicals (III)
Vitamin E (III)

PERINEAL TEARS

Tears of the mother's perineum are common during the birth process. Shipman, Boniface, Tefft, and McCloghry (1997) studied the effects of antenatal perineal massage on subsequent perineal outcomes at delivery. Their single-blind, randomized study included 861 pregnant women with single pregnancies. After adjusting for the mother's age and the infant's birth weight, their findings included a statistical signifi-

cant result for mothers in the perineal massage group, compared to the control, no massage group. The effect was stronger in mothers who were 30 years old or older.

CAROLYN CHAMBERS CLARK

PREECLAMPSIA

There is evidence that oxidative stress accompanies preeclampsia (high blood pressure during pregnancy). Ascorbic acid (vitamin C) salt levels (ascorbates) are 50% lower in preeclampsia relative to normal pregnancy. Hubel and colleagues (1997) concluded that ascorbate-oxidizing activity is increased in preeclampsia plasma, which might contribute to vascular dysfunction.

CAROLYN CHAMBERS CLARK

See also
Pregnancy (II)

PREGNANCY

Scholl and colleagues (1997) examined the relationship between prenatal multivitamin/mineral supplement use during the first and second trimesters of pregnancy by 1,430 low-income, urban women and preterm delivery and infant low birth weight. Compared with women who did not use prenatal supplements, supplement use was associated with a twofold reduction in risk of preterm delivery and infant low birth weights. For very low birth weight infants, there was a sevenfold reduction in risk with first trimester supplementation and a greater than sixfold reduction when supplementation was started in the second trimester. The researchers concluded that prenatal multivitamin and multimineral supplementation has the potential to diminish infant morbidity and mortality.

High blood pressure in the mother can lead to maternal and fetal death. Bucher and colleagues (1996) used a meta-analysis of 14 randomized trials involving 2,459 women to examine the effect of calcium supplements during pregnancy on blood pressure reduction and preeclampsia (sudden rise in blood pressure late in pregnancy, excessive weight gain, generalized swelling, headache, visual disturbances, and other complications). The researchers found that calcium supplements during pregnancy lead to an important reduction in systolic and diastolic blood pressure and preeclampsia.

Exercise during pregnancy is also protective for mothers and does not appear to increase infant risks (Sternfeld, Quesenberry, Eskenazi, & Newman, 1995). Bed rest, though, has been associated with weight loss, muscle atrophy, headache, and depression in the mother. Weight loss is especially troubling because it may increase preterm birth (Land, 1994).

CAROLYN CHAMBERS CLARK

See
Exercise (IV)

See also
High Blood Pressure (II)
Preeclampsia (II)

PREMATURE RUPTURE OF FETAL MEMBRANES

Premature rupture of the fetal membranes (PROM) is a major contributor to fetal and infant death. Nutritional status may play a role. Low levels of vitamin C have been identified as a risk factor. Smoking also depletes vitamin C and may be a risk factor in mothers who smoke.

Despite the cause, low levels of vitamin C can lead to impaired integrity of the amniotic sac because of reduced collagen content or increased susceptibility to damage by free radicals. Barrett (1994) examined the role of vitamins C and E, beta-carotene, and retinol in PROM. The amniotic fluid of 80 pregnant women was analyzed. There were lower fluid levels of vitamin C and beta-carotene in the women with PROM but not in a group of controls. These two nutrients may work together to maintain the health of amniotic membranes.

CAROLYN CHAMBERS CLARK

See also
Vitamin C (III)
Vitamin E (III)

PREMENSTRUAL SYNDROME (PMS)

It is estimated that some 90% of women in the United States suffer from a complex of symptoms called premenstrual syndrome, or PMS. The syndrome is characterized by physical and mental tension, tenderness and swelling of the breasts, depression, irritability, fatigue, aching, menstrual cramping, migraine headaches, cravings for sweets or carbohydrates, and abdominal bloating.

Several factors are known to affect PMS symptoms. Ingesting carbohydrates increases the plasma ratio of tryptophan, affecting central serotonin pathways that regulate mood and modulate eating patterns.

Cravings and their response may be a self-treatment that temporarily relieves PMS symptoms (Moller, 1992). Bloating during the menstrual cycle appears to be more a redistribution of fluid than water retention (Tollan, Oian, Fadnes, & Maltau, 1993), although Marean, Cumming, Fox, and Cumming (1995) found that their sample of eight women with validated PMS consciously or unconsciously restricted their fluid intake. Moderate to severe PMS has also been linked to drinking 10 or more alcoholic beverages per week (Caan et al., 1993). In one study, women with PMS experienced more negative life events, had more difficulty with anger, and more concerns with self- and social control than women with low-severity symptoms (Woods et al., 1997).

Symptoms of PMS are variable and last from 1 to ten days. Although there is no widely accepted medical treatment for PMS, there are some complementary practices that offer hope.

Exercise

Steege and Blumenthal (1993) evaluated the effect of aerobic exercise and strength training on premenstrual symptoms in 23 healthy middle-aged women. Symptoms were assessed at baseline and after 3 months of an exercise program. Both groups were associated with general improvement in many premenstrual symptoms, but women in the aerobic exercise group improved in more symptoms, particularly premenstrual depression.

Food and Supplements

Calcium Supplementation Relieves PMS Symptoms

Thys-Jacobs and colleagues (1989) used a randomized crossover trial to study the efficacy of calcium supplementation in women with PMS. Thirty-three women in a clinic at a large hospital completed the trial. Initial evaluation included a physical exam, routine lab tests, psychiatric evaluation, and dietary assessment. Each participant received 6 months of treatment involving 3 months of supplementation daily with 1,000 mg of calcium carbonate and 3 months with a placebo.

Efficacy was assessed by changes in daily symptom scores and by an overall global assessment at the end of the study. Seventy-three percent of the women reported fewer symptoms while taking calcium supplements. Calcium significantly alleviated water retention, pain, and negative affect.

Carbohydrate Beverage Relieves Symptoms

Sayegh and colleagues (1995) used a specially formulated carbohydrate-rich beverage known to increase the serum ratio of tryptophan to test its effect on PMS symptoms. Twenty-four women with confirmed PMS participated in a double-blind, crossover study that compared the special formula with two other isocaloric products. Standardized measures of mood, cognitive performance, and food cravings were taken before and 30, 90, and 180 minutes after consumption of the treatment and placebo beverages. All were given during the late luteal phase of the menstrual cycle. The carbohydrate-rich beverage significantly decreased self-reported depression, anger, confusion, and carbohydrate craving 90 and 180 minutes after ingestion. Memory word recognition was also improved significantly.

Flavonoids May Reduce PMS Congestion

Serfaty and Magneron (1997) reported a national multicenter study evaluating the use of a micronized purified flavonoid to treat PMS symptoms. Daily assessment diaries and weight and circumferential measurements (twice per cycle) were taken on all 1,473 women who completed the trial. The duration of PMS decreased on average by 2.6 days, and symptoms of congestion and weight gain gradually lessened in both frequency and severity by approximately 60%.

Magnesium Used for Negative Mood Changes

Rosenstein and colleagues (1994) demonstrated decreased red blood cell concentrations of magnesium in women with PMS. Facchinetti and associates (1991) used a double-blind, randomized design with 32 women with PMS confirmed by the Moos Menstrual Distress Questionnaire. Cluster "pain" was reduced in both treatment and control groups after 2 months of baseline recording of symptoms. In the women who received magnesium following baseline, total scores on the Menstrual Distress Questionnaire and negative affect subscale rating were significantly affected. The data suggested that magnesium supplementation could be an effective treatment for negative mood changes during PMS.

Stewart (1987) reported on the effect of a double-blind, placebo-controlled study at high and low dosages of supplementation. Laboratory evidence showed significant deficiencies in vitamin B6 and magnesium, among other nutrients. The multivitamin/multimineral supplement used in the study corrected the deficiencies and improved the symptoms of PMS.

Using a double-blind, randomized design, Facchinetti and colleagues (1991), evaluated the effects of oral magnesium on a sample of 32 women age 23 to 39 years with confirmed PMS (Moos Menstrual Distress Questionnaire). In the study, 360 mg of magnesium pyrrolidone carboxylic acid or a placebo was administered three times a day, from the 15th day of the menstrual cycle to the onset of menstrual flow. Blood samples measuring magnesium content were drawn premenstrually, during the baseline period, and in the second and fourth months of treatment. The score of cluster "pain" was significantly reduced during the second month in both groups (baseline recording). Magnesium treatment significantly affected both the total Menstrual Distress score and the negative affect subscale rating.

Vitamin E May Prove Helpful

London, Sundaram, Murphy, and Goldstein (1983) used a double-blind, randomized dose-response design with 75 women with benign breast disease who used a written questionnaire to score the severity of PMS symptoms before and after two months of treatment with placebo or alpha-tocopherol (vitamin E) of 150, 300, or 600 IU per day. After age and pretreatment were controlled for, vitamin E had a significantly greater effect than placebo, improving three of four classes of PMS symptoms, suggesting that vitamin E supplementation can be of value to women with severe PMS symptoms.

London, Murphy, Kitlowski, and Reynolds (1987) repeated their study to confirm their findings. They performed another randomized, double-blind study using vitamin E and placebo on the 41 participants who completed the clinical trial. A significant improvement in certain affective and physical symptoms was noted in women treated with vitamin E.

Zinc Levels Low in PMS Sufferers

Chuong and Dawson (1994) studied the effect of zinc and copper levels on symptoms of premenstrual syndrome. Ten women with PMS and 10 controls gave blood at 2- or 3-day intervals through three menstrual cycles. Serum zinc and copper were measured by flameless atomic absorption spectrophotometry.

In the controls, zinc values were not significantly different between the follicular and luteal phases. In the women suffering from PMS, the values were significantly lower during the luteal phase than during the follicular phase. Copper levels were higher in the women with PMS during the luteal phase compared with the controls. Since copper competes with zinc for intestinal absorption, the zinc to copper ratio can reflect the available zinc in the body. Computations showed that the ratio was significantly lower in women with PMS than the controls during the luteal phase. The researchers concluded that zinc deficiency occurs in PMS during the luteal phase and is further reduced by an elevation in copper.

Ginkgo Biloba Reduces Breast and Neuropsychological Symptoms

Tamborini and Taurelle (1993) reported the use of a standardized *Ginkgo biloba* extract to treat congestive symptoms of PMS in a multicenter, double-blind study. One hundred sixty-five women age 18 to 45 who had at least three cycles of congestive premenstrual symptoms during at least 7 days per cycle comprised the sample. Characteristics of women in the treatment and placebo group were similar. Women were observed for one menstrual cycle to confirm the diagnosis of PMS. For the following two cycles, each woman received either *Ginkgo biloba* or a placebo from the 16th day of the first cycle until the 5th day of the next cycle. Women used a daily rating scale, and the practitioner also evaluated each woman during visits. Gingko results were statistically significant for congestive symptoms of PMS, particularly breast symptoms, compared to the placebo.

Guided Imagery Reduces Menstrual Distress

Groer and Ohnesorge (1993) provided preliminary evidence that menstrual-cycle rhythmicity and premenstrual distress are amenable to the mind-body intervention of guided imagery. Their sample included 30 healthy college women with regular menstrual cycles. Participants completed the Moos Menstrual Distress Questionnaire at the beginning of the study and after 6 months. They recorded their menstrual cycles for 3 months on an investigator-developed calendar recording sheet. Participants were then given an audiotape with a progressive muscle relaxation exercise followed by guided imagery with a suggestive message focusing on lengthening the menstrual cycle and delaying the onset of menstrual bleeding. Fifteen women completed the study, and all had significant increases in cycle lengths during the 3 months of imagery. Total premenstrual distress scores also declined significantly, as did subscales measuring behavior and negative affect.

Positive Reframing and Social Support Decrease Impairment

Morse (1997) reported the use of reframing of perceptions of menstrual cycle experiences to diminish perimenstrual impairment. Through the use of a preexperimental design, social support and a positive reframing component were presented to 18 women. Prospective assessment of perceptions of perimenstrual changes were taken daily. Retrospective assessments of moods (anxiety and depression), social resources, and perimenstrual change perceptions were gathered before, during, and after the treatment. Impairment did decrease as a result of the program, and there were significant changes from baseline to follow-up on state depression and personal resource variables.

Reflexology Relieves Menstrual Symptoms

Oleson and Flocco (1993) studied the use of reflexology. Thirty-five women complaining of previous distress with PMS were randomly assigned to be treated by reflexology or to receive placebo reflexology. All participants completed a daily diary monitoring 38 PMS symptoms on a 4-point scale. Somatic and psychological indicants of PMS were recorded daily for 2 months before treatment, for 2 months during treatment, and for 2 months after treatment. Thirty-minute reflexology sessions were provided for both groups by a trained reflexology therapist once a week for 8 weeks. Analysis of variance revealed a significantly greater decrease in PMS symptoms in women given true reflexology treatment as opposed to the placebo group.

CAROLYN CHAMBERS CLARK

See
Exercise (IV)
Imagery (IV)
Nutrition (IV)
Reflexology (IV)

See also
Calcium (III)
Dang Gui (Dong Quai) (III)
Flavonoids (III)
Gingko (III)
Vitamin E (III)

PRESSURE SORES

Also called bedsores or decubitus ulcers, pressure sores involve ulceration of tissues overlying a bony prominence. Occurs most often in people with diminished or absent sensation, or who are debilitated, emaciated, paralyzed, or long bedridden. Depending on the individual's position in bed, wheelchair, cast or splint, tissues over the sacrum, ischia, greater trochanters, external malleoli and heels are most susceptible. Muscle, bone and more superficial tissues can be affected (Berkow, 1990).

Goode, Burns, and Walker (1992) examined the contribution of specific nutritional deficiencies to the risk of pressure sores. They used an observation cohort study at St. James University Hospital in Leeds. Participants were 21 older adults who presented consecutively to the orthopedic unit with femoral neck (leg) fracture. Their measure was the full thickness epidermal break over a pressure-bearing surface. Forty-eight percent ($n = 10$) developed a pressure sore during their hospital stay. Zinc status and concentrations of albumin, hemoglobin, and vitamins A and E were similar in participants who developed a pressure sore and those who didn't. What did differ was the mean leucocyte vitamin C concentration. The researchers concluded that low concentrations of leucocyte vitamin C was associated with subsequent development of pressure sores in older adults with femoral neck fracture.

Declair (1997) examined the use of topical application of essential fatty acids to see if it improved hydration and elasticity and helped prevent skin breakdown. In a double-blind study, 86 participants were equally divided into two groups. All had a Norton Scale score of 9 and were fed orally a high-protein diet and/or received parenteral nutrition if severely malnourished. Every 8 hours, approximately 20 ml of solution A (1.6 g EFA with linoleic acid from sunflower oil, 112 IU vitamin A, and 4 IU vitamin E) or solution B (1.6 g mineral oil, 112 IU Vitamin A, and 5 IU vitamin E) was applied to the entire body for 21 days. In group A, two participants developed stage 1 ulcers, 98% had hydrated skin, and 76% maintained skin elasticity. In group B, 12 participants (27%) developed stage 2 ulcers, 22% had hydrated skin, and 34% showed scaly skin; 10 (24%) maintained skin elasticity, while 33 (76%) showed a loss of elasticity. The results provide evidence that essential fatty acids can help the skin maintain integrity.

CAROLYN CHAMBERS CLARK

See
Nutrition (IV)

See also
Fatty Acids, Essential (III)

PROSTATE, ENLARGED

Braeckman (1994) reported on the results of an open, multicenter study that corroborates numerous double-blind, controlled studies. All research shows that saw palmetto (*Serenoa repens*) standardized to contain 85% to 95% fatty acids and sterols is an effective treatment for benign prostatic hyperplasia, or enlarged prostate gland.

Saw palmetto demonstrated superiority over finseteride (Proscar). While Proscar takes approximately a year to produce any significant results, saw palmetto extract produced relief of symptoms within the first 30 days of treatment. Physician global evaluations after days 45 and 90 demonstrated 81% to 88% effectiveness, respectively. There were no serious adverse reactions reported.

Maximum urinary flow increased from 9.78 to 12.19 ml/s, and the international prostate symptom score decreased from 19.0 to 12.4. The most impressive improvements occurred in the quality of life scores.

CAROLYN CHAMBERS CLARK

RADIATION POISONING

Gong and colleagues (1991) studied the effect of 23 sodium alginate (seaweed or kelp) preparations from different species of algae (*Sargassum* sp.) and kelp (*Laminaria* sp.) on reducing absorption of the radioactive element strontium. Sodium alginate proved to be a potent agent for reducing strontium absorption, with virtually no toxicity. In human volunteers, strontium absorption was reduced by 78%. No undesirable effects on gastrointestinal function were observed nor were calcium, iron, copper, or zinc metabolism levels changed in either animal or human studies. The researchers concluded that alginate preparations derived from *Sargassum* species are a suitable antidote against radiostrontium absorption on a long-term basis when added to bread at a 6% level. In cases of emergency, they suggested that an alginate syrup preparation may be more suitable because of its rapid action.

Sakagami and colleagues (1997) found that the addition of vitamin E prior to radiation provided a protective effect for body cells.

CAROLYN CHAMBERS CLARK

See also

Heart and Blood Vessel Conditions (II)

Wounds (II)

REPETITIVE STRAIN INJURIES

Moore and Wiesner (1996) examined the effectiveness of behaviorally induced vasodilation (hypnosis with biofeedback and autogenics) in the treatment of upper extremity repetitive strain injuries (RSI). Thirty participants with recent onset of upper extremity RSI symptoms were randomly assigned to hypnotically induced vasodilation or a waiting-list control group. Individuals in the treatment condition had significant increases in hand temperature and pain reduction between pre- and post-treatment, as compared to the control group.

CAROLYN CHAMBERS CLARK

See

Autogenic Training (IV)

Biofeedback (IV)

Hypnotherapy (IV)

SKIN DISORDERS

Zachariae, Oster, Bjerring, and Kragballe (1996) reported the use of stress management, guided imagery, and relaxation in the treatment of psoriasis. Fifty-one individuals with psoriasis vulgaris were randomly assigned to a treatment or a control group. Those in the treatment group participated in 12 sessions, which covered stress management, guided imagery, and relaxation techniques. When analyses were performed for both groups separately, the treatment group showed significant reductions on the Psoriasis Area Severity Index, Total Sign Score, and Laser Doppler Skin Blood Flow, but no changes were seen in the control group.

Sheehan and Atherton (1994) conducted a double-blind, placebo-controlled trial of a specific formulation of Chinese medicinal herbs for atopic eczema. After 12 months, 18 (of 37) children who had not responded to other treatments showed at least 90% reductions in eczema activity, and 5 showed lesser degrees of improvement. Fourteen children withdrew due to lack of response and 4 because of unpalatability of treatment or difficulty in the preparation of treatment. After a year, 7 of the remaining children were able to discontinue treatment without relapse. The other 16 required treatment to maintain control of their eczema, but only 4 required daily treatment. The researchers concluded that Chinese medicinal herbs provided a therapeutic option for children with extensive atopic eczema that failed to respond to medical treatment.

Stewart and Thomas (1995) treated 18 adults with extensive atopic dermatitis that was resistant to conventional treatment. The researchers used hypnotherapy and found their approach produced a statistically significant benefit measured both subjectively and objectively. Results were maintained 2 years later. The researchers also treated 20 children with severe, resistant atopic dermatitis. All but one showed immediate improvement. Eighteen months after treatment, of the 12 children who replied to a questionnaire, 10 had maintained improvement in itching and scratching, 9 in sleep disturbance, and 7 reported mood improvement.

Skaper and colleagues (1997) found that flavonoids are broadly protective for skin subjected to oxidative stress. Quercetin, in particular, when paired with vitamin C, may be of therapeutic benefit in protecting the skin from oxidative damage.

Shukla, Rasik, and Patnaik (1997) investigated the involvement of free radicals in a self-healing cutaneous wound. Vitamins E and C decreased by 60% to 70% post-wounding and do not fully reach prewound levels for 14 days, indicating an increased need for the vitamins.

CAROLYN CHAMBERS CLARK

See
Herbal Therapies (IV)
Hypnotherapy (IV)
Imagery (IV)

See also
Vitamin C (III)
Vitamin E (III)

STRESS

Stress is an elusive concept. For this reason, endocrinological and immunological correlates are often used to study its effects. Infection, trauma, and even martial conflict (Kiecolt-Glaser, Glaser, Cacioppo, & MacCallum, 1997) result in inflammatory stress. Tissue damage, enhanced inflammatory mediator production, and suppressed lymphocyte function are all expected consequences. Deficiencies in vita-

min E, vitamin B6, and riboflavin reduce cell numbers in lymphoid tissue and produce abnormalities in immune function. Vitamins C and E exert anti-inflammatory effects in studies in humans and animals. Dietary supplementation in humans with vitamins C, E, and B6 enhances lymphocyte function. The effect is most apparent in older adults (Grimble, 1997).

Antioxidative Vitamins

Martin and colleagues (1996) studied the effect of d-alpha-tocopherol (vitamin E) on oxidative stress in human aortic endothelial cells. The cells were preincubated with vitamin E at 15, 30, and 60 microM prior to exposure to a free radical generator, AAPH. Vitamin E treatment significantly reduced interleukin production after AAPH exposure, showing the vitamin's antioxidant protection against lipid peroxidation.

Sen and colleagues (1997) also studied vitamin E's effect on lipid peroxidation. They divided rats into two groups and supplemented them with fish oil, fish oil and vitamin E, soy oil, and soy oil and vitamin E. Both groups were divided into corresponding exercise groups. The liver appeared to be relatively less susceptible to exercise-induced oxidative stress in the fish oil and vitamin E group.

Artichoke Extract

Gebhardt (1997) demonstrated that artichoke extracts have a marked antioxidative (stress) and protective potential, at least for animal models.

Biofeedback

Infant crying can produce intense parental stress and can precede physical child abuse or neglect. Biodesensitization is a new technique that teaches people to control the source of stress and develop self-control over their physiological stress responses. Tyson (1996) assigned 15 female participants to either EEG biofeedback pretraining without stress, or pretraining or no pretraining while listening to infant crying. Biofeedback training significantly shifted participant response to infant crying. Tyson concluded that stress management training may help ameliorate aversive responses to infant crying and could prevent child abuse.

Chinese Herbs

Haraguchi, Ishikawa, Shirataki, and Fukuda (1997) evaluated the effect of honokiol, magnolol, and neolignans. The neolignans protected mitochondrial respiratory chain enzyme activity against NADPH-induced peroxidative stress and protected red cells against oxidative hemolysis. Honokiol was more potent in antioxidative action than magnolol.

Meditation

Solberg, Halvorsen, Sundgot-Borgen, Ingjer, and Holen (1995) tested the effect of meditation on immune response after strenuous physical stress. They studied six meditating and six nonmeditating male runners in a concurrent, controlled design. After 6 months, blood samples were taken from the meditating group, immediately before and after a maximum oxygen uptake (VO_2max) test. The increase in CD8+ T cells after VO_2max was significantly less in the meditation group than in the control group. The researchers concluded that meditation may modify the suppressive effect of strenuous physical stress on the immune system.

Astin (1997) studied a type of meditation called mindfulness that emphasizes developing a detached observation and awareness of contents of the consciousness. Twenty-eight volunteers were randomized to either treatment or control group. Compared with controls, the treatment group evidenced a significantly greater reduction in psychological symptoms, an increase in overall domain-specific sense of control and utilization of a yielding mode of control, and higher scores on a measure of spiritual experiences. The results suggest that mindfulness may provide relapse prevention in affective disorders.

Music

Aversive auditory stimuli are commonplace in newborn intensive care units. Standley and Moore (1995) studied the effect of music on 20 oxygenated, low-birth-weight infants in a newborn intensive care unit of a regional medical center. Ten infants listened to lullabies and 10 listened to recordings of their mothers' voices through earphones for 20 minutes across 3 consecutive days. Infants hearing music had significantly fewer occurrences of oximeter alarms during auditory stimuli than those who listened to their mothers' voices.

Yoga

Yoga has become increasingly popular in Western countries as a stress coping method. Schell, Allolio, and Schonecke (1994) examined the effect of hatha yoga and a control group of readers in a comfortable position. The course of heart rate was significantly different: The yoga group exhibited a decrease during the yoga practice. Additionally, the yoga group showed significant scores in life satisfaction, stress coping, mood, high spirits, and extrovertedness, and lower scores in excitability, aggressiveness, openness, emotionality, and somatic complaints than the control group.

CAROLYN CHAMBERS CLARK

See
   Biofeedback (IV)
   Hypnotherapy (IV)
   Music Therapy (IV)
   Transcendental Meditation (IV)

See also
   Vitamin E (III)

STROKE

Strokes occur when brain tissue is deprived of blood supply due to an arterial obstruction. The stroke mortality rate in the United States increased for the first time in four decades in 1993, from 26.2 deaths per 100,000 events to 26.4 per 100,000. This increase may correspond to the aging of the population.

Protective Effect of Flavonoids

Some flavonoids are better platelet inhibitors than aspirin and better antioxidants than vitamin E. Research is beginning to accumulate about the protective effect of flavonoids. One recent study examined a cohort of 552 men age 50 to 69. Keli, Hertog, Feskens, and Kromhout (1996) cross-checked and calculated mean nutrient and food intake on dietary histories for 15 years. The association between antioxidants, selected foods, and stroke incidence was assessed by the Cox proportional hazards regression analysis. Adjustment was made for confounding by age, systolic blood pressure, serum cholesterol, cigarette smoking, energy intake, consumption of fish and alcohol, and antioxidant vitamins. Dietary flavonoids, mainly quercetin, were inversely associated with stroke incidence. Vitamins C and E were not associated with stroke risk, whereas black tea and apples were. Black tea contributed about 70% of flavonoid intake, and apples about 10%. The researchers concluded that habitual intake of flavonoids and their major source (tea) may protect against stroke. Men who drank more than 4.7 cups of tea a day had a 69% reduced risk of stroke compared with those who drank less than 2.6 cups a day.

Fruits and Vegetables

Gillman and colleagues (1995) examined the effect of fruit and vegetable intake on risk of stroke among middle-aged men for 20 years as part of the Framingham Study. All 832 men, age 45 through 65 years, were free of cardiovascular disease at baseline (1966–1969). The diet of each participant was assessed using a single 24-hour recall. The estimated total number of servings per day of fruits and vegetables was the variable used for analysis. Age-adjusted risk of stroke decreased across increasing quintile of servings per day. Adjustment for body mass index, cigarette smoking, glucose intolerance, physical activity, blood pressure, serum cholesterol, and intake of energy, ethanol, and fat did not materially change the results. Manson and colleagues (1994) found similar results for women.

Milk

Since 1965, the Honolulu Heart Program has followed a cohort of men in a study of cardiovascular disease. After 22 years of follow-up in 3,150 older middle-aged men, ages 55 to 68 years, Abbott and colleagues (1996) found that men who were nondrinkers of milk experienced stroke at twice the rate of men who consumed 16 oz or more. Intake of dietary calcium was also associated with a reduced risk of stroke, although its association was confounded with milk consumption. Calcium from nondairy sources was not related to stroke. This suggests that other covariates or constituents related to milk ingestion may be important. For example, milk drinkers tended to be leaner and more physically active and to consume healthier foods.

CAROLYN CHAMBERS CLARK

See also
Flavonoids (III)
Heart and Blood Vessel Conditions (II)

SUBSTANCE ABUSE

Alcohol, narcotics, hallucinogens, and stimulants are the psychoactive substances most frequently abused (Randolf, 1993).

Cognitive Behavioral Approaches

Ouimette, Finney, and Moose (1997) compared a 12-step program to a cognitive-behavioral treatment (changing distorted thoughts and enhancing coping skills) for substance abuse. The researchers used a naturalistic design to compare effectiveness. More than 3,000 men participated in the study in 15 Department of Veterans Affairs substance abuse treatment programs. Covariance analyses were used to control for any pretreatment differences. The two programs were equally effective, either individually or combined, for reducing substance symptoms and substance use. Men in the 12-step programs were likely to be abstinent a year later.

Prayer

Some controlled trials have indicated that prayer can influence health status. Walker (1995) explored the use of prayer to reduce drinking in individuals who entered treatment for alcohol abuse or dependence at an outpatient clinic at the University of New Mexico.

Self-report interview on quantity frequency of alcohol or drug use, retention and participation in the treatment program, participation in Alcoholics Anonymous, psychiatric care, religious/spiritual behavior, and more general adjustment comprised the outcome measures. Neither at baseline nor at any point during follow-up was there any difference in drinking outcome between the group receiving intercessory prayer and the control group. Thirty-five percent of participants in the no-prayer group were not located for follow-up, compared to 9% in the prayer group.

Those who were aware that someone was praying for them drank more heavily at the 6-month follow-up. The findings provided evidence that intercessory prayer exerted no effect. At baseline, participants who indicated no one was praying for them had a greater average reduction in drinking.

Yoga

Shaffer, LaSilva, and Stein (1997) compared hatha yoga with dynamic group psychotherapy as methods for enhancing methadone maintenance treatment in a randomized clinical trial. After a 5-day assessment period, 61 participants were randomly assigned to methadone maintenance enhanced by either traditional group psychotherapy or hatha yoga therapy. After 6 months all participants were primarily evaluated on the Symptom Check List and the Addiction Severity Index. There were no meaningful differences between the two groups. Both programs significantly reduced drug use and criminal activities. Additional research is needed to identify which individuals may benefit from yoga.

CAROLYN CHAMBERS CLARK

See
Cognitive-Behavioral Therapy (IV)
Yoga (IV)

SURGERY, EFFECTS OF

Surgery affects nutrient needs and can increase anxiety and stress. Several complementary procedures have demonstrated their usefulness.

Hypnosis, Guided Imagery, and Relaxation

Hypnosis, guided imagery, and relaxation have been shown to improve the postoperative course of adults after surgery. Manyande and colleagues (1995) explored the use of coping imagery with 26 individuals scheduled for abdominal surgery and compared the results with 25 controls who were given background information about the hospital. Participants who were taught imagery were less distressed post operatively,

felt they coped with the surgery better, and requested less analgesia.

Lambert (1996) examined the effect of hypnosis/guided imagery on the postoperative course of 52 children who were matched for sex, age, and diagnosis and randomly assigned to an experimental or control group. The experimental group was taught guided imagery by the investigator, including the suggestion for a favorable postoperative course. Children in the experimental group experienced significantly lower postoperative pain ratings and shorter hospital stays than the control group.

Rapkin, Straubing, and Holroyd (1991) studied the use of imagery/hypnosis with a sample of 36 people who volunteered for the study and were scheduled for head and neck cancer surgery. Twenty-one people received the usual care and were followed through their hospital charts. Fifteen individuals volunteered for the experimental hypnosis intervention. Hypnotizability was negatively correlated with complications postsurgery, and there was a correlation between hypnotizability and blood loss during surgery.

Massage Therapy

DeGood (1995) explored the use of massage therapy for reducing pain after abdominal hysterectomy. Thirty volunteers were randomly assigned to either standard postsurgical care plus therapeutic massage or standard care only. The treatment group of 15 individuals received a daily 45-minute massage beginning the evening of the first day following surgery. Mean systolic blood pressure was significantly lower, and cortisol was substantially lower and more likely to be in a normal range in the massage group by the fifth postoperative day, compared to the control group. Anxiety, depression, and activity restriction, use of patient-controlled analgesia, and use of additional medical services were all lower, but not significantly, in the massage group.

Micronutrient Needs

Berger (1995) discussed the following role of trace nutrients and vitamins around the time of surgery. After elective surgery and in the absence of specific losses, the micronutrient requirements are linked to the metabolic state of the individual and to the energy-protein intakes. Some of the most-needed nutrients include B vitamins and vitamins A and E. Trace element deficiencies that are common include selenium, chromium, and molybdenum. Deficiencies of copper and zinc can result in infection and prolonged wound healing.

Operating Room of the Future

Mailhot (1996) predicted that the operating room of the future will be in the consumer's home. Computers and robots will assist, and clients will be anesthetized with acupuncture, therapeutic touch, and aromatherapy in a totally bloodless environment.

Reflexology

Kesselring (1994) reported the use of foot reflexology postsurgery. In a randomized study, the intervention group showed a lesser need for medication to enhance bladder tone than did the control group. Kesselring reviewed the literature describing the use of foot reflexology to enhance urination, bowel movements, and relaxation.

CAROLYN CHAMBERS CLARK

See
Hypnotic Preparation for Surgery (IV)
Imagery (IV)

See also
Wounds (II)

SYNDROME X

Syndrome X is a collection of symptoms, including insulin resistance, glucose intolerance, hyperinsulinemia, increased levels of very low density lipoprotein and triglycerides, decreased levels of high-density lipoprotein cholesterol, and high blood pressure. Insulin, a pancreatic hormone secreted by the islets of Langerhans, is essential for the metabolism of carbohydrates.

Syndrome X has been linked to heart and blood vessel conditions, diabetes, and obesity. Insulin resistance, the major symptom, is related to an overconsumption of refined carbohydrates, such as breads, pastas, and sugary foods. Eating too much saturated fat (e.g., beef) and too many omega-6 fatty acids (found in vegetable oils) may also increase the risk of insulin resistance. Sustained weight loss is the best way to reduce insulin resistance and arterial pressure (Mangrum & Bakris, 1997), although lack of exercise and a sedentary lifestyle contribute (Kelley, 1997).

Eating too many refined carbohydrates keeps insulin levels chronically high, making cells nonresponsive and resistant to insulin. This results in relatively little glucose getting burned during metabolism, so levels remain high. Chronically elevated glucose levels are believed to turn insulin resistance into diabetes. Even if diabetes never results, eating too many refined carbohydrates sets the stage for heart conditions and high blood pressure (Daly et al., 1997).

Ferrannini and colleagues (1997) provided evidence on the relationship between insulin resistance, hyperinsulinemia, and high blood pressure. They analyzed the database of the European Group for the Study of Insulin Resistance, made up of nondiabetic men and women from 20 centers. The researchers measured insulin sensitivity by the euglycemic insulin clamp. Using univariate analysis, they found both systolic and diastolic blood pressures were inversely related to insulin sensitivity. They also found that for the homotensive, nondiabetic sample, insulin sensitivity and age were significant, mutually independent correlates of blood pressure. They concluded that the relation of blood pressure to both insulin action and circulating insulin levels was compatible with the influence of insulin resistance on blood pressure.

CAROLYN CHAMBERS CLARK

See also
Diabetes (II)
Heart and Blood Vessel Conditions (II)
High Blood Pressure (II)
Obesity (II)

ULCERS

Research data was available for peptic ulcer treatment. Peptic ulcer sufferers complain of a severe burning, gnawing epigastric pain beginning an hour or two after eating. People who suffer from the condition are frequently addicted to antacids, but complementary measures are available.

Cayenne

Kang and colleagues (1995) studied 103 Chinese people with peptic ulcers and a control group of 87 using a standardized questionnaire. People who deliberately avoided chile use because of symptoms or advice from friends or medical practitioners were excluded. The median amount of chile used per month was 312 units in the ulcer group compared to 834 units in the control group. The data support the hypothesis that chile use has a protective effect against peptic ulcer disease.

Garlic

Cellini and others (1996) explored the antibacterial effect of aqueous garlic extract against *Helicobacter pylori*. Sixteen clinical isolates and three reference strains of *H. pylori* were studied. The concentration needed to inhibit 90% of isolates was 5 mg/ml-1.

Licorice

Baker (1994) reported studies that have been done since the 1950s, showing that licorice-derived compounds have antiulcer effects. These are due to the inhibition of 15-hydroxyprostaglandin dehydrogenase and delta 13-prostaglandin reductase. Licorice-derived compounds have the effect of raising the local concentration of prostaglandins that promote mucous secretion and cell proliferation in the stomach. This action leads to the healing of ulcers. Dehpour, Zolfaghari, Samadian, and Vahedi (1994) found the same result when using liquorice to reduce the number and size of ulcers in gastric ulcers induced by aspirin in rats.

Vitamin E

Aldori and colleagues (1997) examined the effect of vitamin A and fiber on risk for developing a duodenal ulcer. This Harvard School of Public Health study involved nearly 48,000 men. Those with the highest intake of vitamin A had a 54% lower risk of a duodenal ulcer than those ingesting small amounts of vitamin A–rich foods. Men who had the highest intake of fiber had a 45% lower risk for duodenal ulcer than those who followed a low-fiber diet. Eating vitamin A–rich yams and liver and fiber-rich apples provided special protection.

CAROLYN CHAMBERS CLARK

See also
Cayenne (III)
Garlic (III)
Licorice (III)

VARICOSE VEINS

Varicose veins result from abnormal distension in the connective tissue of the vein wall. This ultimately renders the vein wall incompetent, and a backflow of blood occurs. With increased pressure, poor tissue drainage results, with a predisposition to infection, clots, inflammation, and venous ulcers. Histamine and bradykinin may contribute to fluid congestion and increased permeability of the vessels (Murray, 1995).

Butcher's Broom

Butcher's broom (*Ruscus aculeatus*) has been shown to reduce inflammation and narrowing of blood vessels and has been used to treat hemorrhoids, varicose veins, and chilblains. Facino, Carini, Stefani, Aldini, and Saibene (1995) found that the herb does exhibit "remarkable anti-elastase activity," as did Bouskela, Cyrino, and Marcelon (1994).

In a clinical trial, Capelli, Nicora, and DiPerri (1988) tested the effectiveness of a venotropic vitamin-herbal mixture (RAES) of *Ruscus aculeatus*, or butcher's broom (16.5 mg), hesperidin (75 mg), and ascorbic acid (50 mg). The crossover, double-blind trial involved two periods of treatment of 2 months with the capsules or a placebo administered three times a day, followed by a 15-day wash-out period. The participants were 30 females and 10 males between the ages of 28 and 74 years, suffering from chronic phlebopathy of the lower limbs. Symptoms and plethysmographic parameters (in particular, MVIV 40 and 60) immediately changed significantly in correspondence to the administration of RAES.

Compression Stockings and Horse Chestnut

Diehm, Tranpisch, Lange, and Schmidt (1996) studied the edema reduction and safety of compression stockings class 2 and dried horse chestnut seed extract (HCSE, 50 mg twice daily). Two hundred and forty individuals with chronic venous insufficiency participated in a randomized, partially blinded, placebo-controlled, parallel study design. Lower leg volume of the more severely affected limb decreased significantly on average by 43.8 ml with HCSE and 46.7 ml with compression stockings, and increased by 9.8 ml with placebo after 12 weeks of therapy. Both treatments were well tolerated, and no serious treatment-related events were reported.

The results indicate that both treatments are effective for individuals with edema resulting from chronic venous insufficiency.

Greeske and Polhmann (1996) also studied the effect of horse chestnut seed extract. Their case observation study involved more than 800 general practitioners, and more than 5,000 individuals with chronic venous insufficiency. The evolution of symptoms, tolerability, and adverse drug reactions were recorded. Pain, tiredness, tension, and swelling in the leg, as well as itching and the tendency toward edema, all improved markedly or disappeared completely.

CAROLYN CHAMBERS CLARK

See also
Butcher's Broom (III)
Horse Chestnut (III)

WOUNDS

Several complementary treatments have been used successfully to enhance wound healing. Chlorophyll and zinc have been found to accelerate wound healing (Ziegler, 1995; Garrison & Somer, 1995).

Holden-Lund (1988) studied the effect of relaxation and guided imagery (RGI) on wound healing after surgery. Twenty-four people undergoing cholecystectomy were randomly assigned to either RGI or control (quiet period). State anxiety, urinary cortisol levels, and wound inflammatory responses were indexed. An analysis of variance for repeated measures revealed the RGI group demonstrated significantly less state anxiety, lower cortisol levels 1 day following surgery, and less surgical wound erythema than the control group. The researcher concluded that the RGI tapes demonstrated stress-relieving outcomes closely associated with healing.

CAROLYN CHAMBERS CLARK

See
Imagery (IV)
Progressive Muscle Relaxation
    Training (IV)

Part III

Influential
Substances

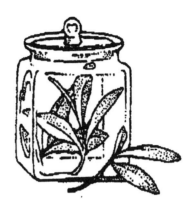

ADAPTOGEN

Any substance that increases resistance to stress or illness. The term was coined by Russian scientists to describe the action of Siberian ginseng, but it is now used to describe other substances that act in a similar fashion.

CAROLYN CHAMBERS CLARK

See
Stress (II)

See also
Ginseng (III)

ALOE

Aloe is the name given to any of over 200 succulent plants of that genus. Related to the lily, aloes grow in warm climates and have been used medicinally for over 2,000 years. Cleopatra is said to have attributed her radiant skin and hair to the use of aloe. The juice is bitter tasting and is used as a purgative and for gastrointestinal complaints, especially colitis and ulcers. It is also used for skin irritations, including insect bites, burns, and sunburn.

CAROLYN CHAMBERS CLARK

See
Skin Disorders (II)

ANTHOCYANINS

Anthocyanins are the purple and blue pigments in grapes and wine. These substances act on the blood vessels and have antioxidant properties. Procyanidins, a subclass of anthocyanidins, are found in grape seeds also. These compounds, among such others as flavonoids, reduce the oxidation process that fosters the formation of atherosclerotic plaque.

Through the ages, parts of the grape plant have been used as medicines. Even Hippocrates used the sap of the young plants to treat eye and skin conditions. Raisins were used to relieve indigestion, and the leaves of grape plants were used to stop bleeding. Recently, anthocyanins have been used successfully to treat vision loss due to diabetes (Boniface & Robert, 1996) and fibrocystic breast disease (Leonardi, 1993).

CAROLYN CHAMBERS CLARK

See also
Antioxidants and Free Radicals (III)
Proanthocyanidins (III)

ANTIOXIDANTS AND FREE RADICALS

Free Radicals: Definition

Increased production of reactive oxygen species is a feature of most, if not all, human disease, including cardiovascular disease and cancer (Jacob & Burri, 1996). Oxygen atoms in the human body contain pairs of electrons. During the course of normal metabolism, a single electron can be lost. The result is a free radical, or unstable molecule, that has a strong drive to replace its missing electron. Free radicals are highly reactive molecules that literally scavenge for an electron, taking one from a neighboring molecule. This process sets off a chain reaction of cellular damage as the free radical binds with and destroys body components.

Sources of Free Radicals

Many free radicals are produced during normal metabolic processes (detoxification, metabolism, and immune defense mechanisms). Besides being produced inside the body, there are free radicals produced in the environment (e.g., cigarette smoke, alcohol, fried foods, air pollutants, aromatic hydrocarbons, pesticides, solvents, ionizing radiation, chemotherapeutic drugs, and formaldehyde). Being exposed to any of these may require additional antioxidant support.

Free Radical Protection

Epidemiologic studies show an inverse relation between coronary artery disease and antioxidant intake, in particular vitamin E supplementation. The oxidative-modification hypothesis suggests that atherosclerosis results due to low-density lipoprotein (LDL) that is resistant to oxidation. There is evidence that plaque stability, vasomotor function, and the tendency to thrombosis can be modified by specific antioxidants (Diaz, Frei, Vita, & Keaney, 1997).

Antioxidants (e.g., selenium and vitamins C and E) are compounds that protect against free radical damage. They can protect against chronic heart disease and cancer and may slow down the aging process. Herbs are some of the most potent antioxidants. Carotenoids and flavonoids protect plants from cellular damage during the process of photosynthesis. Ingestion of plants containing carotenoids and flavonoids affords similar protection for humans.

There are many potent herbal antioxidants, including *Ginkgo biloba* (for the brain and circulation), milk thistle (for the liver), pycnogenols (for the veins), bilberry (for the eyes), and turmeric and *curcumin* from curry powder (for the urinary tract). Green and black tea and cruciferous vegetables (broccoli, cauliflower, brussels sprouts, and kale), along with many other fruits and vegetables, also have antioxidant properties. Recent evidence demonstrated that the amino acid taurine can ameliorate acute lung injury during the systemic inflammatory response syndrome (Wang et al., 1996).

Research Findings

Palozza and Krinsky (1992) examined a membrane model combining fat-soluble antioxidants. A combination of beta-carotene and alpha-tocopherol resulted in an inhibition of lipid peroxidation (important in cardiovascular conditions) significantly greater than the sum of the individual inhibitions. The researchers' data provided the first evidence of these synergistic antioxidants.

Amrita-Bindu, an Ayurvedic salt-spice-herbal health food supplement, can protect against oxidation. Shanmugasundaram, Ramanujam, and Shanmugasundaram (1994) tested the mixture for its effect in maintaining antioxidant defense systems in the blood and liver when exposed to carcinogenic nitrosamine, N-methyl-N'-nitro-N-nitrosoguanidine (MNNG). Amrita-Bindu supplementation prevented MNNG-induced depletion of the antioxidant enzymes and the scavenger antioxidants glutathione and vitamins A, C, and E. The researchers concluded that Amrita-Bindu provides protection against free radical– and reactive oxygen species–induced tissue lip peroxidation and the resultant tissue degeneration.

After exposure to toxic chemicals, natural killer activity (NK) function can be suppressed for prolonged periods of time in some people. Heuser and Vojdani (1997) decided to study the effect of buffered vitamin C on NK activity. After the first blood draw, 55 people who had been exposed to a toxic chemical ingested granulated buffered vitamin C in water at a dosage of 60 mg/kg of body weight. Twenty-four hours later, blood was again drawn. High oral doses of vitamin C enhanced NK activity up to 10 times in 78% of the participants. After vitamin C ingestion, lymphocyte blastogenic responses to T and B cell mitogens were also restored to normal. The researchers concluded that abnormalities in immune system function after toxic chemical exposure can be restored by ingesting large amounts of vitamin C.

Furhman and colleagues (1997) investigated the antioxidative activity of licorice extract against LDL. The study was performed on humans as well as in atherosclerotic apolipoprotein E–deficient mice (because their LDL is highly susceptible to oxidation). LDL oxidation was induced by incubation with copper ions and aqueous or lipid-soluble free radical generators. In an ex vivo study, LDL isolated from the plasma of 10 normolipidemic individuals who were orally supplemented for 2 weeks with 100 mg of licorice/d was more resistant to oxidation than was LDL isolated before licorice supplementation. Dietary supplementation of each Ezero mouse with licorice (200 mcg/d) or pure glabridin (20 mcg/d) for 6 weeks resulted in a substantial reduction in the susceptibility of the LDL to oxidation, along with a reduction in the atherosclerotic lesion area.

The community-based Rotterdam study screened 5,342 individuals with Parkin-son's disease (PD) between the ages of 55 and 95 and administered a semiquantitative food frequency questionnaire. Results were adjusted for age, sex, smoking habits, and energy intake. Those with PD who had a Hoehn-Yahr stage of 2.5 or 3.0 were excluded. The data still suggested that a high intake of dietary vitamin E may protect against the occurrence of PD (de Rijk et al., 1997). Hodis and colleagues (1995) found that vitamin E also protects against the progression of coronary artery atherosclerosis, and Knekt and colleagues (1994) found that vitamins C and E lowered the risk of coronary heart disease mortality for women but not for men.

Girodon and colleagues (1997) used a double-blind, placebo-controlled study to analyze the effects of low-dose supplementation of antioxidant vitamins and minerals on biological and functional parameters of free radical metabolism in 81 hospitalized older adults. All participants were randomly assigned for 2 years to (1) placebo, (2) mineral group (20 mg zinc and 100 mcg selenium), (3) vitamin group (120 mg vitamin C, 6 mg beta-carotene, and 15 mg vitamin E), or vitamin-mineral group (20 mg zinc, 100 mcg selenium, 120 mg vitamin C, 6 mg beta-carotene, and 15 mg vitamin E). At baseline, a large frequency of vitamin C, zinc, and selenium deficiencies were found. A significant increase in vitamin and mineral serum levels occurred in the corresponding vitamin and mineral groups. The results provided experimental evidence that a low-dose supplementation with vitamins and minerals normalized biological nutrient status as early as 6 months of treatment and improved antioxidant defense in elderly adults with low doses of vitamins C and E and beta-carotene (as measured by functional testing utilizing red blood cells challenged in vitro with free radicals).

Knekt and colleagues (1997) examined the effect of antioxidants called flavonoids. The relation between the intake of antioxidant flavonoids and subsequent risk of cancer was studied among 9,959 healthy Finnish men and women age 15 to 99 years. Food consumption was estimated using the dietary history method. During a follow-up from 1967 to 1991, 997 cancer cases and 151 lung cancer cases were diagnosed. The association between flavonoid intake and lung cancer incidence was not due to the intake of antioxidant vitamins, other confounding factors were smoking and vitamin E or C or beta-carotene intake. Of the major dietary flavonoid sources, the consumption of apples showed an inverse association with lung cancer incidence. Other studies have shown a relationship between dietary antioxidants and lung function (Britton et al., 1995), asthma and vitamin C (Hatch, 1995), and vitamin E (Troisi et al., 1995).

CAROLYN CHAMBERS CLARK

See
Aging (II)
Cancer (II)
Heart and Blood Vessel Conditions (II)
Lung Disorders (II)
Skin Disorders (II)

See also
Flavonoids (III)
Gingko (III)
Licorice (III)
Tea (III)
Vitamin A (III)
Vitamin C (III)
Vitamin E (III)

BEE POLLEN

Bee pollen is recommended by many practitioners to desensitize the body against local pollens. It provides 22 amino acids, 27 mineral salts, vitamins, minerals, fructose, glucose, lecithin, hormones, carbohydrates, all the essential fatty acids, and more than 5,000 enzymes and coenzymes.

CAROLYN CHAMBERS CLARK

BRASSININ

Brassinin is a component of cabbage. It is probably also found in radishes and mustard seed. In animal studies, brassinin has induced the production of enzymes that can detoxify carcinogens in cells and excrete them. Brassinin occurs as a molecule called a glycoside. The glycoside is broken down into brassinin from the heat or from enzymes produced by microflora in the digestive tract.

CAROLYN CHAMBERS CLARK

See
Cancer (II)

BURDOCK

Burdock (*Arctium lappa*) is an herb used to treat skin conditions, allergies, arthritis, and kidney and bladder infections, and to bring down fever by increasing perspiration. Believed to be a blood purifier, it has also been used to treat burns, eczema, acne, psoriasis, poison ivy and poison oak, bruises, and sprains.

Lin et al. (1996) demonstrated the anti-inflammatory and radical scavenging ability of burdock. The effects of the root extract included decreasing carrageenan-induced paw edema in rats and protection against acute liver damage. The researchers concluded that both these findings could be due to the scavenging effect of *A. lappa*.

CAROLYN CHAMBERS CLARK

See

Allergies(II)
Arthritis (II)
Bladder Problems (II)
Burns (II)
Skin Disorders (II)

BUTCHER'S BROOM

Butcher's broom is an evergreen with spine-tipped flat, leaflike stalks, tiny violet flowers, and shiny red berries. The whole plant reduces inflammation and narrowing of blood vessels and has been used usually in capsule form for treatment of hemorrhoids, varicose veins, and chilblains.

CAROLYN CHAMBERS CLARK

CAFFEINE

Caffeine is the world's most commonly used mood-altering drug. In low doses, it increases feelings of well-being, the ability to concentrate, and energy levels. At high doses, it produces jitteriness, restlessness, anxiety, and insomnia.

Caffeine is so ubiquitous in American culture that many people are caffeine-dependent and don't recognize the extent to which their preference for foods and beverages is being guided by the pharmacology of caffeine. The drug is widely consumed in coffee, tea, cocoa, soft drinks, and chocolate. It is also a component in hundreds of prescription and over-the-counter drugs, ranging from cold medicines to analgesics.

When ingesting caffeine, calcium and magnesium are excreted, which may increase the risk of osteoporosis (Kynast-Gales & Massey, 1994). Caffeine was found to increase blood pressure (systolic and diastolic) and to suppress heart rate and cardiac output. The effect was greatest in borderline hypertensive participants who experienced a 2 to 3 times greater change in postdrug (caffeine) diastolic blood pressure compared to a control group (Pincomb et al., 1996).

Dim light treatment combined with caffeine condition suppresses nighttime melatonin levels and attenuates the normal decrease in temperature during sleep. Combining caffeine ingestion with bright light exposure suppresses melatonin and attenuates the normal nighttime drop in temperature (Wright et al., 1997).

Curtis, Savitz, and Arbuckle (1997) demonstrated a decrease in the monthly probability of conception due to caffeine consumption. Decreases were observed among women who were coffee drinkers and men who were heavy tea drinkers, regardless of caffeine content. Bolumar, Olsen, Rebagliato, and Bistanti (1997) found similar evidence. Women in the highest level of consumption had an increase in the time leading to the first pregnancy of 11%.

Vlajinac (1997) demonstrated that pregnant women who drink two or more cups of coffee a day may deliver infants who weigh less than babies born to mothers who don't consume caffeine. The researchers theorize that caffeine constricts the placental blood vessels, thereby inhibiting the infant's growth.

CAROLYN CHAMBERS CLARK

See
   Anxiety/Panic (II)
   Heart and Blood Vessel Conditions (II)
   High Blood Pressure (II)
   Insomnia (II)
   Osteoporosis (II)
   Pregnancy (II)

See also
   Calcium (III)

CALCIUM

There is equivocal evidence that high intakes of calcium may forestall development of osteoporosis, hip fracture (Meunier, 1996) and other chronic conditions, including hypertension, and colon cancer (Whiting, Wood, & Kim, 1997). Dietary calcium intake for Americans (U.S. Department of Agriculture, 1995) is less than the recommended dietary allowance. Although calcium is available in dairy products, green vegetables, canned fish, and tofu, most Americans have not met the optimal levels of calcium now suggested by the National Institutes of Health Consensus Development Conference on Optimal Calcium Intake.

Calcium carbonate contains the highest proportion of elemental calcium by weight, but only 5 of 15 brands of calcium carbonate marketed in the United States passed the dissolution test. Further study showed that of 29 U.S. brands, only 18% met the USP specifications (Brennan et al., 1991).

Canadian studies had similar findings (Gorecki, Richardson, Wallace, & Pavlakadies, 1989).

The most soluble (and available) forms of calcium are calcium citrate, calcium lactate, calcium gluconate, and calcium citrate maleate (Smith, Heaney, Flora, & Hinders, 1987). Recker (1985) found that people with reduced hydrochloric acid (a function of aging) can only absorb calcium carbonate with meals. Most people are able to absorb calcium citrate with or without meals. Calcium chelates and refined calcium carbonate contain low levels of lead similar to that found in milk, but dolomite, oyster shell calcium carbonate, and bone-meal supplements may contain very high levels of lead (Bourgoin et al., 1993).

Recommendations to restrict calcium are no longer made because taking moderate amounts of calcium with meals can protect against calcium-oxalate kidney stone formation (Curhan, Willett, Rimme, & Stampfer, 1993). Blumsohn and colleagues (1994) suggested that calcium be taken at bedtime to prevent the bone loss that occurs overnight.

CAROLYN CHAMBERS CLARK

See
   Aging (II)
   Fractures (II)
   Heart and Blood Vessel Conditions (II)
   High Blood Pressure (II)
   Kidney Stones (II)
   Osteoporosis (II)
   Premenstrual Syndrome (PMS) (II)

See also
   Nutrition (IV)

CAPSAICIN

Capsaicin, a nonenadmide derived from the *Capsicum* plant, has proven useful in the treatment of a number of conditions. Marabinni and colleagues (1991) used a spray delivered to the nasal mucosa to treat people with vasomotor rhinitis. The mean symptom score involving nasal obstruction and nasal secretion was markedly reduced by capsaicin treatment. The researchers theorized that the beneficial effect of the treatment may be due to its specific action on the peripheral endings of primary sensory neurons, leading to their functional blockage.

Topical capsaicin may also be useful in painful diabetic neuropathy. Tandan and colleagues (1992) conducted a controlled study with long-term follow-up. Approximately 50% of subjects reported improved pain control or were cured, and 25% were unchanged or worse. A burning sensation at the application site was noted by some participants, but the duration and magnitude decreased with time. The researchers concluded that topical 0.075% capsaicin may be of value in people with diabetic neuropathy and intractable pain.

CAROLYN CHAMBERS CLARK

See
Diabetes (II)

See also
Cayenne (III)

CAROTENOIDS

Carotenoids are the yellow, orange, and red pigments (as carotenes) found in fruits and vegetables. There are some 500 of them available. About 10% of the naturally occurring carotenoids provide vitamin A. They act as antioxidants and anticarcinogens. There is evidence they reduce heart disease risk, prevent cataracts, and other oxidative damages in the eye and enhance immune response. Trans-beta-carotene is one of the major carotenoids and is the most active vitamin A form.

CAROLYN CHAMBERS CLARK

See also
Antioxidants and Free Radicals (III)
Cancer (II)
Cataracts (II)
Heart and Blood Vessel Conditions (II)

CAYENNE

Cayenne pepper's name comes from the city of Cayenne, located on Cayenne Island at the mouth of the Cayenne River in French Guiana. Capsaicin is the principal component of *Capsicum* fruits, used widely as a food additive.

Cayenne has been used as an anesthetic and as a treatment for blindness, gunshot wounds, poor circulation, headache, toothache, difficult childbirth, hangovers, right-sided abdominal pain, flatulence, sore throat, colds, bruises, mucus accumulation in the lungs, frostbite, snakebite, angina, mumps, leg ulcers, sprains, constipation, allergies, arthritis, asthma, arteriosclerosis, blood clots, bowel conditions, cancer, diabetic neuropathy, duodenal ulcers, elevated cholesterol and triglycerides, fatigue, scavenging free radicals, heart arrhythmias, heart attack, heart disease, heatstroke, hemorrhaging, herpes zoster, high blood pressure, indigestion, infection, itching, lumbago, motion sickness, mouth sores, neuralgia, night blindness, obesity, pain, peptic ulcer, poor appetite, psoriasis, respiratory disorders, shingles, stomach ulcer, bursitis, cuts and abrasions, nagging cough (as a gargle), insect invasions, food poisoning, irregular menses, morning sickness, pleurisy, nosebleeds, sinusitis, and tonsilitis (Bernstein et al., 1989; Cordell & Araujo, 1993; Govindarajan & Sathyanarayana, 1991; Heinerman, 1997; Kawada et al., 1986; Palevitch & Craker, 1995).

Capsaicinoids are the naturally occurring compounds in cayenne pepper that give it its pungency and a delayed, but strong burning and numbing sensation. Chile peppers, which belong to the genus *Capsicum*, include cayenne (hot red pepper), jalapeño, serrano, habanero, scotch bonnet, mild paprika, bell, and virtually all other peppers except black pepper. While other chiles are used in whole fresh or dried forms, cayenne is almost always used in powdered form for culinary and medicinal purposes.

Cayenne pepper is an enigma. It can burn the tongue yet cool the body. It promotes blood circulation yet stops hemorrhaging. Its anti-inflammatory action has been used to reduce the pain of arthritis and diabetic neuropathy. With its high vitamin C content, it is able to fight bacteria and possibly some viruses.

Antimicrobial Properties

Cichewicz and Thorpe (1996) surveyed the Mayan pharmacopoeia concerning *Capsicum* species. Using a filter disk assay, plain and heated aqueous extracts from fresh *Capsicum* samples were tested for their antimicrobial effects with 15 bacterial species and one yeast species. All were found to exhibit varying degrees of inhibition against *Bacillus cereus*, *Bacillus subtilis*, *Clostridium sporogenes*, *Clostridium tetani*, and *Streptococcus pyogenes*.

Antimutagenic and Anticarcinogenic Properties

Miller and colleagues (1993) studied the effects of capsaicin on the vitro liver microsomal metabolism of the tobacco-specific nitrosamine NNK, a potent carcinogen in tobacco and tobacco smoke. Liver microsomes from saline-injected, phenobarbital-induced, and beta-naphthoflavone-induced hamsters were used. Capsaicin inhibited the formation of all metabolites of NNK by all microsomal fractions and inhibited alpha-hydroxylation by phenobarbital-induced microsomes more than either of the other two treatments. The results suggest that capsaicin possesses antimutagenic and anticarcinogenic properties and works through the inhibition of xenobiotic metabolizing enzymes.

Homeopathic Use: Acute Otitis Media

Friese, Kruse, and Moeller (1996) compared 28 children on conventional therapy (decongestant nose drops, antibiotics, secretolytics, and/or antipyretics for acute otitis media with 103 children, using homeopathic treatment (*Aconitum napellus*, *Apis mellifica*, *Belladonna*, *Capsicum*, *Chamomilla*, *Kalium bichromicum*, *Lachesis*, *Lycopodium*, *Mercurius solubilis*, *Okoubaka*, *Pulsatilla*, and *Silicea*).

Comparisons consisted of symptoms, physical findings, duration of therapy, and number of relapses. The median duration of pain in the homeopathic group was 2 days; in the conventional group, 3 days.

Conventional therapy lasted 10 days, 4 days in the homeopathic group. In the homeopathic group, 70.7% were free of relapses within 1 year, and 29.3% had a maximum of three relapses. In the convention therapy group, 56% went without relapsing and 43.5% had a maximum of six relapses.

Pain Erasure Effects

Cordell and Araujo (1993) provided an overview of the chemical history, analysis, nomenclature, biology, pharmacology, and pharmacotherapy of capsaicin. They concluded that capsaicin acts specifically by depleting stores of substance P from sensory neurons, making it a successful treatment for the pain of rheumatoid arthritis, osteoarthritis, and peripheral neuropathies.

Tandan and colleagues (1992) conducted an 8-week controlled study with topical 0.075% capsaicin for 22 individuals with chronic severe painful diabetic neuropathy who were unresponsive to or intolerant of conventional therapy. Either capsaicin or vehicle cream was applied to painful areas four times/day. Pain measurements were recorded at baseline and at 2-week intervals for 8 weeks. As measured by physician global evaluation and by a categorical pain severity scale, capsaicin treatment provided a significantly better result than the vehicle cream. Mean pain relief on the visual analogue scale was 16% in the capsaicin-treated group and 4% in the vehicle-treated individuals. Mean pain relief was 45% for the treatment group and 23% for the vehicle cream group. During follow-up, 50% of the participants reported improved pain control or were cured. The results suggest that topical capsaicin may be of value for people with diabetic neuropathy and intractable pain.

Protection Against Peptic Ulcer

Kang and colleagues (1995) studied the frequency and amount of chile taken by 103 Chinese individuals with peptic ulcer and 87 controls, using a standard questionnaire. People who deliberately avoided chile use because of symptoms or advice from friends or health care practitioners were excluded. The ulcer group used less chile, 8 to 24 times per month for the control group. When adjusted for age, sex, analgesic use, and smoking by multiple logistic regression, the odds ratio of having peptic ulcer was .47 for individuals who had a higher intake of chile. The data support the hypothesis that chile has a protective effect against peptic ulcer.

Yeoh and colleagues (1995) expanded on the gastroprotective effect of capsaicin on the digestive system. Although the effect has been found for the gastric mucosa of animals, it had not been documented in humans. The researchers studied 18 healthy volunteers with normal index endoscopies. Each individual took 20 g chile orally with 200 ml water (in one study) and 200 ml water in another study. In each case this was followed in half an hour by 600 mg aspirin with 200 ml water. Endoscopy was repeated 6 hours later to assess gastroduodenal mucosal damage. Using a previously validated scoring system, the researchers found the median gastric injury score after chile consumption was 1.5 compared to 4.0 in the control group, demonstrating a statistically significant gastroprotective effect of chile in human subjects.

Reduction of Vasomotor Rhinitis

Marabini and associates (1991) studied the effects of 15 mcg of capsaicin suspended in 100 microliters solutions for individuals with known vasomotor rhinitis. The treatment was applied three times a day for 3 days by means of a spray delivered to the nasal mucosa. Painful sensation and secretion of nasal fluid occurred on initiation but ended at the last capsaicin application. Participants recorded their symptoms over a 1-month period. The mean symptom score involving nasal obstruction and nasal secretion was markedly reduced by capsaicin treatment. The researchers explained that the beneficial effect of capsaicin may be due to its specific action on the peripheral endings of primary sensory neurons, leading to their functional blockage.

CAROLYN CHAMBERS CLARK

See also
Capsaicin (III)

CHELATE

A compound is a chelate if the mineral is bonded to both the nitrogen and the nitrogen in the ligand that surrounds the mineral and protects it from interacting with other compounds. Supplements containing mineral chelates may increase mineral absorption. Two amino acids can form a chelated structure that is resistant to intestinal enzymes and gastric acid and bypass competition with other minerals. Because of their action, chelated minerals are believed to have greater bioavailability, but many studies show no difference in absorption between chelated and nonchelated forms of minerals (Heaney, Recker, & Weaver, 1990; Scholmerich et al., 1987; Scholmerich et al., 1987b; Solomons, Juswigg, & Pineda, 1984). Chelated minerals include zinc gluconate, selenomethionine, calcium malate, and ferrous fumarate.

A number of studies have demonstrated that there is a significantly greater uptake of organically bound selenium (L-selenomethionine) than there is using inorganic selenium salts such as sodium selenite (Janghorbani, Kasper, & Young, 1984; McAdam et al., 1985).

CAROLYN CHAMBERS CLARK

See also
Bioavailability (I)

CHROMIUM

Chromium is an essential nutrient (trace mineral) required for sugar and fat metabolism. Dietary intake of chromium for humans is suboptimal (Anderson, 1997). Most diets contain less than 60% of the minimum suggested intake for adults of 50–200 mcg. Insufficient intake of chromium leads to signs and symptoms similar to those observed for diabetes and cardiovascular conditions. There is an age-related decrease in chromium levels in hair, sweat, and serum samples. This decrease has implications for the prevention of cardiovascular disease and adult-onset diabetes mellitus (Davies et al., 1997).

Supplemental chromium of 100 mcg a day given to individuals with impaired glucose tolerance or diabetes led to a significantly improved blood glucose, insulin and cholesterol levels (Anderson et al., 1997). Chromium may also improve lean body mass in humans (Anderson, 1993), especially when combined with exercise training (Grant et al., 1997).

Supplementation will only be of benefit to those deficient in the nutrient, however there is a very large safety range and there have been no documented signs of toxicity in any nutritional studies of levels up to 1 mg per day (Anderson, 1997).

Chromium supplementation lowers total cholesterol, LDL-cholesterol, and apolipoprotein B while elevating apolipoprotein A. Lipid profiles were found to improve with chromium supplementation for individuals diagnosed with atherosclerosis (Abraham et al., 1991). It could be that chromium increases insulin efficiency, thereby reducing elevated lipid levels (Garrison & Sommer, 1995).

Good food sources of chromium are wholegrain breads and cereals, brewer's yeast, pork kidney, meats, and cheeses. Most chromium is removed from grains when they are refined. Low chromium levels of highly refined foods combined with an increased intake of sugars and other processed carbohydrates could be predisposing factors to chromium deficiency and aggravation of adult-onset diabetes (Somers & Garrison, 1995).

Hard water can supply from 1% to 70% of the daily intake (Garrison & Somer, 1995). Cooking acidic foods in stainless steel cookware leeches chromium into food, creating an additional source of dietary chromium, while aluminum cookware lowers the chromium levels in cooked foods (Kuligowski & Halperin, 1992).

CAROLYN CHAMBERS CLARK

See

Diabetes (II)
Heart and Blood Vessel Conditions (II)
Insulin Sensitivity (II)

DANG GUI (DONG QUAI)

Dang gui (*Angelica sinensis*), or *dong quai*, is an important Chinese tonic herb, used in many patent remedies as a nourishing blood tonic and regulator of the menstrual cycle. Many over-the-counter preparations based on dang gui are available in the West.

Its character is pungent, warm, sweet, and generally drying. The herb contains vitamins A and B, tannins, bergapten, valerianic acid, resin, volatile oil, and bitter iridoids.

The actions of dang gui are reported to be calminative, antispasmodic, sweat-promotive, anti-inflammatory (topical), expectorant, diuretic, and anti-rheumatic. The herb is to be avoided during pregnancy (because it is a uterine stimulant), and by people with diabetes (because of its sugar content).

CAROLYN CHAMBERS CLARK

ECHINACEA

Echinacea is an immunotonic first introduced by the Native Americans to early European settlers. The roots of *Echinacea purpureu* and *augustifolia* were used externally for the healing of wounds, burns, abcesses, and insect bites. Taken internally, it was used to treat infections, toothache, joint pains, and snake bites.

By the first decade of the 20th century, echinacea had become a mainstay of American medicine. Early researchers determined that echinacea had a profound effect on the number and kind of blood cells. The herb kept the ratio of red to white blood cells in an acceptable range, by promoting or suppressing the production of white blood cells. Researchers also learned that echinacea behaved like a tonic, improving waste elimination and increasing the destruction of foreign substances in the blood. With the advent of antibiotics, however, interest in echinacea waned (Murray, 1995).

There is growing interest in echinacea. See, Broumand, Sahl, and Tilles (1997) demonstrated the in vitro effects of echinacea on natural killer cells. They concluded that *Echinacea purpurea* enhances cellular immune function both in normal individuals and people with depressed cellular immunity.

Some practitioners recommend its use for only up to 8 weeks as a protection against viral infections, such as colds (Graedon, 1997). Others maintain it is perfectly safe to use small doses intermittently and larger doses for an ongoing infection (Mowry, 1993). Graedon (1997) cautions against any use for those with multiple sclerosis. Echinacea's active constituents include polysaccharides, glycoproteins, caffeic acid derivatives, and alkylamides (Bauer, 1996).

CAROLYN CHAMBERS CLARK

See
Cold Symptoms (II)

FATTY ACIDS (ESSENTIAL)

Decades ago, physicians working in the Arctic noticed that the Inuit Eskimos rarely developed heart disease, even though their diets consisted primarily of whale meat, seal meat, and fish, all of which were high in fat and cholesterol. Epidemiological studies confirmed that heart disease rates were much lower than those of Westerners (Dyerberg et al., 1979; Bang et al., 1980).

The difference was not due to the amount of fat in the diet, but to the source of fat. Inuits get their fat almost exclusively from marine mammals and fish, while Westerners generally obtain theirs from land animals and plants. This finding prompted research on omega-3 polyunsaturated fatty acids (PUFA), a type of fatty acid that is present in fish oils. The omega-E PUFA have a variety of effects that may influence heart and blood vessel conditions.

PUFA effect platelets, probably decreasing the tendency toward blood clotting, thereby reducing the risk of an acute heart attack (Zhu et al., 1990). They also reduce blood levels of triglycerides (Fehily, Burr, Phillips, & Deadman, 1983), and may have a beneficial effect on HDL2 cholesterol (Mori et al., 1994; Sacks et al., 1994). They may also reduce blood pressure to a modest degree in some high-risk individuals (Morris et al., 1993). Limited evidence also shows a reduction in cardiac arrhythmias (Christensen et al., 1995; Sellmayer, Witzgall, Lorenz, & Weber, 1995). Epidemiologic data show an inverse relationship between fish consumption and death from heart disease, especially nonsudden death from myocardial infarction (Daviglus et al., 1997).

CAROLYN CHAMBERS CLARK

See
Heart and Blood Vessel Conditions (II)

FIBER

Dietary fiber is a complex mixture of plant materials that are resistant to breakdown by the human digestive system. There are two major kinds of dietary fiber—insoluble (cellulose, hemicellulose, and lignin) and soluble (gums, mucilages, and pectins). Insoluble fiber is most frequently found in whole-grain products. Foods containing soluble fibers are fruits, vegetables, dry beans and peas, and some cereals such as oats.

Insoluble fiber promotes normal elimination by providing bulk for stool formation, hastening the passage of the stool through the colon. Insoluble fiber also helps to satisfy appetite by creating full feelings.

Soluble fibers may play a role in reducing the level of cholesterol in the blood. Jensen and colleagues (1997) randomized a sample of 31 healthy men and 27 healthy women (stabilized on a self-selected low-fat and low-cholesterol diet) and fed them a mixture of psyllium, pectin, guar gum, and locust bean or placebo-controlled powder. By week 8, there was a significant decrease in mean plasma total cholesterol in the treatment group. This decrease was sustained for 24 weeks.

Dietary fibers lack the risk of side effects that sometimes occur with cholesterol-lowering medicines (Dishong, 1994). Cerda (1994) revealed that adding 15 grams of grapefruit pectin to the daily diet reduced cholesterol levels by an average of 11% within 4 weeks. The study, conducted with 27 volunteers with high cholesterol at the Clinical Research Center of Shands Hospital at the University of Florida, showed that this amount of dietary fiber reduced cholesterol levels even when study participants did not alter their regular diet or lifestyle (Dishong, 1994).

Aldoori and colleagues (1994) studied a cohort of 47,888 men. Total dietary fiber intake was inversely associated with risk of diverticular disease. Especially risky was a high intake of total far or red meat and low dietary fiber.

Giovannuci and colleagues (1992) found that dietary fiber was inversely associated with risk of cororectal adenomas, which are precursors of cancer. Fiber may also help protect against cardiovascular disease and, in high amounts, the amount of insulin needed by diabetics (Dohn, 1996).

Adding fiber to the diet in the form of bran cereal or psyllium supplements and drinking plenty of water is the recommended treatment for irritable bowel syndrome (Bonis & Norton, 1996). Extensive medical tests are considered wasteful by these clinicians.

CAROLYN CHAMBERS CLARK

See
Diverticular Disease (II)
Heart and Blood Vessel Conditions (II)
Irritable Bowel Syndrome (II)

FLAVONOIDS

Fruits and vegetables have therapeutic properties and substances that are just beginning to be well studied. These nutrients include pigments, called flavonoids, which give plants their color. Flavonoids are found in vegetables, fruits and beverages, especially tea, and give fruits and flowers their vibrant hues.

Flavonoids help restore health to cell membranes and blood vessels. The most well-known flavonoids are rutin, bioflavonoids, and quercetin. They are a class of dietary phytochemicals with anticarcinogenic properties (Zhair et al., 1998; Huk et al., 1998; Barotto et al., 1998).

Gottlieb (1995) summarized the available research on the use of flavonoids: A five-year Dutch study of 805 elderly men found that those who regularly consumed fruits and vegetables high in flavonoids were less likely to die of heart disease than those who ate fewer flavonoids. Intake of other nutrients did not significantly affect heart-related deaths. Clinically, shingles may respond to a combination of 2,000 mg of vitamin C, 400 international units of vitamin E, and 1 gram of citrus bioflavonoids twice daily. Animal and human trials demonstrated that milk thistle, which contains a mixture of flavonoid derivatives called silymarin, works directly on liver cells.

CAROLYN CHAMBERS CLARK

FLAXSEED

Also called linseed, flaxseed is a component of many health foods and may appear as a hidden ingredient in multigrain breads. Studies are just beginning to accumulate information about its powerhouse preventive qualities.

Flaxseed is high in *lignans*, which have antitumor, antimitotic (prevents bad cells from reproducing themselves), antiviral, and antioxidant effects. Flaxseed also helps the body get rid of "bad" estrogens or convert them to "good" estrogens (in the liver), and is crucial in enhancing the ratio of "good" to "bad" estrogen levels. Rich in omega-3 fatty acids and a number of other phytochemicals, flaxseed has become celebrated for its cholesterollowering cardiovascular benefits. A study by Hamadeh (1992) showed that elderly participants who consumed two flaxseed muffins per day had lower total cholesterol and a significant increase in bowel movements during the treatment period, compared to the nontreatment period. Animal studies have provided the first direct evidence that con-

sumption of flaxseed may play a role in cancer prevention. Flaxseed is a potent source of lignans, one of the many plant compounds with estrogenlike qualities that may interfere with the development of breast, colon, prostate, and other cancers.

Flaxseed contains high levels of secoisolariciresinol diglucoside and matairesinol, compounds intestinal flora convert into the lignans enterodiol and enterolactone. Flaxseed, a rich source of lignan precursor secoisolariciresinol-diglycoside (SD) and alpha-linolenic acid (ALA), has been shown to be protective at the early promotion stage of carcinogenesis.

Thompson, Rickard, Orcheson, and Seidel (1996) studied whether supplementation with flaxseed (in either lignan or oil fractions) would reduce the size of established mammary tumors present at the start of treatment and the appearance of new tumors. In their study after 7 weeks of treatment, established tumor volume was over 50% smaller in all treatment groups, whereas there was no change in the group receiving corn oil alone.

The researchers suggested that the effect of flaxseed oil may be related to its high ALA content. The SD in flaxseed appears to be beneficial during early stages of carcinogenesis (promotional phase), while the oil component has more effect when tumors have become established.

In another study, Thompson and colleagues (1996) researched the antitumorigenic effect of flaxseed. SD was isolated from flaxseed and tested for its effect on mammary tumorigenesis. There was a 46% reduction in the number of tumors. This study showed that SD has an antitumor effect when provided in the early promotion stage of tumorigenesis and may explain the health benefit of high-fiber foods.

CAROLYN CHAMBERS CLARK

See
Cancer (II)
Heart and Blood Vessel Conditions (II)

See also
Antioxidants and Free Radicals (III)

GARLIC

Onion and garlic contain many sulfur containing active principles, mainly in the form of cysteine derivatives, which decompose into a variety of thiosulfinates and polysulfides. Allicin, one of the active principles of garlic, has the ability to inhibit *Entamoeba histolytica* troophozoites, which can destroy kidney cells. Cysteine proteinases, which are important contributors to amebic virulence, as well as alcohol dehydrogenase, are strongly inhibited by allicin (Ankri et al., 1997).

Artery Wall Protection

Animal models have shown that garlic causes direct preventive effects at the level of the artery wall. It is possible that garlic reduces lipid content in arterial cells and prevents intracellular lipid accumulation (Orekhov & Grunwald, 1997).

Epidemiological studies have also suggested that garlic may protect against heart and blood vessel conditions. Breithaupt-Grogler, Ling, Boudoulas, and Belz (1997) used a cross-sectional observational study to see if garlic would delay the stiffening of the aorta known to occur with aging. They investigated 101 healthy adults, age 50 to 80 years, who were taking 300 mg per day of standardized garlic powder for 2 years and compared them with age- and sex-matched controls. Pulse wave velocity (PWV) and pressure-standardized elastic vascular resistance were the measures used. The study found that PWV increased less in the garlic group than in the control group. The researchers concluded that chronic garlic powder intake reduced age-related increases in aortic stiffness in humans.

Cancer

The chemoprotective effects of garlic are related to diallyl sulfide (DAS), a flavor component of garlic (Jin & Baillie, 1997). Hatono (1994) reported on the chemopreventive activities of garlic and its derivatives. Glutathione-S-transferase activities in the liver, small intestine, and colon were increased significantly by the administration of a garlic derivative. This strongly suggests that S-allylcysteine decreased the risk of carcinogenesis by enhancing the detoxification system not only in the liver but also in the small intestine and colon.

Milner (1994) reported on the delay of tumors and suppression of the number of tumors as the quantity of garlic is increased in the diet. Several other investigations (Milner, 1996) indicated that garlic and its organic allyl sulfur components inhibit the cancer process. Oil-soluble compounds such as diallyl disulfide are effective in reducing the number of new tumors, while the water-soluble compound S-allyl cysteine is not.

Pinto and colleagues (1997) studied the use of garlic derivatives on human prostate cancer cells. Their data provided evidence that garlic derivatives may modulate tumor growth.

Cholesterol

Garlic preparations standardized for allicin content have been shown to prevent oxidation of LDL cholesterol (Lewin & Popov, 1994; Popov, Blumenstein, & Lewis, 1994).

In a meta-analysis of 16 trials and 952 participants, Silagy and Neil (1994) concluded there was a significant reduction in total cholesterol (12%) for the garlic groups compared to the placebo groups, but it took between 3 and 4 months to see a stable decline in cholesterol.

Warchevsky, Kamer, and Sivak (1993) studied 325 people, using five trials in three different countries. They concluded there was a net decrease in the total cholesterol attributable to garlic (one half to one clove per day).

Adler and Holub (1997) examined the effects of garlic and fish oil supplementation (alone and in combination) on lipoproteins and fasting serum lipids in men with hypercholesterolemia. Fifty men were randomly assigned to one of four groups: (1) 900 mg of garlic placebo per day, (2) 900 mg of garlic per day plus 12 g of oil placebo per day, (3) 900 mg of garlic per day plus 12 g of fish oil per day, or (4) 900 mg of garlic placebo per day plus 12 g of fish oil (3.6 g n-3 fatty acids) per day. Mean group total cholesterol was significantly lower with garlic plus fish oil and with garlic after 12 weeks, but not with fish oil alone.

Garlic supplementation significantly decreased both total cholesterol and LDL-C, whereas fish oil supplementation significantly decreased triacyglycerol concentrations and increased LDL-C. The combination of garlic and fish oil reversed the moderate fish oil–induced rise in LDL-C.

Free Radical Damage Protection

Ide, Nelson, and Lau (1997) examined the effect of aged garlic extract on oxidative modification of LDL in vitro. The extract inhibited oxidative modification of LDL.

Memory Improvement

Nishiyama, Moriguchi, and Saito (1997) investigated the effects of aged garlic on learning and memory. Although not confirmed in humans, their mouse study showed that aged garlic extract increased the survival of participants, ameliorated the memory acquisition deficit and memory retention impairment that occurs with age, and prevented the normal atrophy of the frontal cerebrum.

Moriguchi, Saito, and Nishiyama (1997) also studied the use of aged garlic extract on age-related changes in a novel strain of senescence acclerated mouse with age-related brain atrophy. They had similar results. The extract improved learning and memory deficits and prevented decrease in brain weight and the usual atrophic changes in the frontal brain.

Thrombus Formation

Garlic indirectly affects atherosclerosis by reduction of hyperlipidemia (Mader, 1990), hypertension, and (probably) diabetes and prevents thrombus formation (Augusti, 1996).

CAROLYN CHAMBERS CLARK

See

Aging (II)

Cancer (II)

Diabetes (II)

Heart and Blood Vessel Conditions (II)

Infection (II)

GINGKO

The *Ginkgo biloba* tree is believed to pre-date the last Ice Age. Some trees have lived over 1,000 years. Found in the leaves, the active constituents are flavoglycosides (heterosides and quercetin). The product is only effective when extracted and concentrated. Gingko has a tonic action on several aspects of neural functioning: stabilization of neural and muscular membranes, removal of toxic metabolites, normalization of transmitter concentrations, and maintenance of appropriate levels of important electrolytes (Mowry, 1993).

Gingko activates beta receptors in muscles and organs, including the brain, and dilating airways in the lung and blood vessels (Racagni, Brunello, & Paoletti, 1986). Because of its capacity to release catecholamines, gingko could affect the heart, blood vessels, and nervous system (Auguet, DeFeudis, Clostre, & Deghenghi, 1982).

Ginkgo biloba is one of the best-studied and most popular herbs in Europe. It is prescribed more than 5 million times a year in Germany alone. The evidence of its safety is solid. The dose ranges from 120 to 124 mg daily, but it may take 6 weeks to see results (Bilger, 1997).

Gingko has been used in the treatment of peripheral blood vessel conditions and heart/blood vessel insufficiency in older adults. Maitra, Marocci, Droy-Lefaix, and Packer (1995) provided in vitro evidence that gingko acts as an antioxidant.

Taillandier and colleagues (1986) studied the effectiveness of gingko in the treatment of cerebral disorders due to aging in a multicenter, double-blind drug versus placebo trial. In the study 166 individuals were divided into treatment (with gingko supplementation) and control groups. The results confirmed that gingko was effective against cerebral disorders due to aging. The difference between treatment and control groups reached statistical significance at 3 months and increased in the following months.

Lanthony and Cosson (1988) reported on the use of gingko in a double-blind trial with 29 individuals with diabetic retinopathy. The treatment group showed a statistically significant improvement in the condition, whereas the control group had evidence of aggravation.

Bauer (1984) studied the use of gingko versus placebo in a 6-month randomized clinical trial using 40 mg of *Ginkgo biloba* extract. Gingko was significantly superior to placebo in two groups of people with peripheral arterial insufficiency.

Grassel (1992) reported on the used of gingko to improve mental performance using a double-blind study and computerized measurements of cerebral insufficiency for 72 outpatients at three test centers. Statistically significant improvement in the short-term memory occurred after 6 weeks and the learning rate after 24 weeks in the gingko group, but not in the controls.

Cano Cuenca, Marco Algarra, Perez del Valle, and Pellicer Pascual (1995) studied the use of *Ginkgo biloba* extract (4 ml/12 hours by mouth) for a group of 70 individuals complaining of vertigo. Six months later, statistically significant changes occurred in terms of ringing in the ears and vertigo. Besides favorable changes in the peripheral blood vessels, hearing improved.

Gingko may also have beneficial effects for relatively healthy individuals. Gessner, Voelp, and Klasser (1985) and Hindmarch (1986) reported studies of healthy young females. In both, memory improved significantly on a memory test within an hour of ingesting gingko.

CAROLYN CHAMBERS CLARK

See
Alzheimer's Disease (II)
Heart and Blood Vessel Conditions (II)
Memory Problems (II)

See also
Antioxidants and Free Radicals (III)

GINSENG

According to Mowry (1993), all the major species of plants that go by the name of ginseng have similar effects on the immune system. They act as tonics that increase resistance to organisms and restore normality when other changes present a threat to health. Ginseng is basically an adaptogen, that increases the ability of individuals to adapt.

Ginseng appears to influence the immune control centers of the central nervous system. It affects adrenocortical hormones, by toning, increasing output, or simply restoring equilibrium. In this way, blood pressure, glucose levels, insulin levels, and white blood cell count are stabilized. Ginseng also has analgesic, antipyretic, and anti-inflammatory actions. It is believed to strengthen the heart, stimulate recovery from surgery and debilitating infectious disease, and assist the body in overcoming physiological stress (Mowry, 1993).

Lim and colleagues (1997) provided evidence of the scavenging activity of red ginseng powder, validating the empirical usage of ginseng root over thousands of years for the prevention of cerebrovascular diseases. See, Broumand, Sahl, and Tilles (1997) demonstrated the in vitro ability of ginseng to significantly enhance the natural killer cell function.

CAROLYN CHAMBERS CLARK

See
Heart and Blood Vessel Conditions (II)
High Blood Pressure (II)
Surgery, Effects of (II)

See also
Adaptogen (III)

HOMOCYSTEINE

Homocysteine is an amino acid found in the blood. It can double the risk for vascular (blood vessel) disease, taking it to a level similar to smoking or hyperlipidemia.

Graham and colleagues (1997) used a case-control study of 19 centers in 9 European countries. A total of 750 individuals diagnosed with atherosclerotic vascular disease (heart, brain, and peripheral) were compared to 800 controls of both sexes, 60 years of age and younger. Plasma total homocysteine was measured while participants were fasting and once again after a standardized methione-loading test. Red blood cell folate, serum cholesterol, smoking, blood pressure, plasma cobalamin, and pyridoxal 5-phosphate levels were also measured. Folic acid and vitamins B6 and B12, known to modulate homocysteine metabolism, were found inversely related to total homocysteine levels. The small number of participants taking these vitamins appeared to have a substantially lower risk of vascular disease.

CAROLYN CHAMBERS CLARK

See
Heart and Blood Vessel Conditions (II)

HORSE CHESTNUT

The horse chestnut tree (*Aesculus hippocastanum*) is fragrant with creamy flowers in summer. In autumn, spiny green fruits are prominent, and the leaves turn yellow orange. The fruit mash has been used as fodder, and the protein-rich seeds can be made into coffee and flour.

In extract form, horse chestnut has anti-edema and anti-inflammatory properties. It also has antiradical action in both in vitro and in vivo studies. The extract inhibits both enzymatic and nonenzymatic in vitro lipid peroxidation (Guillaume & Padioleau, 1994).

CAROLYN CHAMBERS CLARK

See
Varicose Veins (II)

IRON

See
Iron Overload (II)

LAVENDER OIL

Lavender is a woody evergreen shrub that usually grows to a height 3 or 4 feet. The ancient Greeks and Romans prized lavender as a perfume and for its cleansing properties. Romans added lavender to their baths to relieve fatigue and stiff joints. For centuries, lavender has been used as a remedy for ailments as diverse as insect bites, muscular aches and pain, lice, nervous disorders, headaches, scabies, and sprains. Herbalists prescribed it to relieve respiratory ailments, to soothe stomachaches, and to fight fatigue. Early in the 20th century, medications for coughs, headaches, colic, hoarseness, sore joints, toothaches, and nervous palpitations contained lavender oil. During World Wars I and II, medics and soldiers carried lavender oil with them on the battlefield to disinfect wounds (Wilson, 1995).

One study (Cornwell, 1994) investigated the effect of lavender oil as a bath additive postnatally to reduce the mother's perineal discomfort. A blind randomized clinical trial divided 635 new mothers into three groups: One used pure lavender oil, another used a synthetic lavender oil, and the third used an inert substance in their bath for 10 days after childbirth. Although there were no statistically significant differences between groups (based on daily discomfort scores), women using lavender oil recorded lower mean discomfort scores on days 3 and 5. These are the postpartum days new mothers tend to feel the most discomfort, so lavender oil may be useful at these times.

CAROLYN CHAMBERS CLARK

See
Aromatherapy (IV)

LICORICE

Nearly half a century ago Revers reported that administration of a paste prepared from succus liquiritiae, dried watery extract of the roots of *Glycyrrhiza glabra*, resulted in a reduction in abdominal symptoms and provided radiographic evidence of healing in people suffering from gastric ulcer. Subsequent studies showed this preparation could prevent the formation of gastric ulcers in experimental animals, confirming the effect. However, about 20% of those treated developed facial and dependent edema, headache, shortness of breath, stiffness, and pain in the upper abdomen. These appeared to be allergic reactions that subsided with a reduction in dose for most people, but for others, the treatment had to be discontinued. For this reason, licorice as a remedy for peptic ulcers fell out of favor.

The popularity of licorice in candy and other products still exists, despite electrolyte and blood pressure homeostasis that can occur with the ingestion of large quantities of licorice-containing products (Schambelan, 1994).

In 1979, Pompei and colleagues (1979) found that glycyrrhizic acid inactivates herpes simplex virus particles irreversibly and inactivates other viral growth. Badam (1997) found purified glycyrrhizin to be a potent antiviral agent against Japanese encephalitis virus.

Kuo, Shankel, Telikepalli, and Mitscher (1992) found that *Glycyrrhiza glabra* was capable of intercepting *E. coli*, acting as a scavenger or antioxidant. Shenkel, Kuo, Haines, and Mitscher (1993) provided further evidence that *G. glabra* is an antioxidant that intercepts mutagens/carcinogens.

Vaya, Belinky, and Aviram (1997) found that licorice root contains potent antioxidants toward LDL oxidation. Because LDL oxidation is a key event in the formation of the early atherosclerotic lesion, the use of these natural antioxidants may attenuate atherosclerosis.

Zani and colleagues (1993) found that *Glycyrrhiza glabra* inhibited the mutagenicity in *Salmonella typhimurium*. Boscaro and Armanini (1994) found that licorice ameliorates postural hypotension caused by diabetic autonomic neuropathy.

CAROLYN CHAMBERS CLARK

See
Chronic Fatigue Syndrome (II)
Constipation (II)
Diabetes (II)
High Blood Pressure (II)

LYCOPENE

Lycopene is one of the most powerful antioxidants. It is a non–provitamin A carotenoid. Its activity is about double that of beta-carotene. Franceschi and colleagues (1994) conducted a case-control study of tomatoes, which are rich in lycopene. Data were obtained from a series of hospital-based studies (1985–1991) on various cancers of the digestive tract. Results showed a consistent pattern of protection by high intake of raw tomatoes in all examined cancer sites of the digestive tract. The degree of protection was similar, but more marked, than that afforded by green vegetables and fruit salads. There was a 40% reduction in the risk of esophageal cancer for eating one raw tomato per week, and a 50% reduced rate for cancers in all sites among elderly Americans reporting a high tomato intake. Increasing dietary lycopene levels may provide a significant protection against cancer.

Lycopene is found in very few fruits and vegetables (Mangels et al., 1993) but is retained in food processing. Milligrams of lycopene per 100 grams of vegetables and fruits are tomato juice, canned, 8.6; tomato paste, canned, 6.5; tomato sauce, canned, 6.3; watermelon, 4.1; grapefruit, pink, 3.4; guava juice, 3.1; tomato, raw, 3.1; apricot, dried, 0.8; apricot, canned, 0.06.

CAROLYN CHAMBERS CLARK

MILK THISTLE

Milk thistle (*Carduus marianus*) is an herb whose aerial parts and seeds are used as a liver tonic and stimulant, as an antidepressant and demulcent, and to promote milk flow.

CAROLYN CHAMBERS CLARK

PHYTOCHEMICALS

Some food compounds may provide health benefits beyond the traditional nutrients they contain (American Dietetic Association, 1994). Phytochemicals are naturally occurring nonnutritive chemical substances in plants that have a beneficial role in health and wellness. The word *phytochemical* is derived from the Greek word for "plant," *phyto*. Phytochemicals probably evolved to promote the growth of plants and to protect them from sunlight and insects. The class of phytochemicals that possesses biological activity to block cancer processes includes the plant phenol compounds, such as flavenoids. These sub-

stances, ubiquitous in nuts, fruits, whole grains, vegetables, even tea and certain spices (e.g., curry and turmeric) and essential oils (e.g., rosemary), have been shown to prevent or significantly reduce a variety of conditions.

Whole grains, nuts, fruits, and vegetables contain great quantities of phenolic compounds, pigments, terpenoids, and other natural antioxidants associated with protection from and treatment for cancer, diabetes, heart disease, hypertension, and other conditions. Foods with the highest anticancer activity include soybeans, garlic, ginger, licorice, and the *Brassica* class of vegetables (broccoli, cauliflower, cabbage, brussels sprouts, and kohlrabi).

In addition to providing a good supply of vitamin C, citrus fruits contain folic acid, potassium pectin, and a host of active phytochemicals. Grains also contain phytochemicals that reduce the risk for cancer and heart disease.

Sulforaphane and other isothiocyanates that stimulate the production of anticancer enzymes bolster the body's natural ability to ward off cancer and stimulate enzymes that make estrogen less effective (thereby possibly reducing cancer risk). They are found in the brassica vegetables.

Allyl sulfides are found in the *Allium* class of vegetables, including garlic, onions, leeks, and chives. They may block cancer-promoting chemicals. Limonene found in citrus fruits increases the production of enzymes that may help the body dispose of carcinogens. Protease inhibitors (which suppress enzyme production in cancer cells to slow tumor growth), phytosterols (which hinder cell reproduction in the large intestine, possibly preventing colon cancer), isoflavones (which block estrogen from entering cells, possibly reducing the risk of breast cancer), and saponins (which interfere with DNA replication, preventing cancer cells from multiplying) are all found in soybeans and legumes (dried beans and peanuts). Phytic acid (which binds to iron, possibly preventing the creation of cancer-causing free radicals) is found in grains. *Caffeice acid* (which aids in the production of an enzyme that makes it easier for the body to get rid of carcinogens) and ferulic acid (which binds to nitrates, possibly preventing them from converting to cancer-causing nitrosamines), is found in fruits.

CAROLYN CHAMBERS CLARK

See
Antioxidants and Free Radicals (III)
Cancer (II)
Diabetes (II)
Heart and Blood Vessel Conditions (II)
High Blood Pressure (II)

PHYTOESTROGENS

Classes of plant compounds that have estrogenic effects are called phytoestrogens. Soy is one example, flaxseed another. Phytoestrogens are among the dietary factors affording protection against cancer and heart disease in vegetarians. Incidences of breast, colorectal and prostate cancer are high in the Western world compared to countries in Asia, where the semivegetarian diet may alter hormone production, metabolism, or action at the cellular level.

Two important hormonelike phytoestrogens of dietary origin are the lignands and the isoflavonoids. Both are abundant in the plasma of people living in areas with low cancer incidence. The precursors of these protective elements are soybean products, whole grain cereal foods, seeds, and berries. Because of their estrogenic activity,

these foods reduce hot flashes and vaginal dryness in postmenopausal women and may inhibit osteoporosis.

Animal experiments provide evidence that both lignans and isoflavonoids may prevent the development of cancer and atherosclerosis. Ingrahm, Sanders, Kolybaba, and Lopez (1997) interviewed women with newly diagnosed breast cancer by means of questionnaires. They also collected 72-hour urine and blood samples before starting treatment. Controls were randomly selected from the electoral roll after matching for age and area of residence. One hundred forty-four pairs were included in the analysis. After adjusting for age at menarche, parity, alcohol intake, and total fat intake, the researchers found that both the phytoestrogen equol and the lignand enterolactone were associated with a substantial reduction in breast cancer risk. They concluded that there was a substantial reduction in breast cancer risk among women with a high intake of phytoestrogens (as measured by excretion), particularly equol and enterolactone. These findings could be important in the prevention of breast cancer.

CAROLYN CHAMBERS CLARK

See
Cancer (II)
Heart and Blood Vessel Conditions (II)

See also
Flaxseed (III)

PROANTHOCYANIDINS

Proanthocyanidins are one of the most beneficial groups of plant flavonoids. The most potent proanthocyanidins bind to other proanthocyanidins and are called procyanidolic oligomers, or PCOs. PCOs trap free radicals and lipid peroxides, delay the onset of lipid peroxidation, inhibit superoxide production, and inhibit the damaging effects of enzymes (hyaluronidase, elastase, collagenase, etc.) that can degrade connective tissue structures (Facino et al., 1994). PCOs exist in many plants, red wine, grape seeds, pine bark, peanuts, cranberries, and citrus peels. Once called pycnogenols, that term is now reserved for extract of the bark of the French maritime pine (Murray, 1995).

The importance of foods containing PCOs is seen in the following anecdote. In 1534, French explorer Jacques Cartier led an expedition up the St. Lawrence River. He and his crew were forced to eat only salted meat and biscuits on the journey. Scurvy in the group was rampant due to the severe deficiency of vitamin C. A Native American told the group to make a tea from the bark and needles of pine trees. They did, and the scurvy was controlled (Switters & Masquelier, 1993).

PCOs increase intracellular vitamin C levels, decrease capillary permeability and fragility, scavenge oxidants and free radicals, and inhibit destruction of collagen (Switters & Masquelier, 1993). The importance of collagen is quickly grasped when it is remembered that the substance provides the support structure of skin and blood vessels and maintain the integrity of tendons, ligaments, and cartilage.

CAROLYN CHAMBERS CLARK

See
Anthocyanins (III)
Antioxidants and Free Radicals (III)

PROBIOTICS

Yogurt contains beneficial bacteria called probiotics that reside in the intestinal tract and are decreased or eliminated by antibi-

otics, environmental toxins, poor nutrition, and excessive amounts of alcohol. When wiped out, an overgrowth of harmful bacteria and yeast organisms can occur, including yeast infections.

Probiotics maintain balance in the bowels, promote overall health, and help fight off yeast infections. There are more than 20 identifiable types of probiotics, the most common being *Lactobacillus acidophilus*, *bulgaricus*, and *Bifidobacteriium bifidum*. Frozen yogurt and many store-bought fruit-containing yogurts may not have viable live probiotics in them.

CAROLYN CHAMBERS CLARK

ST. JOHN'S WORT

St. John's-wort (*Hypericum*) is the most popular antidepressant in Germany and has been used for centuries by herbalists to heal wounds and treat depression.

CAROLYN CHAMBERS CLARK

See
Depression (II)

SAW PALMETTO

The saw palmetto (*Serenoa repens*) is a palm tree native to the South Atlantic coast. It has emerged as a useful treatment for enlarged prostate. Shimada, Tyler, and McLaughlin (1997) isolated two mono-acylglycerides, 1-monolaurin and 1-mono-myristin. Both compounds showed moderate biological activity against renal and pancreatic human tumor cells, and borderline cytotoxicity was exhibited against human prostatic cells.

CAROLYN CHAMBERS CLARK

See
Prostate, Enlarged (II)

SELENIUM

Selenium (Se) is an essential micronutrient that is unevenly distributed in the earth's crust. Dietary intakes vary over a wide range and are frequently inadequate. Selenium is found in the form of selenocysteine in several enzymes and proteins but also occurs in other organic and inorganic forms in the organism. The *glutathione peroxidases* form a group of selenium-dependent enzymes that protect cells against oxygen radical damage by preventing the accumulation of lipid hydroperoxides and of hydrogen peroxide in tissues and body fluids. Other selenium-dependent enzymes regulate thyroid hormone metabolism and assist in electron transfer reactions of physiologically important compounds. At least 12 other selenium containing proteins have been detected in different organs and tissues. *Selenoprotein P* contains as many as 10 selenocysteine residues and is believed to play a role in selenium transport. A selenium-containing protein is found in the mitochondrial membrane of sperm, another in the prostate gland. The functions of these and several other selenoproteins are as yet unknown. In addition to its enzymatic functions, selenium detoxifies a variety of heavy metals, drugs, and environmental poisons.

Selenium is required for the maintenance of all immune functions, including lymphocyte proliferation, the macrophage-induced cytodestruction, and natural killer cell activity (Kiremidjian-Schumacher & Stotzky, 1987; Koller et al., 1986). Extreme selenium deficiency accordingly produces symptoms and conditions resembling those in advanced HIV-infection, including a cardiomyopathy resembling that occurring in advanced cases of AIDS.

Studies have demonstrated that AIDS patients exhibit subnormal plasma and blood selenium levels which further decline with the progression of the disease (Dworkin et al., 1988; Look et al., 1997). The administration of selenium at nutritional levels, in adults typically 200 to 400 µg Se/day, was suggested as a supportive measure (Schrauzer & Sacher, 1994), the purpose being to prevent selenium depletion, increase host resistance and antibody production, and stimulate other natural defense mechanisms. Supplemental selenium, along with vitamin E and other antioxidant vitamins, should also be one of the support measures in AIDS patients receiving total parenteral nutrition (TPN), especially when lipid-based parenteral formulas are employed to prevent weight loss (Singer et al., 1992). An adequate supply of selenium and of antioxidant vitamins may also be important for the protection of the fetus against the placental transmission of HIV. As selenium is known to stimulate antibody production, selenium supplementation holds promise as a means *of potentiating the efficacy of AIDS vaccines* and of other biological therapeutic or prophylactic agents. Supplemental selenium could furthermore prevent or reduce toxic side effects and synergistically potentiate the action of drugs such as AZT and ZVD.

The importance of selenium is underscored by recent analyses of the genomic structure of HIV, which indicate the presence of genes that have the potential to encode selenoproteins (Taylor, Nadimpalli, & Ramanthan, 1997). It is accordingly assumed that *infected cells require more selenium than normal cells* to accommodate the virus and to moderate the rate viral replication, as selenium, in general, acts as an antiproliferative agent. Selenium is also required *to prevent the excessive generation of oxygen radicals during viral replication.* In selenium deficiency, increased levels of malondialdehyde (MDA), a marker of lipid peroxidation, are accordingly observed. Other agents that stimulate oxygen radical production include sperm, nitrites, opiates and, in the case of hemophiliacs, factor VIII (Papadopulos-Eleopulos, 1998; Revillard et al., 1992).

Oxygen radicals not only damage the virus-infected host cell but also cause damage to the viral genome, resulting in the production of mutants with higher pathogenicity, as was demonstrated in studies with an nonpathogenic strain of Coxsackie B4 virus. When grown in selenium-deficient cultures, that virus changed into a variant with high pathogenicity (Levander & Beck, 1997). Supplemental selenium furthermore protects the host against opportunistic viral infections, notably hepatitis B, and reduce the associated primary liver cancer risk (Yu, Li, Zhu, Yu, & Hou, 1989).

As to the supplemental use of selenium in HIV-infected patients, it is necessary to take into account that gastrointestinal functions may be impaired, diminishing the uptake of selenium. In addition, hepatic, adrenal, pituitary, and splenic functions may be impaired to varying degrees, resulting in complex endocrine abnormalities that require the supplementation not only of selenium but also of other nutrients.

Initial data indicate that selenium in organic forms normally contained in foods (mainly selenomethionine) is absorbed by HIV-infected subjects with intact gastrointestinal function. In a study with 19 symptomatic HIV-antibody-positive male patients with AIDS and ARC (AIDS related complex), the daily administration of 400 µg Se in form of selenium yeast increased blood Se levels to 0.280 ± 0.08 µg/ml in 70 days. During the period of supplementation, 14 patients (74%) reported subjective improvements, such as diminished recurrent illness, improvement of gastrointestinal function, improved appetite, and positive neurologic and psychologic changes. Four patients noted a diminution of their oral candidasis, and only one patient developed the condition during the study (Olmsted, Schrauzer, Flores-Arce, & Dowd, 1989). In another observational study, 15 AIDS patients (13 in stage III and 2 in Stage IV), none of whom had been treated with AZT, received sodium selenite orally at dosages of 100 to 300 µg of Se per day for 3 to 8 months. Selenite was well tolerated, patients reported improvements of appetite and intestinal function (diminished cramping and diarrhea), their weight remained constant or increased, and skin conditions cleared up. The CD4 blood cell numbers still tended to decline, although often only slightly, and CD8 counts tended to decrease more often than to increase, causing the CD4/CD8 cell ratios to increase. Plasma Se was not correlated with CD4 cell counts, and an inverse association of plasma Se with the number of CD8 cells was observed. A pilot study with 10 AIDS patients with nonobstructive cardiomyopathy, the administration of 800 µg per day of Se as sodium selenite for 15 days followed by 400 µg per day for 8 days produced improvements of heart function, notably, increases of the ventricular shortening fraction (Zazzo et al., 1988). An improvement of cardiac function was also observed in a pediatric AIDS patient with virally induced cardiomyopathy (Ruff et al., 1991).

GERHARD N. SCHRAUZER

See
AIDS/HIV (II)

TEA

Several polyphenols called cathechins, which are thought to have anticancer activity, are present in green tea. They are destroyed in the brewing of black tea but are present in green. One cathechin found in green tea, epigallocathechin-3 gallate, or EGCG, may prevent cancer or reduce tumor size by binding to and inhibiting urokinase, a proteolytic enzyme frequently found in human cancer tissue. When EGCG binds to urokinase, invading cells and metastases to other body areas are prevented. A single cup of green tea provides a safer and more effective dose than other known urokinase inhibitors (Jankun, 1997).

CAROLYN CHAMBERS CLARK

THYME

Thyme is a much-branching subshrub with woody stems and numerous small, pointed, strongly aromatic green leaves. Culinary thyme aids in the digestion of fatty foods and is ideal for stews and soups. Lemon thyme is delicious with chicken and fresh fruit dishes. Distilled from the leaves and flowering tops, thyme is used as a stimulant and antiseptic. It has been used as a nerve tonic to treat depression, colds, muscular pain, and respiratory problems. Research is accumulating to show that thyme does have therapeutic action.

Using bioassay-directed fractionation, Haraguchi and colleagues (1996) isolated a biphenyl compound and a flavonoid, both antioxidants, from the leaves of *Thymus vulgaris*. The flavonoid inhibited mitochondrial peroxidation and oxidative hemolysis. Both compounds were shown to be effective in protecting biological systems against various oxidative stresses.

Panizzi, Flamini, Cioni, and Morelli (1993) found thyme to have antimicrobial and fungicidal properties. Van Den Broucke and Lemli (1983) studied the action of thyme in vitro for spasmolytic activity on the smooth muscles of the ileum and trachea in the guinea pig. The flavones in thyme induced relaxation of the carbachol contracted tracheal strip.

CAROLYN CHAMBERS CLARK

See
Antioxidants and Free Radicals (III)
Flavonoids (III)
Mediterranean Diet (IV)

VITAMIN A

Vitamin A prevents eye problems such as night blindness and some skin disorders. It may also heal ulcers in the digestive tract and protect against pollution and cancer formation.

Vitamin A analogs, called retinoids, suppress mouth and lung cancer in animal models and prevent the development of secondary problems of the head, lung, and neck in individuals diagnosed with lung cancer (Lotan, 1997). The vitamin and its analogs also have a role in the prevention of heart and blood vessel conditions (Hinds, West, & Knight, 1997).

CAROLYN CHAMBERS CLARK

See
Macular Degeneration (II)
Skin Disorders (II)

VITAMIN C

Vitamin C, or ascorbic acid, is an antioxidant. It is needed for tissue growth and repair, healthy gums, and proper adrenal gland function. It also protects against infection, enhances immunity, protects against damage caused by pollution, increases the absorption of iron, protects against bruising and blood clotting, and promotes wound healing and repair after burns. Additionally, it may have a role in the prevention of cancer, the reduction of cholesterol levels and high blood pressure, and the prevention of atherosclerosis (hardening of the arteries).

Vitamin C is needed to metabolize tyrosine, folic acid, and phenylalanine and works synergistically with vitamin E. Both attack free radicals.

Because the body cannot manufacture it, vitamin C can only be obtained through foods or supplements. Scurvy results from extreme deficiency of the vitamin. Symptoms of lesser degrees of deficiency include increased susceptibility to infection, joint pains, lack of energy, poor digestion, prolonged healing time, tendency to bruise easily, gums that bleed when brushed, and tooth loss (Balch & Balch, 1997).

Heuser and Vojdani (1997) studied the effect of buffered vitamin C on natural killer (NK) function in individuals who had been exposed to toxic chemicals. Blood was drawn on 55 participants prior to giving them granulated buffered vitamin C in water at a dosage of 60mg/kg of body weight. Blood was drawn again 24 hours later. Vitamin C was capable of enhancing NK activity up to 10-fold in level after ingestion. The researchers concluded that immune function can be restored after toxic chemicals by oral ingestion of vitamin C.

CAROLYN CHAMBERS CLARK

See
Burns (II)
Cancer (II)
Cold Symptoms (II)

See also
Antioxidants and Free Radicals (III)

VITAMIN E

Vitamin E (alpha-tocopherol) is a fat-soluble vitamin that assists in blood circulation, helps prevent atherosclerosis (hardening of the arteries), provides free radical scavenger protection after burns, and may stimulate immunity and enhance healing. Vitamin E occurs naturally in egg yolks, nuts, vegetable oils, butter, and wheat germ.

CAROLYN CHAMBERS CLARK

See
Alzheimer's Disease (II)
Burns (II)
Cystic Fibrosis (II)
Heart and Blood Vessel Conditions (II)
High Blood Pressure (II)
Wounds (II)

See also
Antioxidants and Free Radicals (III)

ZINC

Zinc is a mineral that is distributed in all tissues, with substantial concentrations in the eye (especially the retina, iris, and choroid), kidney, brain, liver, muscle, and male reproductive system (prostate, prostate secretions, and spermatozoa). The two to three grams of zinc found in the body act as cofactors in more than 20 enzymatic reactions. They also bind with some nonenzymatic molecules including histidine, cysteine, and the albumins. Zinc is also important for insulin activity, for protein and DNA synthesis, for normal taste and wound healing, to maintain normal vitamin A levels and usage, in the structure of bones and the immune system, in the treatment of acne, and to reduce infant morbidity and mortality.

Zinc Deficiency

Individuals who eat little or no red meat or who are on restrictive diets often consume two-thirds to one-half of the amounts recommended for zinc intake. Zinc absorption is impaired when large amounts of calcium in the diet bind with phytates (found in spinach, for example) and form an insoluble complex. A diet high in cereal and low in animal protein has produced zinc deficiency in Middle Eastern populations. Other populations where zinc deficiency may exist are preschools, hospitals, low-income groups, and the elderly. Athletes and strict vegetarians are also at risk. Low meat consumption combined with refined grains, convenience foods, and high-fat, high-sugar intake add additional risk. Individuals suffering acute or chronic infections, pernicious anemia, alcoholism, cirrhosis of the liver, renal disease, cardiovascular disease, some malignancies, protein-calorie malnutrition, and parenteral (IV) feedings are all at risk of deficiency. Maternal zinc deficiency can result in retarded fetal growth and maturation, including cleft palate and lip; brain and eye malformations; abnormalities in the heart, lung, skeleton, and urogenital system, reduced brain DNA and survival in infants (Scholl et al., 1993; Keen et al., 1993; James, 1993).

Animals in a low-zinc state exhibit impaired learning, hypersensitivity to stress, and increased aggression. Pregnant women are at high risk for deficiency, increasing their chances of a spontaneous abortion, pregnancy-related toxemia, extended pregnancy, premature delivery, or prolonged labor (Sandstead, 1991).

If the deficiency occurs during a high fetal growth period, failures of sexual development are more severe. Testicular degeneration is not reversible, while prostate gland, seminal vesicle, and sperm degeneration from deficiency are reversible. Growth can be stunted and immunity impaired. Increasing zinc intake can reverse these symptoms (Nakamura et al., 1993; Schlesinger et al., 1992).

Serum zinc declines with increases in dietary fiber. Zinc is needed daily since body stores are not readily available. Elevated temperatures in certain environments can lead to zinc deficiency when the mineral is lost through sweat.

Short-term zinc deficiency is responded to by the body by absorbing a greater amount of dietary zinc and reducing excretion. Inadequate zinc intake will affect a wide variety of functions including protein synthesis, energy production, collagen formation, alcohol tolerance, changes in hair and nails, sterility, skin inflammation, lethargy, poor wound healing, and a loss of taste and smell (Gibson, 1991; Lee et al., 1993).

Suppressed immune systems recover with the addition of zinc and vitamin A supplements to the daily diet. Supplementation also improves immune function in children with Down syndrome (Singh et al., 1992; Stabile et al., 1991).

Uses

Low serum zinc levels have been noted in individuals diagnosed with AIDS/HIV. Vomiting and reduced appetite may contribute to the problem by reducing zinc availability. Zinc deficiency may be responsible for secondary symptoms including anorexia, digestive malfunctions, diarrhea, impaired immunity, and central nervous system malfunction. As a result, Odeh (1992) suggests zinc supplementation for this population.

Zinc deficiency damages the integrity of blood vessels and the blood. Zinc enhances the barrier between deep layers of blood vessels and the blood, reducing the risk of atherosclerosis, and heart and blood vessel disease (Hennig & McClain, 1992).

Individuals diagnosed with anorexia and bulimia have low urinary zinc levels. Depressed zinc status might be a factor in eating disorders. Zinc supplementation has proved effective in reducing eating disorders (McClain et al., 1992; Varela et al., 1992).

Inadequate zinc could reduce fertility in men (Hunt et al., 1992).

Daily Requirements and Food Sources

Healthy adults require 12.5 mg of dietary zinc every day. Adequate secretion of gastric acid is important for optimal zinc absorption.

Good food sources of zinc include oysters, herring, milk, meat, egg yolks, and breast milk. Although not well absorbed, zinc in wholegrain breads and cereals supplies a ready source for vegetarians with reduced protein intake. Including as little as 3 ounces of beef in the daily diet can significantly improve zinc status (Zheng et al., 1993).

Toxicity

Fifty milligrams for high bioavailable forms and 100 mg for low bioavailable forms of the mineral are safe doses. Toxic doses are more than 2 grams. High doses of zinc are ingested from food stored in galvanized containers (Prasad, 1993).

CAROLYN CHAMBERS CLARK

See
AIDS/HIV (II)
Diabetes (II)
Eating Disorders (II)
Heart and Blood Vessel Conditions (II)
Lung Disorders (II)
Skin Disorders (II)
Wounds (II)

See also
Bioavailability (I)
Vitamin A (III)

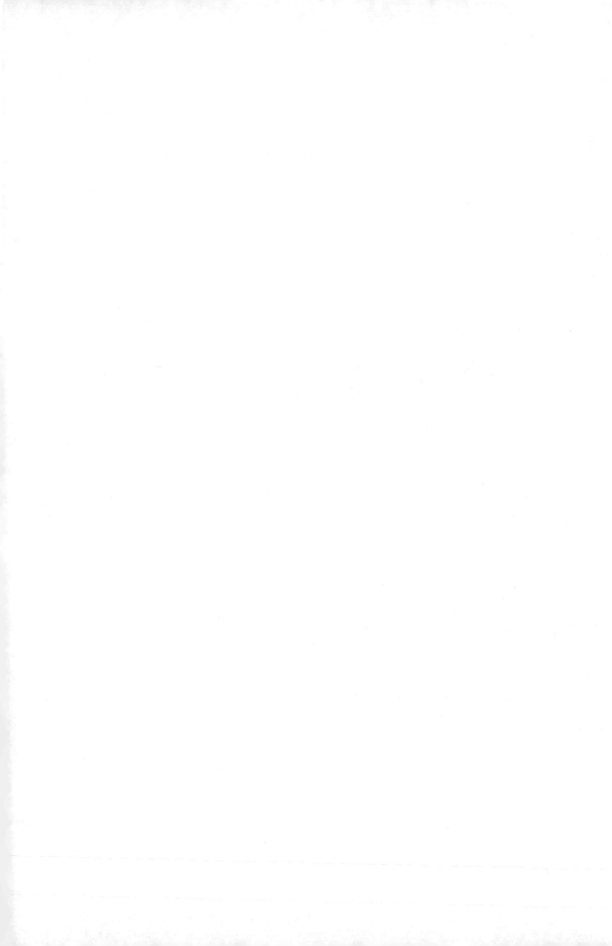

Part IV

Practices and Treatments

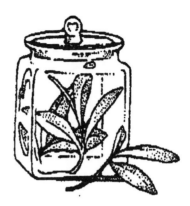

ACUPUNCTURE AND CHINESE MEDICINE

The term *acupuncture* refers to a family of procedures within Chinese medicine that are used to prevent and treat disease. Acupuncture itself involves the insertion of thin, solid, usually stainless steel needles at precise anatomic locations. These locations are classic acupuncture points, motor points, and areas of tenderness (Ahshi points). Insertion depth averages from 1 mm to several inches, depending on point location and desired effect. Inserted, needles may be manipulated by hand or through attached electrodes. Various waveforms and intensities of voltage may be applied. Needles may be stimulated through moxabustion, the local and focused application of heat (by the burning of the herb *Artemisia vulgaris*), and cupping, a suctioning of the skin through the application of small jars in which a vacuum is created. Magnets of various strengths may also be used.

A Brief History of Chinese Medicine

The roots of Chinese medicine, of which acupuncture, massage, and herbal medicine are the principle components, reach back as early as the Shang dynasty (c. 1000 B.C.). Archeological discoveries from this period include acupuncture needles and texts on the discussion of medical problems. By the Han dynasty (206 B.C.–220 A.D.) the basic tenets of Oriental medicinal theory and practice were in place. Prominent developments of this period were the treatment paradigms of yin and yang, the Five Phases, and the Channels. Needling methods and a comprehensive herbal pharmacopoeia were also in place. *The Yellow Emperor's Inner Classic*, a most significant text, was written during this time. It was composed of two parts: "Simple Questions" and "Spiritual Axis."

Major contributions of later dynasties include the following: in the Western Jin dynasty (A.D. 256–316), *The Comprehensive Manual of Acupuncture and Moxibustion*, by Zhen Jiu Jia Y. Jing; in the Ming dynasty (A.D. 1368–1644), *The Great Compendium of Acupuncture and Moxibustion*, by Zhen Jiu Dei Cheng. During these periods the use of acupuncture spread throughout Asia.

Acupuncture was introduced to the West in the 17th century by Jesuit missionaries who had been sent to Beijing. The first European reference to the topic was not until 1671, in *Secrets of Chinese Medicine*, by P. Harviell. In the 20th century sinologist Soulié de Morant, writing in the 1940s, provided a basis for serious study. *Auriculotherapy* (ear acupuncture) was developed by the French physician Paul Nogier, in 1958. By the 1970s acupuncture was being taught in many medical schools throughout Europe. Veterinary acupuncture was also well established.

In the United States references to the topic are found as early as 1825, with the publication of *Case Illustrative of Medical Effects of Acupuncture*, by Franklin Bache, M.D. In 1892 William Osler's textbook, *The Principles and Practice of Medicine*, cited acupuncture for the treatment of lumbago.

Recent U.S. history begins with the account by the *New York Times* reporter James Reston of his experiences with acupuncture at the Anti-Imperialist Hospital in Beijing, in 1971. In 1973 the Food and Drug Administration (FDA) required acupuncture equipment to be labeled as investigatory. The first licensed acupuncture school opened in Boston in 1976. In 1996 the FDA reclassified acupuncture needles as class 2 medical devices.

Today there are over 8,000 licensed or certified nonphysician acupuncturists in the United States. In California alone there are over 3,000. Thirty-three states currently permit the practice of acupuncture by nonphysician acupuncturists, who act as independent health care providers or under the supervision of a medical doctor. Practitioners attend 3- to 4-year postgraduate-style programs. Schools may receive accreditation for Master's degree programs through the National Accreditation Commission of Schools and Colleges of Acupuncture and Oriental Medicine (Washington, DC). A certification examination is offered through the National Certification Commission for Acupuncture and Oriental Medicine (Washington, DC). A minimum of 1,300 hours of training is required to sit for this exam. The state of California requires a minimum of 2,348 hours. The largest and oldest professional association is the American Association of Oriental Medicine (Catasauqua, PA). The American College of Addictionology and Compulsive Disorders (Miami, FL) offers 120- and 300-hour specialization training and certification programs in addiction medicine.

Presently in the United States there are over 1,000 medical doctors and dentists practicing acupuncture. Few states require specialized training or any form of certification for medical doctors and dentists to perform acupuncture. The American Academy of Medical Acupuncturists (AAMA, Los Angeles) is a professional association for medical doctor acupuncturists who are trained in acupuncture by members of the AAMA. Training consists of 200 hours of instruction, much of which is nonclass-room. No proficiency exam is presently given, however, one is reported to be in development.

Acupuncture continues to become more accepted by the general public. A 1991 *Time* magazine/CNN poll indicated that 6% of Americans (15 million) had been treated with acupuncture. It is estimated that 90 million acupuncture treatments are given each year (Helms).

There are various approaches to diagnosis and treatment in contemporary acupuncture practice in the United States. Cultures that have influenced the practice include Japan, Korea, France, England, and Germany. All have made contributions that have moved the practice of acupuncture in new directions.

Theory and Practice

The Chinese ideogram for *energy*, pronounced *chi*, or *qi*, depicts the lid of a pot being raised by steam. What is shown is not the steam but rather the energy of the steam. Good health is a state of energy balance within the body. Body tissue and structures are seen primarily in relation to the energy activating and maintaining them. Energy is the primary component of all physiological activities. It varies quantitatively and qualitatively, manifesting in the polar forms of yin and yang energy. Energy in its basic undifferentiated state, as a potential rather than an active force, is termed the *Tao*. This is understood as the One underlying all phenomena. Tao is manifested in all things through the dynamic interaction of the two polar energy forces called yin and yang. The Nei Ching indicates that "the universe is an oscillation of the forces of yin and yang." As with the universe, the chi of the body is constantly circulating by means of the meridian system. This movement is essential for life.

Disease is thought to arise out of imbalances or disharmonies in the natural flow of the body's energies. Symptoms of disease, both emotional and physical, are reflections of these imbalances. In and of themselves, symptoms are only meaningful in the context of a particular patient at a particular time. Signs and symptoms are pieced together and synthesized until a picture of the whole person appears.

Although there are several different assessment and treatment paradigms from which the practitioner may choose (five elements, eight principles, etc.), treatment is centered on correcting the energetic patterns of disharmony. In correcting energetic imbalance, the practitioner of Chinese medicine is facilitating the body's inherent capacity to heal. Treatments have a cumulative effect and are often curative.

The Western scientific investigation of acupuncture has had a number of inherent problems. The very nature of the practice of Chinese medicine does not lend itself easily to the needs of the traditional Western model. From a Western perspective, physiological mechanisms that mediate the beneficial effects of acupuncture are not completely understood. Despite these limitations, research by Pomerance and Stux with neural mechanisms has brought about some illumination. The Office of Alternative Medicine of the National Institutes of Health is currently sponsoring nine pilot projects and had sponsored a Consensus Development Conference in November 1997.

JAMES D. MORAN

See also

Addiction Treatment (IV)
Auriculotherapy (IV)

ACUPUNCTURE IN GYNECOLOGICAL DISEASE

An in-depth study of acupuncture offers a practitioner with Western medical or surgical training, a different way of approaching cases, one that is not purely symptomatic. Qi is believed to circulate in the body through a series of meridians or invisible channels flowing under the skin. Acupuncture points lie on each meridian and are regarded as the entrances and exits for vital energy (see below for key definitions).

Certain etiopathogenic conditions (underlying causes) of an illness (e.g., *cold* or *heat* in the blood, accumulation of *damp-heat* in the *urinary bladder*, congenital excess of *phlegm*, disharmony between the *heart* and *kidney*, ascending of *liver fire*, etc.) may seem unusual to someone unfamiliar with acupuncture, and italicized words (organs, cold, heat, damp) used here refer to energetic structure, rather than the actual anatomic organs or physical properties. This is because the terminology has no correspondence in western medical language. For an acupuncture practitioner, recognition of these conditions is indispensable to choosing an adequate treatment.

In Chinese traditional medicine, a woman's development and evolution are a succession of stages represented by the number 7 and its multiples (Bossy, Guevin, & Yasui, 1990). The woman is under the Chinese sign of Yin (as in Yin and Yang), so there is a *blood* predominance as a characteristic. Gynecological physiology and pathology are under the influence of Qi/*blood* dynamic balance. Qi (life energy) and *blood* have a reciprocal relationship, as "Qi is *blood* commander and *blood* is the mother of Qi." When Qi controls *blood*, menstruation is regular, of normal aspect and quantity (Beijing, Shanghai, & Nanjing Colleges of Traditional Chinese Medicine, 1980; Liangyue, Yijun, Shuhui, et al., 1987). But if there is a Qi stagnation, it may cause excessive menstrual flow, amenorrhea, dysmenorrhea, infertility, and uterine prolapse in cases of sinking of the Kidney Qi (Auteroche, Navailh, Maronnaud, et al., 1986; Liangyue et al., 1987; Tureanu & Tureanu, 1994).

Considering the concept of Qi, it can be said that the state of health and illness reflects the human body's energetic balance or imbalance. Acupuncture treatment is based upon needling acupoints along the channels and regulating Qi and *blood*. General principles of treatment include Yin and Yang regulation, removal of the pathogenic factors and increasing the body's resistance. Individual condition (e.g., age, sex, constitution), season variation, and different geographic conditions are also taken into account.

Selection of acupoints and therapeutic method is based upon the differentiation of syndromes according to the eight principles of diagnosis, the theory of Qi and *blood*, the theory of Zang-Fu organs, and the theory of channels. For example, if *blood* stagnation (due to the invasion of *cold* as pathogenic factor) occurs, it is necessary to dispel *cold* and remove stagnation; acupuncture is then given with the reducing method.

Menstruation is governed by the uterus, an extraordinary organ named Baozang or Zigong. It is also related to the five Zang organs—*heart, liver, spleen, lung*, and *kidney*—and with the three Yin channels of the foot, but mainly with the extraordinary vessels Ren Mai and Chong Mai. When Chong Mai is disturbed it may cause lumbar and abdominal pain, infertility, uterine

retroversion, uterine prolapse, vaginitis, and abnormal hair growth. When Ren Mai is disturbed, the following symptoms may appear: infertility, leukorrhea (discharge), pelvic tumoral masses, menopause disorders, dysmenorrhea (painful menstruation), and pains of external genitalia. Ren Mai is also related to the thyroid, adrenals, and pancreas. Dysfunctions of Dai Mai, Du Mai, Yin Wei Mai, and Yin Qiao Mai can also be involved in menstrual cycle disorders, infertility, leukorrhea, and sexual dysfunctions (Auteroche et al., 1986; Ionescu Tirgoviste, 1992; Tureanu & Tureanu, 1994).

Establishing a precise diagnosis is based upon careful attention to past history, inspection, palpation, and tongue and pulse diagnosis. Possible etiopathogenic conditions can be overstrain, stress, excessive sexual activity, constitutional deficiency, or exogenous pathogenic factors such as *heat, cold*, or *damp* (Auteroche et al., 1986; Liangyue et al., 1987; Tureanu & Tureanu, 1994). The next step in establishing the diagnosis is the differentiation of the syndromes to which an adequate therapy is related.

Numerous syndromes are involved in gynecological illnesses and possible relations can be established as follows (Auteroche et al., 1986; Liangyue et al., 1987; Ross, 1983; Tureanu & Tureanu, 1994):

1. According to Qi and *blood* theory

   • Deficiency of Qi—menstrual cycle disorders (antedated menstruation with bright red, excessive flow), uterine bleeding
   • Stagnation of Qi menstrual cycle disorders, amenorrhea (absence of

menstruation), dysmenorrhea, infertility, ovarian cyst, etc.

- Sinking of Qi—uterine, vesical prolapse, urinary incontinence
- Deficiency of *blood*—disorders of menstrual cycle (postdated menstruation with bright red, scanty flow), dysmenorrhea, infertility, menopause disorders (e.g., insomnia)
- Stagnation of *blood*—disorders of menstrual cycle (postdated menstruation with dark-colored fluid, with clots, scanty flow), pelvic inflammatory disease, amenorrhea, dysmenorrhea, uterine leiomyomata (benign tumor)
- *Heat* in the *blood*—disorders of menstrual cycle (dark red excessive menstrual flow), metrorrhagia (irregular flow), vicarious menstruation (as in endometriosis, i.e., blood flow outside the uterus), vulvar pruritus (itching)

2. According to Zang-Fu organs theory

- *Kidney* Qi deficiency—leukorrhea, menopause disorders, urinary incontinence, uterine prolapse (displacement), urinary tract infections
- Yang *kidney* deficiency—leukorrhea, infertility, frigidity, uterine retroversion (tilting), urinary retention, edema (swelling), etc.
- Yin *kidney* deficiency—metrorrhagia, dysmenorrhea, leukorrhea, menopause disorders, vulvar pruritus
- *Damp-heat* in the *urinary bladder*—urinary disturbances, urinary tract infection, urinary retention

- *Liver* Qi stagnation—irregular menstrual cycle, premenstrual syndrome, dysmenorrhea, infertility, insomnia, fibrocystic breast disease
- Ascending *liver fire*—vicarious menstruation
- *Liver blood* deficiency—oligomenorrhea (abnormally frequent menstruation), amenorrhea
- *Damp-heat* in the *liver* and *gall bladder*—vulvar pruritus, leukorrhea, urinary disorders Spleen Qi deficiency—hypomenorrhea
- Spleen dysfunction in controlling blood—uterine bleeding

3. According to complicated syndromes of Zang-Fu organs, usually involved in uterine bleeding of perimenopause and menopause disorders:

- Disharmony between *heart* and *kidney*
- Yin deficiency of *liver* and *kidney*
- Yang deficiency of *spleen* and *kidney*
- Deficiency of *spleen* and *heart*

Acupuncture can be useful for the following conditions: premenstrual syndrome, dysmenorrhea, menstrual cycle disorders (even after oral contraceptives), menopause disorders (e.g., hot flushes, psychological disorders, insomnia, etc.), leukorrhea, and uterine bleeding (Auteroche et al., 1986; Ionescu-Tirgoviste, 1992; Liangyue et al., 1987; Ross, 1983; Tureanu & Tureanu, 1994).

From the perspective of Chinese traditional medicine, there are other cases where acupuncture can be useful: pelvic inflammatory disease, ovarian cyst, uterine leiomyomata, uterine prolapse, fibrocystic breast disease. In Western medicine, all these have well-established treatments, including surgical procedures (Auteroche et al., 1986; Quan, 1985; Tureanu & Tureanu, 1994).

For sexual dysfunctions, such as decrease or absence of libido, anorgasmia (failure to reach orgasm), dyspareunia (painful intercourse), vaginismus (vaginal spasms), or frigidity, acupuncture treatment can also be used as adjuvant or alternative therapy (Deroc, 1991).

In many cases, women with gynecological diseases do have urinary complaints such as urinary tract infections or urinary incontinence. Acupuncture can help in these cases, unless there is an established need for antibiotic therapy or a surgical procedure (Auteroche et al., 1986; Sheng, 1986).

From the perspective of Chinese traditional medicine menstrual disorders are described as follows, with etiopathogenic conditions for each:

a) Amenorrhea due to *blood* stagnation and *blood* deficiency
b) Irregular menstruation
    —antedated menstruation due to heat in the *blood* and Qi deficiency
    —postdated menstruation due to *blood* deficiency, *cold* in the *blood*, and Qi stagnation
    —irregular menstrual cycles due to stagnation of *liver* Qi and *kidney* deficiency

The acupuncture prescription aims to improve and restore the energetic imbalance, either of excess or deficiency type, or to remove pathogenic factors.

In Figure 1 are displayed many of the frequently used acupoints (located in dif-

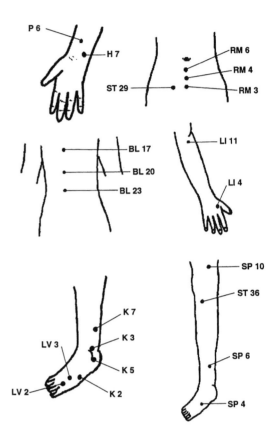

FIGURE 1   Frequently used acupoints essential to gynecological disease

ferent areas of the body), which are essential to gynecological diseases, including: SP 6 (Sanyinjiao), SP 4 (Gongsun), SP 10 (Xuehai), RM 4 (Guanyuan), RM 3 (Zhongji), RM 6 (Qihai), ST 36 (Zusanli), ST 29 (Guilai), K 3 (Taixi), K 2 (Rangu), K 5 (Shiquan), K 7 (Fuliu), LV 3 (Taichong), LV 2 (Xingjian), BL 20 (Pishu), BL 23 (Shenshu), BL 17 (Geshu), LI 4 (Hegu), LI 11 (Quchi), H 7 (Shenmen), P 6 (Neiguan) (Auteroche et al., 1986; Ionescu-Tirgoviste, 1992; Jiansan, 1988; Kefu et al., 1982; Liangyue et al., 1987; Ross, 1983; Tureanu & Tureanu, 1994). Other points can be associated in different prescriptions. The needle stimulation, with reducing, tonifying, or even movement method, and the number of sessions are related to each case (a session duration is about 15–20 minutes; generally speaking few sessions, three to five on average, are needed in acute cases and eight to ten in the chronic ones—their repetition may be necessary).

In the Chinese approach, other factors, such as diet, physical exercise, massage, mental discipline, and lifestyle modification are also taken into account when establishing the therapy. Thus, the approach is much less symptomatic but mainly based upon correcting etiopathogenic circumstances. This is understandable, if it is remembered that a certain disease can be caused by: the invasion of the six etiopathogenic exogenous factors (e.g., wind, heat, cold, damp, fire, dryness), the seven emotional factors (e.g., fear, worry, grief, joy, anger, melancholy, and fright), and other varied factors (e.g., strain, stress, inadequate diet or lack of physical exercise, traumatic injuries, etc.). Thus, the care is not only about treatment; it is also about prevention and a more prophylactic approach.

Case Study

P.M., a 32-year-old patient, presented with amenorrhea (absence of menses) with sudden onset. Associated clinical manifestations were: pain with cold and heavy sensation in the lower abdomen, alleviated by warmth, cold limbs, dark complexion, red tongue with white coating and string-taut or wiry, deep pulse. Using bimanual examination and ultrasound examination, possible organic causes were excluded and amenorrhea was considered to be of a functional nature. The case was considered amenorrhea due to *blood* stagnation caused by invasion of cold as an exogenous pathogenic factor. Points were selected to regulate Qi, promote *blood* circulation and remove stagnation, as follows: RM 4 (Guanyuan), SP 6 (Sanyinjiao), SP 10 (Xuehai), LV 3 (Taichong) and ST 29 (Guilai). Acupuncture was given with the reducing method. After five sessions of acupuncture, each of 15–20 minutes, the patient reported the onset of menstrual flow. In the following month, four days before the supposed time of menstruation, the same points were stimulated again and after three sessions her period began.

Key Definitions

Pulse Diagnosis. Pulse diagnosis, or pulse palpation, is a method of diagnosis based upon feeling the pulse on radial artery at the wrist. Because of the relationship to the Zang-Fu organs their physiologic or pathologic condition can be interpreted by feeling the pulse. Normal pulse is smooth and forceful and there are physiological variations related to age, sex, individual constitution seasons. Several types of pathological pulses are described and they indicate the etiopathogenic condition and the possible progression of the disease.

Qi. Qi is derived from Chinese traditional medicine. The concept of Qi refers to fundamental substance of the universe. Thus Qi is energy at the same time it is matter. With regard to the human body and the activity of each organ, physiology and physiopathology are explained mainly within the concept of Qi. Qi is the source of any change and movement. Several categories of Qi have been described: congenital (Yuan Qi) and acquired (Hou Tian Zhi Qi), defensive (Wed Qi), and nourishing

(Yin" Qi). There is a normal Qi (Zheng Qi, or correct) and a pathologic Qi. Qi has different functions: growth and development, supporting the activity of Zang-Fu organs, promoting blood circulation, distribution of body fluids, but also warming, defensive, nourishing and regulating functions. As there is no equivalent term for Qi in western medicine it is rather difficult to provide a precise definition.

Reducing Method. The reducing method is used as a treatment method in cases with excess syndromes. It is able to enhance the body's resistance and so the ability to fight illness. By using this method one can dispel the exogenous pathogenic factors that have entered the body (i.e., cold, wind, heat).

Tongue Diagnosis. Tongue diagnosis is an important part of establishing the diagnosis, it is based upon tongue inspection. From the perspective of Chinese traditional medicine the Zang-Fu organs are related to the tongue and so pathological changes of Zang-Fu organs will find their expression at tongue level. Information concerning the tongue proper (color, form, motion) and its coating (color, quality) are related to etiopathogenic condition and the evolution of disease towards alleviation or aggravation.

Yin and Yang. The theory of Yin and Yang reflect the dual aspect of all phenomena that take place in the universe. The relationship between Yin and Yang is a complex one, under several aspects, of opposition, interdependence, interconsuming-supporting, intertransforming and infinite divisibility. Thus each phenomenon or condition is relative and expresses itself as these two aspects of opposite but complementary at the same time, named Yin and Yang. *Cold* and heat, inside and outside,

down and up, winter and summer, moon and sun, night and day, rest and movement, female and male, and the examples can go on, are all Yin and Yang. The theory of Yin and Yang is an approach or characterization of each phenomena, thus health and illness condition are also expressed under Yin and Yang.

Zang-Fu. In the Chinese approach, the body organs are named Zang-Fu. There are five Zang organs—*heart, liver, kidney, spleen,* and *lung*—and six Pu organs—*gall bladder, stomach, large intestine, small intestine, urinary bladder,* and *San Jiao.* The task of the Zang organs is to maintain a full and vital supply of Qi. If Qi becomes stagnant, illness occurs. The theory of Zang-Fu organs is based upon observation of correlations between illness-symptoms and the affected organ, considering physiology and pathology together with their relationships. The theory of Zang-Fu organs is also used in the differentiation of syndromes; it is a comprehensive way to establish a precise diagnosis and select an adequate prescription.

VALENTIN TUREANU
LUMINITA TUREANU

See also
Premenstrual Syndrome (PMS) (II)

ADDICTION TREATMENT

Substance Misuse

Substance misuse affects millions of individuals of nearly all age groups, may result in many physiological ailments, and is a leading preventable cause of death in the United States. According to the American Medical Association (AMA), between 25% and 40% of general hospital inpatients are being treated for complications resulting from alcoholism (Brady, 1995).

The term *substance misuse* will be used to refer to the consumption of psychoactive substances that results in serious impairment in major role functioning and is characterized by such features as tolerance for the substance, intoxication, withdrawal, craving, and a pattern of continued or recurrent use over time. This discussion will be restricted to alcohol, nicotine, and illicit substances (opiates, cocaine). Inclusion of a treatment modality in this review does not imply endorsement of the therapy.

Alternative Medicine in Addiction Treatment

The field of addiction medicine has integrated complementary and alternative medicine (CAM) to a greater degree than have most other medical specialties. There are several CAM treatments that are in use as and in combination with conventional treatments. For example, traditional 12-step programs such as Alcoholics Anonymous emphasize spiritual awareness (Culliton, Boucher, & Carlson, 1997).

After spirituality, *acupuncture* is the most widely used CAM modality for the treatment of substance misuse, offered to patients at over 700 chemical dependency programs in the United States. The influx of crack cocaine users in the 1980s overburdened urban treatment centers, and acupuncture has served to fill this treatment need. Citing the lack of efficacious conventional treatments, practitioners asserted that they could effectively treat large numbers of patients at minimal cost. The National Acupuncture Detoxification Association, formed in 1985, has taught more than 4,000 U.S. acupuncturists, counselors,

nurses, and physicians how to perform acupuncture for substance misuse. Encouraged by early clinical successes, numerous courts across the nation have started to mandate acupuncture for the treatment of offenders. To date, no significant negative side effects have been reported (Culliton & Kiresuk, 1996).

Acupuncture

The use of acupuncture and electroacupuncture (the addition of mild electricity to acupuncture needles) is based on the belief that small needles inserted into the skin at points consistent with the major energy pathways of the body, can help rebalance the flow of energy, or chi (qi). These pathways, called meridians, are the basis of Oriental medicine, and a balanced flow of energy corresponds to good health.

Opiate-dependent patients in China were the first to receive acupuncture as substance misuse treatment. Electroacupuncture was administered to diminish symptoms of withdrawal and accelerate detoxification. In the United States acupuncture is used to treat all forms and stages of addiction, although electrical stimulation is less frequently administered.

Treatment Encounter

There are significant variations in treatment provision. Patients receiving acupuncture through chemical dependency programs are typically treated concurrently in a common room. Comfortable chairs, low lighting, soft music, and tea may be incorporated into the environment. Less common for the treatment of addictions are private treatment sessions, which are more costly and time consuming for both the patient and the practitioner. The difference in treatment outcomes resulting from these variations is unknown.

In order to acquire useful treatment outcome information, several basic treatment and research procedures should be considered and recorded. Among these considerations are accurate recording of treatment processes, informed consent for treatment, consistent use of accepted measures of symptoms and complaints, the points used, patient response, number of treatments, and duration of treatment outcomes. Of central importance is the distinction between treatment of withdrawal and maintenance of recovery.

Mechanism

Western scientists have proposed that prolonged drug use may interfere with the body's natural production of *endorphins*. One hypothesis suggests that craving may be linked to the deficiency of endorphins and other endogenous opioids, as well as to other neurochemical deficits. Research indicates that acupuncture may stimulate the peripheral nerves to send messages to the brain to release endorphins. Acupuncture has also been shown to alter levels of other neurotransmitters, such as serotonin, and to affect hormonal regulation. These findings form the basis for a preliminary model for the efficacy of acupuncture in the treatment of opiate and alcohol addiction (Boucher & Kiresuk, in press).

Efficacy

Literature on the use of acupuncture is more prevalent than for any other CAM modality used to treat substance misuse. This literature is characterized by descriptive and controlled studies regarding the efficacy of acupuncture. However, findings have been mixed, and with few exceptions, the quality of research has lacked adequate statistical power and assurances of reliability and validity. Overall, research has not confirmed clinical reports and patient testimonies, although it should be noted that research protocols typically have differed from clinical applications (Culliton & Kiresuk, in press; McLellan, Grossman, Blaine, & Haverkos, 1993).

Other Therapies

Numerous other therapies have been used for the treatment of addictions; however, none has received scientific or popular attention to the same extent as acupuncture (see Table 1). As with acupuncture, clinical

TABLE 1   CAM Therapies for the Treatment of Addictions

	Alcohol	Cocaine	Nicotine	Opiates
Acupuncture	x	—	x	x
Aromatherapy	—	—	—	—
Biofeedback	x	—	x	—
EMDR	x	x	—	—
Hallucinogens	x	x	—	x
Herbal therapies	x	—	—	—
Homeopathy	x	—	—	—
Hypnosis	x	—	—	—
Light therapy	x	—	x	—
Massage	—	—	x	—
NET	x	x	—	x
Nutrition therapies	x	x	x	x
Relaxation	x	—	x	—
REST	x	—	x	—
Spirituality	x	—	—	—
Transcendental meditation	x	x	x	x
Yoga	x	—	—	x

x = academic/research literature available (Boucher & Kiresuk, in press; Culliton, Boucher, & Bullock, in press; Culliton et al., 1997) and patient testimonies have been positive for the majority of these therapies, although there are insufficient or inadequate research data to support the assertions. History has established justifiable skepticism of all new treatments, conventional or CAM. Medicine is replete with treatments initially applied with enthusiasm but later discovered to be ineffective (Shapiro & Morris, 1978). Research is thus an integral part of the process of confirmation or refutation.

Table 1 summarizes CAM treatment for substance misuse for which academic literature is available (Boucher & Kiresuk, in press; Culliton, Boucher, & Bullock, in press; Culliton et al., 1997). The quality of literature varies widely but provides a starting place for further discussion.

Conclusion

In summary, CAM therapies appear to hold promise for the treatment of substance misuse. Proper research will help clarify preliminary clinical reports and determine whether a given therapy is efficacious. Therapists and physicians should assist patients by providing information regarding both the potential dangers and benefits of a chosen therapy.

THOMAS J. KIRESUK
TACEY ANN BOUCHER

See also
Acupuncture and Chinese Medicine (IV)
Spirituality and Psychotherapy (IV)
Spiritual/Religious Approaches (IV)

AFFIRMATIONS

Affirmations are positive thoughts people give to themselves or others to counter negative thinking or enhance performance.

Chakalis and Lowe (1992) studied the effect of subliminally embedded auditory material on short-term memory recall. Sixty volunteers took a face-name-occupation memory test before and after a 15-minute intervention. Participants were randomly assigned to one of three groups: no sound, supraliminal presentation of relaxing music, or subliminal presentation of memory improvement affirmations embedded in relaxing music. After intervention, only members of the subliminal group significantly improved their performance on recall of names.

Gruenfeld and Wyer (1992) asked participants to read either affirmations or denials of statements from either newspapers or reference volumes. They found that affirmations of fact affected participant attitudes toward the described situations. Although theirs was a laboratory study, they theorized that such statements might stimulate even more attitude change if they were encountered in a more meaningful communication context.

CAROLYN CHAMBERS CLARK

ALEXANDER TECHNIQUE

Prevention

Many people suffer from the deleterious effects of poor posture and excess bodily tension. Everyday movement habits, such as slumping or forcing the arch in the back in an effort to be more erect, produce compressive forces and muscular imbalance that can precipitate such maladies as back pain, disk problems, sciatica, and osteoporotic deterioration. Without intervention, the downward force of gravity and the ongoing force of habit perpetuate postural misuse and painful muscular tension. The Alexander Technique is a highly effective noninvasive antidote to this dilemma. It can alleviate pain and prevent further deterioration when the postural component is the cause or exacerbating factor in an existing condition. Reversing the compensatory effects of spinal compression, students of the Alexander Technique acquire fluid integrated movement mechanics, improved breathing coordination, vocal clarity, heightened proprioception and balance, and greater functional strength and mobility. This is accomplished without prescribed exercise. The technique focuses instead on the student's ability to identify, alter, and prevent harmful tension, movement, and breathing patterns in any activity. In addition, students of the technique learn to recognize a variety of sources triggering bodily tension. Thus harmful responses to stress, such as tightening the muscles of the head, neck, and back and straining the vocal mechanism in speech, can be prevented before they cause pain or disease (Reiser, 1994).

Theory

Frederick Matthias Alexander (1869–1953), founder of the Alexander Technique, theorized that many human ailments, pain, and injuries were related to poor postural habits. He discovered what he termed *primary control*, a dynamic, reflexive relationship of the head and neck to the torso that reactivates postural reflexes and facilitates a general freedom and fluidity of movement. Furthermore, he specified the habitual malalignment of the head and neck in relation to the torso as the primary cause of malcoordination limiting human function and movement potential.

Alexander's theory of primary control preceded investigations by his contemporary, Rudolf Magnus. Magnus confirmed the existence of a central neural control that mediates the body's dynamic postural balance and alignment in space through experiments on vertebrates in 1925 and later on humans. As early as 1918 Alexander wrote about the effects of postural use on human function, specifically the primary control mechanism of the head, neck, and back and its influence on the performance of particular functions. He demonstrated that certain habits of muscular response can interfere with the proper functioning of this control mechanism and discovered the importance of thinking in the process of effecting new muscular responses and of reliable propriocetion to achieve optimal motor control. He suggested widespread application of his ideas and discoveries to many fields of inquiry to prevent painful conditions and improve human function.

Methodology

The Alexander Technique is the practical method Alexander developed to reverse the compensatory muscular imbalance that results from postural misuse. A teacher of the Alexander Technique, a highly trained professional, transmits the skills to the student through a process of psychophysical reeducation. The role of the teacher is essential in the initial stages of the learning process, when the student lacks the subtle observation skills necessary to identify harmful habits of muscular tension or movement coordination. The teacher promotes cognitive and experiential awareness by offering verbal feedback and manual guidance while the student performs familiar activities such as sitting, standing, walking, bending, lunging, squatting, reaching, and lying down. The movement quality begins to change as the student learns to inhibit, or consciously quiet muscular tension prior to and during activity. The student then learns to direct, or mentally project the preferred relationship of head, neck, and torso. This thought process interrupts the habitual muscular response of excess tightening and, instead, engages the appropriate muscular response. In each lesson these new patterns are reinforced through verbal instructions and feedback, and the student becomes more adept at using the Alexander Technique thought process to effect change in muscle tension, movement mechanics, and breathing coordination. The number of lessons to achieve satisfactory results will vary from 10 to 30 according to the goals and initial physical condition of the student. With continued practice of the technique in daily activity, the student attains greater kinesthetic awareness and level of skill, approaching even the most novel and specialized tasks with safety and intelligence.

Medical Rehabilitation

Medical scientist Nikolaas Tinbergen, Nobel laureate for physiology, referred to the Alexander Technique in his 1973 acceptance speech: " . . . many types of underperformance and even ailments, both physical and mental, can be alleviated, sometimes to a surprising extent, by teaching the body musculature to function differently." The Alexander Technique enables people with neurologic and/or musculoskeletal injury or disease to maximize their movement potential and decrease pain (Barlow, 1990; Caplan, 1987). Ambulation, transfers to and from chairs, and bed mobility become less effortful, and improved head-neck-back integration provides increased stability that enables some patients to dispense with assistive devices such as canes or walkers (Leibowitz & Connington, 1990). The technique also addresses habits of muscular tension in the neck, back, and shoulders, offering the person with chronic pain highly effective pain management skills (Fisher, 1988). Persons with disability from stroke and other neurologic, postural, and balance disorders increase independence when they gain conscious control of movement and improve the performance of daily activities. In the case of repetitive stress or traumatic injuries, the improved coordination and dynamic postural control result in a practical self-management process to prevent reinjury, facilitate mobility, and effectively decrease joint and muscle pain.

Training of Athletes, Dancers, Singers, Actors, and Musicians

The Alexander Technique is an integral part of the specialized training of performing artists and athletes in university and professional settings, conservatories, and acting studios. Due to its emphasis on awareness, conscious motor control, and experiential learning, a study of the Alexander Technique can refine and enhance focus, speed, dexterity, balance, and, in the case of the actor or singer, potential for vocal clarity (deAlcantra, 1997; Macdonald, 1997). Through heightened self-awareness, the performer can achieve greater spontaneity, virtuosity, and expression, while simultaneously applying principles of self-care to prevent injury during practice and performance.

History of the Alexander Technique

F. M. Alexander developed the technique's premise from experimental observations of his own movement habits. An Australian actor and solo Shakespearean orator, his performance career was interrupted at the age of 19 by chronic vocal strain and restricted breathing. When doctors could not identify the source of his affliction or offer a cure, Alexander began an investigation of what he termed the "use of the self" (Alexander, 1996). In the process of solving his vocal problems, Alexander discovered basic principles about how the mind and body interact, which became the foundation of his technique.

Alexander's story did not end in personal self-discovery. Although he returned to the stage after regaining control of his voice, he continued to experiment with his newly formulated technique, testing its application to other areas of human endeavor. Alexander brought his work from Australia to Great Britain in 1904 and introduced his technique in the United States in 1914. Among his clientele were the philosopher and educator John Dewey, who wrote the introduction to two of his books, and the writers Aldous Huxley and George Bernard Shaw. After studying with Alexander, the renowned anatomist and physiologist George E. Coghill (1941) provided the introductory remarks to Alexander's fourth volume, *The Universal Constant in Living*. The anatomist Raymond A. Dart and the neuroscientist C. S. Sherrington also endorsed the technique after studying with Alexander (Dart, 1959; Jones, 1997).

Over the years of his teaching career, Alexander refined his methodology for conveying his procedure to others. In 1934, at the age of 62, he initiated his first teacher-training course. Currently there are numerous teacher certification programs in the United States and around the world. There are 10 affiliated societies for teachers of the Alexander Technique, one in the United States and others in Australia, Brazil, Great Britain, South Africa, and Israel. Members of these societies have codified and enforced standards for training teachers and participated in global conferences for professional development, presentation of research, and further refining of training course standards. Teacher certification requires 1,600 practical hours over a 3-year period.

Related Fields of Inquiry

In praising the life work of F. M. Alexander, Dewey (1918) remarked, " . . . there is no aspect of the maladjustments of modern life which does not receive illumination." Alexander's work continues to arouse interest in the diverse fields of education (Dewey, 1918), skill learning and athletics (Gelb, 1994), psychology and behavioral science (Jones, 1997), performing arts (deAlcantra, 1997), speech pathology, vocalization (McDonald, 1997), childbirth education (Machover, Drake, & Drake, 1993), ergonomics (Oliver, 1997), pain management (Fisher, 1988), and rehabilitation medicine (Caplan, 1987).

IDELLE PACKER

See also
Back Pain (II)
Repetitive Strain Injuries (II)

AMAZON RAINFOREST AND MEDICINAL USES OF PLANTS

For generations indigenous peoples of the Amazon have effectively used their plants for food, housing, and survival. Their herbal medicine is based on social, cultural, medical, and religious traditions, and without prescriptions, modern physicians, and laboratories. The Amazonians have used these medicinal herbs for regulating blood sugar levels, strengthening the immune system, restoring hormonal balance, enhancing nervous system functioning, and other physiological applications. Ongoing research on the functions, capabilities, and benefits of Amazon medicinal herbs will undoubtedly render remedies and/or cures for several ailments in the near future. Because world trade has expanded so rapidly, other cultures can now experience the health benefits from the use of these herbs.

The Rainforest

The Amazon rainforest houses more species of plants and animals than all other ecosystems combined. Estimated plant numbers range between 35,000 and 80,000 species. The compendium of plants includes those used for food and others used for their medicinal properties. Without animals or the use of modern agricultural machinery, the peoples of Amazonia discovered and domesticated more than half of the world's seven major food crops, including corn, potatoes (both sweet and cassava), tomatoes, peanuts, chile peppers, chocolate, vanilla, pineapples, papayas, passion fruit, and avocados. Cashews, Brazil nuts, figs, and guava are also found in the rainforest.

One eighth of all U.S. prescription drugs contain active ingredients that are plant chemicals derived from the tropical rainforest. Modern-day anesthetics, now synthetic, were originally derived from curare, extracted from woody vines growing in the Amazon. Quinine was derived from cinchona bark from a Peruvian tree.

Medicinal Uses

It is not uncommon to find plants that grow in the Amazon rainforest in the other rainforests of the world. However, this article will focus on plants endemic only to Amazonia.

Amazonian herbs that have been used in the United States for at least 5 years include jaborandi (*Pilocarpus jaborandi*), suma (*Pfaffia paniculata*), pau d'arco (*Tecoma impetiginosa*), quebra pedra (*Phyllanthus niruri*), and una de gato, also known as cat's claw (*Uncaria tomentosa*). Jaborandi has been used in pharmaceutical preparations; all the others are used as herbs. A short description of their medicinal properties follows.

Jaborandi is the main plant source of pilocarpine, the drug used for glaucoma patients. It is also used in a pharmaceutical preparation to increase salivation in patients receiving chemotherapy. Active ingredients in this herb have many effects, including increasing metabolism. Contraindications for the use of this herb are similar to that of ephedra.

Suma, high in electrolytes and trace minerals, especially germanium, has both adaptogenic and immune-enhancing properties. Active ingredients include pfaffic acid sugar compounds, which inhibit cultured tumor cell melanomas, and sitosterol and stigmasterol, which encourage estrogen production and reduce high serum cholesterol. It is effective in the treatment of hot flashes.

Pau d'arco is used topically or orally for wounds, infections, and boils and to control fungus and yeast overgrowth. It has a reputation for being extremely useful in cancer to decrease pain and increase red blood cell production. It is also a diuretic and sedative.

Una de gato has been shown in research studies to increase white blood cell production by at least 34%. Its active constituents are oxindole alkaloids. It is effective in the prevention of chemotherapeutic side effects, the reversal of ulcers, acne, and viral diseases, especially herpes, and has been found to contain an active ingredient known to be helpful in cases of depression. This herb, also known as cat's claw, is thought to be an immunomodulator and can be used on a long-term basis. Its use is contraindicated in those who have had organ transplants. It also contains an anti-leukemic factor. Studies by Keplinger have shown it to be extremely beneficial to patients in various stages of HIV virus symptomatology.

Other herbs from the Amazon have only recently been used in the United States. These include muira-puama (*Ptychopetalum oficinale*), catuaba (*Erythroxylon catuaba*), guarana (*Paullinia cupana*), chuchuhuasi (*Maytenus krukovit*), and jatoba (*Hymenaea courbaril*).

Muira-puama has aphrodisiac properties and is a tonic for the nervous system. A recent study done at the Institute of Sexology in Paris showed it to be effective in cases of impotency. It also has been used for depression, and for the treatment of menstrual cramps and premenstrual syndrome.

Catuaba is a strong tonic and fortifier of the central nervous system. It is an aphrodisiac and is used with muira-puama for the treatment of impotency.

Guarana is best known for its caffeine and caffeine derivatives theophylline and theobromine. However, its saponins counterbalance the stimulant action, producing more of a sustained type of energy than that experienced with coffee.

Chuchuhuasi contains active constituents that are highly anti-inflammatory. This herb has been used for decades in the treatment of arthritis and rheumatism.

Jatoba is used by the natives of South America to keep energy levels high all day long. It has strong antifungal properties and is used for many lung conditions. It has been known to alleviate the symptoms of prostatitis.

The list of Amazonian herbs contains hundreds more that have been used medicinally. These include manaca (*Brunfelsia uniflora*), iporuru (*Alchornia caastaneifolia*), samambaia (*Polypodium lepidopteris*), espinheira santa (*Maytenus ilicifolia*), boldo (*Peumus boldo*), and tayuya (*Cayaponia tayuya*).

A direct result of the modern synthetic chemical criterion for treatment of disease and illness has kept the benefits of medicinal plants, in particular, Amazon herbs, in obscurity. However, the proven record of rainforest herbal products has turned the tide in favor of further research, development, and use of Amazon herbs in medical treatments.

DONNA SCHWONTKOWSKI

See also
  AIDS/HIV (II)
  Arthritis (II)
  Cancer (II)
  Depression (II)
  Diabetes (II)
  Lung Disorders (II)
  Premenstrual Syndrome (PMS) (II)
  Prostate, Enlarged (II)

ANIMAL-ASSISTED THERAPY

The history of animal-assisted therapy has evolved since the time of early cave dwellers. Dogs were first tamed from the wolf species using food as a reward. Early humans gradually assumed responsibility for domesticated animals' survival.

Animal ownership became widespread in the late 18th century. Dogs, cats, and horses provided both companionship and useful functions such as hunting and transportation. Animals and humans continued to develop a multiplicity of relationships. One unique human and animal relationship that has evolved is identified as therapeutic. Beck and Katcher (1996) reported the following therapeutic chronology: In the 1700s, horses and farm animals were used in therapy, at the York Retreat in England, to treat emotionally disturbed residents. In 1867 pets were part of the treatment program for epileptics at the Bethel facility in Germany.

Later, the American Red Cross used animals, from 1944 to 1945, as diversional therapy for airmen undergoing intense therapeutic programs in Pawling, New York.

In 1969 Boris Levinson, a child psychologist, involved dogs in his practice. Levinson used companion animals in diagnostic and therapeutic techniques with children. Results were published in a 1969 book, *Pet-Oriented Child Psychotherapy*. Levinson is considered to be the modern-day founder of animal-assisted therapy.

Definitions

Animal-assisted therapy (AAT) is a goal-directed intervention in which an animal, which meets specific criteria, is an integral part of the human treatment process. AAT is directed and/or delivered by a health/human service professional with specialized expertise and within the scope of his or her professional practice (Delta Society, 1992). These professions include

Nursing
Occupational therapy
Speech therapy
Social work
Psychology
Physical therapy
Counseling
Recreational therapy
Education
Medicine

Additionally, animal-assisted activities (AAA) provide opportunities for motivational, educational, recreational, and/or therapeutic benefits to enhance the quality of life. Activities are delivered by trained professionals, paraprofessionals, and/or volunteers with animals that meet specific criteria. A credentialed therapist, however, is not required to guide these activities (Delta Society, 1992).

Functions

Both AAT and AAA sessions may be conducted individually or in groups. Clients may be either children or adults with special needs. Programs are conducted in hospitals, homes, schools, nursing homes, prisons, and other community facilities. An animal is present for all or part of planned AAT sessions. Animals may be visiting or live in the facility. The focus of AAT is to facilitate change in a client through interactions with an animal. Therapeutic goals, interventions, and an evaluation are important parts of the treatment process. All AAT animals and their handlers must be screened, trained, and meet specific criteria (Gammonley et al., 1996). Participation in

AAT must be voluntary by the client. All animals must be monitored carefully for signs of stress and/or illness. All interactions should be mutually beneficial for both the client and the animal.

Categories of AAT

According to Nebbe (1995), there are five categories of AAT that may be prescribed, depending on human needs. Following each category is an example of an AAT application.

1. *Instrumental.* A nursing home resident assumes care for a caged parakeet, which results in increased mobility and coordination.
2. *Relationship.* An adult male, with paraplegia, enjoys visits by a social therapy dog. The client then applies for a service therapy dog to assist him at home.
3. *Passive.* Two depressed clients have fun and laugh while watching an exotic bird show. Increased stimulation and social interactions then occur.
4. *Cognitive.* A group of adolescents with behavioral problems visit a city aquarium. Several clients learn to establish a home aquarium. A positive leisure activity is developed.
5. *Spiritual.* An animal provides a sense of oneness with creation and a sense of well-being. A hospice client experiences feelings of comfort and a closeness to nature while stroking an elderly cat.

Theories of AAT

Currently, there is no one single theory that has been accepted as a basis for therapeutic human-animal interactions. Repeated anecdotal reports state that nurturance, pet attachment, security, touch, and social lubrication are positive human outcomes associated with AAT. Social support and attachment theories are most often cited in the literature.

More recently, the biophilia hypothesis proposes that humans are drawn to a tendency "to focus on living things" and that this disposition has a partly genetic basis (Kellert & Wilson, 1993).

Related Research

Several AAT research studies conducted in the 1970s focused on the psychosocial outcomes of human-animal interactions. Results generally demonstrated that institutionalized residents seemed happier and less socially withdrawn during and after animal interactions, as cited by Beck and Katcher (1996).

Other studies conducted in the 1970s and 1980s demonstrated the importance of companion animals to human health and longevity. Results demonstrated that such activities as watching aquarium fish or stroking a dog or cat can reduce human blood pressure and stress levels, as cited by Beck and Katcher (1996).

Thomas (1994) studied the human habitat approach as reported in the Eden Alternative model. Birds, dogs, cats, and rabbits were placed in a nursing home. Results indicated a significant reduction in the usage of psychotropic drugs, as well as a 15% reduction in residents' deaths. A comparison was made to a control group nursing home (without pets) 18 months after full program implementation (Thomas, 1994).

Trends

Animal-assisted therapy is considered to be a complementary therapy using an interdisciplinary approach. This emerging profession is in the process of developing national certification requirements, improved standards, and increased public awareness of the role of AAT in health care.

JUDITH GAMMONLEY

ANTHROPOSOPHICAL PHILOSOPHY

Definition

Anthroposophy (*Anthropos* = human, *Sophy* = wisdom), or spiritual science, is an extension of natural scientific thought that proposes to increase one's supersensible conceptions to develop a holistic understanding of the human being's unfolding sequential development in health and disease. It seeks to understand the mind-body-spirit relationship and its connection to nature. It is an investigational process for the practitioner, healer, teacher, therapist, and individual to develop spiritual sight, and in cooperation with physical sight, to enhance the observation of the spiritual nature distinguishable from the physical nature of life. The application of this philosophy was formally inaugurated by its founder, Rudolf Steiner, a philosopher, research scientist, and clairvoyant, and presented to the medical community of Dornach, Switzerland, from March 21 through April 9, 1920, in a series of 20 lectures constituting the first course for physicians and medical students (Steiner, 1989). It has led to the development of formal training for educators, physicians, and nurses, along with art, movement, massage, speech, and other therapists, and to the establishment of schools (Waldorf Schools), clinics, and extensive practices throughout the world.

Theory

Anthroposophy operationalizes the "wisdom of man" in an ecological and process-oriented health paradigm. Steiner's model of spiritual insight includes two fundamental theories: the process of the physical nature of man, which Steiner called the threefold nature of the physical human being, and the hierarchical environmental realms of man, which Steiner called the fourfold human. These spiritual insights lead to an understanding of the totality of the human organism as primary to health and disease, and "invading organisms" as secondary. Therapeutics, described as "curative processes," reflect this holistic perspective and allow for a more accurate application of current scientific knowledge.

Steiner described the process of the physical nature of man (threefold nature) as the incarnation, transformation, and molding of the ego, or individuality, within hereditary structures and environmental influences as the reality of the soul and spirit. Physical existence as an expression of supersensible systems at work can be observed in the formation of living substances. Earthly elements must combine with empyrean or spiritual elements, as in plant formation through the process of photosynthesis. What is expressed is not the nature of the individual elements involved in creation but the essence of the predetermined structure as influenced by the metabolism of these forces.

The process of anabolism and catabolism, necessary for physical life, can be observed as well in spiritual life through the expressions of the three supersensible systems in bodily organ functions. The first is the nerve-sense system whose combined functions allow impulses from the external and internal environment to penetrate the organism. This system expresses a nature that is itself immobile, associated with rest, cold, catabolism, and death, and deals with the process of the formation of images. The second is the metabolic-limb system whose combined functions include metabolic processes. This system expresses a nature that is associated with motion, warmth, anabolism, and life and deals with the transformation of matter. As is apparent, these two systems express opposites. The third is the rhythmic system, which mediates between the two and expresses compensation, harmony, and health. In compression is expressed the dynamics of the nerve system, and in expansion is expressed the dynamics of the metabolic system.

The theoretical construct of the human hierarchical environmental realms (fourfold human) describes human's relationship to the life kingdom, as well as developmental and reciprocal relationships. The physical environment is reflected in the mineral kingdom and incorporates substances and dynamic workings from this perspective. The etheric environment is reflected in plant life and its cycles, growth, and regeneration. The soul environment represents the activities of the animal kingdom and is associated with expression. The ego or astral environment brings about consciousness and creative thinking, permeates all environments, and is unique to human beings as the sum of individualization.

Use/Therapeutic Modalities

Understanding health and illness as a natural and meaningful aspect of the process of individualization is essential in contemplating the totality of the human being. Identifying the predominant tendency, how it relates to development, in terms of time, age, and functional ability, as well as understanding the nature of these systems as they relate to and balance each other, serves as the basis for practitioners to develop insights for curative therapeutics and medicinal remedies on an individual basis.

Curative Education

The Waldorf School system, established in 1919 under Steiner's original anthroposophical pedagogic direction, has since flourished as an approach to prevent the development of disease from premature and precocious educational stressors. The shaping of the soul environment is the school-age child's supersensible "developmental task," first, through the rhythmic system and the etheric environment during ages 7 to 14 as the predominant area of formative activity for future functioning, then through the metabolic-limb system from ages 14 to 21, while the nerve-sense system matures (Holtzapfel, 1989). Educational activities are designed to support this growth, development, and balance.

School Health

The role of the school health practitioner is to assess the balance of the process of ego development in tandem with education to promote health and prevent disease. Recognition of standard childhood illness as part of the normal, healthy, progressive progress of ego development is essential.

Imbalances in this process have been attributed to the development of chronic illnesses (Holtzapfel, 1989; Incao, 1997; Steiner, 1989). Children who have developmental disabilities and chronic illnesses benefit greatly from this method of intervention. Camphill Village, with residential treatment communities worldwide, successfully continues these methods through adulthood.

Anthroposophically Extended Medicine

Physicians with contemporary medical education backgrounds can learn how to bridge Steiner's spiritual concepts of the human being to understand the totality of the human organism as primary to health and disease. Treating the individual with constitutional remedies and curative processes, alone or with conventional or complementary therapeutics, requires physicians' own development of spiritual insight as to the individual manifestations of illness. Therapeutics may include potentized plant substances, diet, external applications, and other curative therapies.

Curative Nursing

Dr. Ita Wegman began the first formal training for nurses while practicing as Steiner's personal physician. The health-oriented paradigm she developed complements Florence Nightingale's theories on nursing practice and can be utilized by advanced practice nurses. In conjunction with their contemporary education and practice, nurses learn the application of the elements—warmth, air, water, and earth—for creating healing environments. Some nurses work independently in home health care settings and teach family self-care.

Research Base

The foundation for practice is built on the current scientific base for each health-related discipline as seen from the practitioner's view of anthroposophy. Current research studies can be found in the quarterly *Journal of Anthroposophical Medicine*.

MARGO DROHAN

See also
Spirituality and Psychotherapy (IV)

APITHERAPY: HISTORY AND THEORY

Apitherapy is the medicinal use of various products of the common honeybee (*Apis mellifera*). Applications include therapeutic use of bee venom, raw (unheated) honey, pollen, royal jelly, beeswax, and propolis. All have been used medicinally by humans.

The historical use of honey bee products may be traced at least as far back as Hippocrates, Pliny the Roman naturalist, the writers of the Bible and the Koran, and to present-day scientists and physicians throughout the world. All bee products were used to treat colds and sore throats. Bee products were continually observed to possess medicinal properties that in today's language would be considered antibacterial, anti-inflammatory, and antifungal, among other medical virtues.

The use of bee products (specifically bee venom) for medicinal purposes is considered by many an alternative form of medical treatment, and for this reason it has received little funding in the United States for scientific or medical research. This is not the case in Asia (Japan, Korea, and China), Eastern Europe (Bulgaria, Czechoslovakia, and Romania), and Western Europe (Germany, Switzerland, and France). More than 1,500 articles on bee venom alone have been published in the scientific literature since 1930. The number of articles on all bee products is far more extensive. In the United States, many physicians privately suggest bee venom therapy (BVT) as a treatment for a variety of diseases for which traditional methods of therapy have proven ineffective.

Bee Venom

Bee venom, available from live bees or in a purified, injectable form, enjoys a long tradition as a folk remedy for arthritis and other degenerative diseases. More recent interest indicates that bee venom possesses significant anti-inflammatory, analgesic, and immunostimulant properties. It is these demonstrated therapeutic attributes that lead to claims of value in treating a wide variety of diseases.

There are no reported incidences of symptoms resulting from stimulation of the hypothalamic-pituitary-adrenal system by BVT. In contrast, exogenous equivalent doses of corticosteroids have well-known and documented discouraging side effects.

Honey

The use of raw (unheated) honey to treat burns can be traced back almost 2,000 years to China. Honey has been recognized as a powerful medicine that can be used both internally and topically. It has been used to treat insomnia, obesity, and constipation, among other internal complaints. Today, it is included in many over-the-counter pharmaceuticals because of its pleasant taste and its medicinal action. Lesser known, but more significant, is its use as a sterile and painless wound dressing. Raw honey is hydroscopic (draws water from its environment). It kills bacteria by converting the antibacterial enzyme glucose oxidase to hydrogen peroxide, which aids in healing. Only a few bacteria have been shown to be capable of living in honey; all are harmless to humans. As a result, bacterial growth in the presence of is greatly reduced, making it easier for a wound to stay clean and thus promoting healing. Honey is considered by many to be the perfect sterile wound dressing. Medical professionals in many countries, including France and Germany, recommend its use in treating burns and superficial or deep lesions.

Bee Pollen

One of the oldest known bee products is bee pollen, the male element of the flower, which consists of very fine grains of powder containing substantial nutritive and medicinal properties. Bees gather pollen, mix it with nectar to form a pellet, and carry that pellet to the hive. A teaspoonful of bee pollen, the recommended dose, contains approximately 1,200 pellets.

Pollen is extremely complex, containing nitrogenous materials in the form of proteins, minerals, free amino acids, and small amounts of trace elements. On average, pollen is comprised of more than 20% proteins and 12% amino acids, more than grains, cereal, or any product of animal origin.

Although these amino acids are indispensable for our diet, the human system is incapable of manufacturing or synthesizing them. Bees somehow select the pollens rich in nitrogenous matter and ignore those pollens poor in this material.

Here again, it may be seen that pollen contains all the vital minerals that are so important to human metabolism and is the reason why it is used as a food supplement. It is considered by many to be nature's most nearly perfect protein food source.

Finally, the rutine in pollen helps reduce the deposits that collect in veins, thus helping more oxygen reach the brain and cells of the body.

Propolis

Propolis, the thick, tarlike material produced by bees from tree resins that helps to keep their hives sterile, is used medicinally in salves, ointments, chewing gums, lozenges, and creams. In dentistry, it is used in tinctures. It is commonly used to treat sore throats and has been employed as a topical medication for nonhealing lesions of the skin. Russian and Chinese physicians have conducted clinical trials to test it as an internal treatment of hypercholesterol. In vitro laboratory tests indicate it is a potent antibacterial, antiviral, and antifungal agent (Broadman, 1958).

At least 25 factions have been identified in propolis, and more than 40 major flavonoids and phenolics have been isolated. Some studies claim the anti-inflammatory and antiviral activities of propolis include inhibiting the growth of melanoma and carcinoma tumors.

Beeswax

Beeswax is the base of better facial creams because it is the finest natural emulsifying agent. When taken internally, it serves as a "vaccine" against pollen allergies, because the wax has tiny amounts of pollen trapped in it.

Royal Jelly

Royal jelly can be considered the world's best example of "you are what you eat." Royal jelly, which is fed to the queen bee larva, allows the queen to develop into a genetically complete (fertile) insect. This may explain the difference between the life expectancy of a queen bee (3 to 6 years) and an infertile worker bee (6 to 8 weeks).

In summary, bees synthesize a variety of proteins that are generally helpful, not harmful, to human beings. It may be said with more than a little accuracy that bees were, are, and should continue to be one of humankind's greatest allies.

STEVE SHAPIRO

See also
   Allergies (II)
   Arthritis (II)
   Bee Pollen (III)
   Cancer (II)
   Cold Symptoms (II)
   Wounds (II)

APITHERAPY: RESEARCH AND CLINICAL USE

It has been observed since the earliest times that the application of venoms secreted by bees produces powerful effects in human beings. Mesolithic drawings from India and Paleolithic cave paintings in Spain document human collection and use of honeybee (*Apis mellifera*) products. Hesiod (800 B.C.), Aristophanes (c. 450–388 B.C.), and Varro (166–27 B.C.) were all reputed to be familiar with the cultivation of bees and beehives.

Other early researchers include Galen (A.D. 131–201), who was among the earliest to write about the use of venoms; in 14 B.C. Pliny the Elder chronicled venom use in a text entitled *Natural History*. It is documented that Charlemagne (A.D. 742–814) received beestings, and Monfat (1566–1634) prescribed bee stings as a treatment for kidney stones and to improve the flow of urine.

Current belief is that the practice of apitherapy began in ancient Greece. Curative properties of venoms were documented by Hippocrates (460–377 B.C.), who described it as "Arcanum," a mysterious remedy whose curative properties he did not understand.

Several modern studies on bee venom have shown it contains at least 18 pharmacologically active components. Whole bee venom can be divided into low molecular weight factions (melittin, apamin, adolapin, and fraction Oa) and high molecular weight factions (phospholipase A2, hyaluronidase, and mast cell degranulating peptide), to name a few.

Research shows that melittin possesses known powerful anti-inflammatory and antibacterial properties. Adolapin is active at doses 100-fold lower (on a molar basis) than some currently used pharmaceutical agents. It has more anti-inflammatory and analgesic properties in some ways than aspirin. Apamin produces anti-inflammatory effects without compromising the body's immunologic defense system. In addition, it is thought to be the operational component in the treatment of multiple sclerosis. Apamin is also known to have antiarrhythmic effects in patients with intrinsic arrhythmias. Other components contribute

therapeutically in specific biochemical ways that are beyond the scope of this discussion.

Chemically, the components of bee venom are known to be complex compounds. They include apamin, histamine, dopamine, melittin, mast cell destroying peptides, minimine, the enzymes phospholipase A and hyaluronidase, and at least eight protein factions.

Professor V. Tsitsin, in the April 1946 issue of the *Bee Journal*, reported that a study of Russian centenarians revealed that most of them were beekeepers. Further research revealed that the old beekeepers' diet included regular doses of honey and pollen, in addition to the literally thousands of stings they received from years of keeping bees. Tsitsin attributed the beekeepers' longevity in part to the action of these products.

Since his studies, researchers at laboratories and hospitals throughout the world have discovered new components, new uses, new reactions, and new applications for bee products, principally in the catalytic and metabolic pathways of the human system. For example, a 1975 study of severely arthritic dogs conducted at Walter Reed Army Hospital focused on the actual physical improvement of the animals as a result of bee venom injections. One advantage of this study was the elimination of any human psychological effects or subjective evaluations on the results.

Two measures of activity were recorded in both the treated and control saline-injected dogs in this doubly controlled experiment. The first was the level of plasma cortisol, a major endogenous anti-inflammatory agent of the body; the second was actual voluntary movement (cage activity) by the dogs.

Bee venom therapy (BVT) dogs exhibited both prolonged increases in cortisol levels and, after a 7-day lag, a significant and meaningful increase in cage activity. In this trial, bee venom was determined to manifest pronounced antiarthritic effects. The study has since been quoted in journals throughout the world.

Studies show bee venom to possess both local and systemic therapeutic effects. Experiments have demonstrated bee venom is far more potent an anti-inflammatory agent than some currently used anti-inflammatory drugs.

Important differences between bee venom and currently used anti-inflammatory drugs include the following: Bee venom acts indirectly on the problem by encouraging the body to do its own healing. This is different from drugs that act directly on the problem (i.e., by attacking the invading germs or bacteria). Thus drugs actually teach the body dependence (immune apathy), whereas bee venom encourages system self-reliance.

A comparison of the side-effect profile of bee venom versus other anti-inflammatory drugs shows, for example, that cortisone, one of the most potent anti-inflammatory drugs on the market, produces side effects that include irritable moods, fatigue, hypertension, weight gain, and water retention. Bee venom has a surprisingly different effect. BVT patients feel increased energy and experience normalization of blood pressure and mood elevation. The amount of bee venom needed for anti-inflammation is 100 to 10,000 times lower than the required doses of other membrane stabilizers (e.g., glucocorticoids).

Since the 1930s studies have been conducted that show bee venom to be a therapeutic agent. Medical conditions documented to respond to bee venom injections include chronic rheumatoid arthritis (Burt, 1937), atrophic arthritis (Kroner, 1938), chronic polyarthritis (Fellinser, 1954), neuralgia (Fichkov, 1954), peripheral radiculitis (Artemov, 1959), and trigeminal neuralgia (Krivoloutskaya, 1958–1960). Additionally, bee venom has been shown to treat ankylosing spondylitis, thrombophlebitis, trophic ulcers, and slowly granulating wounds (Zaitsev & Poriadin, 1958–1959). Clearly, then, there appears to be a substantial body of anecdotal evidence that bee venom effectively treats a variety of inflammatory conditions.

In June 1997 the Multiple Sclerosis Association of America announced the awarding of a $250,000 grant to Georgetown University Hospital to conduct the first Food and Drug Administration–approved double-blind, placebo-controlled scientific study of bee venom to determine its value as a treatment for multiple sclerosis. Results of the first phase of the study (i.e., the determination of the safety of bee venom injections on human beings) is expected shortly.

STEVE SHAPIRO

See also
Arthritis (II)
High Blood Pressure (II)
Infection (II)
Multiple Sclerosis (II)

AROMATHERAPY

Aromatherapy, the use of plant oils, is a part of herbal medicine. The distilled essences of various herbs and flowers are not actually oils, however. These substances, made from steaming plant materials, have molecules so small they can pass through the skin and produce sometimes powerful effects on the emotions as well as on the physical plane. These volatile essences may be used in massage oils, in baths, or in steamers for inhalation. Memories may be triggered by certain smells; thus these aromas can have deep psychological and spiritual effects as well as physically healing properties.

The use of oils for healing, religious ceremonies, and perfumes dates back thousands of years. Many references to oils occur in the Bible and in historical texts of ancient Egypt, Greece, and Rome. Mummies were embalmed with oils, and famous seductions, such as Mark Antony by Cleopatra, were secured by using oils. Hippocrates, the father of medicine, believed the fragrant fumes of certain herbs would protect people from a plague, and ancient soldiers carried myrrh with them into battle to help heal their wounds.

Herbs are the basis of most modern medicines, and by the 1800s Western chemists were discovering how to synthesize them. Physicians employed essential oils until the latter part of the 18th century. In 1887 a Dr. Chamberland performed the first documented research into antiseptic qualities of essential oils by spraying and thereby killing various airborne disease organisms. Modern synthetic pharmaceuticals, however, pushed herbs and their oils to the back shelf. In 1937 the French chemist René Gattefosse began research anew and published a book entitled *Aromatherapy*. A French army doctor, John Valnet, also published books based on his experiences using oils to treat soldiers during the Indochina war. One book, *The Practice of Aromatherapy*, is now a standard text in the field.

The use of oils with massage and for beauty was popularized by the biochemist Marguerite Maury, who received recognition for her work on the oils' healing and rejuvenating properties. Other uses have been the subject of broad studies. Japanese plant managers have even shown that lemon oil in the air can improve productivity in the workplace. Today, aromatherapy is one of the fastest growing alternative healing modalities.

Oils are derived from herbs and other plants and are either absorbed through the skin or inhaled. In using oils, it is important to remember that certain oils are not for direct use on the skin, such as in a bath; it is equally important to know that very small quantities are therapeutic, whereas larger quantities could be toxic or have adverse effects. Some individuals may have allergic reactions to plant derivatives such as oils, just as they are allergic to pollens or certain standard medications. Just as many drugs today are available in topical forms to be absorbed through the skin, such as heart medications, analgesics, and hormone therapies, and must be carefully titrated, so essential oils should not be overused. Being "natural" does not mean an oil is not potent.

Oils that are applied to the skin directly either in massage or in bath form may require several hours to absorb and reach their therapeutic level. Generally, the amount of body fat will mitigate the absorption—the more fat, the slower the absorption rate. Essential oils are rarely used full strength on the skin but should first be diluted in water or in a carrier oil. The exceptions are lavender and tea tree, which can be used in minute quantities directly on the skin. A patch test, such as diluting a small amount and dabbing an area of skin (e.g., inside the elbow), is recommended before using any oil. If a rash or other untoward reaction occurs within 24 hours, the oil should not be used. A stronger caution is made for persons sensitive to central nervous system stimuli. Persons with epilepsy should not use rosemary, sage, fennel, or hyssop. Persons with respiratory problems such as asthma, as well as persons known to have skin conditions such as eczema, should consult with an aromatherapist before buying or using any essential oils. Most books on essential oils or aromatherapy will have recipes for the mixing and use of oils, and it is recommended that these be closely followed.

Essential oils are used in a variety of ways—to perfume rooms, to invigorate the senses or stimulate the mind, to banish fatigue, and to calm and assist with sleep. In medicinal uses, certain scents have been used to treat depression and agitation, even some confused states. Fear and anxiety, problems relating to childbirth, skin irritations, and minor wounds, as well as infections, colds, and flu symptoms, have all benefited by the use of specific oils. Often oils are used instead of stronger medications with unwanted side effects. There are numerous books and references available today on the subject, but readers are encouraged to consult trained practitioners regarding the suitability of any treatment.

Some commonly used oils are lavender, chamomile, and clary sage to help induce sleep; neroli, sandalwood, and jasmine to help calm anxieties; rose, patchouli, and geranium for depression; and lemon, sage, and pine to relieve nausea and invigorate or enhance mental alertness. Although synthetic oils may smell the same as essential oils and are less expensive, they do not have the same therapeutic effects. Because of the expense of essential oils, therefore, it is wise to consult qualified therapists or check reference sources regarding correct use.

LESLIE AGUILLARD

See also
Anxiety/Panic (II)
Asthma (II)
Chronic Fatigue Syndrome (II)
Cold Symptoms (II)
Infection (II)
Insomnia (II)
Pregnancy (II)
Wounds (II)

AROMATHERAPY RESEARCH

Aromatherapy is a modality that is more firmly rooted in traditional rather than modern Western medicine. Therefore, there is very little scientifically based research on the subject. Most of the information about chemical composition of essential oils can be found in the cosmetic industry literature, but in this application, the studies do not speak to the use of aromas as therapeutic intervention with humans.

In one study conducted on an intensive care unit in England, 122 patients were randomly assigned to receive either massage aromatherapy using essential oil of lavender, or a period of rest. Pre- and post-therapy assessments were completed, including measurements of psychological distress and self-perception of anxiety, mood, and coping ability. While there were no significant differences between the groups relative to physiological stress factors, the patients who received aromatherapy reported greater improvement in their mood and perceived levels of anxiety over the other groups. They also felt less anxious and experienced an upbeat attitude following the therapy, although the effect was not sustained or cumulative (Dunn, Sleep, & Collett, 1995).

Another study determined the anesthetic effects of lavender on perineum in reducing pain after giving birth (Dale & Cornwell, 1994). In this study, 635 women were randomly assigned to one of three groups: one using pure lavender oil, one using synthetic lavender oil fragrance, and one using an inert substance. It could not be concluded that postnatal delivery discomfort was reduced. However, women receiving lavender oil treatment as a bath additive reported lower mean discomfort scores.

There is also some documented concern in the research literature. One study found an increased incidence in confusion and respiratory impairment in elderly confused people receiving aromatherapy treatment (Savage, 1996). Also, in the dermatology literature there is a study concerning an increased incidence of contact dermatitis. One percent of the total population is allergic to fragrances and only 70% of perfume allergies can be accurately detected by testing skin sensitivity to premixed floral combinations (deGroot & Frosch, 1997).

A Japanese study introduced scents into the workplace to boost productivity and create a more relaxed atmosphere. Lavender, jasmine, and lemon oils were diffused through the air-conditioning ducts. Employee accuracy increased dramatically (Sucov, 1994). At Memorial Sloan-Kettering Cancer Center in New York, doctors are studying the impact of using vanilla scent to ease anxiety during magnetic resonance image testing (Sucov, 1994).

Qualitative evidence in the form of case reports is reported by Price and Price (1995). However, the cases are not formally analyzed and therefore the value of the scenarios described, from a research frame of reference, must be questioned.

ANN BURKHARDT

ART THERAPY

Art is the oldest form of communication. In prehistoric times primitive painters expressed life events on cave walls with scenes of hunts, domestic activities, and natural surroundings. These images are a link to modern people thousands of years later from a place before language. In the future, art may be the link to other generations or even other species in much the same way.

Since the time of cave painters, art was included in and on many of the items used in daily life, from ceremonial masks and walking sticks to pottery and wall murals. The sculptures of the ancient Greeks and Romans, the ceramics of the early Chinese and Japanese dynasties, African woodcarvings, and Persian textiles are just some examples of the prolific level of artistic expression in the world as different civilizations rose and fell. With the establishment of trading, the arts of various lands began to spread and in turn be copied, imparting a language anyone could understand. It was the language of beauty and mystery. Even today, these works of art speak of those same attributes.

As occupations such as painter, potter, architect, and metalsmith developed, art moved away from the everyday to the realm of the professional. Society became more complex and sophisticated, and a delineation separating the folk arts from the fine arts appeared. An important aspect during this period was renumeration for production. The professional artist was supported by a patron, who paid money but often exerted influence and control over the artworks produced. This was sometimes to the detriment of the artist's creative expression. However, the artist was able to master the technical aspects of a particular trade, which often led to more patrons, more work, and more money.

Over time artists began to rebel against how art had evolved, and the state of the world along with it. After several wars, famines, and other assaults on humanity, some artists felt that art had lost its ability to communicate. There was a lack of connection with the everyday. A variety of art movements came into being that were given names that either described the artists or the type of artwork. Impressionism, Dadaism, and Expressionism are examples of these movements. Some art was a direct statement about the inhumanities witnessed. Some was a direct blow to the master artists then long gone but whose works were still supported by patrons, galleries, and museums. If nothing else, art and artists would never be the same.

Art is not the same. How can it be? Today there are studies being done that show that humans are not the only species to attempt "art" as a means of expression. For example, there is an elephant that paints and apes that take a stick and draw a line in the dirt. There is even an octopus that squirts blobs of ink onto its underwater canvas, making a statement about its need for safety and survival. Art is the process used by living beings to make a connection when words or anything else cannot. Although studies are being conducted in music (sound) and dance (movement), the old-est and the most widely used form of communication has been art.

Art Theory

Art is the process of bringing forth images and colors. It is a form of communication that is universal. The most amazing thing about art is how the process unfolds. The images, symbols, and colors that the individual brings out can be those that he or she has seen visually and is literally copying, or they can be those that the mind has formulated on its own from feelings or emotions rather than objects. This is a form of communication that every living being has the potential to explore. Art theory, then, is not about the technical aspects but about that process that makes each creative interpretation as individual as the person who is doing it.

Uses of Art

During World War II, art therapy was developed and was used in treating victims of "shell shock," a term now referred to as posttraumatic stress syndrome. It was used to help patients express their feelings when words were insufficient. Following the war, the uses of art therapy were broadened. It is now used in many different populations, including traumatized children and adults, self-improvement groups, and people with chronic illnesses.

An art therapist often has both an art and a psychology background. The media used range from those with very tight handling properties, like markers and crayons, to those with very loose properties, like fingerpaints and clay. Color, shapes, symbols, and relationships of objects in the artwork are some of the aspects the therapist will evaluate when working with a client.

Color therapy is a specific way in which art is used to promote health. Colors are considered energies and have vibrational frequencies. Each color is a part of white light; as a part of this whole, any disharmony can lead to an imbalance and subsequent illness. This type of therapy is incorporated in ancient Chinese and Eastern Indian philosophies. There are colors associated with yin/yang, the seven chakras, and the inner eye. A variety of techniques are appropriate for applying color therapy: color lamp treatment, the application of colored film or material, healing flower cards, and color visualization. Working in conjunction with the energy points, or chakras, *acupuncture*, or acupressure points; wearing particular colored clothing; and eating specific foods based on their color are all examples of the employment of color therapy.

Artistic creative expression in art therapy can help the individual focus on the process and thereby add to his or her sense of well-being. The creative process can be as simple as pencil drawings or as grand as giant swaths of cloth encircling an island. It can be as minimal as black ink calligraphy or as complex as multicolored mosaics. Doing repetitive actions shuts down the left side of the brain, associated with logic, and allows the right side, associated with emotional expression, to spring to life. Creative expression in art therapy includes sculpting in plaster, clay, or plasticene; developing photographs; painting or drawing; making jewelry; printing on clothing or paper; and sewing, knitting, and crocheting. By immersing the individual in the process, the conscious mind rests, leaving dreams, images, colors, and symbols to surface and be utilized.

KATHLEEN M. IWANOWSKI

See also

Acupuncture and Chinese Medicine (IV)

Color Therapy (IV)

ASIAN LIFESTYLE

Asian cultures are known for their healthful foods. Although each culture uses distinctive spices and seasonings, each cuisine is rich in grains, vegetables, and other plant foods. Each also includes very little fat and animal products. As a result, the people of Asia share a low incidence of cancer, heart disease, and other chronic illnesses so prevalent in the United States.

In China, for example, people get only 14% of their calories from fat. (The current U.S. average is 34%.) Asians in general consume three times the amount of grains and vegetables as the average American. The Asian diet also includes soybeans, garlic, onions, and tea, all of which contain phytochemicals, which are linked to cancer prevention.

Not all of the Asian cuisine is healthy. Deep-fried foods, such as egg rolls and temperas, and pickled and smoked products may increase the risk of certain types of cancer.

For the most part, though, the Asian cuisine is healthy. The typical Asian lifestyle is also healthier. People in this region tend to be less sedentary, depending on walking and bicycling as their main forms of transportation. This type of lifestyle can lower the risk of certain cancers.

Carolyn Chambers Clark

See also

Cancer (II)
Heart and Blood Vessel Conditions (II)
Garlic (III)
Phytochemicals (III)
Tea (III)
Vegetarianism (IV)

ASTON-PATTERNING

Aston-Patterning is a sophisticated approach to the human body—its structure, its movement, and its relationship to the earth's gravity field. Its founder and developer, Judith Aston, uses a new math for interpreting the body structure. By factoring in three dimensionality, asymmetries, and movement patterns and limitations, equations for change are created. The ease and flow that are the trademark of these techniques are uncharacteristic of traditional therapeutic practices and take advantage of gravity and ground reaction forces.

Aston is a former college instructor of dance and movement for actors, dancers, and athletes (1963–1972). She has also worked in the field of psychology, helping therapists and their patients to identify and evolve individual patterns of expression. At Ida Rolf's request, Aston developed and taught the movement program for the Rolf Institute (1968–1977).

The basic components of Aston-Patterning are bodywork, movement education, fitness, and ergonomics.

Bodywork

Bodywork involves three forms of *touch therapy*.

Aston Massage

This massage utilizes a detailed assessment and customized sequence to affect specific change in the tissue. Each stroke considers the direction of the tissue in its three-dimensional design and works in a spiral pattern to unwind its tension. The tension, however, is treated in relationship to the other tensions of the body, and the goal is to honor the body's natural integrity by achieving a balance that allows each part its truest form. The stage is then set for cooperative movement throughout the structure.

Myokinetics

This form involves working with the connective tissue more specifically and is applied to smaller areas than the broader strokes of the Aston massage. The goal here is to assist in rehydration of specifically restricted layers of tissue, again to restore flexibility and balance to the overall structure.

Arthrokinetics

In this form, the three-dimensional touch and movement of tissue between the hands of the practitioner allows powerful change in the tissues as they connect to the bones and comprise the joints of the body structure. The alignment of the skeleton and the joint surfaces are addressed to ensure accurate weight bearing throughout the upright body and to allow unrestricted movement, accessing the forces of gravity and ground reaction to enhance function.

Movement Education

Neurokinetics

The principles of movement are explored to achieve more comfortable, effortless, and efficient motion, beginning with the basics of sitting, standing, walking, bending, and reaching. By breaking down everyday functions into simple steps, movement patterns can be progressed all the way from common daily activities to the specialized skill needed for athletics. Aston-Patterning combines the accuracy of balance and alignment with the natural asymmetry of the body, using gravity to set the structure in motion, then drawing from the power of ground reaction force to perpetuate the motion. All movement incorporates the three dimensions combined into spiral patterns, which match the body structure and enhance the fluidity of the entire human system.

Fitness

Loosening

Aston-Patterning techniques are based on the premise that specific sequences of motion, with the assistance of the forces of gravity and ground reaction, can create a softening of tension. These techniques are done both in the upright position and horizontally. Each individualized program of loosening is designed around the patterns of tension in that particular person. The techniques are often different from one side of the body to the other, factoring in the natural asymmetries of the body. Loosen-

ing is recommended at the beginning of a workout to lengthen the body prior to toning.

Toning

The strengthening work of Aston-Pattering utilizes the total body in its best dimension to exercise each specific muscle group. The entire structure is always considered when working a part, so that the body works cooperatively to accomplish the strengthening while maintaining the optimal shape and dimension of the parts around the area of focus. The result is a heightened sense of balance and coordination, with increased strength drawn from the power of the push off the ground.

Stretching

Once the tissues are softer and the joints have been loosened, the structure is more amenable to stretching, which again is accomplished through the whole body and with the aid of gravity and ground reaction forces.

Facial Toning

This sophisticated combination of the above techniques is designed to maintain the healthy tone of the delicate muscular system of the face, head, and neck, as well as the more balanced movements of the eyes, mouth, and jaw.

Summary

Aston-Patterning truly considers the person as a whole. In our tissue, we carry the sum total of our experiences, and so the psychological impact of changes in the body can be profound. Aston-Patterning does not purport to include psychological therapy, but it can be a valuable adjunct to verbal counseling or other growth work.

Aston-Pattering can help each person achieve an ideal state of expression that is flexible depending on the environment, circumstances, and emotions of the moment. The movement of energy through the body allows for constant renewal in terms of the individual's personal expression, balance, physical efficiency, and capacity for change.

Differentiating Aston-Pattering from other somatic therapies are its focus on three-dimensional asymmetry; its degree of integration between the bodywork, movement education, and environmental tools; and its level of client education, which involves teaching the client to become his or her own teacher.

LAURA SERVID

See also
Rolfing: Structural Integration (IV)

AURICULAR RESEARCH: HISTORY

When Dr. Paul Nogier developed his theory of *auriculotherapy*, he recruited interested physicians and organized them into geographically based study groups for further research. These groups reported back to Nogier with their findings, which were then communicated to the other research groups. Nogier formed GLEM, the Groupe Lyon D'Etudes Medicales (Lyon Medical Study Group), which holds classes and conferences and trains practitioners to this day.

In 1956, at the Mediterranean Society of Acupuncture, Nogier presented his findings to a large audience. This information was published in a German acupuncture journal that reached China (Nogier & Nogier, 1985). The Chinese medical researchers at this time were renewing their interest in acupuncture. Nogier's findings sparked original research based on traditional Chinese medicine. Dr. H. Huang (1974), in the first English translation of the Chinese work, stated that in 1958 "there was a massive movement to study and apply ear acupuncture across the nation." The Chinese learned what the French already knew: Some people "spread erroneous ideas such as Chinese medicine is unscientific and insertion of the needle can only kill the pain but not cure disease. . . . Since the Cultural Revolution has dispelled the erroneous ideas, ear acupuncture has been again broadly applied all over the country."

The Nogier discovery led to the systematization of somatic points. For the Chinese, this led to a type of auricular diagnosis and guide for herbal formulas. At the Pain Management Center at the University of California at Los Angeles (UCLA) in 1980, a double-blind study revealed a statistically significant level of scientific accuracy of 75% in diagnosing the musculoskeletal pain problems in 40 patients. Palpable tenderness and a change in skin conductivity correctly predicted pain and dysfunction in musculoskeletal areas (Oleson, Kroening, & Bresler, 1980). A review of the literature from this time (especially the UCLA studies) shows that this is a viable repeatable system for pain control and various addictions. Further interest was sparked, as indicated by the various studies published in the *American Journal of Acupuncture*, the *British Journal of Acupuncture*, and other physical medicine journals.

German researchers discovered many functional points (Bahr, 1978) in addition to the French and Chinese findings. Dr. Frank Bahr of the German Acupuncture Society, in a paper given at the 1994 Auriculomedicine Congress in Lyon, France, reviewed his work, which consisted of localizing the regular acupuncture meridians on the ear.

Research in China

The current research and therapeutic approaches in the People's Republic of China are outlined in *Auriculotherapy, Diagnosis, and Treatment* (Huang, 1996). Comprehensive, if somewhat political, this treatise reveals the philosophical split between East and West. The Chinese relate everything back to traditional Chinese medicine, including the finding, selection, diagnosing, and treatment of points. In contrast, European researchers have been examining results by looking at them through the lens of Western scientific medicine and anatomy, then adding some Chinese theories when they prove useful.

Currently, European practitioners are pursuing studies in auriculomedicine, which uses the vascular autonomic signal (VAS) pulse and is very precise in locating new points, diagnosis, and treatments.

Research in the U.S.

In the United States, most researchers have focused on the use of auriculotherapy in the treatment of addictions and in smoking cessation and weight loss programs, less interest in the other qualities of the technique. Researchers at UCLA and a few other lone researchers are the exceptions. In just the past few years, however, prac-

titioners have started to realize the powerful healing potential of auriculotherapy.

About 1980 it became apparent that a common ground—or map—was needed in order to translate research results regardless of the differences in approach, technique, or history. The World Health Organization (WHO) mediated committees from many countries, including France, the United States, and China, and finally settled on basic standards and auriculomappings (WHO, 1985, 1987, 1990). In 1994 the final nomenclature report was presented to Paul Nogier at the Lyon conference by Terry Oleson, who was on the U.S. team and had written numerous groundbreaking articles about auriculotherapy.

The current trend in auriculotherapy research is the use of electricity to stimulate points. The Electrotherapy Association (Tulsa, OK) has been instrumental in setting up a study group system in the United States and Europe. Because there is no corporate money behind auriculotherapy research, many studies are done on a one-to-one or clinical basis, with information shared through journals and conferences. Perhaps this will change when research proves the effectiveness of this technique.

STEVE MEEKER

AURICULOTHERAPY

Auriculotherapy is the technique of diagnosis and treatment of disease and pain using the auricle, or pinna, of the ear. It was developed in 1952 by Paul Nogier, a French physician. Nogier noticed that sciatic pain had been eliminated in some of his patients by a local lay healer who had cauterized a spot in the ear. The pain was immediately controlled by manipulating the point and did not return. Knowing the origin of sciatic pain, he postulated that the ear held a map of the body. By stimulating or evoking pain in an area, like a finger, he could find its reflection in the ear. This led to the prototype of the upside-down fetus in the ear. The head correlates with the lobe of the ear, and the spine travels along the semicircular ridge in the center of the auricle (the antihelix). Arms and legs are logically distributed along the posterior and upper part of the ear. Nogier shared his findings with his colleagues and published his results in a German acupuncture journal, which was then sent to China. Chinese researchers saw its value and implemented their own successful trials, which yielded different but complementary results.

Nogier and his study group in Lyon, France, were able to map the intricacies of the musculoskeletal system and define treatments for pain control and healing. These included needling, implanted needles, magnets, laser, massage, and electricity. Nogier designed special instruments for the detection and treatment of ear points that are still being used today.

Along with anatomical points, special areas were found called master points. These master points are active all of the time, even postmortem, as opposed to the regular points, which are active only when they are sick or pathological. Master points globally control certain functions. For instance, the autonomic point controls the sympathetic nervous system, whereas the thalamic point controls parts of the thalamic motor group.

It was established that the sensory nerves were on the front of the ear and the motor nerves on the back, or mastoid, surface. In 1966 another serendipitous event occurred. Nogier noticed that while taking a pulse, the lighting hitting the patient changed, and the pulse changed with it. This led to the introduction of auriculomedicine, which gave a new insight to the ear. By using the pulse filters containing substances and colored photographic filters that pass only one frequency, the map of the ear was filled in with the missing anatomy—internal organs, hormones, neurotransmitters, and so on. Everything in the body was now visualized on the auricle.

New Discoveries

New detection and treatment modalities were devised to take advantage of this new form of therapy. Two major discoveries led the way. First was the finding that, along with the upside-down fetus map, there were two more important maps imposed on the first, now called the first phase. The upright man, or man facing right, was called the second phase and addressed problems of the chronic degenerative type, or yin in Chinese medicine. The third phase was the standing man. The top of his head is depicted on this particular auricle map. This man consists of the yang, or hot inflammatory burning pains, which are usually more acute than the second phase.

The second advance was finding that there are seven frequencies in the ear, each one representing a higher organized tissue. These start at 2.5 hz for amorphous-type tissue (neoplasm) and double each step to 160 hz for the frontal lobes. These frequencies are the threshold firing rates for their respective cells. Add to this the fact that the ear is only one synapse away from the brain, and you have a quick and effective technique for the treatment of *pain*.

Treatment

Auriculotherapy has been used in smoking cessation and *addiction* control therapy. Lesser known in the United States is its use in musculoskeletal pain control and healing. Because almost everything in the body, according to auriculotherapy, has its reflection in the auricle, auriculotherapy very precise diagnoses and treatments are possible.

Microcurrent electricity, low-powered frequency laser (infrared or visible), needles, and massage are all part of auriculotherapy treatment. Sometimes these are combined for further effectiveness. For example, when treating pain, treatment continues until the pain diminishes or goes away completely, which take only a few seconds to a minute or two. When treating joint/movement problems, the patient moves the affected part while treatment is given. As the range of motion increases, the pain decreases over a few minutes. Regular acupuncture body needles can then be placed—always after the ear is treated.

Some *acupuncture* protocols are followed—a standard course of treatment is 10 treatments, with appointments two or three times a week. The pain typically recedes, then returns, then slowly fades after each treatment. Knowing both Western and Chinese auriculomappings is an advantage for the practitioner, since both modalities can be used simultaneously.

Auriculotherapy/auriculomedicine are not well known in the United States today. This is slowly changing, however, as research and the training of practitioners continue and as these techniques are proven to be effective.

STEVE MEEKER

See also
Acupuncture and Chinese Medicine (IV)
Pain (II)
Substance Abuse (II)

AUTOGENIC TRAINING

Autogenic training is a systematic program that teaches the body and mind to respond quickly and effectively to one's own verbal commands to relax. It helps the mind and body quickly return to a balanced, normal state. It is one of the most effective and comprehensive reducers of chronic stress.

"Autogenic" means "self-regulation" or "self-generation." Autogenic training (AT) uses the power of the trained mind to influence the body in a healthy fashion. In AT, relaxation is accomplished by passively paying attention to verbal cues for relaxation. In a sense, in AT involves reprogramming the subconscious mind to create a state of internal calm. Unlike progressive muscle relaxation, which uses an active tensing and releasing of the muscles, AT involves no direct muscle relaxation exercises. In AT, the body is conditioned to respond to verbal cues that reduce physiological arousal and tension.

AT is thought to help balance the body's self-regulating systems or "homeostatic" mechanisms (i.e., it regulates what goes on inside the body). AT helps to control stress by training the autonomic nervous system to be more relaxed when the person is facing a fearful or anxiety-producing situation. In essence, AT helps to regulate or counter the "fight or flight" response by controlling the sympathetic nervous system and its responses (heart rate, breathing, muscle tension, etc.). For many, AT is the treatment of choice to teach self-regulation of the autonomic nervous system. The goal of AT is to normalize physical, mental, and emotional processes that get out of balance due to stress.

Autogenic training was conceived in 1910 by Berlin psychiatrist Johannes Schultz and his colleague, Wolfgang Luthe. Schultz and Luthe were intrigued with the work of Oskar Vogt, a brain physiologist who practiced and did research in the area of hypnosis in the last part of the 19th century. Vogt studied the hypnotic trance phenomenon and began to experiment with having subjects put themselves in the trance state by the use of autosuggestion. Schultz and Luthe, stimulated by Vogt's work on hypnosis, began exploring the potentialities of autosuggestion. They wanted to eliminate what they saw as one of the major unfavorable aspects of hypnosis—reliance on the therapist or hypnotist for trance induction and therapeutic gain.

In their work, Schultz and Luthe noticed that subjects under hypnosis exhibited some fairly "standard" reactions when going into trance, such as heaviness in limbs, warmth in limbs, etc. Eventually, Schultz and Luthe found that they could create a state much like the hypnotic trance by having patients give themselves the suggestion of heaviness and warmth in their extremities. In 1932, Schultz and Luthe combined their techniques with some techniques from yoga and presented their system in the book *Autogenic Training* (1959).

Schultz's autogenic training consisted of a series of autogenic phrases that patients would repeat to themselves to induce a state of deep relaxation and healing. Schultz thought this state to be much like the hypnotic trance. Schultz's system includes autogenic phrases from six main themes: heaviness in the limbs, warmth in the extremities, regulation of cardiac activity, regulation of breathing, warmth in the abdomen, and cooling of the forehead.

As Schultz's system became more fully developed, it came to include four different types of exercises: (1) standard exercises, which focused mainly on the physical activities of the body; (2) meditative exercises, which focused on mental activities; (3) organ-specific exercises, which targeted specific symptoms or organs (e.g., bronchial asthma); and (4) intentional formula, which targeted specific mental functions. The standard exercises are by far the most commonly known and used of the exercises and are most commonly associated with AT.

AT consists of a series of exercises that patients are asked to repeat over a specified period of time. The exercises cover six basic "themes": (1) heaviness, which promotes relaxation of the voluntary muscles in the arms and legs; (2) warmth, which brings peripheral vasodilation, or relaxation of the muscles that control the diameter of the blood vessels; (3) normalization of cardiac activity; (4) regulation of respiratory activity; (5) regulation of abdominal activity; and (6) regulation of blood flow to the head. In AT, the client is instructed to silently repeat specific autogenic phrases (e.g., "my right arm is heavy") that relate to the various themes. The client works with Theme One (heaviness) until that theme is mastered. At that point, the client moves on to Theme Two, and so on.

AT clients are instructed to sit or lie down in a quiet place, close their eyes, and then begin silently repeating the autogenic phrases. Visual imagery sometimes is encouraged (e.g., imagining heavy weights attached to one's arms) if relaxation is not attained via the verbal cues. Each phrase is said slowly, followed by a pause, and then repeated again. Each phrase is repeated three to five times. When doing the exercises, clients are encouraged to have an attitude of passive concentration.

Instruction concerning how long and how often to practice AT varies. Some AT trainers suggest practicing for 1 to 4 minutes 4 to 7 times per day, while others suggest longer practice periods for fewer times each day. Session length will increase (while frequency decreases) as a client gains experience and skill in the method. It usually takes 3 to 10 months to master all six themes.

AT often follows training in progressive muscle relaxation, in which clients learn to induce a general state of relaxation by learning to control tension in major muscle groups. In AT, those clients learn to control, or regulate, the more subtle muscle groups and the functions of the autonomic nervous system. AT also is often used with biofeedback; the biofeedback equipment can provide immediate feedback to clients concerning their ability to regulate their biological functions. This can be a very powerful training method.

AT has been shown to be effective in treating disorders of the respiratory tract (e.g., bronchial asthma, hyperventilation), gastrointestinal tract (e.g., constipation, diarrhea, ulcers), and circulatory system (e.g., racing or irregular heart beat, high blood pressure, cold extremities), as well as migraines and other types of headaches.

It also is effective in treating a variety of psychosomatic disorders, stuttering, nocturnal enuresis, anxiety, and phobias. In addition, it decreases general anxiety, irritability, and fatigue. AT can also be used to modify reaction to pain, increase resistance to stress, and reduce or eliminate sleeping disorders.

One advantage of AT is that patients carry out their therapy on their own. It requires relatively little time each day, and 80% to 90% of adults respond positively to it. Adolescents can also be treated with AT, though often with less success than adults. It is difficult to use AT successfully with subjects under the age of 10.

There are a few cautions to be heeded before treating with AT. Prior to AT, patients with any physical problems should have a physical exam and/or consult with their physician about the effects of AT. Clients with serious diseases (e.g., diabetes, hypoglycemia) should be under a doctor's care while in AT. Persons with high or low blood pressure should also consult a physician before and during AT treatment. Persons who lack motivation do not do well with AT; nor do people with severe mental or emotional disorders. During AT exercises, subjects may experience "autogenic discharges"—feelings of irritability, crying, pain, stiffness, headache, nausea, tingling, even hallucinations. These symptoms are usually transitory and will pass as subjects continue with the program.

Common problems with AT include: (1) patients moving too fast with the exercises or phrases and not thoroughly learning each theme; and (2) the inability of subjects to maintain an attitude of passive concentration or to keep their mind from wandering. Patients reporting such problems should simply be encouraged to return to the exercises and the verbal formulas.

MICHAEL C. MURPHY

See also
   Asthma (II)
   Constipation (II)
   Diarrhea (II)
   Headache (II)
   High Blood Pressure (II)
   Insomnia (II)
   Pain (II)
   Stress (II)
   Ulcers (II)

AYURVEDA

Ayurveda is a Sanskrit word that combines two roots: *ayus*, which means daily living, and *vid*, which means knowledge. It is both a system of health and healing and a philosophy of life. Ayurveda is ancient, yet also modern. It had its origins on the Indian subcontinent anywhere from 3,000 to 5,000 years ago. Ayurvedic knowledge is considered to originate from divine sources. Numerous references to healing are found in the *Veda*, a sacred Hindu collection of hymns and songs that dates back to 1200 to 800 B.C. Two Vedas are of special importance in the development of Ayurveda, the *Rig Veda* and the *Atharva Veda*, both of which give detailed information about longevity, healing, and surgery.

Later, in the few centuries before and after the beginning of the common era, two influential Sanskrit medical treatises appeared: *Charaka Samhita* and *Sushruta Samhita*. Both are considered to have had

a great influence on the development of Ayurvedic knowledge. The combined wisdom of the *Vedas* and the later treatises resulted in the classical paradigm of Ayurveda.

Around the 16th century, this classical paradigm was influenced by Islamic medical systems. For example, during this time frame diagnosis by examination of pulse and urine was added to the body of Ayurvedic knowledge. Ayurveda continues to be influenced as it adapts itself to modern science. In particular, many precepts of Ayurveda are being more frequently explained in terms of and correlated with mind-body science and quantum mechanics.

To understand Ayurveda, it is important to realize that above all Ayurveda is a system of achieving and maintaining health. However, health is viewed not as the ultimate goal, but rather as an important condition for spiritual growth. In this regard, Ayurveda is truly an integration of mind, body, and spirit and fits readily within a holistic paradigm. Ayurveda is rooted in the belief that the forces of nature operate both within us and outside us; there is a connection between the microcosm and the macrocosm.

The theoretical foundations of Ayurveda begin with an appreciation of the nature of the universe. According to Ayurveda, the cosmos is composed of five basic elements, or *mahabutas*. These are: earth, air, fire, water, and space. In living matter, these five elements come together and give rise to the fundamental physiological energy that regulates the body. This is called the *dosha*, or force. Three *doshas* (*tridosha*) occur. They are *vata*, *pitta*, and *kapha*. *Vata* is a combination of space and air, *pitta* is a combination of fire and water, and *kapha* is a combination of water and earth. Each person is born with a body constitution based on the three *doshas*. Most people are a combination of *doshas*, in which one *dosha* predominates; hence a person can be recognized as predominantly a *vata*, *pitta*, or *kapha* type. This concept of body constitution, determined largely by *dosha*, is referred to as *prakriti*. To maintain health, the *doshas* must remain in balance.

Besides *doshas*, several other factors must be taken into consideration when assessing a person's state of health. These include *dhatus*, or tissues; *malas*, or waste products; *srotas*, or the channels through which substances circulate; and *agnis*, or digestive enzymes. The *dhatus* are responsible for sustaining the body. They include *rhasa* (tissue fluids such as chyle, lymph, and plasma), blood, flesh, fat, bone, marrow, and *shukra* (which includes male and female sexual fluids). There are three principal *malas*: urine, feces, and sweat. A fourth category of *malas* comprises fatty excretions, ear wax, mucus, saliva, tears, hairs, and nails.

Digestion is considered by Ayurveda to be one of the most important functions that takes place in the human body, and when it is not working results in the presence of undigested food (*ama*). *Ama* is a principal cause of maladies.

Gerson (1993) writes that according to the *Charaka Samhita*, health occurs when the following seven conditions exist:

1. all three *doshas* are in perfect equilibrium;
2. all the *dhatus* of the body are functioning properly;
3. the *malas* are eliminated in normal quantities;
4. the *srotas* are unimpeded;
5. *agni* (digestion) is good;
6. the five senses are functioning naturally; and
7. the body, mind, and consciousness are in harmony.

According to Ayurvedic theory, disease occurs when causative factors (e.g., food, drink, regimen, season, mental state) suppress enzyme activity in the body, which results in *ama*. Circulating *ama* then blocks the channels or mixes with one or more *doshas*, eventually coming to rest and afflicting a certain body part. In Ayurveda, internal disease begins with *ama*, and external disease produces *ama*.

In doing an assessment, the Ayurvedic physician seeks to identify (1) the site of origin (e.g., which channels are blocked), (2) the path of transportation (e.g., which *doshas* are involved), and (3) the site of manifestation (e.g., which body part is afflicted). The approach to the patient is a preliminary exam by means of visual observation, touch, and interrogation, followed by the eightfold method of detailed exam. This includes a pulse exam, urine exam, exam of body parts, etiology, early signs and symptoms (those that appear before the onset of the disease), manifestation of signs and symptoms, exploratory therapy (the use of diet, drugs, and other regimens to provide more information), and pathogenesis (determining which *dosha* is in imbalance).

Ayurvedic treatment is both prophylactic (i.e., maintaining a normal condition) and therapeutic. Treatment might include purification (sweating, use of purgatives, enemas) or the use of herbs and foods. All herbs and foods are characterized on the basis of taste (*rasa*), potency (*virya*), post-digestive taste (*vipaka*), qualities (*guna*), ability to increase or decrease *vata*, *pitta*, or *kapha*, and their pharmacological action. The underlying principle is try to correct existing imbalances. Hence if the physician determines that a client's current condition was caused by an excess of *vata*, the client would be given a herb that, by virtue of its properties, can decrease *vata*. The client also would be encouraged to avoid foods that contain space and air.

Above all, Ayurveda emphasizes the maintaining of a healthy state. Many regimens are recommended that can maintain balance and prevent illness. These include meditation, proper diet, periodic fasting, aromatherapy, self-massage, the use of oils, and regularity in daily routines. The emphasis on prevention through adoption of a healthy lifestyle makes Ayurveda an attractive system to investigate and to advocate for clients. It is holistically grounded therapy because of its integration of mind, body, and spirit. Many who embrace Ayurveda also embrace this philosophy of wholeness and desire to attain spiritual goals.

It is important to keep in mind that Ayurveda is a system and cannot be characterized by a single technique or modality. Its philosophy of health and healing is more important than any one of the many modalities it traditionally uses, although time has proven the effectiveness of many of these modalities. The modalities it embraces are low tech and low cost and have little potential for harm. The assessment diagnosis and treatment of illness require a skilled practitioner. To prescribe herbs, according to Ayurvedic principles, requires extensive training and experience. Ayurveda is most appropriate for the treatment of chronic illness, rehabilitation from acute injury, prevention of disease, and maintenance of health. It can be used effectively with many mainstream Western modalities.

The goal of maintaining harmony and balance through diet, meditation, and life-style changes can be particularly beneficial to those motivated to maintain or improve health. Adherence to a daily routine involving attention to diet, meditation, and daily routine in the larger context of Ayurveda theory can reduce stress and increase the feeling of connectedness to a reality larger than the individual.

KENNETH ZWOLSKI

BACH FLOWER REMEDIES

Edward Bach (1880–1936), a physician and graduate of Birmingham University and the University College Hospital, London, became convinced that stress, if unresolved, leads to physical distress. In 1930 he abandoned his practice at the Royal London Homeopathic Hospital and went to live in the country. Once there, he identified medicinal healing agents in wildflowers.

Over a 7-year period, Bach identified 38 flowers with healing qualities and designated them useful for treating emotional conditions. The process by which he developed his remedies included taking the heads off wildflowers, placing them on the surface of water contained in a glass bowl, and leaving them for 3 hours to absorb sunlight and transfer their essence to the water. The flowers were then removed and the water was retained. Blossoms from trees were boiled in a sterile saucepan for 30 minutes (Drury & Drury, 1989).

Bach's 39 remedies were classified using seven categories: fear (cherry plum, aspen, red chestnut, rock rose, and mimulus), uncertainty (cerato, gentian, scleranthus, hornbeam, gorse, and wild oat), disinterest (honeysuckle, clematis, wild rose, olive, white chestnut, chestnut bud, and mustard), loneliness (water violet, heather, impatiens), oversensitivity to influences and ideas (agrimony, centaury, walnut, holly), despair (pine, elm, larch, star of Bethlehem, sweet chestnut, crab apple, oak, and willow), and overcare of others (rock water, chicory, vervain, vine, and beech).

Within each of the seven groupings, there were subcategories of emotions, each with a specific remedy. Today, there are Bach flower remedies ranging from depletion after illness or long-term stress (olive) to victim role (willow). Lavender, peppermint, sage, and yarrow, additional essences beyond Bach's original remedies, have also been developed (Somerville, 1997).

Critics contend that any beneficial effects are due to a placebo effect. Practitioners, however, point to benefits seen in animals and children, two groups supposedly not susceptible to placebo effects. Additionally, there are no known side effects or harmful interactions with drugs or medications.

Bach used his remedies singly, not in combination, and only in a water base. Today, some practitioners combine the essences and preserve them in alcohol. To administer, two to four drops of an essence are placed either under the tongue or in a glass of water and sipped throughout the day, or used topically or added to baths (Somerville, 1997).

The Bach Rescue Remedy is widely used to produce a calming, stabilizing effect. The active ingredients include star of Bethlehem, rock rose, impatiens, cherry plum, and clematis. Rescue Remedy is also available as a cream and is recommended for shocks and nervous upsets, and as an alternative to over-the-counter remedies in an herbal first aid kit (Ody, 1993).

CAROLYN CHAMBERS CLARK

BIOACOUSTICS

The health status of a person may be displayed in his or her voice pattern. According to Edwards (1993), the "norm" for a voice pattern is at least one complete octave of all the notes in the musical scale. Analysis of nonharmonious notes, that is, missing notes or notes outside the person's "normal" octave, may indicate health problems.

Theory

Bio-Acoustics was developed after 20 years of work by Edwards (1995). Bio-Acoustics literally means "life sounds" and involves the study of frequencies that emanate from living organisms. The human body is dense energy that gives off nonverbal sounds. When the body is dis-eased, it produces nonharmonious notes (Edwards, 1989). Low-frequency sounds, similar to a murmur and based on the client's nonharmonious notes, are capable of interacting with the denser energy patterns of the body to stimulate healing. If the low-frequency sounds are inappropriately used, illness instead of wellness can result.

Determining the frequencies the client needs to heal is a three-step process. First, a computer program is used to assess the nonharmonious notes in a person's voice pattern. The recording takes less than a minute and simply requires the client to speak into a microphone. By expanding various portions of the voice recording, the notes outside the person's normal octave (nonharmonious notes) can be identified. These notes will appear extremely high or low depending on whether there is an excess or deficit of the notes.

After the nonharmonious notes are identified, the second step of analysis, podding, is conducted. Podding is a mechanical process of identifying the distressed notes that the individual needs to have replaced so that the body can heal itself. A pod consists of the nonharmonious note and five related notes; each note is multidimensional. An example of the pod for note E is provided in Figure 1. An individual who has three nonharmonious notes (e.g., notes E, C, and D) may actually need the replacement of two or three other notes that are distressed and located within the pods of E, C, and D.

Upon completion of the podding process, the identified distressed notes, their

TABLE 1   Notes of the Musical Scale and Their Reciprocals

Musical Notes	Reciprocals
C	F#
C#	G
D	G#
D#	A
E	A#
F	B
F#	C
G	C#
G#	D
A	D#
A#	E
B	F

reciprocals, or a combination of the distressed notes and their reciprocals, are tested on the client to determine his or her response, the third step of analysis. With some health problems and when the client's right brain is dominant, the reciprocal notes are needed. If the client is whole-brained, a combination of the distressed note and its reciprocal may be needed. Table 1 lists the notes of the musical scale and their reciprocals. This third step fine-tunes the distressed notes so the most effective set of frequencies is provided. For example, although two clients may have note C distressed, one client may need the frequency of 16.20, while the other client needs the frequency of 16.56. A difference of 3/100 of a frequency may affect the way a person responds to a note. When clients are having positive reactions to the note(s), their heart rates will be normal, they will feel relaxed, their oxygen saturation will increase, and they will comment that they like the sound. Conversely, when clients are having negative reactions to the note(s), their heart rate will significantly increase

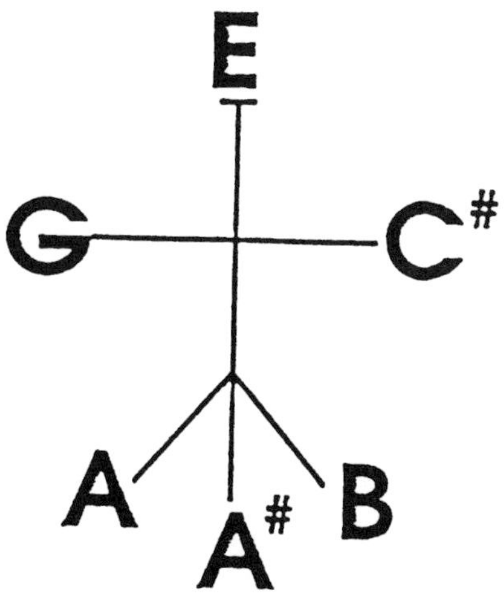

FIGURE 1   Pod E.

or decrease, they will feel dizzy or restless, their oxygen saturation will decrease, and they will be relieved when the sound is turned off. Step three requires special equipment and a controlled environment. All external noises must be controlled while the client is being tested. Health care providers, who are interested in Bio-Acoustics, need to be aware that the training and cost can be extensive.

Previous Research

The research conducted on Bio-Acoustics predominantly consists of case studies. One case study involved an elderly male client who suffered from emphysema. After his voice pattern was analyzed, certain frequencies were tested. When the needed frequency was supplied, his oxygen saturation rose to 98% or 99%. Without the frequency, his oxygen saturation fell to 89% or 90% (Edwards, 1993). After 2 years of working with this client, Edwards stated that he was no longer taking any medications, had returned to work, and was breathing normally. Other case studies involve clients with trauma, stroke, multiple sclerosis, and epilepsy. These case studies are available on video from Signature Sound Works located in Athens, Ohio.

Data collected on 50 clients have shown relationships between health problems and distressed notes (Edwards, 1994). Clients with chronic fatigue, for example, are likely to have notes F and F# in distress or their reciprocals, notes B and C, depending on the clients' brain dominance. Clients with Parkinson's disease frequently have note D# in distress. The molecular weight for dopamine is similar to the numeric frequency of D#. Clients with Parkinson's disease usually have a dopamine

deficiency. Individuals with bone diseases and bone trauma are likely to have notes E and G in distress. These notes have numeric frequencies similar to the atomic weights of calcium and magnesium, respectively. Clients with migraine headaches generally respond well to C#.

Current Research

For the purpose of the study reported below, clients' voices were recorded and analyzed to determine relationships between distressed notes and health problems previously studied with Bio-Acoustics.

Methodology

The study included a convenience sample of 26 nursing home residents (19 females and 7 males). All participants were White and their ages ranged from 59 to 100 years with a mean age of 83 years.

A health assessment questionnaire was used to collect data from the participants' medical records. To record their voices, an unidirectional microphone and a handbook computer (Gateway 2,000) were used.

A list of competent and capable residents was obtained from the director of nursing. The residents were not randomized nor screened for specific diseases. Each resident on the list was invited to participate, and if willing to do so, he or she signed the consent form. The residents were asked to speak into the microphone for 45 seconds on any topic they desired. During the recording, the doors to their rooms were closed, the televisions were turned off, and essentially all external noises were eliminated as much as possible. If the subject had a roommate, the roommate was informed of the recording and asked not to make any sounds during the recording. Medical records were reviewed to obtain data on the subjects' health problems. The study was approved by the appropriate committees and the administrator of the nursing home.

Data Analysis

Each voice recording was analyzed twice by the researcher. Only notes that were identified as nonharmonious in both analyses were included in the study. Determining a nonharmonious note from a harmonious note can at times be a judgment call. The trained practitioner makes the decision as to whether the note is unduly excessive or deficient. Bone diseases, osteoporosis and osteoarthritis, common to this sample, were studied. These medical diagnoses were not known at the time the voice recordings were analyzed. A frequency table and the t-test were used to describe the subjects with and without bone diseases and their distressed notes.

Results

Eight subjects had osteoarthritis and four subjects had osteoporosis. Six subjects with osteoarthritis had both notes E and G distressed, one subject had note E distressed, and one subject had note G distressed. Three subjects with osteoporosis had both notes E and G distressed, while one subject had neither note distressed. The distribution of the distressed notes E and G in relationship to osteoarthritis and osteoporosis is shown in Table 2. A t-test conducted on the data showed a significant difference ($t(23) = 3.52$, $p = .0018$) and the results of the t-test are summarized in Table 3.

TABLE 2 Distribution of the Distressed Notes E and G in Relationship to Osteoporosis and Osteoarthritis ($N = 26$)

| Subjects | Notes Distressed | | | |
	Note E	Note G	Neither	Both
With Osteoarthritis or Osteoporosis	1	1	1	9
Without Osteoarthritis or Osteoporosis	3	3	6	2

TABLE 3 t-Test if Bone Diseases and Notes E (Calcium) and G (Magnesium) ($N = 26$)

Subjects	Distressed Notes E, G, or Both	Non-Distressed Notes E, G, or Both	t
With Osteoarthritis or Osteoporosis	11	1	3.52**
Without Osteoarthritis or Osteoporosis	8	6	

**$p = .0018$

Discussion

The results of this study are significant, in spite of the small sample size, and support the theory of Bio-Acoustics. Osteoporosis frequently causes pathological bone fractures, while osteoarthritis frequently causes joint deformities and the development of bone cysts and bone spurs. Thus, it is not surprising that participants with these bone diseases would have the vibratory rate of calcium (note E) and magnesium (note G) in distress. Jensen (1995) pointed out that everything in life including diseases has a vibratory rate.

Since this is a small study and one of the few conducted on Bio-Acoustics, further research is needed before any conclusions can be drawn. Hopefully, this study will precipitate further research.

Implications

With further research and verification of the relationships between specific distressed notes and health problems, low frequency sounds will be more readily used to create a therapeutic environment that stimulates healing. Currently, there are few alternative health practitioners who offer sound therapy based on the theory of Bio-Acoustics.

RITA HOLL

BIOFEEDBACK

Biofeedback therapy involves the use of electronic monitoring equipment to help clients learn self-regulation over physiological processes that they are not normally aware of, such as heart rate or skin temperature, to reduce or eliminate uncomfortable physical and emotional symptoms. The term "biofeedback" refers to the client's conscious awareness of biological processes becoming part of a "feedback loop," from body to brain and back again.

Initially, the client learns to control these physiological responses voluntarily by learning to manipulate the displayed visual and/or auditory signals. With training and practice, the client learns to control the physiological responses by becoming aware of subtle internal psychophysiological (physical and mental) cues. Relaxation training is often used with biofeedback training to assist in learning self-regulation. This process of learning self-regulation of previously distressing symptoms increases self-confidence and gives the client a sense of personal control. It is the learning of self-regulation by the client that produces therapeutic benefits, not the biofeedback itself.

Because biofeedback teaches regulation of basic physiological functions, it has many applications for a broad array of conditions, including but by no means limited to tension headaches, migraine headaches, chronic pain, Raynaud's disease, attention deficit hyperactive disorders, addictions, anxiety, phobias, panic attacks, hyperhidrosis, irritable bowel syndrome, hypertension, urinary and fecal incontinence, and conditions requiring neuromuscular reeducation, such as strokes or other neurological injuries.

Many of the conditions that benefit from biofeedback therapy, such as tension headaches and panic attacks, result from overactive or excessive physiological activity or arousal. In these cases, biofeedback therapy teaches clients to lower physiological arousal, which results in a decrease or elimination of the uncomfortable symptoms. Other problems that benefit from biofeedback therapy result from reduced physiological activity or inadequate control of physical responses, such as the loss of muscle strength and control in urinary or fecal incontinence or the loss of muscle strength and inadequate coordination that results from stroke or other neurological injuries. In these cases, biofeedback is used to teach clients to increase the strength of their response and gain greater, more appropriate control over physiological functions.

Biofeedback equipment allows for noninvasive monitoring; sensors are placed on the surface of the body rather than inside the body, as is the case with invasive monitoring. The noninvasive approach allows the monitoring to be done without any discomfort for the client. The only minor discomfort that sometimes occurs is when sensors using adhesive are removed from the skin. Some biofeedback equipment monitors and displays only one type of biofeedback signal at a time, while other equipment can monitor and display several different types of signals simultaneously. The most frequently monitored biofeedback signals are skin temperature, muscle tension (electromyographic feedback, or EMG), and galvanic skin response (GRS).

Several types of biofeedback monitoring are currently in use. Here are the most common.

Temperature biofeedback uses an electronic wire called a thermistor, which is usually attached to one of the longer fingers on the client's dominant hand to measure peripheral skin temperature. Skin temperature is an indirect measure of circulation in the extremities. Temperature biofeedback often is used for migraine headaches and Raynaud's disease, a painful condition of poor circulation in the hands and feet. It can be used for any condition that benefits from learning lower physiological arousal.

Electromyographic (EMG) biofeedback uses small metal electrodes attached with adhesive paper or foam placed on specific muscles to measure the electrical activity produced by muscle cells during contraction. Increased contraction causes painful muscle spasms, so EMG biofeedback is frequently used for back and other muscle pain. Surface EMG (sEMG) biofeedback uses electrodes on several muscle sites at the same time and can help a client to correct inappropriate body posture or poor body mechanics, both of which contribute to and aggravate muscle pain. EMG biofeedback also is used to "reeducate" appropriate muscle use and train increased strength after neurological injury (neuromuscular reeducation). Another use for neuromuscular reeducation is for the treatment of urinary and or fecal incontinence.

Heart-rate biofeedback uses a sensor called a photoplethysmograph, which is placed on a finger to measure the variation of the amount of light passing through the small blood vessels. This information is translated and displayed by a computer as an average heart rate. Heart-rate biofeedback is often used to treat anxiety, panic attacks, and phobias.

Blood-volume pulse also uses a photoplethysmograph sensor to measure the volume of blood in the small blood vessels. Blood volume changes more quickly than heart rate and other types of biofeedback in response to emotional changes. It often is used with heart-rate biofeedback for treating anxiety, panic attacks, and phobias.

Galvanic skin response (GRS) measures the activity of the sweat glands on the hands by measuring the salts from sweat that are conductive to electricity. This is also called *electrodermal activity* (EDA) or *electrodermal response* (EDR) monitoring. GRS is particularly useful for clients with hyperhidrosis (excessively sweaty hands) but can also be used for any condition that benefits by learning lower levels of physiological arousal.

Electroencephalographic biofeedback (EEG) measures the electrical activity of the brain by using small metal electrodes that are placed on the surface of the scalp. It is used primarily for attention deficit hyperactive disorders and addictions. Some research is currently under way to determine if EEG biofeedback can improve cognitive (thinking) skills in elderly people with memory problems.

Clients undertaking biofeedback usually attend weekly sessions, although the sessions may be more frequent. Therapy may last for as little as 6 weeks or may last much longer, depending on the severity of symptoms and the client's rate of progress. Fees vary but range from $75 to $125 per session. Biofeedback is covered by many health insurance companies.

The field of biofeedback therapy is an interdisciplinary one, and biofeedback practitioners include general practitioners, psychologists, licensed mental health counselors, registered nurses, physical therapists, occupational therapists, and specially trained biofeedback technicians. Most practitioners belong to the Association for Applied Psychophysiology and Biofeedback (AAPB). Certification is recommended but not required, and practitioners may become certified through the Biofeedback Certification Institute of America. A biofeedback practitioner can be located by calling AAPB for a list of members in a given area or by consulting the Yellow Pages under "Biofeedback."

SUZANNE E. FOSTER

See also
Addiction Treatment (II)
Headache (II)
High Blood Pressure (II)
Memory Problems (II)
Pain (II)

BODY-ORIENTED PSYCHOTHERAPY AND TRANSFORMATION-ORIENTED BODYWORK

Body-oriented psychotherapy and transformation-oriented bodywork refer to the two convergent mind and body therapy genres that combine physical and psychological processes for therapeutic purposes. Reflecting the growing mind-body interface between medicine, bodywork, and psychology, the numerous modalities within both of these categories share a body-focused approach to healing. Both are based on the simple principle that because the body's physiological response is central to a person's overall response to trauma, so too must the body be involved in the therapeutic healing of such trauma—something that "talk therapy" alone cannot adequately address.

Body-oriented psychotherapy, although technically more concerned with the wholeness of the psyche and not a bodywork system per se, often uses direct hands-on contact to further psychological gains. Despite the mainstream taboo of touch in psychological work, in body-oriented psychotherapy touch is believed to enhance the transference process, quicken inner processing, and provide corrective emotional experiences.

Historically, this movement is rooted in the Reichian psychodynamic model of the early 20th century, but it currently includes approaches drawing from diverse fields such as neurology and psychoneuroimmunology (PNI) of Western medicine, acupuncture, and Chinese medicine, as well as all the major schools of psychotherapy. Reichian therapy holds that the body's musculature is a mirror of psychological defense mechanisms: repeated protective muscular contractions in the face of emotional trauma freeze the mind-body system into what Reich called "body and character armoring." Reich's approach to healing involved direct hands-on contact with the supine client, deep breathing, and abreaction, all culminating in a simultaneous loosening of both sets of armor.

Other body psychotherapies that dispense with hands-on contact instead may focus on reflecting the client's awareness to posture or movement to personalize psychological insight. All embrace the notion of internalized blocked physical energy (producing tension and anxiety) as paralleling blocked awareness. The goal of body-oriented psychotherapy is the gradual unraveling and direct release of both physical and psychological aspects of these life-negating barriers, a healthy integration of the past, and a return to the normal uninhibited state in the present.

Examples of body-oriented psychotherapy include Somatic Trauma Therapy, as practiced by Babette Rothchild of Denmark; the neo-Reichian Radix therapy, as presented by Dr. Charles Kelley; Systemic Integration by R. Cascone; Hakomi therapy by Ron Kurtz; the Pesso Boyden System Psychomotor (PBSP); and Centropic Integration by Andy Bernay-Roman and Dr. Camden Clay.

Transformation-oriented bodywork stands as the counterpart of body-oriented psychotherapy within the bodywork field and includes those modalities of body-oriented healing that deal with the whole of a person's experience, yet do not qualify as psychotherapies.

Rolfing, Ida Rolf's system of structural integration and realignment of body posture via a physical manipulation of the fascial sheets surrounding muscle bundles, stands as the grandmother of transformation-oriented bodywork. Rolf introduced her methods at the Esalen Institute of Big Sur, California, in the 1960s, which greatly helped somatosize the psychotherapy movement of the day. Fritz Perls, founder of Gestalt therapy, partook of Ida Rolf's early work at Esalen and said her rolfing saved his life. Unlike its psychotherapy counterparts, transformation-oriented bodywork often does not focus on the verbal or emotional content of the client's experience, but rather lets those elements naturally reintegrate in the wake of the physical realignment and dismantling of the body's armor.

Other modalities in this category include Feldenkrais movement-oriented therapy, Rubenfeld Synergy, Hellerwork, Transformational Bodywork of Fred and Cheryl Mitouer, and Interactive Facilitation.

Both body-oriented psychotherapy and transformation-oriented bodywork aim to achieve wholeness of the mind-body system by facilitating physical, emotional, and mental changes. The work in these different camps often looks identical, involving both physical manipulation of soft tissue and verbal emotional processing. Only the practitioner's credentials and preferences determine whether the treatment is labeled primarily a bodywork or a psychotherapy intervention.

ANDY BERNAY-ROMAN

CENTERING: THE PATH TO HEALING PRESENCE

Illness and disease prompt people to enter the "health care system" in search of healing. Healing goes beyond symptom relief and also beyond cure, though patients are grateful for both. Healing refers to an integrating tendency in an individual which engenders a state of full aliveness. Borysenko (1989) described the central theme of healing as "reunion" between a sense of the separate, limited self and the limitless expression of consciousness. Healing results in a deeper understanding of life's meaning and one's place in it. Healing goes beyond cure: While it can occur along with a resolution of symptoms, healing can also take place when death becomes inevitable, as part of the dying process itself. Healing delivers us to what Taoists refer as the "Eternal Moment," the moment free of past regrets and future fears; that is, the present moment, the only moment in which happiness, contentment and a sense of wholeness are possible.

Healing is not "done to" another, nor is it a result of professional technique. Remen (1989) asserted that one person does not heal another, rather, we invite someone to participate in life with us, to engage in that movement toward wholeness which underlies life. Healing occurs in the context of relationship: relationship with the self, with nature, with others. The health professional has the opportunity to facilitate the patient's growth beyond symptom relief and cure, into healing, by engaging in a healing relationship.

The present "health care system" seems, paradoxically, to work against the experience of healing. Outcome criteria rely on techniques which relate to signs and symptoms; the definition of health is reduced to the absence of illness. Kreiger (1993) asserted that healing requires the practitioner's conscious, full engagement of energies in compassionate interest in helping. Yet, health care settings often stress, impinge upon, and fragment the delicate relationship with the patient within which the healing response emerges. Time and resources are often inadequate to the process of healing. Grinding stress in the workplace can manifest in health professionals who are hurried, harried and "burned out," unable to be fully present with patients in a helpful way.

Healing, that is, restoration to a state of wholeness, vitality and purpose in life, requires a certain environment in which to develop. Healing is incompatible with reactive stress responses, which, when severe or prolonged, deplete organismic reserves. Healing requires that the individual be in a state of rest from which restorative processes emerge. If the health care provider is unable to transcend stress, its effects will contaminate the therapeutic relationship and interfere with the patient's efforts to heal. It seems that the survival of the healing relationship requires strategies in which the possibility of healing is supported.

Hypocrites' admonition: "Physician, heal thyself," is a wise directive for all health care practitioners. Our ability to influence others in healing depends on a familiarity with our own experiences of health and healing. We cannot facilitate healing when exhausted, preoccupied, distracted. Nor can healing occur for a patient when we are merely performing techniques and treatments "on" the patient. The patient is vulnerable to the energetic resonance of the professional as surely as he or she is sensitive to the quality of touch or to the level of technical expertise. Just as it is our responsibility to be professionally competent in the technical aspects of our roles, it is also our task to establish the relational environment within which healing is possible. In order for healing to occur, it is imperative that the practitioner be fully present to the patient's experience. Without this sense of *presence*, the professional relationship is not a healing one.

Healing Presence

The golden thread that unites all healers is the quality of *presence*, and the capacity for *"being there for what is"* (Johnson, 1989, p. 132). Through presence, the healer welcomes and encourages the patient's expectations, fears, and expressions of need beyond the evaluation of symptoms and the prescription of treatment. It requires that the practitioner be in touch with her/his excitement about what is real, and aware of how her/his habitual patterns of automatic "professional" behavior inhibit apperception of what is. What is "real" for the patient often goes beyond the parameters of symptoms and treatments. Patients often remark that their most valued practitioner is the one who takes the time to listen, and who shows interest beyond the presenting complaint. Patients thrive on the full, respectful, caring attentiveness which healing presence provides. Healing presence is, in its essence, an exquisite energetic contact which mirrors, supports, and informs the experience of the patient in the service of her/his personal growth toward wholeness.

Centering

Centering is a conscious process that facilitates a calm, focused state of being where

healing can occur. Being centered is a sense of self-relatedness, a state of inner being, a place of quietude within oneself where one can feel integrated, unified, and focused (Kreiger, 1979). By centering, we take the responsibility which is ours as health professionals for creating the therapeutic relationship.

How to Center

1. Begin by sitting comfortably in a quiet place. Close your eyes if you feel excessively distracted. Inhale and exhale slowly and deeply. Feel the lower belly soften and expand with a few deep breaths.
2. Allow the eyes, jaw, face, back of the neck, shoulders, arms, pelvic floor, joints and limbs to soften and relax. Shift body position and exhale deeply to release any tensions of which you are aware.
3. Notice the breath. Breathe normally, then gradually let your breath slow down until it is quiet, even, and the breath lengths are fairly long. Notice how slowing the breath induces quietness and relaxation.
4. Observe how your thoughts, sensations, and emotions continue in your experience. Allow them without becoming preoccupied with them. Return to your awareness of the breath when becoming distracted.
5. Allow a sense of taking in vital energy when inhaling, and releasing deep tension when exhaling.
6. Maintain awareness of yourself as the center of your own experience, with your inner experience as the main focus and stimulation, sounds, etc. from the external environment

as peripheral to the center of your being.

7. Experience the sense of doing nothing but being with yourself. Allow yourself to enjoy any sense of relaxation, calm and peacefulness that you might feel as you maintain your inner focus. Be aware of how you are breathing as you enjoy being with yourself.

8. When you are relaxed, gradually allow your focus to expand to meet the external environment. Stay connected with your inner focus and bring it along with you as you re-engage in your professional role.

9. Approach your patient with your sustained inner focus, and include your awareness of her within it.

10. When you experience the inevitable distractions of the workplace, sustain your attention within the therapeutic relationship by bringing your attention back to your breathing and to your awareness of your patient.

The Effects of Centering

Centering allows the focusing awareness inward, relaxing and balancing the sympathetic "fight or flight" nervous system response, along with related experiences of anxiety, restlessness, distractibility, shallow breathing, a sense of being under pressure, and fatigue. Attention is shifted from involvement with the external environment toward self observation and experience. Centering engages the functions of the parasympathetic nervous system by facilitating slower, deeper breathing, focused concentration, enhanced perception, and a sense of balanced calmness. This inner quieting allows the practitioner to restore

equilibrium, not unlike the martial artist who gathers in energy before entering into practice and returns to center when off balance.

Conclusion

The centering experience has certain characteristics which clearly differentiates it from ordinary reactive consciousness. First, time seems to slow down, replacing the urge to rush with a sense of spacious opportunity. Second, sharpened concentration makes it possible to differentiate salient from irrelevant information, including the influence of intuition on the critical thinking process. Third, the relaxation which results from centering allows for strain to be transformed into a sense of ease in action. Fourth, centering is a healthy practice which is good for the practitioner as well as an enhancement of the therapeutic relationship. Finally, centering establishes an energetic resonance within the therapeutic relationship which the patient can use for the purposes of her own healing.

Gerber (1988) said that consciousness participates in the continuous creation of either health or illness. Centering is a way in which to transform the stress-reactive consciousness of the workplace and everyday world to an energetic environment for optimal professional practice. By "practicing what we preach," that is, by creating an inner environment which supports our own health and functioning, we model for our patients the process from which healing can develop.

Centering unites the art of caring with the science of caring by organizing the practitioner's focus on the essential processes of therapeutic relationship. Centering reflects a value which returns healing presence to its rightful place: Don't just do something. Be there!

MARY ANNE BRIGHT

CENTROPIC INTEGRATION

Centropic Integration (CI) is a body-oriented psychotherapy modality that features sustained acupressure point holding, evocative music, and emotional facilitation as its core tools. It can be practiced in both one-on-one and group settings.

Centropic, meaning "movement towards the center," refers to the natural tendency of a person to return to core experiences or issues, and *Integration* refers to the reuniting of disconnected parts. Centropic Integration takes its theoretical foundation from the science of psychoneuroimmunology, which postulates and explains the biology of memory storage via the neuropeptide system, and seeks to apply those physiological principles to the realm of real human, personal experience. The work was created by Andy Bernay-Roman and Dr. Camden Clay in the 1980s, synthesizing elements of John Ray's Body Electronics, Stanislav Grof's Holotropic Breathwork, and a unique form of core-feeling counseling.

Theoretical Foundations

For survival's sake, some experiences or portions of experience are "hidden away" in the recesses of the body, biochemically encoded in their entirety on neuropeptide molecules. This network of neuropeptides and receptor sites located throughout the soft tissue of the body makes up what could be called "body memory" at both conscious and unconscious levels of awareness. Empirical investigation shows that all experiences stored in memory can be retrieved, and that memories tagged with higher emotional charge make more of an impact on the psyche. Arthur Janov says that neurosis, or the splitting up of the whole-brain response into its components for the sake of not feeling them, is man's unique survival adaptation in the face of overwhelm or pain. Out of this splitting (and numbing of feeling) is generated the impetus to be whole, the natural centropic impulse to reintegrate that which has been cut off.

Centropic Integration carries a two-fold approach: first, the conscious introduction of a whole-brain, highly charged, desired outcome into the system, and second, accessing and releasing all earlier life-negating programming in the matter by feeling repressed pain. Feeling, with its three aspects of meaning, emotion, and body response, (reflecting the triune nature of the brain) is the key to Centropic Integration, and that which separates it from other emotional release-oriented therapies.

Setting the Banks of the River

Before any reservoir of suppressed or unconscious feeling is tapped directly, it is important to set the "river banks" within which the water is to flow so that not only will blocked energy be freed, it will propel the client in an empowering direction, from current reality (point A) to where he or she wants to be (point B).

A session begins with a face-to-face encounter of the client's relevant past and current situation with primarily open-ended questions to ascertain not only important medical and personal history, but also intensify the focus on emotionally charged material as it shows up in the present moment. Common questions might be: "What are you aware of right now in your body as you tell me about your brother?" or "What's the feeling being expressed in your voice as you mention the hospital?" or "If your heart had a voice right now, what would it say?"

Point A (the unfulfilling aspect of a client's "current reality") inevitably reveals an underlying existential theme or message linked with a core feeling, often rooted in past childhood conclusions that are no longer relevant and which diminish healthy self-esteem, trust, boundary-setting, relationships, etc., in the adult context, and lie at the core of the problem for which the client sought help.

The CI facilitator then helps the client focus on and arrive at an aligned statement of desired and meaningful outcome. "If you could have things any way you wanted, how would you have them be?" Some examples: "I choose to be able to touch others with love without taking their pain" or "I choose to know and feel my own heart even if it means feeling pain and disappointment" or "I choose to consistently stand up for myself even in the face of others' anger and disapproval." Point B choices bring about a sense of possibility of balance and integrity in a particular problematic area of life.

With both Point A and Point B thus fully felt with a meaning, emotion, and body response, the "banks of the river are set." Any additional emotional or tension release in the next hands-on phase of the session serves to catapult the person further along the path to his or her outcome.

Accessing the Memory

Centropic Integration uses sustained point holding along acupressure meridian lines to access the body-component of stored fragmented memories. The acupuncture lines of the endocrine system hook directly in to the circuitry of the limbic "loop" in the brain where emotional memory is processed. The client lies supine, and the appropriate points for the session are determined through a simple system correlating the endocrine glands to different emotional states, or simply by assessing the client's energy field with the hands for points of "interruption," trigger response, or just plain tenderness to touch. Points can be held by one or more participants, with one taking on the role of facilitator.

Breathwork and Altered States

The first 15–20 minutes of point-holding are devoted to deep synchronous breathing by client, facilitator, and other participants, accompanied by evocative and emotional music designed to activate and uninhibit the abreaction process. Tapping into the long tradition in human cultures of using music, ranging from tribal drums to a huge pipe organ in a cathedral, to evoke trance states and deep feelings, this phase of CI elicits both emotion and right-brain, imagery-infused thinking.

Heat, Resistance, and the Body Electric

Just as the electrons in an electric heater generate more heat when we turn the resistance up, so do the acupressure contact points, reflecting the person's resistance to change, manifest as heat. At this time the client may be experiencing images and/or body sensations that either symbolically or directly reflect the spontaneous reemergence of stored unconscious information that may have to do with non-integrated memories. The centropic impulse for resolution, coupled with the client's desire for a new outcome, brings the electrical potential at the resistance points upscale enough to match and finally surpass the resistance. The blocked portions of experience flood forth in emotional catharsis and/or realization, biologically integrating the meaning, emotion, and body response aspects of previously repressed pain. Point-holding and evocative music thus help "flush out" hidden, peripheral features of experience, making the integrative results of CI dramatic compared to conventional "talk therapies." With conscious catharsis, the Gestalt achieves wholeness once more. The life force overcomes internalized blocks and surges into any body part where dysfunction had set in, often initiating a period of intense burning sensations (the *kundalini* of Eastern philosophy?). The electrical flow of nerve conduction soon shifts from an experience of heat to one of light, inundating the client with insight, not only about the original issue, but also about a deeper sense of purpose in life.

The In-Filling

The final phase of the session, the "in-filling," beyond the abundance of insight and the burning inner fire, takes on a spiritual quality hallmarked by peacefulness and deep body relaxation. Clients report this as a time of integration, personal victory, and healing, full of recognition and connectedness. Time elapsed up to this point is two hours, and the session ends with the cooling, pulsing, and releasing of the points, followed by a sense of "afterglow" which can last for hours and sometimes days.

Final Notes

The healing of Centropic Integration begins with a direct bodily encounter with one's own locked-up pain and resistance to feeling, and ends in renewing daily life with empowering choices and revitalized hope. Unlike the cognitive therapies that affect experience by consciously altering the thinking process, in CI, cognition "takes care of itself" as a natural outcropping of deeply processed feelings. Follow-up sharing, especially in the intimate group setting of a Centropic Integration workshop, enhances cognitive anchoring of new learning. Changes and insights facilitated by a natural integration at the body level endure over time.

ANDY BERNAY-ROMAN

CHELATION THERAPY

The Greek word *chele* ("claw") indicates that chelating substances "grab into" or claw offending elements in the body to usher them out of the body, where they do no harm. Although chelating substances occur naturally in plants and in the body (chlorophyll with its magnesium binding and hemoglobin with its clawlike grasp of iron), the treatments that are used to withdraw unwanted toxic elements from the body commonly employ artificial substances. From a practical standpoint today, chelation therapy is available for the treatment of lead poisoning, cadmium excess, aluminum overload, mercury and arsenic poisoning, and iron toxicity. Other toxic metals also may eliminated to some extent in the process of eliminating lead, cadmium, aluminum, and iron.

Because of the extensive and widespread use of intravenous chelation therapy for circulatory disorders today, the term "chelation therapy" has become essentially equivalent to the intravenous administration of EDTA (ethylenediaminetetraacetic acid), an artificial amino acid, for the opening of blocked arteries. EDTA is found in catsup, mayonnaise, frozen Brussels sprouts, salad dressings, and many other food because of its effectiveness in retarding food spoilage. Just as EDTA slows the unwanted breakdown of foodstuffs, it can slow the unwanted breakdown of body cells.

When given according to the protocol of the American College for the Advancement of Medicine and only after a full medical evaluation that engages all aspects of the person's well-being, intravenous chelation therapy, customized to the patient's individual tolerances, can be employed. Customarily seen are a cessation of advance in obstructive arterial plaque, clearing of arterial obstructions, lowering of elevated blood pressures, enhancement of blood flow in capillaries and large vessels, improved venous health, lowering of blood fats, improved digestion and absorption of foods, slowing or cessation of cataract formation, improvement in glaucoma and macular degeneration, lessened arthritic complaints, and an improved sense of well-being. In persons who have received chelation therapy along with regular "boosters," chelating physicians often find a significant paucity of cancer. In view of the fact that a profound fullness of the blood vasculature (vasodilation) can be appreciated during the chelation treatment, it is not difficult to understand that all organs and cells of the body may improve their function. When arterial beds in tissues open up to supply local areas with a greater supply of oxygen and nutrients, beneficial results can be expected. Sexual function commonly improves with chelation therapy.

EDTA, properly combined with magnesium and other ingredients, provides anti–free-radical effects, "mopping up" of unwanted ionic calcium, dissolution of unwanted metastatic calcium deposits in soft tissues and arterial walls, and improvement in the elasticity of arteries. Patients with gangrenous digits or limbs have been spared amputations. Carotid artery obstructions ranging from 100% obstruction to lesser amounts diminish on average by 35%. EDTA chelation therapy, a potent antioxidant, has long been combating unwanted oxidative damage in body cells. Simultaneously, the body burden of toxic metals that inexorably increases with each decade of life on an increasingly toxic planet is lowered by chelation.

Chelation therapy used for circulatory disorders (angina, intermittent claudication, cold feet, cold hands, transient ischemic attacks, heart attacks, strokes, gangrene, etc.) usually results in the decrease of medications and sometimes their complete elimination. Sometimes, however, chelation therapy is ineffective. Properly used, side effects are usually absent. Persons undergoing renal dialysis for kidney failure should not undergo chelation therapy. Close monitoring of chelated patients for proper kidney function is mandatory. Usually the blood supply to the kidneys increases with an improvement in kidney function as measured by the creatinine-clearance test. In all cases, the intravenous chelation combines with the best possible dietary therapy, nutritional supplementation, and exercise program tailored to the needs and capacities of the individual to elicit best results. Smoking, of course, is counterproductive.

The actual process of chelation therapy is accomplished by the slow, intravenous drip of EDTA and magnesium in a suitable carrier solution along with supportive nutrients over the course of 1.5 to 4.0 hours. Treatments are usually administered twice weekly. Twenty to 40 treatments are commonly used, although many more may be needed. Some persons without fixed disease but who wish to use the treatments for antiaging benefits take an initial set of 10 treatments followed by one treatment a month. On a yearly basis, a cluster of 10 or more treatments would be taken. At all times, specific nutrient supplementations are required to prevent nutrient deficits.

A meta-analysis (a study of studies) conducted by Chappell and Stahl (1993) collected 40 published and 30 yet-to-be published studies. Some 25,000 patients with vascular disease were surveyed. All but one of the multipatient studies (that one carried out by Danish cardiac surgeons on patients who, for the most part, continued to smoke) showed positive results. Eighty-seven percent of the patients showed measurable improvement in their vascular disease. More than 10 million chelation treatments have been administered without a single fatality attributable to the procedure. Chapell writes, "This undoubtedly makes EDTA Chelation Therapy one of the safest treatment methods in modern medicine." The cost of coronary artery bypass surgery is often $30,000 to $50,000 and perhaps more. The cost of an average course of chelation therapy over several months is perhaps $2,000 to $3,000.

Chelation therapy does not replace proper diet, exercise, some medications at some times, and some surgery at some times. Properly used and judiciously applied, EDTA chelation therapy has proven a most valuable method of preventing and managing vascular disease, and since the rule of the artery is supreme, in promoting the health of the entire body.

An exciting field of mercury chelation has opened to those physicians who open their minds to the widespread mercury toxicity in the population of developed countries. The combined impact of mercury in dental amalgams, seafood, and environmental exposures appears to have adversely affected the lives of untold numbers. When the body burden of mercury is accurately assessed by means of appropriate use of safe mercury chelators, then steps can be taken to safely eradicate the body (and brain) burden of the toxic metal and to rehabilitate those individuals whose lives may have been compromised by it. Because of the current investigative status of the agents used, more cannot be said at this time. The availability of strong, hard composite materials suitable for long-term use in the teeth now heralds the fast-approaching day when the use of mercury in the mouth shall not be needed.

As a final note in chelation therapy, intravenous vitamin C must be mentioned. When properly used, with close attention to the kidney function and the urinary tract, intravenous sodium ascorbate (with suitable supporting and adjunctive nutrients) acts as a weak chelator for a detoxifying, antiallergic, anti-infectious, and antidepressant effect.

RAY C. WUNDERLICH, JR.

See also
Arthritis (II)
Heart and Blood Vessel Conditions (II)
Macular Degeneration (II)

CHIROPRACTIC: DEFINITION, HISTORY, AND THEORY

Chiropractic is a manual healing art that focuses on the relationship between structure (primarily of the spine) and function (as mediated by the nervous system). Chiropractors analyze structural disrelationships of the spine and other joints and manually adjust or manipulate these areas to restore proper function.

Central to chiropractic theory is the concept of vertebral subluxation. Originally conceived as a spinal misalignment causing direct pressure on a nerve, current thinking describes the subluxation as "a complex of functional, structural, and/or pathological articular changes that compromise neural integrity and may influence organ system function and general health" (Redwood, 1997). Contemporary definitions of the vertebral subluxation place strong emphasis on interruption of proper spinal joint motion as well as bony misalignment.

Daniel David Palmer, a self-educated healer, founded chiropractic in 1895 in Davenport, Iowa. Palmer and many early chiropractors considered the vertebral subluxation to be the cause of virtually all disease and the chiropractic adjustment its cure. This controversial "one cause-one cure" philosophy was a key factor causing antagonism between conventional physicians and chiropractors. With rare exceptions, contemporary chiropractors reject monocausal theories of disease in favor of multifactorial models.

During chiropractic's first century, education and practice standards underwent profound changes. Chiropractic education now consists of a rigorous 4-year curriculum, with in-depth training in anatomy, physiology, pathology, and diagnosis, as well as spinal adjusting, nutrition, physical therapy, and rehabilitation. Surgery and pharmaceutical therapy, which lie outside the chiropractor's scope of practice, are addressed in the classroom so that chiropractors will know when to refer cases to medical physicians. Chiropractic standards of care call for orthopedic, neurological, and chiropractic examination of each patient on the initial visit, the use of diagnostic imaging procedures when appropriate, application of manual chiropractic adjustments as the centerpiece of treatment strategy, and timely referral of patients not demonstrating sufficient clinical progress.

Chiropractic theory includes five common domain principles of natural healing: (1) that the body has an innate healing potential that the healing arts seek to elicit; (2) that addressing the cause of an illness should take precedence over suppressing its symptoms; (3) that natural, nonpharmaceutical measures (including chiropractic adjustments) should generally be an approach of first resort, not last; (4) that a balanced, natural diet is crucial to good health; and (5) that regular exercise is essential to optimum bodily function (Redwood, 1996).

Fundamental chiropractic principles do not directly address the issue of pain relief, focusing instead on the role of the spine and nervous system in restoring overall balance and homeostasis. Nonetheless, nearly 90% of patients seeking chiropractic care do so for pain-related neuromusculoskeletal conditions—most commonly back pain, neck pain, and headaches.

Extensive research on the efficacy of spinal manipulation for these ailments (see entry, "Chiropractic Research"), especially lower back pain, has over the past two decades permitted chiropractic to move significantly toward mainstream status. Based on an extensive literature review and consensus process, the 1994 Guidelines for Acute Lower Back Pain, developed by the

Agency for Health Care Policy and Research of the U.S. Department of Health and Human Services, concluded that of the wide range of therapies in use, only two nonsurgical professional interventions for lower back pain had adequate research support: nonsteroidal anti-inflammatory drugs and spinal manipulation (Bigos et al., 1994). Of the two, only spinal manipulation, 94% of which is provided by chiropractors, was judged to both relieve pain and restore proper function.

Chiropractors are licensed throughout the English-speaking world and in an increasing number of other nations. In the United States, home to more than four-fifths of the world's 60,000 chiropractors, among the significant markers of progress in the last generation are inclusion of chiropractic services in Medicare and federal worker's compensation insurance, approval of the Council of Chiropractic Education as the accrediting agency for chiropractic colleges, and establishment of the Center for Chiropractic Research as part of the National Institutes of Health.

DANIEL REDWOOD

See also
  Back Pain (II)
  Headache (II)
  Pain (II)

CHIROPRACTIC RESEARCH

Research on spinal manual therapy (SMT) has focused on neuromusculoskeletal ailments, which comprise close to 90% of chiropractic cases. Back pain, neck pain, and headaches have been explored most extensively, with data on lower back pain (LBP) by far the most substantial. There are now approximately 40 clinical trials on spinal manipulation; at least 25 controlled trials had been published in English by 1992 (Anderson et al., 1992).

Among the earliest landmarks was the 1985 study at the University of Saskatchewan by W. H. Kirkaldy-Willis, an orthopedic surgeon, and J. D. Cassidy, a chiropractor. This retrospective study, the first joint publication in a medical journal by a medical doctor/doctor of chiropractic team, evaluated 283 subjects who had been totally disabled (unable to work or perform normal daily activities) by LBP for an average of 7 years and had previously undergone the full gamut of standard medical interventions. After 2 to 3 weeks of daily chiropractic adjustments, between 79% and 93% of those patients without spinal stenosis had good to excellent results, reporting substantially decreased pain and increased mobility. Even among those with stenosis, classically a difficult subset, a measurable minority showed substantial improvement. After chiropractic treatment, over 70% of those studied were improved to the point of having no work restrictions. Long-term follow-up demonstrated that the changes were sustained.

The first randomized controlled trial (RCT) on SMT for LBP was published by British orthopedic surgeon T. W. Meade and colleagues in 1990. Over 700 subjects received either SMT or standard outpatient treatment for LBP, which consisted of physical therapy (PT) and wearing a corset. The study yielded demonstrably superior results for the chiropractic group. Meade concluded, "For patients with low-back pain in whom manipulation is not contraindicated, chiropractic almost certainly confers a worthwhile, long-term benefit in comparison to hospital outpatient management."

There have been far fewer trials on neck pain than LBP. Unlike the LBP literature, more of the neck pain studies have focused on subacute and chronic pain rather than acute conditions. Currently there are five RCTs on SMT for subacute/chronic neck pain and none for acute neck pain. In the Netherlands, Koes and colleagues compared SMT, PT, and treatment by a general practitioner (GP) for neck and back complaints (1992). Both SMT and PT proved far superior to GP treatment. Compared with PT, SMT patients on average showed somewhat greater improvement in fewer visits. Another neck pain trial was conducted by Cassidy and colleagues (1992), who studied 100 subjects with unilateral neck pain with referral into the trapezius. SMT proved superior to PT in terms of immediate pain relief. It should be noted that studies that compare SMT with other therapies tend to obscure the full benefit of SMT, which can be judged more accurately when an SMT group is compared with one receiving no treatment.

Six RCTs have studied SMT for headaches. Most dramatic among these is the 1995 study by Boline and colleagues on tension headaches. In that study, 126 patients received either SMT or the tricyclic antidepressant amitriptyline, a widely utilized headache medication. During the 4- to 6-week treatment phase of the trial, pain relief among those treated with medication was comparable with the SMT group. After treatments were completed, the chiropractic patients maintained their levels of improvement, while the amitriptyline group returned to pretreatment pain levels in an average of 4 weeks following discontinuation. A reasonable conclusion is that while amitriptyline suppressed symptoms, chiropractic adjustments addressed the problem at a more causal level. The investigators are now pursuing comparative studies on migraine headaches.

A 1997 RCT by Winters and colleagues compared SMT, PT, and corticosteroid injections for 172 patients with shoulder pain. For patients with "shoulder girdle" pain, those receiving manipulation of the spine and shoulder fared best by far in terms of pain relief. For the "synovial" group—those whose pain focused at the glenohumeral joint—the corticosteroid injection group fared best.

Research on SMT for visceral disorders is currently far less developed than research on musculoskeletal disorders. Pilot studies on conditions including dysmenorrhea (Kokojohn et al., 1992) and duodenal ulcers (Pikalov & Kharin, 1994) have been promising, but further research is necessary before any conclusions on the efficacy of SMT for internal organ conditions can be reached.

DANIEL REDWOOD

COGNITIVE-BEHAVIORAL INTERVENTIONS

Central to cognitive-behavioral therapy is the assumption that individuals contribute to their own psychological problems, by the manner in which they interpret events and situations in their life. The basic premise of cognitive-behavioral therapy is that a reorganization of self-statements can result in a parallel reorganization of behavior.

Borrowed from a learning-theory framework, an individual's thoughts are explicit behaviors that can be modified, in the same way overt behaviors can be modified. Behavioral techniques that have been employed to modify overt, physical behaviors such as operant conditioning, modeling, and rehearsal, can be adapted to the more covert and subjective processes of cognition and internal dialogue. Simply stated, what individuals say to themselves directly influences the things they do. Therefore, primary importance is given to the role of self-talk.

The therapeutic emphasis is on acquiring practical coping skills for problematic situations. The therapeutic process consists of educating clients to modify the instructions they give to themselves so they can cope more effectively with the problems encountered in life.

While cognitive-behavioral therapy is comprehensive and eclectic, there are common denominators. First and foremost, all cognitive-behavioral therapies stress the importance of cognitive processes as determinants of behavior. It is maintained that how people feel and what they actually do are heavily influenced by a subjective assessment of the situation. Since the evaluation of life situations is influenced by beliefs, attitudes, assumptions, and internal dialogue, such thoughts become the major focus of therapy.

Cognitive-behavioral therapists are customarily eclectic in selecting therapeutic interventions. Most concentrate on cognitive and behavioral strategies that are designed to uproot the irrational or unfounded beliefs that guide self-defeating feelings.

Since behavior and emotions are viewed as a product of cognitive processes, the therapist's major function and role is that of a diagnostician and educator. The main goals of the therapist are to expose maladaptive thoughts and to help the client develop new and more productive cognitive and behavioral standards. Therapists have the liberty to develop their own personal style and to exercise creativity within the cognitive-behavior framework. However, it has been suggested that cognitive-behavioral therapists need to master a number of skills. Therapists are encouraged to be diversified in teaching ability and technical skills. Therapists must be good listeners, accurate observers, and effective problem-solvers. While cognitive-behavioral therapists are not bound by fixed techniques for specific problems, Meichenbaum (1975) described a variety of assessment and intervention techniques standard to cognitive-behavioral therapy. A brief overview of specific interventions follows.

The Clinical Interview

The cognitive-behavioral therapist assesses the nature of the client's behaviors and accompanying thought processes in the clinical interview. Attention is directed toward the manner in which these two aspects of the client interact. The clinical setting and interview are viewed as a representation of the client's experiences outside of the therapy session; thus, the clinical interview is seen as a microcosm of the client's perceptions. A theme of experiences associated with the presenting problem may be described by the client, at which time the therapist may explore other situations where similar cognitions, affects, or behaviors were experienced. Thus, the clinical interview becomes a tool to explore the extent of the client's symptoms.

The clinical interview emphasizes the client's elaboration of the areas of concern that led him or her to originally seek counseling. Exploration is usually carried out through direct questioning of the client, in a supportive and encouraging atmosphere. Open-ended questions serve to minimize therapist bias. After a series of direct yet gentle questions, the therapist may begin to help the client state goals for therapy.

In the early phases of therapy, the clinical interview should involve three key objectives. First, the therapist should conceptualize the thoughts, affects, behaviors, and environmental situations cardinal to the client's presenting problems. Secondly, the cognitive-behavior therapist should grasp the manner in which the thoughts, affects, and behaviors interact, resulting in the client's psychological distress, and to increase his or her coping abilities. Thirdly, a determination should be made of which thoughts, affects, behaviors, and environmental cues are missing from the individual's repertoire but if present would decrease the client's distress and increase coping skills.

Imagery-Based Techniques

Meichenbaum (1975) advocated to encourage the client to envision a time when the presenting problem first surfaced. As if viewing a movie or television show, the client may remember details of an event that otherwise would have been forgotten. This technique is especially helpful in emotional situations when important details may be overlooked. Specific consideration should be devoted to the way in which clients perceive the event.

Imagery techniques are also useful in exploring a client's potential for growth. A client may be asked to imagine himself or herself performing more adaptive be-

haviors or repeating positive self-statements in challenging situations (covert behavioral rehearsal). A client may also be instructed to imagine pleasurable or relaxing images to balance out feelings of anxiety (Singer, 1974).

Behavioral Assessment and Situational Analysis

Another way to access the private thoughts and affects of a client is by asking him or her to perform the problematic behavior in a situation that is either realistic or an enactment of the behavior in a therapy session. As part of the behavioral rehearsal, the therapist may probe the client concerning his or her thoughts and self-statements.

If the client is asked to perform a difficult behavioral task outside the therapeutic settings, the behavior may be assessed in either a priori or post-hoc manner. The therapist may instruct the client to devote attention to any self-talk or internal dialogues while performing the behavior; or the therapist may question the client after performing the behavior. In either scenario, the behavior is perceived and assessed in a new way. Of primary importance is the encouragement given to the client. Evaluation of problematic behaviors should be performed in a way to increase the client's sensitivity to previously concealed yet vital aspects of the individual environment/behavioral construct.

Decision-Making and Problem-Solving Strategies

This intervention instructs the clients in specific problem-solving strategies. Techniques may include the ability to acknowledge and define the problem, develop realistic and governable decision maps, assess the pros and cons of decisions, create alternatives to difficult situations, develop a concrete plan of action, and judge the outcome of the decision (Kanfer & Busemeyer, 1982).

Problem-solving skills provide the client with tools to create alternative solutions. The goal of teaching problem-solving skills is for the client to solve problems once therapy has been terminated.

Self-Efficacy Training

How a client feels about himself or herself in any given scenario influences the person's decision to engage or avoid certain activities. Individuals tend to avoid activities that they believe are outside the range of their capability (Bandura, 1982). One of the interventions used in cognitive-behavioral therapy is to create an environment to bolster self-efficacy expectations. This can be achieved by helping the client delineate the past versus the present. A review of the client's progress of behavioral change can increase perceptions of self-efficacy.

The therapist may also encourage a client to become more objective in his or her personal assessment. An objective vantage point helps the client achieve a more accurate and less distorted view of self and of the environment.

Self-Monitoring Procedures

Client-specific, structured self-monitoring sheets can be created to monitor problematic thoughts, affects, behaviors, or environmental circumstances. The self-monitoring procedure is not only helpful for reality testing but also serves to reinforce new behaviors after the completion of therapy.

Coping Skills

Instead of solving each particular problem a client may present, a therapist will concentrate on teaching the client a methodology of productive and effective coping skills that can be generalized to a variety of situations. Generalized coping skills will place particular focus on the client's accurate assessment of self-appraisal and the actual practice of specific coping behaviors.

Cognitive-behavioral therapists can incorporate a rich array of intervention strategies into the course of therapy. All strategies serve to increase the knowledge of the interaction of thoughts, affects, behavior, and the environment for the expressed purpose of greater personal adaptability and productivity. Regardless of the techniques used, the final goal should be a greater understanding of the client's maladaptive self-talk and behaviors.

PAMELA L. HAMILTON

COGNITIVE-BEHAVIORAL THERAPY

Cognitive-behavioral therapy is one of the many and varied techniques mental health professionals employ to help individuals lead more productive lives. Cognitive-behavioral therapy aids the client by exploring the relationship between thoughts, feelings, and behaviors. According to cognitive-behavioral theory, there is a direct correlation between a client's thoughts, feelings, and behaviors. Cognitive-behavioral therapy surmises that difficulties in adjustments, relationships, and general well-being are generated and supported by both cognitive and behavioral factors.

As indicated by the name, cognitive-behavioral therapy subsumes elements of both cognitive and behavioral modalities. Cognitive therapy is a short-term, structured therapy that utilizes active collaboration between the client and therapist to achieve therapeutic goals. Cognitive therapy teaches individuals new, more adaptive ways of thinking and acting, based on the premise that thoughts intervene between events and emotional reactions. Behavioral therapy applies well-established learning principles to eliminate unwanted behaviors. The purpose of behavioral therapy is to replace problem thoughts and maladaptive behaviors with more constructive ways of thinking and acting.

Cognitive-behavioral therapy is an integration of two previous divergent therapeutic perspectives. Cognitive-behavioral therapy claims an interactionist perspective regarding the determinants of human behavior and mental health. The core of this perspective maintains that the interaction between the individual and the environment determines cognitions, affects, and behavior.

Historical Overview

The foundation of cognitive-behavioral therapy was established with the resurgent interest in cognition that popularized psychology during the late 1960s and early 1970s. A review of the research literature suggested a shift from radical behaviorism to cognitive-oriented processes (Mahoney, 1974). Higher mental processes of observational learning, thinking, language use, and problem solving were emphasized by the cognitive perspective. People were viewed as active participants in the processing of environmental stimuli, rather than as passive recipients of environmental consequences. Of central importance to this model was the human ability to explore thought, affect, and behavior, and in particular the interrelationship between the three variables.

Historically, cognitive psychology focused on the irrational and problematic thinking habits that were concomitant with psychological distress. In fact, individuals plagued by psychological disorders were thought to participate in inappropriate and maladaptive cognitive patterns. Simply stated, how an individual thought determined how that individual felt. Thus, the crux of cognitive therapy centered on challenging maladaptive, self-defeating thought patterns and replacing them with healthy, goal-oriented facilitative thinking. Mastery of cognitive strategies provided the client with tools to enjoy a more productive lifestyle. Cognitive interventions have been demonstrated to be especially effective in the treatment of anxiety and depression.

Behavioral therapies were derived from the principles of classical and operant conditioning. As a result of experience or associative learning, individuals responded in predictable ways to stimuli. Contingencies were thought to govern human behavior. Some of the learned responses have been maladaptive or ineffective, leading to discomfort. Instead of trying to alleviate distressing behaviors by addressing an assumed underlying problem, behavioral therapy applied well-established learning principles to eliminate the inappropriate behavior. Behavioral therapy attempted to replace problem thoughts and maladaptive behaviors with more constructive ways of thinking and behaving.

Behavioral interventions have been successful in the management of a wide variety of behaviors, including phobias, maladaptive habits, anxiety, and depression. The overall goal of behavior interventions is to aid the client to develop healthy and supportive behaviors in response to life.

Central to cognitive-behavior therapy is its hybrid origin from the cognitive and behavior schools. The basic tenet of cognitive-behavioral therapy is an interactionist perspective concerning the determinants of human behavior and psychological wellness. A recent survey identified nearly two dozen distinct varieties of cognitive-behavioral therapies (Dobson, 1988). Among the most influential theorists are Albert Ellis (1984) with rational emotive therapy, Maxie Maultsby (1984) with rational behavior therapy, Aaron T. Beck (1976) with cognitive therapy, and Donald Meichenbaum (1977) with self-instructional therapy.

Goals of Cognitive-Behavioral Therapy

The major goal of cognitive-behavioral therapy is to alter clients' interpretation of themselves and their environment, along with the manner by which they create those interpretations. Throughout the course of therapy, therapists challenge the clients' view of themselves and their environment. Clients are instructed in new methods of interpreting themselves and their environment. Specific interventions address new ways of thinking about themselves and their environment.

Goals are obtained by therapeutic confrontations and acquisition of new skills, with particular emphasis on coping mechanisms. Depending on the nature of the therapist and client, a variety of skills may be emphasized. Specifically, relaxation training (Goldfried, 1977), cognitive coping abilities (Goldfried, 1980), imagery (Crits-Christoph & Singer, 1981), self-efficacy (Bandura, 1982), problem solving (Kanfer & Busemeyer, 1982), self-instructional methods (Meichenbaum, 1977), irrational beliefs (Ellis, 1987), or automatic thoughts (Beck, 1976) may be featured as therapeutic interventions.

Cost-effective treatment is another major goal of cognitive-behavioral therapy. Short-term contracts (15 to 25 sessions) are often established to ensure affordable treatment. To this end, clients are expected to rehearse skills, complete homework tasks, and gradually assume responsibility for continued improvement. These methods also serve to increase the probability that therapeutic gains will continue beyond the contracted sessions.

While cognitive-behavioral therapy has generalized goals, specific goals are created as a mutual exercise between the therapist and the client. A skilled cognitive-behavioral therapist will listen attentively, tap into professional and personal resources, and create a therapeutic environment to meet the client's needs in a productive and efficient manner.

PAMELA L. HAMILTON

COLOR THERAPY

Color therapy is the application of colored light to the body for the purpose of correcting disharmony, which may manifest in physical or emotional disease. Color therapists visually assess a client's energy field or aura (*chakra*) for darkness or discoloration over a body part. Colored light is administered through lamps fitted with colored glass plates or plastic gels. Color also can be taken into the body through color meditation and breathing or by drinking color-treated water.

History and Theory

The power of color is described in many ancient texts. In the Bible's book of Genesis, the rainbow is a sign of God's covenant and spiritual protection. In Tibetan yoga, the subtle body of an enlightened yogi is called a rainbow body. Hindu tradition states that each of the seven *chakras* is associated with a specific astral sound and one of the colors of the rainbow. In ancient Egypt, India, and China, there were systems of color science practiced and researched in special color temples or halls.

In the past century, Dr. S. Pan Coast wrote a treatise in 1877 entitled *Blue and Red Light, or Light and Its Rays as Medicine*. Dr. D. E. Babbitt published a book on the power of different colors and the healing effects in 1878. In 1933, D. P. Ghadiali developed color lamps and wrote *The Specto-Chromometry Encyclopedia*, which described color therapy.

All colors represent the energy of light waves in motion vibrating at distinct and measurable rates. Some color therapists believe that color is the visible expression of divinity or the unifying principle manifesting as different light rays. This is based on a belief in the laws of sevenfold nature of humankind and the division of the solar spectrum into seven colors. Some systems teach that each of the seven *chakras* gives off one of the seven colors of the rainbow. When a person is healthy and the *chakras*

are open, all the colors of the rainbow appear in the aura; when there is serious physical, emotional, or spiritual imbalance, colors may appear impure, blotchy, or missing. The vibratory energy of color breaks up blockages, releasing energy and allowing it to flow freely.

Another system of color healing theorizes that all diseases are either acute (hot) or chronic (cold) and that these can be corrected or balanced by the application of cold or warm colors. The hot colors are lemon, yellow, orange, red, and scarlet. Cold colors are turquoise, blue indigo, violet, and purple. Green and magenta are considered neutral colors. Color healing works through the aura to make changes, and only the amount necessary will be accepted. It works by loosening and eliminating toxins from the body.

Many intuitive healers do not "think" a particular color when doing a color treatment but actually try to "be" the color. Instead of controlling the color coming through them, they try to sustain whatever color comes to them spontaneously.

Western science views light and color as being separate from consciousness and as having no inherent spiritual essence or divine qualities. Light behaves both as a wave and as a particle. Color in pigment is a dance of duality between light waves and atomic particles.

Lin Yun's theory of color is both Eastern and Western. Expanding on the system of Feng Shui, the Chinese art of optimal placement, Lin believes that color is a manifestation of cosmic energy (*ch'i*) that can shape an individual's personal energy and destiny. This theory can be applied to simple color cures, such as wearing the right color to a job interview, and to esoteric ideas on color, linking color to both tangible and intangible elements of the universe.

Color Meditation

By visualizing color with the inner eye, one can take in color. Some color therapists believe that color visualization is most effective when combined with color breathing. This is done by visualizing and inhaling a band of color arching up from the earth and flowing into a target *chakra*, exhaling and fixing it there. Or it can be done by imagining soft, oncoming waves of color starting at the feet and reaching overhead. The benefits of healing can be transmitted to another person in the same room or at any distance.

Therapeutic Value of Colors

There is general agreement among the more recently created color systems about the qualities attributed to each of the following colors:

Red controls the first *chakra* and is stimulating and invigorating to the physical body.

Orange controls the second *chakra* and has a powerful tonic effect on body and mind.

Yellow is absorbed through the third *chakra* and vitalizes and stimulates mental activity.

Green is the color of the fourth *chakra* and is a balancing color. It brings a feeling of renewal and new life.

Blue is absorbed by the fifth *chakra* and brings peace to the whole being.

Indigo is used by the sixth *chakra* and clears the psychic currents of the body.

Purple is absorbed by the seventh *chakra* and has the highest vibration of the cosmic energy rays. It soothes processes of the central nervous system and is especially associated with spiritual development.

JILL STRAWN

COOLING AND MULTIPLE SCLEROSIS

It has been shown scientifically that abnormally myelinated nerve fibers are sensitive to changes in core body temperature (Davis, 1970). Researchers demonstrated that a rise in core body temperature can result in failure of nerve conduction and worsening of the symptoms of multiple sclerosis (Watson, 1959). Conversely, it has also been demonstrated the symptoms of MS can be improved by cooling the body (Simons, 1937).

Anecdotal personal accounts and studies involving cold water immersion support the theory that cooling the body does provide temporary symptom relief for MS sufferers. However, it is inconvenient, uncomfortable, and/or impractical to take cold baths several times a day or to sit too close to air-conditioning. Indeed, it may even be dangerous because the body's defense systems produce shivering and vasoconstriction (Basset & Lake, 1958).

The National Aeronautics and Space Administration (NASA) needed to develop pressurized space suits to remove the thermal energy of metabolic heat produced by an astronaut's body when performing activity in space performed outside the protection of a space vehicle. If the thermal energy trapped in the astronaut's pressurized suit is not removed, the body temperature would quickly rise to dangerous levels.

Working with a concept originally developed by the British to cool pilots of high-performance aircraft who needed to wear protective pressurized suits, NASA scientists developed their own version of these liquid cooling garments (LCGs). The units contained a network of small tubes pressed against the body. Water chilled by a cooling reservoir outside the suit is pumped through these tubes. Heat transfer between the skin and the cold water in the tubes removes the body's metabolic heat. The resulting warm water is pumped from the garment to an external cooling reservoir, where it is rechilled and pumped back into the suit in a repeating pattern.

"Cool suits" were first used by NASA in the 1960s and 1970s for the Apollo missions. Since then, LCG technology has been refined for ground use for individuals who must work in hot environments. A number of firms now produce LCGs to address the heating/cooling needs of military and industrial occupations.

NASA scientists used their expertise with LCGs to refine and adapt this technique for the advancement of biomedical research. These developments include cooling systems for cancer patients undergoing chemotherapy, children who suffer from HED (insufficient sweat glands), and MS patients.

Early in 1992, the Multiple Sclerosis Association of America (MSAA) began funding scientific research on the clinical effects of cooling and multiple sclerosis. On May 23, 1994, representatives from MSAA and NASA signed a historic Memorandum of Understanding to develop guidelines for cooperative efforts to enhance the performance of cooling systems for use by MS patients. Spinoff technologies will be analyzed that may prove beneficial to MS patients and others who are physically challenged. To date, MSAA has committed more than $2 million in assets to the advancement of research on cooling and multiple sclerosis.

In the spring of 1996, a clinical study of heat-sensitive MS patients showed that acute, controlled microclimate body cooling at 7° C for 60 minutes could effectively and safely:

1. Decrease body temperature as measured by oral and tympanic methods.
2. Decrease systemic stress.
3. Increase motor function as measured by significant increases in strength of powerful ambulatory muscles, significant increases in static (single leg standing and balance test) and dynamic (tandem gait) coordination, and significant increases in local and systemic endurance activity.
4. Produce heat loss within MS persons that is significantly correlated to motor function changes (i.e., the more heat lost the more motor function gained).

These studies confirmed previous conclusions that cool baths eased the symptoms of MS.

Subjectively and objectively, gains were noticed in the ability of heat-sensitive MS patients to perform repetitive activities. This is an important finding because it is repetitive motor tasks that elicit extreme local and central fatigue in MS patients. Such simultaneous symptomatic relief from fatigue and from strength and coordination loss would be of significant benefit to MS patients who enjoy physical activity and independence.

STEVE SHAPIRO

See also
Multiple Sclerosis (II)

CRANIOSACRAL THERAPY

Craniosacral therapy is a hands-on modality that focuses on the normalization of bodily functions that are either part of or related to a physiological system called the craniosacral system. This body system is composed of the watertight compartment formed by the dura mater membrane and the cerebrospinal fluid within, as well as the bones to which the dura mater attaches, the joints or sutures that interconnect these bones, and other bones that are indirectly connected to the dura mater.

The concept of a functioning craniosacral system is based on the rhythmical rise and fall of cerebrospinal fluid volume and pressure within the dura mater compartment, which is regulated by related inflow and outflow control mechanisms. The changing cerebrospinal fluid volume and pressure cause corresponding changes in dura mater membrane tensions that induce small accommodative movement patterns in these membranes. Research at Michigan State University showed that the bones that directly relate to the dura mater must be in continual, minute motion to accommodate the constant fluid pressure changes within the membrane compartment. This finding is consistent with those published in *Anatomica Humanica* by Guiseppi Sperino, in which he noted that cranial sutures fuse before death only under pathological circumstances. Conversely, British anatomists maintain that human sutures fuse rather early in life, although more recently the 30th American Edition of *Gray's Anatomy* acknowledges that some cranial sutures possess potential for movement throughout life.

The craniosacral system strongly influences the physiological environment of its contents, which include the brain, the spinal cord, the cranial nerves, the spinal nerve roots, and several of the ganglia that are enclosed within the dura mater membrane compartment. Also affected are the pituitary gland and its related structures, the pineal gland, the ventricular system of the brain, the enclosed blood vascular structures including the arterial system, the venous system, and some lymphatic drainage subsystems. The various cisternae of the cranium, the interstitial and intracellular fluids, the arachnoid membrane, the pia mater, and the subarachnoid and the subdural spaces are strongly influenced by the function of the craniosacral system.

When there is impairment of the natural mobility of the dura mater and/or any of its attached bones, the function of the craniosacral system is hindered. More peripherally located bones and connective tissues that attach either directly or indirectly to the craniosacral system also may impair that system's function. Compromise of accommodative motion of the craniosacral system can result in dysfunction of any of the structures within the craniosacral system and/or their related systems.

Restrictions of normal mobility of the craniosacral system can be detected, localized, and corrected by skilled therapists using palpation to evaluate and enhance the optimum function of the craniosacral system. A basic tenet of craniosacral therapy is that each client's body contains information to uncover the cause of health problems. It is the task of the therapy practitioner to communicate with the client's body, primarily through light and gentle touch, to obtain this information and become a facilitator of the client's own self-correcting process.

Inherent in the craniosacral therapy approach is the ultimate integration of the client's body with the mind and, ultimately, with the spiritual aspects of life. Often, there are emotional components to the physical/somatic problems just as there can be physical elements to emotional issues. As therapy progresses, the spiritual aspect generally comes forth. The skillful craniosacral therapy practitioner does not suggest these integrative steps; rather, he or she simply helps the client to accept body-mind-spirit integrative insights as they appear.

Craniosacral therapy is very useful both as a primary treatment modality and as an adjunct. As it enhances the body's own self-corrective mechanisms, the therapy has been useful for a wide variety of problems that are due to physiological imbalances and obstructions. The therapy also is beneficial for many types of visceral dysfunctions. It works well to balance autonomic function and reduce sympathetic nervous system tonus. It has major positive effects in chronic fatigue syndrome, chronic headaches, temporomandibular joint problems, whiplash sequelae, and an assortment of chronic pain syndromes. Craniosacral therapy has been used as intensive treatment for clients rehabilitating from head injuries, craniotomies, spinal cord injuries, post-stroke syndromes, transient ischemic attacks, seizure disorders, and in brain and spinal cord dysfunction problems that have defied conventional diagnosis.

In children, craniosacral therapy has been used effectively in cases of spastic cerebral palsy, seizure disorders, Down's syndrome, and a variety of central nervous system disorders, including problems with the oculomotor system, learning disabilities, attention deficit disorder, speech disorders, childhood allergies, and autonomic dysfunctions, such as colic.

Craniosacral therapy also has been very effective in cases of endogenous depression, often in conjunction with endocrine imbalance. In combination with other body-mind therapies, craniosacral therapy has shown to be very efficacious in cases of post-traumatic stress disorder that is secondary to a wide range of causes from war and abuse to violent acts, such as rape.

Contraindications to craniosacral therapy include any condition in which a subtle change in intracranial fluid pressure could be deleterious. Among these are acute intracranial aneurysm with threat of rupture, cerebral hemorrhage for other reasons, subdural or subarachnoid bleeding, and increased intracranial pressure that could precipitate a medullary or brain stem herniation through the foramen magnum.

The model of craniosacral therapy today represents the refinement of concepts originally put forth by William G. Sutherland, D.O., in the 1930s. John E. Upledger, D.O., O.M.M., worked with Richard Roppell, Ph.D. (biophysics), Ernest W. Retzlaff, Ph.D. (physiology), Zvi Karni, Ph.D. (biophysics) and D.Sc. (bioengineering), Frederick Becker, Ph.D. (anatomy), and Jon D. Vredevoogd, M.F.A. (Design) from 1975 through 1983 in the Department of Biomechanics at Michigan State University, College of Osteopathic Medicine, to research Dr. Upledger's clinical observations and those of other osteopaths. The research produced—much of it published—formed the basis for the modality Dr. Upledger named craniosacral therapy.

A gentle but powerful modality that focuses on problem solving, craniosacral therapy has attained widespread use due to its effectiveness. By following the body, the practitioner often can uncover the source of pain or dysfunction that is key to the client improving quality of life and reclaiming health.

JOHN E. UPLEDGER

DANCE (ETHNIC) AND MOVEMENT

Dance is an inner experience of one's being, as well as a universal means of communicating one culture to another. It is total experience of self and one's ethnicity (Heber, 1993). Folk or ethnic dance within a culture reveals the value system, perceptions, and the aesthetics of movement as expressed by the dancers' cultural personality as a cultural carrier. Also, dance as a universal form of behavior mirrors the culture in which it flourishes and reflects the political, social, and religious nature of its people.

Theoretical Framework of Ethnic Dance in "Wellness"

In the self-theory approach, the therapist or facilitator and clients need to have full inner awareness, as well as an active, open interaction with the environment. That open energy system provides a therapeutic self-process that creates a simultaneous release of tension, anxiety feelings, and rechanneling of anger and frustration through inner expression of movement.

In the therapeutic process of dance/movement, the therapist or facilitator actively listens to one's self, values, and senses and perceives the attitudes, reaction,

and action of the clients. Simultaneously, the clients participate, value, sense, perceive, react, and actualize behavior during the dance interactive process.

Ethnic Dance Movement (EDM)

Ethnic dance movement (EDM) is a medium of individualized activity of body movement with or without music. EDM is a self-coping strategy of adaptation to maintain physical and mental health. It is a self-motivating therapy in which adaptive, expressive, and communicative behaviors are considered therapeutic interventions either for psychiatric or nonpsychiatric clients.

EDM has the following uses:

- It reduces stress and promotes physical and mental health.
- It promotes creativity.
- It voices religion and magic.
- It expresses psychic energy.
- It provides a holistic mind and body approach to wellness.

In one study by the author, 370 clients participated in an average of six to eight sessions of dance movement/therapy (DMT) over a 3-year period at the Hantelman Unit, Royal University Hospital. The participants were predominantly inpatients who were continuing DMT as part of their psychiatric therapeutic regime. The pre-dance chart survey identified the following percentage of client characteristics: 28% of clients were diagnosed with mood disorders; 45% were diagnosed with anxiety-related disorders; 14% were diagnosed with thought-related disorders; 8% were diagnosed with organic mental disorders; 4% were diagnosed with eating disorders; and 3% were undiagnosed.

Evaluation Summary From the EDM, 1988–1991

Mood

There were 14 clients who did not change in their mood or affect. Eleven clients displayed sadness, and some were tearful; 74 were tense; 104 were smiling with some apprehension; and 60 were smiling and their affect was more congruent with their body movement.

Communications

Five participants refused interaction or refused to touch at all; 27 clients interacted on a one-to-one basis with the dance facilitator or therapist; eight clients interacted with two other clients in the group session; 106 clients had more group interaction when prompted; and 82 were spontaneous in their interaction with other clients in the group, during and after the session.

Motivation

There were four clients who were scheduled to attend, but refused to participate (they sat and watched the session); 56 clients attended only half of the session (either they were late coming to the group, or left early); 89 clients attended the DMT session with prompting and 96 clients attended without prompting; 36 clients were actually involved and leading the group when requested or expressed some ideas to the group.

Psychomotor Activity

There were 21 clients who followed with specific instruction and with minimum body movement; 48 clients whose move-ments were identified predominantly with the body trunk area; 40 clients whose movements were predominantly upper extremities, shoulder, and hands; 28 clients whose body movements were predominantly the lower extremities; and 106 clients who were more coordinated with their body, music, and rhythm.

Self-Esteem

There were 37 clients who expressed their low feelings about themselves and had not changed; 57 clients stated they were feeling good but tired; 54 clients were extremely positive about their experience and stated, "I'm feeling relaxed;" 21 clients did not verbalize, but they were observed as happy and more congruent in their movement; 22 clients stated, "I'm really feeling good about myself," during and after the session.

Choe and Heber (1997) did a study of dance/movement training on the wellness of young women. This quasi-experimental study was designed as a nonequivalent control group pretest-posttest study. Ten healthy female subjects, aged between 19 and 31 years, volunteered for an 8-week dance movement program. Ten healthy female subjects, between 19 and 21 years of age, participated as controls. None of the subjects had performed regular physical activity for 6 months prior to the study. Dance movement was created with reference to Heber's movement guide. Following the 8-week dance movement training, body weight decreased significantly, and circumference of mid-thigh and mid-calf increased. The length of time leg-raising could be held tended to increase following the dance movement training. Resting systolic and resting heart rate showed a tendency to decrease. Total mean score of stress response tended to decrease and mean score of habitual pattern, depression, anxiety/fear, anger and cognitive disorganization decrease after dance movement training.

LOURDES HEBER

DANCE/MOVEMENT THERAPY

In dance/movement therapy, the body movement process is the focal point, in healing and growth, being a primary form of communication and a powerful channel for emotional expression. The American Dance Therapy Association (ADTA) defines dance therapy as the "psychotherapeutic use of movement as a process which furthers the emotional and physical integration of the individual." With expressive movement as the medium for change and conscious growth, attention is paid to outer movement processes which simultaneously reflect inner movement, the felt level of experience. This precedes the conceptual verbal level.

The dance movement therapy process is an integrative one of body, mind, and spirit that affects changes in feelings, cognition, physical functioning, and behavior. Mental and emotional attitudes are reflected when viewing the body at rest and in motion. Symbolic language in movement is universal, and used constructively it facilitates the working through of emotional conflicts and unresolved issues.

The ancient roots of dance therapy lie in the dances and rituals of the medicine men and healers in primitive tribes. The total involvement of the self in the dance has been prominent throughout primitive cultures regardless of historical time or geographic place. Dance was used directly in curing the "sick" and indirectly as an outlet for and expression of emotions. From these origins arise many of the therapeutic concepts affiliated with modern-day dance therapy.

With the advent of modern creative dance in the early 1900s, Western civilization rediscovered the therapeutic benefits of the body-mind-spirit integrative process when engaging in self-expression through dance.

We persist in categorizing our experience to create dichotomous realms of mind-body, spirit-matter, psyche-soma, psychological and physical. We have evolved a tendency to relegate physical and sensory experience to a subordinate position and to emphasize those aspects of life dealing with the intellectual, thinking processes. In the dance movement therapy process, the nonverbal bodily expression of underlying charged emotions can become appropriately discharged and integrated on a cognitive level as the individual begins to increase self-awareness and reintegrate disconnected aspects of self.

Dance/movement therapists work with individuals and groups at all levels of psychological and physical functioning. Children, adults, and older people all display positive responses to this treatment modality. Therapists also work with populations with specific problems, such as addictions (alcohol, drugs, eating disorders), affective and anxiety disorders, special education, and rehabilitation.

Common throughout the healing process are goals that include but are not limited to the following:

1. Facilitate appropriate emotional self-expression and incorporate this

into a functional manner in daily living.

2. Focus on body movement to decrease maladaptive behaviors, release aggressive energy appropriately, and decrease excessive body tension and rigidity.

3. Increase the range of movement and improve body alignment and body awareness.

4. Increase awareness of personal nonverbal and verbal communication systems.

5. Promote interactional skills and establish improved communication patterns.

6. Increase self-esteem, assertiveness, and positive body concept.

7. Increase reality orientation, sensory awareness and sensory input, and decrease tactile defensiveness.

8. Confront and explore nonverbal, maladaptive defense mechanisms.

9. Guide for congruence of verbal and nonverbal affective content.

10. Free and appropriately channel repressed affect and explore a broadening range of emotional response.

11. Enhance kinesthetic awareness and increase awareness of a diminished body armoring.

12. Encourage the synthesizing of the movement experience and symbolism into patients' recurrent maladaptive patterns of living and then follow up via exploration of choices.

Research in the field of dance/movement therapy addresses a wide range of clinical issues and can best be examined via referral to the ADTA's American Journal of Dance Therapy, published annually.

NANCY J. TERRY

DEEP TISSUE THERAPY

"Deep tissue bodywork" is a generic term for any type of massage designed to reach deep muscle tissue and often to cause corrective adjustments to the skeletal system to help return a body to its proper alignment. The therapy seeks to restore full range of motion to joints and improve the blood circulation as does other massage forms. It resembles aspects of rolfing (developed by Dr. Ida Rolf, who was familiar with osteopathy and homeopathy) and Reichian therapy, and some forms of it have developed from practitioners trained in those areas but desiring more flexibility in their practices, since both aforementioned therapies are strictly controlled. Persons who suffered chronic pain have spoken of great relief from deep tissue therapy, some patients experience pain during the sessions or have emotional releases, while others say they feel no pain and fall asleep during the therapy. The therapy is versatile, and the experience of the recipient is highly dependent upon the symptoms brought in to the session.

Other forms of deep tissue therapy include deep muscle massage, Pfrimmer deep muscle therapy, connective tissue massage, and myotherapy. Myotherapy has several related therapies as well, including trigger point therapy, myofascial release, and neuromuscular massage therapy. Each has overlapping and also unique techniques and routines; for example, a common massage technique is called cross fiber, and yet Pfrimmer therapy specializes in specific cross-fiber techniques. Deep tissue massage may mean many different things to different therapists.

There has been an understanding between the fields of massage and chiropractic not to infringe upon each other's area of practice. Chiropractic would adjust bones and joints, and massage would work on muscles. Rolfing claims to be in neither camp, and therefore deep tissue bodywork also often falls in the gray area between. Deep tissue bodywork should be considered as a more intense form of therapy as compared with, for example, Swedish-style massage, and the same cautions one considers for vigorous massage should be also considered and underscored.

Among the injuries often treated by deep tissue massage therapies are: whiplash, noninjured but yet damaged muscles of the low back and sciatica; and problems with hiatal hernias, colitis, and circulatory problems of varicose veins. Deep tissue massage may be useful after fractures to regain full rehabilitation of the muscles and tendons involved.

The work should not be done on acutely injured muscles, such as tears. In those cases, the massage needs to be lighter. Medical evaluations are always recommended if blood clots or herniation of a disc might be suspected.

In the various forms of myotherapy and deep tissue bodywork, sensitive areas known as trigger points are sought and treated. A trigger point is an area of pain, usually a hard painful lump, considered to be caused by congested circulation that can also cause pain in distant sites. A pain in the back of the head may have a trigger point in a neck or shoulder muscle, for example. These trigger points are pressed, held, and will then stimulate and identify the distant problem areas they cause. Thus, the sore spot on the neck may trigger a familiar headache pain. Resolve the sore spot on the neck and there will be no more headaches caused from it. Often, a single

session may resolve trigger points, although there may be residual soreness for a day or two after the session. Myotherapists may also make use of implements to enhance their thumbs and elbows, such as small wooden tools with rubber tips and grease pencils to mark areas for easy referral when trigger points are found.

Stretching is often suggested as well as a regime of exercises to help keep muscles limber. Many techniques can be learned by clients, who then can use them at home to help remain pain-free or to treat minor problems rather than using analgesic medicines, which only cover the sensation of the problem. Muscle injuries from sports, accidents, or occupational stresses are commonly treated by myotherapists. TMJ syndrome (jaw pain) is perhaps the one pain that helped launch myotherapy into the forefront of the public's eye. Like many other forms of massage, there are enthusiastic supporters who have been relieved of debilitating pains in backs and limbs generally caused by years of relative neglect. To become pain-free has been their motivation to adopt more active participation in their health care and more active lifestyles to maintain that freedom.

LESLIE AGUILLARD

See also
Chiropractic: Practice Issues (I)
Myotherapy (IV)
Rolfing (IV)

DIET AND MOOD

Recent interest in the effects of diet on mood have centered on the effects of tryptophan (the precursor amino acid of serotonin), carbohydrates (linked to serotonin via tryptophan), and folate (a compound intrinsic to the vitamin B complex) on depression. Christensen and Burrows (1990) studied the effects of eliminating refined sucrose and caffeine from the diet of 20 moderately to severely depressed volunteer subjects. Depression was measured on the Beck Depression Inventory (BDI). Seven subjects in the experimental group completed the study. These subjects reported a continued amelioration in their depressive symptoms 3 months after completion of the study. While the authors do not generalize their findings to the general population of depressed individuals, they do hypothesize that the elimination of refined sucrose from the diet of those experiencing atypical depression (symptoms of increased sleep, inertia, overeating, and rejection sensitivity) has beneficial effects. They make no assertion regarding the underlying mechanism of this hypothesis.

In a review of the literature, Christensen and Redig (1993) noted that individuals with bulimia, seasonal affective disorder, premenstrual syndrome, and those in alcohol withdrawal were found to crave carbohydrates, especially simple sugars. However, those increasing their intake of carbohydrates achieved only a short-term elevation in mood. After 1 or 2 hours, these individuals experienced a substantial decrease in their positive mood, along with feelings of fatigue and decreased energy.

Reid and Hammersley (1995) examined the effects of a sucrose drink on mood and appetite. On the Profile of Mood States, female subjects who received a sucrose drink (19/38 adults; total $n = 58$) reported increased energy at 30 minutes postingestion. However, these data were confounded by the intervening ingestion of a nonneutral beverage that contained calories from other sources. When these subjects were excluded, only one subject (female) reported a substantial increase in energy at 30 minutes. Another female subject reported a small increase in energy. Ingestion of the carbohydrate drink resulted in a significant delay in consumption of the next solid meal. From these results, the authors concluded that the proposal that the ingestion of foods high in sugar content influences mood state in such a way that carbohydrate craving is thereby induced, which, in turn, enhances appetite was not supported.

In a two-experiment study, Christensen and Redig (1993) randomly assigned 27 nondepressed (BDI) female subjects to ingest meals that were either predominantly complex carbohydrates, predominately simple carbohydrates, or predominantly protein. Calorie content of the meals remained the same through the manipulation of fat content. In the second experiment, 38 nondepressed (BDI) female subjects were randomly assigned and given the same types of meals, plus one meal similar to the simple carbohydrate meal but with less protein. Mood was measured by the Profile of Mood States. Blood samples were drawn to determine amino acid composition. Both experiments failed to reveal differential mood effects based upon type of meal. The authors postulate that findings of a tryptophan mood link may be most evident in a distressed adult population rather than in a normal population.

The manipulation of fat to yield same-calorie meals may have affected the Christensen and Redig study. Lloyd, Green, and Rogers (1994) studied mood and cognitive performance in relation to fat and carbohydrate meals. Eighteen subjects completed 16 visual analog scales and computer-based cognitive tasks 30 minutes before and 90 and 150 minutes after low-fat/high-carbohydrate (LF/HC), medium-fat/medium-carbohydrate (MF/MC), and high-fat/low-carbohydrate (HF/LC) same calorie meals. Results indicated that the LF/HC and the HF/LC meals both increased feelings of drowsiness and muddledness and produced longer reaction times compared to the MF/MC meal. The authors hypothesize that, since the MF/MC meal closely approximated the subjects' customary meal, meals that differ from an individual's customary intake may have more noticeable effects than meals that are similar to those the individual generally consumes.

The tryptophan mood link was the subject of a study by Lam and colleagues (1996). Volunteer patients who met criteria for seasonal affective disorder (SAD) were withdrawn from medication prior to undergoing light therapy. At the end of treatment, those who had achieved remission with light therapy were entered into a double-blind, two-session study. These 12 subjects were randomized into a rapid tryptophan depletion group and a control group. Two subjects withdrew from the study. Session 2 consisted of repeat measures with reversals of the study groups. The authors found that tryptophan depletion leads to a recurrence of depressive symptoms in patients previously in remission from SAD symptoms following light therapy.

The role of folate in depression was the object of a brief review by Alpert and Fava (1997). They concluded that, while there is evidence of a folate depression link, causality in either direction, if it does exist, cannot be determined at this time. However, the evidence for a folate antidepressant response link is greater. While research in this area is promising, the use of folate or folate assay in the treatment of depression will not be immediately forthcoming.

Finally, Wardle (1995), whose aim was to review the evidence relating lipids to psychological well-being, discovered a U-shaped relationship between cholesterol and total mortality in males. Up to a certain point, lowering cholesterol levels results in a lowered mortality rate. However, after this point is reached, mortality rates begin to climb. From this point on, adverse health outcomes are due to noncardiovascular-related deaths (e.g., suicide). Such findings have come mostly from studies of drug rather than dietary lowering of cholesterol. While Wardle notes that the case for a causal link between low cholesterol and depression looks weak, she does review studies in monkeys that find a low-cholesterol diet resulting in low or reduced serotonin levels.

While the research does indicate that both carbohydrates and proteins (amino acids) affect mood, at least for some subgroups of depressed individuals, via a carbohydrate-amino acid-neurotransmitter pathway, the use of diet or nutritional supplements in the treatment of mood disorders is not in the near future. However, as microassay of neurotransmitters and nutritional status becomes more sophisticated, it may some day be possible to supplement medical and/or psychological treatment of depression with nutrition therapy. Treatment of depression will then become truly multimodal and open the door further for multidisciplinary collaboration.

MARIE LOUISE BERNARDO

See also

Depression (II)

Nondieting (IV)
Nutrition (IV)

ELECTROCHEMICAL TREATMENT OF LOCALIZED TUMORS WITH DIRECT CURRENT

Electrochemical treatment (EChT) of tumors is a method utilizing direct current (d.c.) to produce chemical changes to kill cancer cells. It involves inserting platinum electrodes into tumors. A constant voltage of less than 8 volts is applied to produce a 40 to 80 milliampere (mA) current between the anodes and cathodes for 30 minutes to several hours, delivering 100 coulombs per cubic centimeter. Due to electrolysis, electrophoresis, and electroosmosis, cells near the electrodes are killed by the microenvironmental changes.

The investigation of electrophysiological phenomena can be traced back 200 years; however, EChT of cancer has been used for only a few decades. Reis and Henninger studied the effect of d.c. on Jensen sarcoma in rats. A platinum anode was inserted in the tumor and a cathode on the leg, 18 to 20 mA at 60 to 70 V was delivered for 15 to 20 minutes. After 8 to 10 treatments, the tumors regressed. Björn Nordenström utilized d.c. for treating human lung tumors in the 1970s. The anode was inserted into the tumor and the cathode at least one tumor diameter away in normal lung tissue. His rationale was that the negative electric field of the cathode could push the negatively charged tumor cells away from the cathode and thereby cause metastasis. This method was later introduced to Slovenia, Japan, and China. In China, Dr. Xin Yu-ling modified Nordenström's method by inserting both cathode and anode platinum electrodes into tumors of conscious patients. More than 10,000 patients, most with malignant tumors and some with benign tumors, were treated with EChT. In the United States, EChT has been developing at the City of Hope National Medical Center in Duarte, California, since 1993. Through in vitro and in vivo studies, EChT has been approved for a Phase I clinical trial by the U.S. Food and Drug Administration.

Clinical Uses

Nordenström was the first in recent years to utilize d.c. for treating human tumors. He treated 26 lung metastases in 20 patients. Twelve of the 26 metastases regressed completely. Two patients were still alive 10 years later. In Japan, Nakayama and Matsushima et al. have treated human cancer with EChT combined with chemotherapy and radiation. They summarized 26 cases (the majority of those cases were inoperable due to poor general condition or advanced cancer stage) treated with EChT, including two cases of breast cancer. There was symptom improvement in almost half of the patients, and a decrease in tumor size, to some degree, was observed in 21 measurable lesions. Two tumors disappeared completely, and in one case it was histopathologically verified that no tumor cells remained. This shows the usefulness of EChT alone, since these two tumors had not responded to other previous treatments, including chemotherapy.

In 1987, Nordenström introduced EChT to China. Xin summarized the results of 2,516 cases on 23 types of tumors (including lung, skin, liver, and breast cancer). Most patients were unsuitable for surgery, radiation, or chemotherapy due to poor health, resistance, and tolerance. Total 5-year survival rate was 46.6%. For superficial tumors, 366 skin cancer cases and 95 malignant melanoma cases were treated. The short-term objective responses (complete and partial response) were 91.8% and 94.7%, respectively. Among the 228 breast cancer cases, 31, 121, 41, and 35 were Stages I, II, III, and IV, respectively. Tumor sizes treated were: 3 to 5 cm (56 cases), 5 to 7 cm (99), 7 to 9 cm (61), 9 to 11 cm (9), and greater than 11 cm (3). An overall 62.7% (143/228) 5-year survival rate was achieved, and it was comparable to conventional treatment.

EChT could also be used for deep-seated tumors. Xin reported EChT results on 386 patients with non-small cell lung cancer. The short-term (6 months after EChT) effectiveness of those lung cancer cases were: complete response (CR), 25.6% (99/386); partial response (PR), 46.4% (179/386); no change (NC), 15.3% (59/386); and progressive disease (PD), 12.7% (49/386). The total effective rate (CR + PR) was 72% (278/386). The 1-, 3-, and 5-year overall survival rates were 86.3% (333/386), 58.8% (227/386), and 29.5% (114/386), respectively. The clinical results show that EChT provides an alternative method for treating lung cancers that are conventionally inoperable, not responsive to chemotherapy or radiotherapy, or cannot be resected after thoracotomy.

EChT produces minimum trauma compared with surgery. It preserves the patients' body integrity, functions, and appearance. Furthermore, unlike chemotherapy and radiation, this method has no serious side effects and can be repeated. The local control rates were considered satisfactory compared with conventional therapy. Chinese physicians concluded that EChT is a simple and effective local therapy. This method has been approved by

the Chinese Ministry of Public Health and is used in about 1,000 hospitals in China.

In the United States, a clinical trial conducted at the City of Hope has been approved by the FDA. Five late-stage patients have been treated as of October 1997. Three patients developed complete response, one partial response, and one no response (tumor reduced less than 50%) due to incomplete treatment. All patients tolerated treatment well.

Research Bases

Although a number of laboratory studies have shown that EChT has an antitumor effect, it is not widely used in clinics. The reason is that EChT is not a well-established therapy due to the lack of a standardized method and unclear mechanisms. At this time, different electrode placements have been used in Europe and China. The dosage guideline is arbitrary. Optimal electrode distribution has not been determined. Dose-response relationships are not established. Although it is known that EChT involves electrolysis, electroosmosis, and electrophoresis, the detailed mechanisms of cell killing induced by EChT remain uncertain. It is necessary to conduct basic studies and clinical trials to verify EChT's value. The basic scientific research will help formulate a standardized EChT method for cancer treatment and provide a better understanding of EChT mechanisms. A standardized method will enable physicians to treat those cancer patients who are untreatable with conventional therapies in a consistent and confident manner.

CHUNG-KWANG CHOU
RU-LONG REN

See also
Cancer (II)

ELECTROMAGNETIC HEATING FOR CANCER TREATMENT

Electromagnetic (EM) heating is a major method of cancer hyperthermia treatment. It involves depositing EM energy in a tumor to raise its temperature either locally, regionally, or whole body to a therapeutic level. The EM energy used in hyperthermia is usually classified by frequency as either microwave energy or radiofrequency (RF) energy. Microwaves occupy the EM frequency band between 300 MHz and 300 GHz; RF, between 3 kHz and 300 GHz. In hyperthermia, RF usually refers to frequencies lower than microwaves.

Various forms of hyperthermia were used in the treatment of cancers at a wide range of anatomical sites. Heating methods included whole body heating by hot wax, hot air, hot water suits, or infrared radiation, and partial body heating by either RF EM fields (including microwaves), ultrasound, heated blood, or fluid perfusion. Among those heating methods, EM heating plays a major role. EM heating became very popular after the German physicist Heinrich Hertz demonstrated the physical nature of EM waves and described their characteristic features. D'Arsonval, a French physician-physiologist, reported that such currents could also affect physiological mechanisms in muscles and nerves, and the Croatian physicist Tesla recognized the heating capability of high-frequency currents in various biological tissues. As technology developed, higher frequency EM fields were used. By 1920, shortwave diathermy became the standard approach, with frequencies of up to 100 MHz, and by 1930 with frequencies of 100 MHz to 3,000 MHz. At present, frequencies of 13.56 and 27.12 MHz have been widely used in diathermy and hyperthermia. However, the most commonly used microwave frequencies in hyperthermia are 433, 915, and 2,450 MHz. Frequencies higher than 2,450 MHz have no practical value due to their limited depth of penetration. At lower frequencies, penetration is deeper, but the applicator must be larger and focusing is difficult.

Clinical Uses

Although EM heating methods have been developed for whole body hyperthermia, most are used for local hyperthermia. Applicators in phased arrays have been used for regional heating.

External Heating

The cooling mechanism of superficial tissues makes deep heating difficult by conductive methods. Two basic RF methods have been used to provide subcutaneous heating. First, tissues can be placed between two capacitor plates and heated by displacement currents. This capacitive heating method is simple, but overheating of fat, which is caused by the perpendicular electric field, remains a major problem for obese patients. The second RF method is inductive heating by magnetic fields that are generated by solenoidal loops, or "pancake" magnetic coils, to induce eddy currents in tissue. Because the induced electric fields are parallel to the tissue interface, heating is maximized in muscle rather than in fat.

In microwave frequency range, energy is transferred into tissues by waveguides, dipoles, microstrips (antennas that consist of a thin metallic conductor bounded to a thin grounded dielectric substrate), or other radiating devices. The shorter wavelengths of microwaves, as compared with longer wavelength RF, provide the capability to direct and focus energy into tissues by direct radiation from a small applicator. Engineering developments have focused on the design of new microwave applicators. A number of applicators of various sizes operate over a frequency range of 300 to 1,000 MHz. Most of them are dielectrically loaded and have a water bolus for surface cooling. Low-profile, lightweight microstrip applicators, which are easier to use clinically, have also been reported. Methods based on high-permittivity dielectric material, electric-wall boundary, and magnetic materials have been used to reduce applicator size and mass. These applicators are used, for the most part, for treatment of tumors a few centimeters below the skin. Pain and thermal burns are usually the major problems.

Intracavitary Heating

Certain tumor sites in hollow viscera or cavities may be treated by intracavitary techniques. The advantages of intracavitary hyperthermia include (1) better energy deposition due to the proximity of an applicator to a tumor, and (2) reduction of normal tissue exposure compared with externally induced hyperthermia. There have been clinical and research studies on hyperthermia and radiation or chemotherapy of the esophagus, rectum, cervix, prostate, and bladder cancers. Both RF energy and microwaves (13.56 to 2,450 MHz) have been used for intracavitary hyperthermia. The main problem is that tumor temperature is unknown. Most temperatures were measured on the surface of the applicators,

which can be very different from those in the tumor.

Interstitial Heating

Tissues can be heated by alternating RF currents conducted through needle electrodes. The operating frequency should be higher than 100 kHz to prevent excitation of nerve action potentials. The advantage of this technique includes better control of temperature distributions within the tumor compared with those of externally induced hyperthermia, and sparing of normal tissue, especially the overlying skin. Also, microwaves can be used for interstitial heating; small microwave antennas inserted into hollow plastic tubing can produce satisfactory heating patterns at frequencies from 300 to 2,450 MHz. A common frequency used in the United States is 915 MHz. A small coaxial antenna can irradiate a volume of approximately 60 cc. With a multinode coaxial antenna, the extent of the heating pattern can be extended to approximately 10 cm in a three-node antenna. For large tumors, it is necessary to use an array of microwave antennas. As in resistive RF hyperthermia, the degree of control of microwaves radiating from these antennas is important in achieving homogeneous heating. Because the antennas couple to each other, the spacing, phasing, and insertion depth affect the heating patterns of array applicators. Ferromagnetic seed implants is another kind of interstitial heating. This technique is applicable for delivering thermal energy to deep seated tumors. When exposed to RF magnetic fields (100 kHz), the implants absorb energy and become heated. When a Curie point is reached, absorption stops. Temperature control can be achieved by selecting proper seed material.

Current Status and Future of Hyperthermia

Although several thousand cancer patients have now been treated with hyperthermia, it has not become part of the routine cancer treatment modalities. Particularly in the United States, interest in the application of hyperthermia to cancer treatment has steadily declined during the past five years due to two negative results of Phase III clinical trials. Clinical hyperthermic oncology is having a difficult time.

Despite the slow pace of investigation into thermal effects in U.S. clinics, several important studies are ongoing and strong interest persists in Europe and Asia. Recently, positive clinical results have emerged from well-controlled Phase III randomized trials (including melanomas and head, neck, and breast tumors), where good quality assurance has been implemented. According to the literature, there is no doubt that hyperthermia would provide a significant and worthwhile improvement in cancer control. Future basic studies should give more attention to the following areas of research: (1) better biological knowledge with regard to effects of thermal cytotoxicity in normal and tumor tissue, sequencing of modalities and impact of thermotolerance, etc.; (2) better physics and engineering support with regard to homogeneity of the power deposition, improved methods of treatment planning, and better ratio of power deposition to tumor volume, noninvasive thermometry control, etc.; and (3) better pain control.

CHUNG-KWANG CHOU
RU-LONG REN

ESALEN MASSAGE

Esalen massage establishes a functional intersection of sensory awareness and massage, interweaving tactile sensitivity, breath awareness, and heartfelt communication as the conscious threads that unite its eclectic approach to bodywork. Sometimes known as "intuitive" or "environmental" massage, Esalen massage's emphasis, unlike other hands-on treatment modalities, is less on stimulating physiological processes than on creating an environment to heighten a naturally therapeutic self-awareness. Slow, lengthening, and unifying strokes, rhythmic rocking and stretching, passive range-of-motion joint movement, deep muscle bundle manipulation, subtle cranial balancing, and Chinese acupressure-like precision are blended into a primarily meditative approach to somatic work.

Esalen massage is defined as "a way of exploring, person-to-person, a matrix of physical, psychological, energetic and spiritual awareness united by the balm of touch" (Ostrom, 1997). Central to the approach are the attitudes of respect for the whole person and an active rather than passive client participation. Known for its mindfulness and sensuality, Esalen massage builds its therapeutic outcomes not by working on areas of dysfunction or pain but by eliciting pleasurable feelings and sensations to override and relieve sore areas. Its goal is to ground the client in the natural therapeutics of the body.

Esalen massage comes as a direct outcropping of the Esalen Institute in Big Sur, California, where it originated 35 years ago and where it remains rooted both geographically and philosophically. The massage style reflects Esalen's goals of integrating body awareness into an ongoing educational program dedicated to unlocking and exploring human potential.

The Institute was founded by Michael Murphy and Richard Price in 1962, in the form of a residential educational center on 27 acres of the Big Sur coastline. Esalen soon became a showcase for cutting-edge approaches in psychology and personal growth, and a mecca for philosophers, scientists, religious teachers, therapists, and artists seeking to balance the mainstream's focus on intellectual and vocational education with sensory, kinesthetic, emotional, interpersonal, and spiritual training. The format of residential experiential workshops, retreats, and ongoing classes dedicated to self-enrichment continues to this day.

The recognition of the innate unity of psychological and somatic processes, paramount in the Esalen approach as a whole, spilled over into the arena of its evolving bodywork style. Esalen massage over the last 35 years has been equally influenced by psychotherapeutic and bodywork innovations presented to the public at the Institute. Notables include giants like Gestalt therapy's Fritz Perls, family therapy's Virginia Satir, and psychosynthesis's Roberto Assagioli, and bodywork greats like Ida Rolf with her structural realignment and Moshe Feldenkreis with his facilitated movement work. Sensory awareness was introduced and popularized by Bernard Gunther. Elements of meditation, ritual, dance, drumming, yoga, *t'ai chi*, and, more recently, sports massage have since been added and blended together to form a holistically oriented, unified, yet eclectic bodywork offering. Freeing the blocks of the body as a pathway to knowing and freeing

the self was popularized via Esalen massage.

As the demand for Esalen's bodywork approach grew, the Institute had its massage program accepted by the state of California in 1984, and it currently offers its unique massage training, integrating basic Swedish massage-type skills, anatomy, meditation, movement, and sensory awareness, in classes ranging from 2 days to 3 months in duration. A newly formed Esalen Massage and Bodywork Association provides a forum for information exchange regarding practitioners and classes worldwide.

ANDY BERNAY-ROMAN

EXERCISE

Physical exercise is movement of the body that promotes the health and fitness of the individual. There are three primary components of fitness: muscular strength, flexibility, and cardiorespiratory endurance. For each of these components, there are a wide variety of physical exercise options.

Cardiorespiratory endurance exercises are better known as aerobic activity. Aerobic activity consists of continuous movement for a minimum of 20 minutes within a range of exertion that can benefit an individual's heart, lungs, and vascular system. The American College of Sports Medicine recommends that individuals participate in aerobic activity for 20 to 45 minutes 3 to 5 times a week. This type of exercise includes walking, running, swimming, and bicycling. The range of intensity should be between 60% and 85% of an individual's maximum heart rate. A stress test by a physician can most accurately identify this information. An estimated target heart rate can be calculated by subtracting an individual's age from 220, multiplying that by .60 and then .85. This will identify the rate of beats per minute necessary to strengthen the cardiorespiratory system. It is recommended that an individual should consult a physician before beginning any exercise program. F.I.T.—frequency, intensity, and time—are three important variables in an exercise program. An exercise program should begin slowly, and as the body accommodates gradually increase these variables.

Muscular strength and endurance are acquired through resistance-oriented physical exercises. This form of training is beneficial in developing lean muscle tissue and increasing the body's metabolic rate (the number of calories the body requires in a 24-hour period). Strength training is beneficial for the musculoskeletal structure of the body and is most effective for both weight loss and health promotion when combined with aerobic activity. Various forms of resistance can be used for strength training, such as water, weights, and rubber tubing. Most individuals are encouraged to participate in some form of strength training 2 to 3 times a week.

Flexibility is developed through specific stretching exercises. Flexibility is an important component of fitness. Stretching the muscle tissue can increase an individual's range of motion, reduce the risk of musculoskeletal injury, and offer relaxation benefits for both the body and the mind. Stretching exercises designed to increase flexibility are most effective when the body is warmed up, such as following aerobic activity. Muscle-specific stretches can be beneficial before beginning a workout or other athletic activities, such as golf or tennis. There are a variety of stretches and techniques to choose from.

Physical exercise can extend beyond the three components of fitness addressed above. Taking stairs instead of elevators, parking further away from shopping destinations and walking the extra distance, going for a short stroll during lunch breaks, or even involving oneself in activities and interests that include movement such as dancing and gardening are also health promoting activities.

In years past, everyday life required plenty of physical exertion. Exercise was experienced through daily labors for survival. The urbanization and industrialization of the 1800s started to change society's daily behavioral patterns. Health and fitness became more of a societal concern during World War II, when approximately one third of all draftees failed the physical and mental examinations (Nieman, 1986). Health problems of heart disease and obesity were also on the rise. However, the adult "fitness" movement did not really take affect until the late 1960s. With the change in lifestyle habits, regular physical exercise has become a necessary requirement for our mental and physical well-being.

Exercise has many benefits for the body. Most research has been with a specific focus on aerobic exercise. Benefits include reducing blood pressure and resting heart rate, improving cardiovascular efficiency, promoting healthy weight loss, and improving sleep patterns. Moreover, it can help prevent and treat coronary heart disease, osteoporosis, diabetes, hypertension, and depression (Harris & Associates, 1989).

In regard to emotional health, physical exercise has been associated with a sense of accomplishment, improved mood, decreased tension, and enhanced self-image. Clinical benefits in combining exercise and psychotherapy have also been noted (De Angelis, 1996).

Exercise not only is helpful in ridding the body of stress hormones, resulting in mental and physical relaxation, but also through exercise the body can be strengthened to respond more effectively to mental and physical stress. The benefits of physical exercise tend to support and complement each other: improved health, enhanced emotional state, and better ability to respond to stress. As the interest and research in the body-mind connection and psychoneuroimmunology continue to grow, the benefits of physical exercise will be further defined.

KIMBERLY SIBILLE

FELDENKRAIS

Moshe Feldenkrais, D.Sc., stated, "Movement is life. Life is a process. Improve the quality of the process and you improve the quality of life itself." The method named after him is a path to improving the quality of life for anyone, young or old, physically fit or physically challenged. The Feldenkrais method utilizes the exploratory type of movements we experienced as babies and children learning to crawl, walk, and talk. The results of the method are not only immediate but also cumulative and far reaching. Although flexible bodies are a direct result of practicing the method, Feldenkrais asserted, "What I am after is not flexible bodies, but flexible brains. What I am after is to restore each person to their human dignity."

Dr. Moshe Feldenkrais (1904–1984) gained his D.Sc. in the fields of mechanical engineering and physics. He studied for his doctorate at the Sorbonne and worked with Fredric Joliot-Curie in nuclear research. He was the first European to gain his black belt in judo and formed the first judo club in France, which today has upward of 1 million members. When a knee injury threatened to cripple him for life, he focused on learning how to walk again, without pain. The success of his personal discovery led him to originate the method we now call the Feldenkrais method. Among his students were David Ben-Gurion, Yehudi Menuhin, Helen Hayes, Julius Erving, and Margaret Mead, who stated, "the Feldenkrais work is the most sophisticated and effective method I have seen for the prevention and reversal of deterioration of function."

Feldenkrais Method

The method concerns itself mainly with function of movement rather than focusing on structure. The body is moved in specific sequences that enhance awareness by evoking changes in the brain. The education is accomplished by carefully designed movement sequences either one does for oneself, such as in an Awareness Through Movement class (where the student is verbally guided by a teacher in a noncompetitive environment), or through a Functional Integration lesson, which is a one-on-one experience provided with precise, gentle touch. Both of these aspects of the Feldenkrais method work by improving the way movements are organized. Through movement, the nervous system is offered alternatives to the old habitual patterns and relearns or remembers increased flexibility and freedom. The focus of the lessons is on how to do the movement, not on how much, how hard, or how fast. Lessons are accomplished comfortably clothed while sitting, standing, kneeling, or lying down on a floor or padded table.

Here is an exercise that demonstrates a Feldenkrais movement: Interlace your fingers together. Before you read further, take a moment to notice how you do this and how it feels. Now interlace all your fingers the other way, starting with your other thumb on top. Initially you may even experience confusion regarding the instruction, simple as it may be. Notice how this second way (the nonhabitual organization of your hands and fingers) feels. Habituating movements can limit choice and resiliency on many levels. The Feldenkrais method offers release from the rigidity of unconscious habits. The results are a multilevel increase in comfort and flexibility, eliminating any division between body and mind.

The challenges and cautions of doing this work are unique. Alon (1990) states that "some people are willing to invest any effort and pay any price to be free of back pain, except for this one thing: they are unwilling to give their full attention to themselves, to look inward and communicate patiently and kindly with their body." Belief systems can be of much greater limitation than body structure. In the Feldenkrais method, the slower, softer, and lighter the movement of a lesson, the greater awareness and clarity can be generated. The physical repercussions of a lesson are the easiest to notice and talk about. But because the kinesthetic sense of movement is closer to the unconscious than any other of the five senses, repressed emotions and memories are freed to the conscious realms, and emotional abreactions and releases are not uncommon. In a society where so much money is invested in maintaining emotional equilibrium through denial (drugs, alcohol, TV, etc.), emotional equilibrium through direct experience and release can be daunting and cause subconscious resistance to continuing the work.

Outcomes

The most prevalent experience after doing a Feldenkrais lesson is a feeling of lightness and grace. People often feel taller, breathe easier, and have a sense of release and relaxation. Athletes, dancers, and musicians report greater ease and skill of performance. Those interested solely in personal growth find that the method evolves them toward what Feldenkrais called the "authentic self." Lessons can be done sitting at a desk. Repetitive stress injuries at a computer can be alleviated or prevented. Persons traveling can do lessons as they sit and arrive at their destinations more refreshed and comfortable than they otherwise would. Persons who have suffered strokes or other nervous system damage frequently are able to regain function far beyond what was predicted possible by their original care givers. Those who have lost limbs or were born with severe imbalances in their structures learn to better accommodate this challenge and move with greater efficiency and sense of security. Women can experience less effort with managing the change in their center of gravity during pregnancy, often alleviating back pain and other common discomforts. Persons suffering from chronic fatigue are able to do the lessons solely in their imagination and still gain benefit. When fatigued people move through life, if it is with less exertion, their energy is then economized and they can be more effective in the world. People who are restricted to wheelchairs or beds can improve; transferring and activities of daily living become easier and comfort increases. Shelhav-Silberbush (1986) writes that children with cerebral palsy can improve their ability to function. Women who have had mastectomies or others who have suffered disfiguring surgeries are assisted not only by the increased recovery of movement but also by the correction of the self-image. Feldenkrais (1972) wrote that "in reality our self image is never static. It changes from action to action." There are four components of any action; feeling, thought, sensation, and movement. Movement is the most direct path to change and correction of the self-image. With improved self-image, we gain better coordination and are better able to prevent injuries. However, "the Method can speed the rehabilitation of those who are injured" (The Feldenkrais Guild of North America, 1996).

The Feldenkrais Guild of North America is a nonprofit organization dedicated to the advancement of the Feldenkrais method. It approves and regulates professional training programs through the Guild Training Board. All Feldenkrais practitioners must complete 800 to 1,000 hours of training over a 3- to 4-year period. Continuing education is required, and recertification every 2 years is mandatory for authorized practitioners. The guild maintains a directory of practitioners and makes available numerous other resources. It also provides information concerning accredited professional trainings, workshops, and classes. The F.G.N.A. is a member of the International Feldenkrais Federation (I.F.F.) headquartered in Paris, France.

Since the 1940s, thousands of people worldwide have used the Feldenkrais method. The method teaches individuals how to autonomously improve themselves so that they are not left dependent on any program or practitioner.

PAMELA S. LEWIS

FENG SHUI: HONORING THE SACREDNESS OF SPACE

Feng Shui is the 5,000-year-old Chinese art of placement. Pronounced "fung schway," it literally means "wind and water." Feng Shui is derived from ancient observations of how wind and water energies circulate on earth and how people learned to place themselves in such a way as to benefit from those energies. The term Feng Shui is derived from this ancient poem, which describes the ideal site.

> *The wind is mild,*
> *The sun shines,*
> *The water is clear,*
> *The vegetation, lush.*

Early man recognized and honored the interdependence and connectedness with the landscape, immediate environment, the earth, and heavenly forces. Positioning of home had everything to do with safety, survival, and potential prosperity.

There are many schools of Feng Shui. Feng Shui evolved in the East out of the observations that health, balance, and prosperity were affected by one's environment and that being in balance and oneness with nature contributed to good luck. Early Feng Shui was a product of Taoism, Buddhism, the Five Element theory, and the Yin-Yang theory, a Taoist concept that unifies all opposites. The term used to describe this intuitive study of man's connection to the earth is known as geomancy—"geo" means earth, "mancy" means the divination or messages from the earth. Early geomancers used a compass-like tool, or Lo Pan. The Lo Pan combines this knowledge, including attention to cardinal directions that would most benefit an individual.

An early mystical text of divination, *I-Ching, The Book of Changes*, is a system of 64 hexagrams that offered additional wisdom regarding man's fate—the discovery that the laws of nature are also the laws of humanity and that since nature and humanity are one, harmony is the key to life.

A new school of Feng Shui, known as *Tibetan Tantric Buddhism Black Sect Feng Shui*, was brought to the West by Professor Lin Yun. It incorporates modern technologies and Western knowledge of medicine, psychology, architecture, ecology, and the social sciences. This school of Feng Shui evolved out of the journey of Buddhism from India through Tibet and into China. It absorbed the indigenous ancient teachings from these cultures, incorporating observations of tangible, observable environmental factors of the land, home site, and floor plan known as "sying." In addition, this new school of Feng Shui incorporated *yi*; invisible, mystical, and transcendental influences that give additional power and results to the individual. *Yi* is a blessing, a wish, or an intention that is a way of adjusting and enhancing the energy of the space. Another important component of Black Sect Feng Shui is following the ancient tradition of transmitting the mystical knowledge orally from master to pupil.

Feng Shui is about living more harmoniously with earth and heavenly forces. It is about finding and creating in life the same principles that create the miracle of the balance in nature and in the universe. Thousands of ancient insights, known as the rules of good Feng Shui, are pillars of Chinese culture and may be used in setting up home and workspaces. When people are in personal alignment with the flow of natural cosmological rhythms, connected to their environment, they can be transformed.

Homes and workspaces are sacred spaces that are meant to shelter, nourish, and support. No less alive and vibrant than the physical body, spaces are alive with energy, known as *ch'i*, or the cosmic breath. Feng Shui helps people create a balance and harmony in their spaces by improving the flow of *ch'i*. *Ch'i* and *ch'i* cultivation are the heart of Feng Shui. We are familiar with the term *ch'i* through the study of acupuncture. Acupuncture uses needles to stimulate the *ch'i* flowing through the body along invisible lines known as meridians. *Ch'i* also exists in spaces, environments, towns, cities, countries—everywhere in the cosmos. Rivers, roads, doors, windows, and hallways are purveyors of *ch'i* in our environments, just as circulatory and nervous systems bring nutrients and messages to organs and muscles in the physical body. As gardeners, people can create spaces planted with seeds of change and empowerment with proper Feng Shui placements just as needles stimulate and balance the body in acupuncture.

Feng Shui is becoming recognized as the art and science of healing spaces. Feng Shui principles teach ways to create a new sense of harmony and life balance through proper placement of objects and furnishings in home and workspace. The purpose is to create an environment that enables the *ch'i* to circulate and spiral freely. Moving a bed, changing the direction faced while sitting at a desk, creating a welcoming entrance, or adding mirrors, plants, color, or brighter lights are simple changes that can dramatically affect how one feels regarding one's place in the universe. Feng Shui is a way to manifest sacred spaces that can empower by correcting imbalances in room or house design or to deflect ill-fortune by using transcendental cures as suggested from the Tibetan Tantric Buddhism Black Sect School of Feng Shui.

Applying Feng Shui helps individuals align with their life's purpose, opens the limitless possibilities of the universe, and helps create spaces as sacred and empowering gardens of *ch'i*. Spaces create a metaphor for who people are, how they respond to the world, and where they can manifest their goals and intentions. Living and working in spaces that delight and resonate with one's essence can contribute to health, harmony, and sense of balance, thereby affecting one's destiny.

Feng Shui helps us create our own sacred space by giving us a format for change and personal growth. The first part of Feng Shui begins with a **conversation**, with oneself or with a consultant. The conversation determines where one stands and wishes to travel with respect to nine energies or aspects of life. These nine life situations are derived from the *Bagua*, an octagonal symbol containing the eight trigrams of the I-Ching and eight characteristics energies relating to nature, man, and relationships. In Tibetan Tantric Buddhism Black Sect Feng Shui, these energies are expressed as nine life situations: **career, wisdom, health/family, prosperity, fame, rela-tionships, creativity/children, helpful people/travel, and mental health/total balance** as exemplified by the *t'ai chi* symbol in the center of the *Bagua*. Understanding which of these areas of one's life is balanced or out of balance is the place to begin.

Creating sacred space begins with **clearing** the energy of the space. Who lived there before—also known as the Predecessor Law—is an important question. Did they prosper? Did they experience difficulty there? Did they experience serious illness there? That energy may still be affecting you. Feng Shui uses transcendental clearings; but sage, sound, bells, clapping, spritzing with lemon water, sweeping, especially at the end of the year and throwing away the broom as is the Chinese custom, may be used.

Creating sacred space begins with **cleaning** the space. A meal always starts with a clean plate. The same applies to life. When spaces are kept clean and uncluttered, life will be orderly.

Creating sacred space begins with **correcting** for negative energy flow or cutting *ch'i*. Feng Shui consultants are trained to look at external factors on the property and landscape that may or not be contributing to a proper flow of *ch'i*. External factors include the *ch'i* of the land and the shape of one's property. Other external factors that may be considered are the road, bridges, trees, roof shape, churches, graveyards, telephone poles, transformers, electromagnetic fields, and others. Once inside the home or workspace, interior factors to evaluate include the shape of the home or building, floor plan, and structural elements such as exposed beams, pillars, or columns, doors, windows, and brightness. Position and placement of bed, desk, stove, and foyer are critical elements. How one positions oneself with respect to one's personal environment is about creating a place where one is positioned in a place of empowerment and energetic balance. The "cures" used to balance a space are colors, light, sound, life force, moving objects, heavy objects, fragrance, your own imagination and artistry, and transcendental "cures" such as bamboo flutes. Lin Yun states that these transcendental cures and the ceremonies used to reinforce their influence can account for 110% of the power of Feng Shui.

Creating sacred space means **creating** new intentions. Moving objects or furnishings with intention may activate an energy that is out of balance, such as career or relationships when one understands where that *ener-ch'i* exists in the home. Crystals may be placed with intention to activate an energy, while a heavy stone sculpture may be placed to stabilize a life situation. This is the fun part of Feng Shui. The changes or "cures" are about creating sacred spaces that reflect individuals as creative, empowered beings—creating a temple for the soul while moving individuals toward their karmic future.

Another suggestion for incorporating Feng Shui principles in designing a space are to work with the concept of the Five Elements or Transformations, the central theme in Oriental culture about the balance in nature. The five elemental energies are fire, earth, metal, water, and wood. Why is the kitchen such a satisfying place to be? Possibly because all of the elemental energies are present there. The stove represents the energy of fire; sink and refrigerator the energy of water; pots, pans, and utensils the energy of metal; wood cabinets, butcher block, wood spoons, and

plants the energy of wood; fresh fruits, vegetables, and ceramic the energy of earth. People can begin by combining these energies in all rooms to create the experience of being in balance with the primary forces of nature.

Having a **ceremony** can honor and reinforce the placement of objects and furnishings that have been made with new intentions for the future. For example, moving one's bed to a different position can have powerful results in placing oneself in a new position of empowerment in one's universe. In Tibetan Tantric Buddhism Black Sect Feng Shui, there are many powerful and beautiful ceremonies to reinforce new placements.

Creating sacred space is cause for **celebration.** Honor the space that allows the unfolding of the self. Expressing one's individual uniqueness within personal environments can be like dressing a space as one would dress oneself for a party. Dress your space as a celebration of self. One's space can reflect joy in the gifts of life and of nature. Fresh flowers, nine new lush plants, or a mirror to reflect an exterior scene are good ways to begin.

Finally, **courage.** Occasionally it takes courage to gather, to reflect, and move boldly into new areas of life and life situations. Profound changes can happen in one's life when small changes are made in one's space, when courage cannot be found to move in other ways.

Feng Shui deals with concepts intuited by our ancient ancestors. In *Awakening the Buddha Within*, Lama Surya Das states, "The wisdom traditions tell us that we can afford to slow down, take a breather, turn inwards, to master ourselves is to arrive HOME, at the center of being—the universal mandala."

Feng Shui is about creating spaces as sacred. Individuals have what they need. Feng Shui offers a format to put what they possess in the right places. The process of healing one's own spaces may begin with conversation, clearing, cleansing, correcting imbalances, ceremony, celebration, and courage. However, the most sacred space that is affected by improving the *ch'i* of our spaces is one's own **inner space**, "the universal mandala." When one creates spaces that cultivate one's *ch'i* according to Feng Shui principles, creating a metaphor for who and what one wants to become, individuals affect their destiny, the ultimate potential of Feng Shui.

LURRAE LUPONE

FIBROMYALGIA: COMPLEMENTARY TREATMENT APPROACHES

There have been numerous reports of trials with various nutritional supplements, such as Chinese herbs, and alternative physical techniques, such as acupuncture, for individuals with fibromyalgia. Unfortunately, many of these reports are anecdotal, with very few controlled, double-blind studies in the use of complementary treatment approaches for the treatment of fibromyalgia.

Of the few actual studies that have been done, there have been several treatment approaches that have been found to improve functioning and lessen pain in the individual with fibromyalgia. The single most effective complementary treatment that has shown significant improvement in the number of trigger points and lessening of myalgic pain scores in people with fibromyalgia is the use of cardiovascular training (Goldenberg, 1989; Martin et al., 1993).

Cardiovascular exercise should be started slowly and be based on the physical condition of the individual. Exercise should include warm-up and cool-down periods with initial stretching exercises so that damage to muscles from overuse or excessive use is avoided. When exercise is increased in slow increments, individuals with fibromyalgia can obtain sustained cardiovascular workouts for 30 or more minutes plus a 10-minute warm-up and 10-minute cool-down period. Water aerobic exercises have been especially effective because water provides support for joints while lessening stress on the body.

When education about fibromyalgia was combined with physical exercise, the quality of life improved significantly, pain was reduced, and a decrease in the "number of days of feeling bad" was found (Burckhardt et al., 1994).

Physical modalities such as electroacupuncture and trigger point injection have been shown to provide some relief of myalgic symptoms. Electroacupuncture, used with 62 fibromyalgia patients in an open trial and 70 fibromyalgia patients in a controlled trial, resulted in 70% of patients claiming some relief of pain for periods of 1 to 12 months duration (Wilke, 1995).

Several studies have investigated the use of trigger point injections and, interestingly, have found that dry needling, saline injection, and procaine injection were equally effective in reducing pain. The effectiveness of treatment was positively correlated with the initial intensity of pain at the treated site and the precision of the needling procedure, and not the substance injected (Lewit, 1979; Jaeger & Skootsky, 1987; Wilke, 1995).

Electromyography (EMG) biofeedback training has been studied with fibromyalgia patients and resulted in significant improvement in tender points, subjective pain reporting, and morning stiffness (Furacciolo et al., 1987). Cognitive-behavioral psychotherapy that focused on the sensory, affective, cognitive, and behavioral elements associated with fibromyalgia have also resulted in improvement in pain severity and psychological variables (Bradley, 1989).

In one study, a supplement of 200 mg of malic acid and 50 mg of magnesium, marketed under the brand name of Super Malic, was found to provide "significant reductions" in the severity of pain and tenderness when given in doses of up to 6 tablets of Super Malic for at least 2 months. Improvement in energy, concentration, depression, memory, pain sleep, and headaches has also been found in a study that tested glyconutritionals (Ambrotose capsules), phytonutritionals (Phyt.Aloe capsules), dioscorea complex (PLUS and MVP caplets), and vitamins and minerals (profile caplets) for fibromyalgia (Dykman, Tone, & Dykman, 1997).

Pain reduction has been achieved with the use of capsaicin ointment rubbed on painful trigger points. It is thought that the capsaicin, a derivative of a hot pepper, interferes with pain transmission by reducing the amount of substance P in the muscle. To achieve maximum effectiveness, the capsaicin must be used consistently and applied several times a day.

Moist heat applied to painful areas and soaking in a hot bath, shower, or hot tub have been demonstrated to reduce muscle pain and are effective when used on a regular basis with exercise and supplements. Encouragement of restorative sleep by the development of healthy sleep patterns and the avoidance of caffeine and nicotine has also been shown to be helpful in pain reduction. Finally, myofascial massage performed regularly by a trained massage therapist who is experienced in identifying trigger points and knows how to release them can reduce muscle pain and aid in maintaining a pain-reduced state.

Perhaps the best complementary treatment approach to ameliorating the various symptoms associated with fibromyalgia is a comprehensive approach. This includes a good basic nutritional program with full vitamin and mineral supplements such as Super Malic, stress reduction and relaxation response training (possibly with biofeedback), massage, routine stretching and cardiovascular water exercises, good sleep hygiene, use of topical capsaicin, and cognitive-behavioral therapy for dealing with medically related issues, depression, and stress management. Taken together, these components will go a long way in helping individuals with fibromyalgia manage their symptoms.

LESLIE ELLIS

See also
Capsaicin (III)
Exercise (IV)
Myofascial Release (IV)

FIBROMYALGIA: RESEARCH AND THEORY

Since the mid 1980s there has been a surge of research into identifying the causes of fibromyalgia (FMS). Investigators have studied neurochemical transmission, the histology of muscle fibers, neuroendocrine disturbances, cardiovascular abnormalities, psychological profiles, and immunologic components. Researchers have uncovered a number of pathological findings in their search for identifying an etiology of FMS.

Research Findings of Pathologies Associated with FMS

- Neurologic—Migraine, neurologic inflammation, increased release of substance P, decreased regional cerebral blood flow, increased activity of cholinergic, and decreased activity of adrenergic components of peripheral nervous system, altered nociception, increased incidence of alpha EEG NREM sleep.
- Neuromuscular—Empty sleeves of basement membrane, lipofuscin bodies, degenerative muscle changes, metabolic deficiencies, lowered exercise tolerance.
- Autoimmune—Defined autoantibody pattern consisting of antibodies to nucleoli, gangliosides, and phospholipids, defect in T-cell activation.
- Infectious—Epstein-Barr virus (found in CFIDS patients), cytomegliavirus.
- Cardiovascular—Mitral valve prolapse.
- Endocrinological—Perturbed hypothalamic-pituitary-adrenal axis, disturbance in the growth hormone-somatomedin C axis.
- Psychological—Hysteria, depression, hypochondriasis, psychosocial problems, schizophrenia, panic disorders and anxiety, irritable bowel syndromes, cognitive deficits.

First in 1994 and then again in 1995, Daniel J. Clauw, M.D. at Georgetown University School of Medicine in Washington, D.C., proposed that by looking at the totality of conditions that occur along with FMS, an understanding could be obtained as to the nature of the condition. In an article entitled "The Pathogenesis of Chronic Pain and Fatigue Syndromes, with Special Reference to Fibromyalgia" (*Medical Hypotheses*, 1994), Clauw proposed that there exists a genetic susceptibility for "one or more abnormal proteins that are normally responsible for downregulating the central nervous system" in 2% to 6% of the population.

With the occurrence of a "triggering event" that could either be psychological (i.e, extreme stress or abuse) or physical (i.e., an automobile accident), "an adaptive stress response" activates the HPA axis and the sympathetic system. CNS hyperactivity occurs, and any or all CNS symptoms can become manifest. Clauw further postulates that "an elevated ratio of excitatory to inhibitory neuromodulators is responsible for the genesis of this entire spectrum of conditions, and when this occurs in a region of the central nervous system that controls one of these effector functions, the symptoms of syndromes noted result" (Clauw, 1994). This hypothesis presents a unified field theory that would account for the various independent research findings that have been reported within the last 10 years, but it does not address the FMS mind-body connection.

Fibromyalgia: Mind-Body Interaction

The pathways identifying the physiological response to stress and causal connections between occurrences in our environments and the way human physiology responds to stressful environmental circumstances have been well documented. Ernest Lawrence Rossi and Steven Dubovsky are two researcher-writers who have extensively identified the mind-body pathways as they pertain to cancer and cardiac and immunological problems. These physical pathways are unconsciously activated by the mind's perception of a stressor (Rossi, 1992; Dubovsky, 1997).

There is current research to indicate that under conditions of stress, there occurs an HPA axis dysfunction in the FMS patient. Because this stress response is aberrant, the CNS disregulation proposed by Clauw is most likely activated. Research has shown high levels of anxiety in FMS patients. When approached from the vantage of mind-body interactions, stress-induced HPA axis and CNS dysfunction explains two things about FMS.

First, it explains the psychological/physiological mechanism by which primary FMS develops and through which secondary FMS can be exacerbated. Secondly, if stress-generated physiological changes in the body can stimulate the HPA changes that cause CNS disregulation, then therapy directed to helping the individual attend to the repressed issues that cause stress should assist in the alleviation of some of the symptomology of FMS and make it more controllable. Indeed, this is what is seen in comprehensive treatment programs that deal with FMS patients. Without such intervention, it would seem that other treatments are symptom versus cause treatments that can only address the manifestations of the CNS dysfunction.

LESLIE ELLIS

HEALING RETREAT FOR PEOPLE WITH HIV

Retreats have been used for centuries to strengthen the spiritual life of individuals and empower Christians. Usually this means retreat to a retreat center, but it can be as simple as taking "retreat time" and going to the park, backyard, woods, lake, or some place nice (Rademacher, 1991). Review of the health literature presented examples of the use of retreats to empower people with cancer (Lane & Davis, 1985; Walsh-Burke, 1992); hospital personnel (Galbraith and colleagues, 1992); families (Bender, Eastop, & Keller, 1994; Burke, Kauffman, Costella, & Dillon, 1991; DePompei, Whitford, & Beam, 1994); children (Hanna & Jacobs, 1993; Shannon, 1986); and stress management for men with HIV (Coates, McKusick, Keno, & Stites, 1989). Psychosocial support groups for people with HIV have been studied by Riddle (1989) and Ramsey (1992). The purpose of both studies was to investigate the effect of support group participation on the individual's ability to adapt. The studies used a nonexperimental design. Results indicated that community support groups were most effective for those who were symptomatic for HIV infection.

Hay (1987, 1988a, 1988b) has written extensively about creating positive approaches for people with HIV for healing their body. Use of relaxation, meditation, visualization, alternative therapies, support systems, and healing circles, among other activities, are suggested.

Planning the Retreat

Kentucky has divided its state into regions, and within each region, one or two HIV care coordinators work with those people with HIV and AIDS. The Barren River District HIV Care Consortium, which changed its name in 1994 to River Trail ARC (AIDS Resource Council), encompasses 25 counties in Kentucky. The purpose of the consortium is to plan, develop, and deliver comprehensive support services to meet the identified needs of individuals with HIV disease within the geographic service area. Within this region there is one community-based AIDS service organization and that is AIDS Southern Kentucky (ASK). ASK is staffed by volunteers and provides prevention education and services for people with HIV.

At approximately the same time, both the care consortium and ASK began to question the feasibility of a healing retreat for people with HIV. Representatives from both organizations met, and a committee composed of a nurse, social worker, minister, two volunteers, health educator, and three people with HIV was formed. An announcement of a Healing Weekend in Ohio was reviewed, and a member of the committee was sent to attend this weekend and bring back information. The committee member that attended the weekend in Ohio reported that the Ohio AIDS Coalition has held Healing Weekends for several years.

The committee decided to try and implement a healing retreat for people with HIV and AIDS within the service region in Kentucky. Goals identified for the retreat included to:

- Expose participants to a number of complementary and alternative healing approaches.
- Provide both informational and experiential workshops to help meet the needs of participants.
- Provide free time for socializing with other participants and time for rest and relaxation.
- Increase self-empowerment and self-control in our lives.
- Learn more ways to survive.

The planning committee looked for a location where a retreat could be held that would provide privacy and security for people with HIV. Several locations were visited and the committee settled on a secluded conference center located along a small river. There was a 5,000-square-foot conference center building that could accommodate 100 people as well as an area providing 14 bunk beds for men and 14 bunk beds for women attached. In addition there were six cabins, each accommodating eight people. The location blended beautifully with the outdoors. The conference center had a complete institutional kitchen, loft meeting room with a cozy fireplace and sitting area, and an extensive outdoor deck overlooking the river and a separate picnic pavilion. No hunting was allowed on the site, and therefore deer, fox, raccoons, wild turkey, coveys of quail, and many other birds and animals could be seen. Recreational activities included two beautiful swimming pools, a softball field, horseshoes, basketball courts, sand volleyball, and a playground. People could be free to explore the 150 acres of wooded hillside. It was an idyllic location.

The planning committee developed a flyer to be mailed to clients of the HIV care coordinator; developed a budget and set the fee for the retreat ($50.00); identified organizations to provide $25.00 scholarships if the individual could not afford the fee; developed a registration form, confidentiality statement, logo, and mailings for speakers and clients; contacted potential speakers; developed the schedule of activities; arranged for a member of the committee to prepare a list of healing modalities, list of abbreviations, and a glossary of terms to be given to participants; selected printed material to be handed out; planned for the meals and arranged for a caterer; appointed someone to coordinate volunteers to serve and assist at mealtimes; arranged for off-site physician coverage and 24-hour-a-day on-site nurse coverage; developed an evaluation instrument; and made assignments for committee members during the time of the retreat. The individual responsible for planning the meals recommended turkey and spinach as the basic components for both lunch and dinner and continental food for breakfast.

During the Retreat

Registration for the retreat began at noon on Monday and was followed by a brief welcome and a session on positive living. The purpose of the positive living session was to help people become acquainted and to provide an opportunity to empower individuals, help them claim their space, their right to be present, and help affirm their self-worth. Retreat participants were requested to write down all their negative thoughts and concerns during the retreat on a piece of paper and told this would be utilized on Day 3 in an experiential activity. Sessions were scheduled for 1 to 2 1/2 hours each. The next session was on stress management, providing an opportunity to learn ways to cope with the stressors of life. Small group sessions were scheduled once a day for 30 minutes to an hour just prior to the evening meal. The small group sessions provided a time to discuss individual concerns with a smaller number of people. The evening of the first day included two presentations. The first was on safer sex and the second on coping with depression in a positive manner. The session on safer sex included a discussion of the point in a new relationship to discuss HIV status, and ways to find appropriate, healthy, and safe means to express sexuality. A comedy movie was scheduled at the end of the day.

Day 2 started with a morning workout with tai chi using a video. Tai chi was selected because it is a low-impact exercise that helps to increase energy. Tai chi includes graceful flowing movements that tone muscles, firm the body, and enhance flexibility. Use of a video was not a good idea because people wanted to work with someone. After breakfast a healing circle was held in order to open to the healing power inside oneself, as well as to the healing energy from others. The healing circle was experiential and used various forms of meditation, visualization, and relaxation to begin the day. Two sessions were held in the morning: Philosophy, Attitudes, and Spirituality, stressing an opportunity to explore individual philosophies and beliefs about surviving and thriving with HIV and how spirituality can enhance life; followed by Coping with the Social Service System. Knowing more about the social service system can help to reduce the stress of navigating the system. This session included exploration of social security, Supplemental Security Income, Medicare and Medicaid, and food stamps. Both the session on spirituality and social services had been recommended by people with HIV. After lunch, 2 hours were free for walking, talking, or whatever. Beginning at 3:00, two sessions were then held prior to the evening meal. Nutrition and the Immune System included information on how to enhance the immune system with food, nutritional supplements, and herbs in order to replenish those nutrients lost because of the hard, fast, nonstop metabolism in the HIV-infected person. This was followed by Reflexology, Hypnotherapy, and Massage as therapies to help unlock the stress in the body. Small breakout group discussions led by a facilitator followed. After the evening meal there were two sessions. The first session was on Addictive Behaviors, HIV, and 12-Step Programs and included discussion on how to deal with the challenge of HIV infection as it relates to recovery from alcohol/drugs/compulsive sex, food, or gambling behavior or growing up in a dysfunctional family. This was a time to share stories and receive support. The last session for the day was Use of Therapeutic Touch. Therapeutic touch is derived from an ancient cross-cultural practice of restoring balance and harmony to another's being and body, thus achieving reduced anxiety, increased psychological relaxation, and decreased pain. This session was experiential and the speaker demonstrated therapeutic touch and taught the individuals to perform therapeutic touch on each other. A healing circle similar to that held at the beginning of the day closed the day. Comedy movies were available for those who wished to view them.

Day 3 began much like Day 2, with a morning workout and breakfast followed by a healing circle. The two topics covered during the morning included Medical Aspects of HIV. This session was presented by a nurse practitioner who worked with people with HIV and AIDS and focused on current medical developments. The complete cycle of the disease from diagnosis to death was explored. The need for a living will and designation of a health care surrogate as defined by Kentucky law were discussed as they related to people with HIV. An Intimacy Workshop, providing an opportunity to begin to develop a feeling of intimacy with each other, including emotionally and physically intimate ways of becoming close, was held. The afternoon again brought time for relaxation for 2 hours and then a session on Grief, Death,

Dying, and Loss. To live is to grieve, to live is to die, to live is to lose. This experiential session sought to utilize techniques to learn to deal with that which is a part of all our lives—death. Following this there was small group sharing time. After dinner, one session was held on the topic of Clinical Trials presented by a person with HIV who had participated in a clinical trial. This session emphasized what to consider when deciding to participate or not participate in clinical trials. This day was closed with a healing circle "We Remember," where a meditation was followed by lighting of candles and remembering the names of loved ones or friends lost through HIV disease. In procession, the group then went to a bonfire where an opportunity was provided for them to burn all the negative thoughts and ideas they had written down during the retreat followed by singing and a time for sharing. People seemed to really get a lot from the experience.

The last day started with exercise, breakfast, a healing circle, and two presentations. The presentations were on Resources and Getting Your Needs Met, which discussed some of the practical tips for getting in and around the system, how to obtain a case manager, and ensuring that the individual is considered a member of the health care team. The final session was The Healing Continues as We Go Home and included a chance for sharing any thoughts and feelings prior to leaving the safe space of the retreat, ideas for continuing in a positive manner when outside the retreat environment, and a healing circle.

Evaluation and Follow-Up

Evaluation of the first retreat gave excellent or very good marks to the following sessions: Positive Living, Stress Management, Safer Sex, Coping With Depression, Social Services System, Use of Therapeutic Touch, Medical Aspects of HIV, Grief, Death, Dying, and Loss, and Clinical Trials. Spirituality, Addictive Behaviors, Nutrition, Reflexology, and Intimacy received fair reviews.

People liked the location and felt it was great. Food was a problem. Participants wanted more variety for the lunch and dinner meals and some hot food for breakfast.

Overall comments about the retreat were very positive. The quiet and location received numerous comments. People commented that the retreat brought hope and good feelings of not being alone with the disease. Centering was a plus for many and just taking time for the self. People liked the opportunity to meet others and to be around people who shared the same or similar problems. The atmosphere was soothing all the way around and people felt accepted by participants, staff, and volunteers. Informal talking and "being able to let down your hair and be yourself" were enjoyed by all. Participants felt they had an opportunity to meet the goals of the retreat.

Some of the negative aspects included: need for fewer speakers, more group work, programs on finding inner peace, more on alternative treatments, more hands-on activity, more depth in some areas, more food, and more free time.

With the completion of the first healing retreat, plans were begun for the second healing retreat to be held in 1994. The committee also booked for the third annual retreat to be held June 1–4, 1995, to allow the participants to be able to swim. Keeping in mind the positive and negative comments from the first year, presentations were held to 2 hours and were to be inter-

active, more time was allowed for group work, the healing circles were continued, and more free time was allowed. Two people who had attended the first retreat planned the meals for the second and decided to prepare the food on-site because we had a kitchen. The fee was again set at $50.00 per person. Scholarships were again obtained for half of the fee by participants if they needed partial funding. The planning committee decided to invite people with HIV and AIDS from throughout the whole state of Kentucky. The invitation to clients occurred through community-based organizations and the HIV care coordinators.

The opening session was on Expressive Therapy, focusing on self-development through expressive therapy utilizing group activities, and the evening program was on Therapeutic Touch. This year, participants had the opportunity to sign up for individual sessions of Therapeutic Touch on Friday and Saturday during free time. A healing circle started and ended each day. On Day 2, sessions included Stress Management, Massage Therapy, and Spirituality. Day 4 sessions included Tai Chi and Loss and Grief. We had intended to go outside for tai chi; however, it was raining and it had to be done inside. Much more time was allowed for free time; however, people wanted more organized activities. The healing circle, remembrance, and bonfire concluded this day. On the last day there was a healing circle, brunch, and one session on intimacy. In addition to individual sessions with therapeutic touch, there was an opportunity for individual sessions with massage on Saturday.

Evaluations indicated people continue to want therapeutic touch with more history and more interaction, stress management for dealing with the day-to-day stresses, massage therapy (especially if the speaker would have participants pair off and learn to give each other a neck and shoulder massage), spirituality (but the person needs to be down to earth and have experiential activities), exercise (preferably done outside), and intimacy (and would have liked it earlier in the program). Participants wanted to learn how to give their spouse/partner a massage or be able to tell their spouse/partner how to give them a massage at home. The healing circle seemed to be accepted but the response was not as great as for the first year; however, they wanted it continued. Variety seems to be the key and allowing participants to experience a variety of healing activities.

Stress, coping, and relationships are problems faced by people with HIV disease and they are seeking ways to empower themselves. The health care system has not empowered them; therefore, other means need to be utilized to assist them in living life to the fullest. Use of retreats and support groups seems to be of value. It is important that people living with HIV disease be included on any planning committee because they provide insight into what is needed to increase dignity and self-worth, empowerment, and self-help.

MARY E. HAZZARD

See also
Hypnotherapy (IV)
Lymphatic Massage (IV)
Nutrition (IV)
Reflexology (IV)
T'ai Chi (IV)
Therapeutic Touch: Uses, Research, and Standards for Practice (IV)

HEALING TOUCH

Healing Touch is a multilevel program of healing techniques with multicultural origins. The human energy field is manipulated by adding energy, subtracting energy, or moving energy around to obtain a balance and promote healing. Therapeutic Touch, which was developed by Delores Krieger and Dora Kunz, as well as selected concepts and/or interventions of Rosalyn Bruyere, Brugh Joy, and Barbara Brennan, are better-known components of the program. Practitioners may be certified by Healing Touch International following the successful completion of five classes as well as practice and academic requirements. Healing Touch International sets standards of practice and a code of ethics for the delivery of Healing Touch techniques. Healing Touch classes are offered throughout the world by certified instructors.

History/Theory

Energy therapies have been used by cultures for healing throughout the world for as long as humans have existed. Hieroglyphics drawn on the walls of caves illustrate healers using their hands for energy transfer and healing. Energy therapies such as the laying on of hands are sometimes associated with spiritual cultural traditions. Modern native cultures around the world include energy work in their collection of healing modalities.

The underlying scientific basis for Healing Touch is electromagnetic field theory. Kirlian photography has been used to provide evidence of the human energy field since the 1970s.

In the 1960s, Martha Rogers, Ph.D., R.N., a nursing theorist, brought to nursing the concept of humankind as an open energy field interacting with the environment. Janet Mentgen, B.S.N., R.N., is a nurse who has been practicing energy based care since 1980. Healing Touch as a program was formally assembled by Mentgen beginning in 1989. The program was then piloted and accepted by the American Holistic Nurse's Association in 1990 as a certificate program. The responsibility and authority for Healing Touch was transferred to Healing Touch International in 1996 to continue to offer Healing Touch education and certification to a wide range of health care professionals as well as the lay public. Healing Touch continues to be endorsed by the American Holistic Nurse's Association. Classes are currently taught throughout the United States. Healing Touch classes have most recently been taken to Canada, New Zealand, Australia, and Africa through Healing Touch Partnerships Inc.

Uses

Healing Touch techniques can be used successfully in combination with other body-oriented modalities in any clinical setting. They are effective in decreasing the perception of pain, decreasing wound healing time, and eliciting the human relaxation response that promotes a feeling of well-being. Healing Touch has been used successfully with patients with depression, anxiety, and pain syndromes. Healing Touch has been taught in prenatal classes to deal with the challenges of birthing and used in the hospice setting to deal with the challenges of dying. Healing Touch techniques have been effective anecdotally in acute illnesses and trauma situations when used with standard Western medical treatment.

Research Base

Research on the efficacy of energy-based therapies has been conducted since the 1970s. Studies on changes in human enzyme function, immune function, pain and stress reduction, increase in wound healing, and effects of the relaxation response have been done by a variety of researchers in a variety of disciplines. Over 300 research studies have been conducted to date on healing in the energy field. The majority of the recent research studies have been done using Therapeutic Touch.

As of the publication date, there have been 10 Healing Touch studies completed, and there are 55 in process. The majority of the studies are done by nurse researchers. Most of the studies completed used questionnaires and self-report techniques pre- and post-treatment. Studies using objective statistical methods found (1) a statistically significant decrease in blood pressure measurement post treatment; and (2) faster return to work in a group of employees with job-related injuries compared to those who had not received Healing Touch.

Studies in process deal with the use of Healing Touch techniques in the areas of depression, pain, and the decreased need for narcotic analgesia, and the effect of Healing Touch in the prevention of cardiac restenosis postcardiac surgery, to name a few.

LINDA HEIN

See also
Therapeutic Touch: Definition, History, and Theory (IV)

HELLERWORK STRUCTURAL INTEGRATION

Hellerwork Structural Integration is a preventive health modality that brings together three components: (1) deep tissue bodywork, which aims to reduce the tension and rigidity that accumulates in the myofascial tissues as a function of time and which moves these tissues to produce an improved alignment of the physical structure with the field of gravity; (2) movement reeducation, which teaches individuals how to use their bodies more efficiently and how to avoid putting unnecessary stress on their structure; and (3) dialogue to make individuals aware of how emotional and psychological stresses affect body structure and movement.

Hellerwork is performed as a series of 60- to 90-minute sessions, each session addressing a different part of the body in sequence. The minimum number of sessions to go over the whole body is 11, but quite often additional sessions are needed to take care of troublesome or traumatized areas.

Hellerwork was founded in 1978 by Joseph Heller, a former aerospace engineer for NASA, who was trained by Ida Rolf in her technique in 1972 and became the first president of the Rolf Institute in 1975. He expanded the scope of his work by adding the components of movement and dialogue and began training practitioners in 1978. Currently there are about 330 Hellerwork practitioners in the United States, Canada, Japan, New Zealand, Australia, and Europe.

Theory

The theoretical framework of Hellerwork is based on the concept that the connective tissues of the body are a continuous tensegrity structure in which the bones act as the compressional elements and the fascia, tendons, and ligaments act as the tensional elements. These tensional elements are designed to be elastic and flexible, being mostly fluid. However, due to physical and emotional trauma and under the influence of stress (whether structural, physical, or psychological), these fluid connective tissues become increasingly dehydrated and rigid. This progressive rigidity causes a loss of function in the form of reduced flexibility, impaired blood and lymph flow, and increasing tension, which can result in mild to severe myofascial pain. The effectiveness of Hellerwork comes from the release of this tension and rigidity, producing better flexibility, disappearance of pain, and better alignment with gravity, which reduces structural stress. This in turn increases the efficiency of movement, and clients report a greater feeling of energy and well-being.

The second component of Hellerwork, movement reeducation, is based on the idea that individuals learn to overexert their bodies in certain habit patterns, which usually contribute to stress. Without any new input, clients will tend to go back to their old patterns. The movement reeducation teaches new ways of moving that are more efficient and less stressful and which support the benefits obtained from the bodywork.

The movement education deals with everyday uses of the body, such as standing, sitting, walking, driving, lifting things, and the various activities that the clients engage in, such as work, hobbies, sports, and exercise.

The theoretical bases of the dialogue work comes from the fact that the expression of emotions that are not acceptable in our social environment (such as anger or fear) are repressed and the musculature that is involved in that expression is tightened. If the repression is an ongoing pattern, it begins to accumulate in the myofascia in the form of rigidity. Tempero mandibular joint (TMJ) disorder is an example of such a condition. Through the dialogue work, Hellerwork makes clients aware of these patterns and teaches them to release tight muscles.

Applications

Hellerwork is particularly successful in relieving musculoskeletal pain and tension. It is also good at releasing rigidity caused by past trauma and reducing scar tissues from injuries and surgeries. It is particularly effective in balancing the structure of the body and improving performance and endurance in athletic activities.

The most intelligent use of Hellerwork is in reducing the effects of stress on the organism and as preventive maintenance. Although we are aware of the benefits of preventive maintenance when it comes to automobiles and other machinery, we tend to wait for the breakdown when it comes to our bodies.

The cost of Hellerwork sessions varies among practitioners in different areas, from $65 to $120 per session. Practitioners undergo a rigorous training program lasting 18 months to 2 years and are certified by Hellerwork International.

JOSEPH HELLER

HERBAL THERAPIES

Herbology is the study of the science and artful use of healing plants or herbs. Every culture has at some point used healing plants as the basis for its medicine and had a basic healing flora from which remedies were selected. Herbal remedy use is found within the Indian Ayurvedic system, in Chinese medicine, in Native American herbalism, in European phytomedicines, and more recently, in American complementary medicine. As the range of plants varies from area to area depending on the local ecosystem, the therapeutic philosophy for plant use varies from culture to culture (folklore). It has been found that scientific data often corroborate with folklore usage and that divergent cultures discovered the same uses for the same or chemically similar plants (Mowrey, 1986).

Modern American medicine has its roots in the use of herbs. Until 50 years ago, nearly all the entries in the pharmacopeias describing the manufacturing of drugs indicated an herbal origin (Hoffman, 1996). These entries were based on numerous published studies on the effects of herbs on animal and human physiology. In an era when debilitating and fatal diseases summoned the advancement of science and technology to promulgate research activities, modern drug research launched the exciting arena of synthetic medicines without preservation of the fundamental value of botanical medicines. Medical botany and the masters who historically handed down the art and science of herbology were abandoned. Today, most of the important herbal research is being done in Europe. America is just beginning to understand the deep wisdom of traditional herbal medicine and is making some effort to focus on plant medicine research.

As the field of plant medicine research is challenged, consideration is given to the manner in which orthodox and herbal medicine views the human being in relationship to health and healing. Each view differs significantly and formulates the basis for the use of conventional or herbal therapies. Orthodox medicine views humans as having compartmentalized units of the body and has created medical specialists who contribute to the proliferation of this viewpoint. In modern medicine, attention is given to the heart (cardiologist), lungs (pulmonologist), hormonal system (endocrinologist), mind (psychiatrist), to name a few, and not to the whole functioning person. Researchers follow this framework and continue to produce synthetic drugs to treat specific, separate human systems. In essence, traditional medicine does not commonly view or treat a human as a "whole" person, where the body-mind-emotion-spirit are integral to a balanced state of health.

Contrary to modern medicine, herbal medicine recognizes that the body is a whole, integrated system, greater than the sum of its parts. Further, the whole of an herbal remedy is vastly greater than the sum of its parts (Hoffman, 1996). The art and science of herbal medicine is based on the premise that thought, emotions, and spiritual flow are as important to health as is the state of organs and tissues within the body. It is the delicate balance of body-mind-emotion-spirit consciousness that creates a positive state of health.

To facilitate the integration of ancient practice and modern research, it must be understood that each plant and each human is a unified, bioenergy field. Ancient cultures have been aware of an organizing power of nature, a unified or bioenergy field that exists at the deepest level of nature (Scalzo, 1994). This dynamic energy field is a life-promoting vital field considered to be a wellspring of intelligence within and around plants and humans that nourishes and fortifies life energy. Modern research has a difficult time accounting for, qualifying, and quantifying this vital energy life-supporting force. However, research can account for human physiology involved when medicinal plants are used; it is known that neuroreceptors respond to biological substances found in plants. Medicinal plant chemistry targets specific receptors within the body, restoring health and balance by the interacting chemistry and organizing power of nature. When humans use plants as herbal medicine, the obvious human-plant chemical physiology must be understood within the context of the human-plant unified energy field. It is the influence and interaction of the human-plant unified bioenergy field, all within the organizing power of nature, that the pure intelligence of healing is expressed.

Herbs are medicines and have medicinal properties used to therapeutically mobilize a person's own capacity for self-healing. In review of herbal medicine literature, it is found that herbs are applied to the systems of the body with the body-mind-emotion-spirit aspects of healing not outwardly being discussed. Perhaps this is inherently understood and not written. The human-plant unified bioenergy field, however, is more openly addressed in the literature pertaining to the use of Bach flower essences (Scheffer, 1996; Wigmore Publications, 1993).

It is worthy to mention Bach flower essences in more detail since the majority of the people today who are self-prescribing focus on the physical aspects of their health, reflected in the form of body symptoms. Without the understanding and application of Bach flower essences, concentrating on balancing body health alone remains aligned with the essence of modern medicine, where repeating patterns of physical imbalances or disease continue to proliferate.

Edward Bach (1886–1936) was an English physician who believed that personality and attitude have a bearing on their state of physical health (Wigmore, 1993). He studied the medicinal and energetic properties of single flower essences and their applications to human health. As a result of many years of research, he developed Bach flower essences, a form of natural medicines based on single wildflowers and tree blossoms. The essences work specifically on unifying the physical body with mental/emotional/spiritual condition of the person concerned. The effect of taking the essences is to transform negative attitudes (attitudes known to contribute to the distortion of health patterns in the body) into positive ones, stimulating the person's own potential for self-healing, thereby freeing the physical system to engage fully in fighting stress and disease. Each flower or plant used has a specific mentally/emotionally/spiritually healing effect. The action of these essences is to raise the person's vibrations and open up to channels for the reception of the spiritual self (Scheffer, 1996). Since the role of energy in medicine is becoming more widely accepted, practitioners who use the essences have found that the plant essences' very pure vibrations interact with the subtle energy system of the person, healing and harmonizing at the physical-mental-emotional-spiritual levels (Wigmore, 1993).

Herbal preparations are only as vital as the quality of the herbs used to prepare the remedy (Green, 1990). Fresh living plants as well as dried plants contain strong organic fixed principles and are considered active constituents responsible for healing properties of the plant. These principles must be known before attempting to extract medicinal properties from plants. For example, volatile oils are aromatic and susceptible to depreciation when exposed to drying, so fresh living plants are used for extraction purposes. In some cases where plants have very strong fixed principles, as in seeds or resins, drying and aging the plant renders the plant less irritating. Artful, intuitive knowledge along with scientific knowledge of the plant's principle constituents directly affects the method chosen to extract medicinal properties from plants.

In general, herbal usage is categorized into two distinct systems—specifics or tonics. These systems are based on whether the single herbs or formulas (more than one herb) are used for a short or long period of time. Specifics are herbs commonly used to alleviate acute conditions or to do a specific job. They are discontinued when they are not needed. Tonics are herbs used to support and nourish body processes and energy systems; they are used for a longer period of time (4 to 6 months). The person rests or ceases to use the herbs at specific intervals during the treatment period. Each period of rest allows for the effects of the herbs to become integrated into the physiology and bioenergy fields (Scalzo, 1994).

Tonics are divided into two categories: nutrient tonics and stimulant tonics. Nutrient tonics provide nutrients the body can use for its function. Foods and spices are nutrient tonics, aiding the structural form and functional activity of the tissues and organs. Stimulant tonics, which are gentle, slow the stimulants that invigorate the body's energy. An adrenal tonic is an example of a stimulant tonic. In modern and herbal medicine, it is known that the adrenal glands are responsible for secreting hormones as a result of the rapid bodily response to stress. Repeated stress results in the adrenal gland's constantly having to keep up with the demands of the body-mind. Eventually, the glands weaken and are rendered insufficient. In herbal medicine, there is a possibility of nourishing and renewing the adrenal glands, promoting activity and reintegration in body function (Hoffman, 1996). A combination of herbs, such as borage, licorice, Siberian ginseng, and Saint-John's-wort, are found to promote adrenal gland health (Tierra, 1988). Whether stimulant or nutrient in nature, all tonics "tone" the systems and play a fundamental role in maintaining a state of dynamic equilibrium or balance.

Individual choice of using plant medicines (phytomedicines) for therapeutic or preventive purposes is one of consumer awareness. Herbs are medicines and have active chemical constituents used to therapeutically mobilize a person's own capacity for self-healing. Since the quality and processing of herbal medicines are not standardized, individuals who are self-prescribing should use caution. Self-prescribing is commonly found among various cultures and is encouraged; however, when the individual is uncertain about herbal medicine use, it is wise to seek the advice of a competent health practitioner trained in pathology and herbology. An herbalist spends years getting to know the qualities, energies, and properties of the herbs so he or she can effectively match the herbs or combinations to the person and the situation. Whether the person follows the guidance of a trained herbalist or practices self-prescribing, it remains an individual responsibility to heal the whole self through making informed choices.

BONNIE T. MACKEY

See also
Bach Flower Remedies (IV)
Phytochemicals (III)

HIPPOTHERAPY

Hippotherapy means "treatment with the help of the horse." Although it is new to the United States, hippotherapy has been used as a form of treatment in Europe, particularly West Germany and Switzerland, since the 1940s. The treatment refers to the use of the horse as a therapeutic modality. The child or adult sits on the horse and accommodates, with automatic reactions, to the swinging motions of the horse's gait.

Hippotherapy does not try to teach riding skills. The focus instead is on the individual's response to the horse's movement. Therapeutic riding, another kind of session used with children and adults, focuses on developing riding skills but requires that the instructor be knowledgeable in the limitations that the rider might have.

It is believed that hippotherapy helps through the combination of the horse's body warmth, which loosens tight muscles, and the rider's attempts to accommodate to the movement. Particularly in therapy with children, there is a real bond between the child and the horse. The horse, for instance, may move to straighten if a child is losing balance.

The horse's movement has a therapeutic effect because it is precise and repetitive, similar to that of the movement of the pelvis during a normal human gait. Studies conducted in Germany have shown that a large horse can transmit 90 to 110 multidimensional impulses per minute to its rider during a walking gait. As the horse walks, the rider's center of gravity is displaced three-dimensionally with back-and-forth, up-and-down, and side-to-side movements.

Physical therapists use a variety of neurophysiological treatment methods when working with children to provide them with the sensation of normal movement. In a similar way, the horse's rhythmical movement transmits symmetrical sensory input to the rider, who then tries to accommodate.

The size of the child is more important than his or her age. The pelvis must be large enough for the child to straddle the horse comfortably. Usually that's about 3 to 4 years of age.

To benefit from a hippotherapy session, the client has to have the ability to follow directions. There are some contraindications, such as severe scoliososis and active rheumatoid arthritis. Many children come to hippotherapy in wheelchairs and go home walking.

The primary goals of hippotherapy are to enhance posture, balance, mobility, and function. The benefits hippotherapy can provide include mobilizing the pelvis, lumbar spine, and hip joints, thus modifying and making muscle tone more efficient. It also develops head and trunk postural control and improves symmetry. Additionally, because of the tactile, proprioceptive, and vestibular input, sensorimotor integration is improved. Righting and equilibrium are also facilitated. Body awareness, spatial orientation, endurance, and strength are also improved. Hippotherapy has a positive effect on respiration, circulation, and neurogenic bladder and intestinal function disorders. Psychological benefits include improved self-esteem, confidence, motivation, attention span, and human-animal bonding.

The horse's body warmth is part of the treatment. A child rides bareback with no saddle or stirrups to hold him or her in place. Before the child ever gets on the horse, he or she is evaluated for strength, balance, range of motion, and coordination. Problems are evaluated, and a program is then designed using the motion of the horse.

Problems for which hippotherapy has proven effective include cerebral palsy, Down's syndrome, and spinal muscle atrophy. Many children with Down's syndrome and cerebral palsy were born prematurely. Often children with cerebral palsy cannot sit up. With hippotherapy, they can learn to sit by themselves.

Children with Down's syndrome may have huge potbellies and waddle when they walk. After riding for 6 months, potbellies disappear and the children walk with a normal gait. To continue the effect, sessions must continue and riding should become a lifelong activity.

Sometimes children start out riding with someone riding behind them. Once the children can sit up and balance, however, they are placed on the horse by themselves and are accompanied by two sidewalkers.

Before being placed on a horse, children participate in a period of therapeutic movement. Children play games, like basketball, to incorporate the movements they will need to make once on the horse. They are eager to join in. In the physical therapy clinic, they often run away, claiming exercise hurts them; but at the stables, they love working with the horses.

Youngsters with spinal muscle atrophy have difficulty with balance and maintaining trunk control. In these cases, the horse is moved very slowly. The rhythmical movement of the animal requires the child's trunk to respond to it. A horse for hippotherapy is chosen based on its anatomy, structure, and temperament. The ideal horse must be sound, gentle, and tolerant. It also has to be able to do "tracking up," which means its hind hooves must land where the front hooves just stepped.

Children need a doctor's prescription to participate in the therapy. Hippotherapy has also been used successfully with adults. It has been used in the treatment of multiple sclerosis and stroke.

CAROLYN CHAMBERS CLARK

See also
Animal-Assisted Therapy (IV)

HOMEOPATHY: MOLECULAR BASIS

Homeopathy is the oldest complementary medical therapy in the United States with its own official pharmacopoeia, *The Homeopathic Pharmacopoeia of the United States* (HPUS). Even with a pharmacopoeia having over 1,000 monographed drugs, homeopathy has not been taken seriously as a therapy by most health care providers. Homeopathy, used by 1% to 2% of the U.S. population, has been underutilized by the vast majority of medical professionals, consumers, and the pharmaceutical industry.

This lack of belief in homeopathy has many causes, but the prime one is that scientists never could find anything in *ultrahigh dilutions* to measure that was increasing the more the *homeopathic medicine* solutions were potentized by shaking and dilution. Homeopathic theory believes that as the homeopathic drug source molecules *decrease*, the potency of a homeopathic medicine *increases*.

Clinicians who prescribe homeopathic medicines and patients who have experienced their healing effects have done so on blind faith that there is something more than just water in high-potency homeopathic drugs. Current research corroborates that it's more than a placebo response as shown by research on hay fever and diarrhea using ultra-high dilutions.

Because allopathic drug strength (potency) is related to the number of molecules or weight of the drug, scientists assume that homeopathic drug potency should, too. But the homeopathic drug spectrum is different because it consists of molecules and no molecules, depending on the potency. At low potency, it's like allopathic molecular pharmacy; at potencies of 6X and higher, few or no molecules exist, but information is present.

Low-potency homeopathic drugs have enough active drug molecules to cause physiological effects. Depending on the homeopathic drug and the molecular dose, there is the possibility of causing anaphylactic shock, organ toxicity, serious adverse reactions, drug interactions, and possible cocarcinogen effects.

Where the homeopathic pharmaceutical knowledge becomes unique is for potencies 6X and higher, where drug toxicity is no longer a problem. Here it becomes difficult to measure molecules, and after 24X potency or 12C potency, there are no more drug molecules by calculation.

New research in basic physics can explain this homeopathic pharmaceutical paradox of the more you shake and dilute a drug the more potent it becomes despite a decrease in drug molecules. A physicist and visiting professor at California Institute of Technology, Dr. Shui-Yin Lo, and his collaborators (1996) have discovered that the molecular basis of two very dilute homeopathic medicines is a new form of ice made from stable water molecules at room temperature and normal atmospheric pressure. This research shows that a new type of ice forms when sodium chloride and nitric acid are shaken and diluted in pure water serially six times, the equivalent of a 6X potency. Lo named this new ice "Ie crystals," for Ice with an electric field. Lo did not check solutions at 24X, those in alcohol, or commercially prepared homeopathic drugs, but he believes they will not behave any differently than the researched lower dilutions 6X to 12X in pure water.

Scientists know that water molecules form stable rigid structures like Ice VI at room temperature and at high pressure over 7 kB. Such a high pressure could exist between an ion and its nearby water molecules due to the electrostatic attraction between the charge of an ion and the electric dipole moments of a water molecule (Lo, 1996).

For 5 years, Lo and his colleagues have experimented with various solutions of Ie crystals found in sucussed dilutions over 6X of homeopathically prepared dilutions of acid, base, and salt solutions in reverse osmosis water. As the number of molecules decreases during dilution plus the shearing force of shaking (sucussion), the water around the initiating substance (the homeopathic drug) reorganizes into clusters. These clusters range from 15 nm to several microns in size and can be seen with some difficulty with a light microscope using high-power magnification. While the molecules continue to decline by shaking and diluting after 6X, 2-micron Ie crystals formed by vigorous shaking begin to appear in the water drug-solution.

These Ie crystals, which are very heat stable to 121° C, are easily visible using both the electron microscope and the atomic force microscope. The crystals evaporate and condense like normal water. They decrease both the surface tension and dielectric constant and increase the refractive index and change the absorption peaks of water molecules.

Ie crystals also have effects outside of medical therapeutics. When an Ie preparation made from a fuel catalyst is added to methane in an engine, methane combustion increases by 100%.

Lo showed that the Ie crystals do not increase linearly the more they are shaken and diluted but increase and decrease in rhythmic alterations with peaks and valleys every dilution or two as measured by UV absorbance at wavelength 190 nm. This measurement of rhythmic alterations in experiments using homeopathic solutions in different potencies has been repeatedly reported in the homeopathic research (Chou, 1986; Stephenson, 1955). This rhythmic alteration of Ie crystal amount dependent on the potency is similar to other rhythmic variations of bodily functions, such as heart-rate variability and electroencephalogram waves.

Always characteristic of our bodies, these rhythmic fluctuations, seen in Lo's research and in other homeopathic research, may be another reflection of the homeopathic simile principle. This wave-like similarity may be one of the main reasons that ultra-high homeopathic potencies can communicate with the body and effect change even in the absence of original molecules.

Measurement of highly potentized drugs is essential if homeopathic pharmacology is to develop fully and contribute more widely to healthcare. Whether Ie crystals are the key to the mechanisms of action of homeopathic medicines will be left to future research. However, there is new basic knowledge about the homeopathic potency process that will enable research to flourish not only in the healthcare field but in the wider arena of healing the planet, including the air.

JACQUELYN J. WILSON

HOMEOPATHY: DOSAGE FORMS

Homeopathic products are produced in a variety of dosage forms. Some are unique to homeopathy, others are more conventional. These dosage forms are described in the Homeopathic Pharmacopoeia (8th edition) Revision Service of the United States (HPRS), Section on General Pharmacy.

Globules, also called pellets or pilules, are made of pure sucrose, lactose or other appropriate polysaccharide. They are formed into small globular masses of different sizes designated according to their diameter in millimeters. Globules are impregnated, or medicated, by fixing a homeopathic liquid attenuation on their matrix. Globules made of lactose will absorb alcoholic solutions containing a much larger percentage of water than will those made of sucrose. The final medicated form of these globules is perfectly white and odorless. They are labeled according to the potency of the liquid attenuation used in their preparation. Globules are uniquely homeopathic and are still a very popular dosage form. They are administered sublingually.

Tablet triturates are defined as tablets produced from moist materials on a triturate mold which gives them the shape of cut sections of a cylinder. These tablets, like the globules, dissolve completely and rapidly when placed under the tongue. The moist starting material used in producing tablet triturates contains the active homeopathic substance in the appropriate attenuation or potency. This is a very popular dosage form in homeopathy and is still used for certain conventional medication such as nitroglycerin.

Compressed tablets are tablets formed by compression of a dry material and contain no special coating. They are compressed from powdered or crystalline solids and as with tablet triturates may contain binders, excepients, lubricants, and disintegrators. Compressed tablets are a more conventional dosage form that has been embraced by the homepathic community. In homeopathy, they are primarily used sublingually.

Tinctures are a very popular dosage form used in homeopathy. They contain ethyl alcohol as both a solubilizer as well as a preservative. Lower potencies and mother tinctures will usually have a higher concentration of alcohol (60% v/v), while higher potencies (more dilute) require less alcohol, a minimum of 20% v/v, for preservation. Tinctures are administered in dropper dosages. A drawback to the use of tinctures is the alcohol content which can pose a problem for alcohol-sensitive individuals even in dropwise volumes. This effect can be minimized by placing the drops in hot water in hope of evaporating off the alcohol.

Oral solutions are a contemporary way of delivering homeopathics in an alcohol- and sugar-free aqueous vehicle. A major advantage is the absence of alcohol. These solutions are also administered in a more traditional teaspoonful dosage for oral administration. A suitable preservative system, such as the food stabilizer potassium benzoate, is used in place of ethyl alcohol. This dosage form is becoming more popular with homeopathic practitioners and consumers.

Suppositories are a popular homeopathic dosage form in Europe. They are beginning to be used in the U.S.A., particularly for vaginal insertion. Most conventional suppository bases are used in production with the aqueous phase being the medicated vehicle containing the homeopathic ingredient(s).

Ophthalmic solutions, containing homeopathic ingredients, are also available. These solution must be isotonic with tear fluid and suitably preserved. Like suppositories, they are becoming a more popular dosage form in the U.S.A.

Nasal solutions are similar to ophthalmic solutions in their composition. They are available in both liquid drops and nasal sprays containing the appropriate homeopathic component(s).

Parenteral products are homeopathic solutions intended for injection. They are prepared in accordance with appropriate specifications of the current Unites States Pharmacopoeia and must bear the federal legend of prescription medication. Injectables are little used in homeopathy in this country, they are somewhat more popular in Europe. One of the major advantages of homeopathics are their oral and topical absorption and efficacy; this may explain the lack of popularity of injectable preparations.

Topical products for external application of homeopathics are becoming more widely used. Ointments, creams and lotions of appropriate active ingredients, usually in lower homeopathic potencies, are useful in a variety of dermatological conditions as well as first aid in sprains, strains, and bruises. These externally used formulations are becoming much more popular with informed consumers seeking alternatives to anti-inflammatory steroids.

ALLEN M. KRATZ

HOMEOPATHY: MIASM

Definition

MIASM/MIASMATIC means a noxious influence. Miasm, as defined by Hahnemann, is the infectious principle, which, when taken into the organism, may set up a specific disease. Miasms may be inherited, acquired or acute. The principle miasms are: psora, sycosis (gonorrhea), syphilis and tuberculosis. It is said that cancer may be a combination of all of these miasms.

Commentary

Modern day homeopathic practitioners view miasms as inherited. This is a difficult concept to embrace . . . let alone prove! It is thought that exposure to these diseases in earlier generations can result in cellular "taints" or imperfections that can be passed along genetically. These genetic imperfections act as toxins to the body, predisposing it to chronic illnesses. Many classically trained homeopaths routinely use homeopathically prepared formulations of these miasms. These formulations are termed nosodes.

Nosodes of miasms are used to "cleanse" the body on a cellular level. They have a constitutional effect; they detoxify on a very "deep" perhaps *intra*cellular, level. Homeopathy is an energetic approach. Nosodes resonant with existing toxins (miasma) adding energy to them and causing them to be expressed or excreted from the body. The question that homeopathic practitioners are often asked is: What happens when we suppress, rather than express, the symptoms of an infection or illness? Homeopathy views symptoms as the body's attempt to clear, repair, or adapt ... to reach homeostasis ... to heal! Should these symptoms be suppressed just to feel better? Does suppression fool the body into thinking that the job is complete? Does the body become retoxified, since the clearing of toxins is incomplete? In my opinion, this retoxification does occur and leads to imperfect cellular regeneration. When enough cells are imperfect, the tissue is compromised and may actually become "foreign" to the body. This is autoimmunity, a contributing factor to many diseases.

Many homeopathic practitioners are convinced that we are actually creating new miasms by suppressing the symptoms of our modern day "infections," i.e., herpes virus. They feel that this genetic predisposition can be passed on to future generations. This is certainly an upsetting hypothesis.

Contemporary practitioners of complementary/alternative medicine (CAM) recognize the need for clearing and detoxification. Some will utilize the classical homeopathic approach with miasmatic nosodes. Others employ the homeovitic approach of clearing, specific cellular detox in conjunction with organ/system support. Both approaches work on an energetic basis to cleanse the body on a cellular level, thus eliminating the potential for problems created by inherited miasms and other cellular toxins such as chemicals and metals. Clearing and cellular detox are the first steps on the path to wellness. Clean the foundation before rebuilding.

ALLEN M. KRATZ

HOMEOPATHY: POTENCY

Definitions

Potentize (dynamization): The process of repeated dilution with succussion (shaking) is how the homeopathic remedy is prepared.

Potency chord (potency accord, PC, homaccord, potency complexes, multi-attenuations): Several potencies of a substance(s) mixed to form one medicinal entity, i.e., Echinacea PC is a homeopathic product containing Echinacea purpureau 6X, 12X, 30X, 200X and Echinacea angustifolia 6X, 12X, 30X, 200X. Though not popular until the 1970s, early work was done by Cahis of Barcelona, who presented his findings at the International Homeopathic Congress in London in 1911. He likened such mixtures to musical melodies or chords and believed the sum total therapeutic effect to be quite different from the individual potencies themselves. Others who did research in this area were: Kroner, Nebel, Reckeweg, Zimmerman, Fuhry, Sunder, Junker, Kolisko, Konig, and Vosgerau.

Commentary

The two most popular potentization approaches are the decimal scale and the centesimal scale. The decimal potency is a 1 to 10 dilution with succussion. It is indicated by an X or D after the number, ex. 6X, 12X. The centesimal potency is a 1 to 100 dilution with succussion. It is indicated by a C after the number, ex. 2C, 12C. A 6X potency is actually a 1 part per million (1 ppm) molecular concentration that has been diluted and succussed six times.

The concept of energetic potency is a primary tenet of homeopathy. It is also the main paradox . . . how can less be more? It is also the major controversy in that beyond a 24X potency, Avogadro's number kicks in . . . no more molecules! Does water have the ability to remember? Scientists confirm that there are many properties of water that remain to be discovered.

The question may be asked: when does the dilution/succussion create a true homeopathic product? At what potency level? Based on my experience, I sense that at the 6X (or 3C) potency, the energetic phase tends to predominate over the molecular (i ppm) phase. At this potency, we are adding energy to the body, rather then requiring energy from the body for digestion, assimilation, and elimination that occurs at lower, more molecular, potencies.

I have also found that a basic rule in using or recommending potencies is: the more acute the condition, the lower the potency and the more frequently the administration. In chronic toxicities, I recommend a potency spectrum of 9X through 200X. These are considered middle-range potencies. Constitutional prescribing by a classically trained practitioner is usually above 200X, often given in a single dose.

Why use a mixture of potencies, or potency spectrum? As a person heals, potency requirements change. If you provide the body with a spectrum of potencies, it can then choose from this spectrum at the appropriate time. BHI and HoBoN were the first two homeopathic companies to mix potencies in their formulations. In the last few years, many other companies have followed suit.

Homeopathy works on an energetic level. It adds energy to the body to intensify the body's innate healing and repairing efforts. The body is always trying to heal and repair itself. In 1994, the respected journal *Science* reported that a system of enzymes, the DNA repair enzymes, have been named the "molecules of the year" for their importance in biochemistry. This discovery will be one of the keys to the mystery of aging and healing.

In conclusion, energetic potency is the key to the efficacy of homeopathy. The dilution level creates the safety record that is unrivaled. The paradox of "less is more" is being revealed to scientists as our technology grows in the area of detecting subtle energies. Stay tuned!

ALLEN M. KRATZ

HOMEOPATHY: USE IN FAMILY PRACTICE MEDICINE

With over 150 years of clinical use, homeopathy is today the safest and the second most widely used medical therapeutic system in the world. This affordable, natural system has over 1,000 extremely safe over-the-counter (OTC) homeopathic medicines and many prescription homeopathic drugs, both of which can be helpful for many acute and chronic problems encountered daily.

These gentle drugs, made from plant, animal, mineral, and human sources, are regulated by the U.S. Food and Drug Administration. Homeopathic medicines can be tailored for individualized treatment of many conditions, often without or refractory to conventional care, such as hepatitis or other viral illnesses and functional illness. Homeopathy is also a good choice for the client who does not tolerate chemical drug treatment because of allergic reactions or intolerable side effects.

Homeopathic drugs are used according to a holistic philosophy based on three principles: (1) *individualization,* including drug selection using the principle of similars or "likes cure likes"; (2) the promotion of self-healing using the *minimum dose* of a drug; and (3) the use of the *totality of symptoms* for assessing patterns of healing.

Therapeutic outcomes are enhanced by the process of serial drug potentization, a vigorous shaking and diluting with water/alcohol, or grinding with lactose. Basic physics research shows that a new form of very stable ice crystal is created in the water during this potentization process.

Official homeopathic drugs have rigorous quality control set by the *Homeopathic Pharmacopoeia of the United States.* Drugs are available in many potencies and various forms. These include lactose/sucrose sublingual tablets or pellets, sublingual or oral liquids, topical creams and ointments, eyedrops, nasal sprays, and suppositories. Injectable homeopathic drugs always require a prescription, as do drugs in certain potencies that have toxicity or are labeled for serious indications. Drug names are in Latin, and expiration dates and National Drug Codes are optional.

Homeopathy came to the U.S. from European general practice roots over 150 years ago. From its beginning, American homeopathy has always been used both for self-care and by practitioners. Since the majority of homeopathic drugs are labeled with OTC indications, patients may empower themselves by doing homeopathic self-care, thus reducing unnecessary doctor visits. There are many self-care educational materials available including books, audio- and videotapes, and computer software.

Homeopathic Prescriptions

Homeopathy, an emerging science, is evolving along several paths: The two main paths are single-drug prescribing and combination-drug prescribing. Clinical research shows that both are equally effective.

Homeopathy's major challenge for family doctors is learning how to use these medicines effectively. For the doctor who cannot take the 1,000 hours needed to study classical single-medicine homeopathy, successful treatment may be accomplished with combinations of homeopathic medicines that have proven clinically efficacious for over 150 years.

One rapid way to learn combination homeopathic prescribing is to understand the basics of 15 commonly used single homeopathic drugs. Start by reading several introductory books recommended to your clients for use in self-care. Try prescribing *Arnica montana* 6X or 6C up to 200 X or 200 C every 4 hours as needed in pellets, tablets, or oral liquid for any injured client who still has the painful effects of trauma recent or distant. Usually 1 to 3 days of *Arnica* treatment will be effective in removing all soreness and pain.

Also search out homeopathic combinations for acute and chronic disease in a local pharmacy or health food store and in the 1997 *PDR for Nonprescription Drugs.* Call the homeopathic pharmaceutical companies for their drug product catalogs that detail homeopathic combination protocols. Consult the resource directory of the National Center for Homeopathy for listings of homeopathic pharmaceutical companies, courses, and seminars in basic homeopathy. About 20 hours of basic homeopathic study is needed for family practitioners to have good outcomes with combination prescribing.

A few combination medicines may be prescription drugs, such as those for heart disease or injectables for pain from inflammation. Common OTC combination formulas include those for arthritis, allergy, colds and flu and other infections, colic, teething, constipation, bladder irritation, menstrual problems, emotional problems, and trauma. Also OTC are hemorrhoidal or fever suppositories, nasal sprays for allergies and sinusitis, and eyedrops.

By starting with combination homeopathic prescribing, chances increase for improved clinical outcomes because there is an increased chance of giving the similar drug. This is especially true for treating clients with acute disease but often holds true for treating those with chronic disease. Certainly, there will be patients who won't respond to specific homeopathic combinations. These patients need different treatment and maybe single-medicine prescribing.

Clinicians who want to use only single homeopathic medicines for acute and chronic disease need to study 500 to 1,000 hours to acquire the skills needed for classical prescribing. One needs to become familiar with hundreds of different prescribing indications looking for those that are most similar to the patient's presentation.

A classical practitioner's client time even with software aids will be 1 to 2 hours for a new visit involving chronic ills, with 30 minutes needed for monthly follow-up visits or acute care prescribing.

Outcomes

Whatever homeopathic method is used, improvement in clients with acute disease can happen within hours, and within days to weeks in chronic disease. Restoration of health is a gradual process. Gradual change and gradual reduction of allopathic maintenance drugs such as antihypertensives, antihistamines, or anti-inflammatories plus objective monitoring is necessary.

Homeopathy has had major success treating clients with various infections, like chronic otitis media, recurrent URIs, sinusitis, pneumonia, hepatitis, enteritis, gastritis, colitis, vaginitis, urinary tract infections, childhood diseases, and tuberculosis. Other areas where homeopathy can help are asthma, attention deficit disorders, mental illness, insomnia, migraine headaches, arthritis, neuralgia, problems of pregnancy, failure to thrive, hormonal imbalances, and skin disorders.

Almost every diagnosis known has been helped at times with homeopathy; the key to success is individualizing the treatment and finding the similar drugs that match the illness while bringing awareness to the client. To help individualize treatment, two reference books are often used: a materia medica and a repertory.

Whatever the homeopathic treatment method, classical or combination, homeopathic medicines 6C or 6X and higher do not cause drug interactions with regular chemical drugs. Some lower potencies, especially 1X to 2X, may have drug interactions or serious drug reactions, including anaphylactic shock.

If a child ate an entire bottle of 6X OTC homeopathic medicine tablets, poisoning would not happen. Homeopathic drug dosage is simple and does not depend on body weight, kidney, or liver function.

Additional benefits of homeopathy include improved compliance from pleasant-tasting pills and reduction of both afterhours calls and unnecessary office visits, when families are educated in safe self-care. Family practices that use homeopathy have a marked decrease both in antibiotic and nonsteroidal anti-inflammatory drug use as well as adverse drug effects.

JACQUELYN J. WILSON

HOSPITAL-BASED MASSAGE THERAPY

As stated by Karen Gibson, R.N., C.M.T., hospital-based massage therapy author, educator, and consultant, "Hospital-based massage therapy is defined as the application of skilled, sensitive, and compassionate touch by professionally trained massage therapists in medical environments with the specific intention of promoting the healing process, improving clinical outcomes, and encouraging higher levels of wellness both in patients and those who care for them."

The term "hospital-based massage" may refer to massage therapy administered in medical settings outside the hospital, such as through hospice or in nursing homes. Hospital-based massage techniques include bodywork and touch therapies other than massage, which often is thought of as rubbing. They may include very gentle techniques, such as placing the hands lightly on the body without moving the hands, or "energy work" therapies in which the physical body is not touched, but rather the therapists' hands are moved around the body, in the space beyond the skin.

Sometimes hospital-based massage therapy programs draw on the assistance of laypeople who are not trained in massage therapy but who are trained to provide touch, which is therapeutic under the guidance or direction of a trained hospital-based massage therapy practitioner.

In the 4th century B.C., Hippocrates is quoted as having stated, "The physician must be experienced in many things, but assuredly also in anatripais, the art of rubbing."

Historically, nurses massaged patients as part of their general duties to ease patients and help them relax. In just the last few decades, hospitals have become more technologically focused, and nurses are now busy with equipment, medications, and documentation and are often too busy to spend any additional one-on-one time with patients. Today's hospital-based massage therapist is often viewed by the rest of the staff as the member of the health care team who has the time to nurture and comfort patients one-on-one. Due to this, massage therapists are often seen as playing the role of bringing caring touch back into today's highly technical and mechanized hospital environment.

Several nurses are obtaining massage therapy training to incorporate caring touch into their work. Nurses who also are massage therapists have the title nurse massage therapist, which is now recognized as a specialty in nursing practice. Many are members of the National Association of Nurse Massage Therapists. Some occupational therapists and physical therapists also are obtaining massage therapy training to add this to their therapeutic tools.

The creation of a hospital-based massage therapy program first requires the approval of the hospital administration. A detailed proposal must be drawn and presented to the appropriate committees. An active proponent within the hospital administration can be of immeasurable assistance in this process. Approval of a program may depend on one or more of the following factors: financial feasibility; belief in the potential benefits of massage therapy for the patients and/or staff; the perception that the public desires massage therapy services in the hospital; and the belief that massage therapy may even provide a marketing edge for the organization.

Hospital units on which massage therapists work include pre- and postsurgery, obstetrics and gynecology, antepartum and postpartum, neonatal intensive care, geriatrics, oncology (including bone marrow transplant), physical therapy, occupational therapy, orthopedics, cardiopulmonary, rehabilitation, outpatient pain management, speech therapy, HIV/AIDS, and hospital fitness and wellness centers. Patients may be self-referred or referred by any interdisciplinary team member, including nurses, doctors, physical therapists, or patient advocates such as the chaplain or social worker.

Massage therapy is used with acute care patients to help alleviate many symptoms, including nausea, cramping, and headaches, and to help improve circulation and lymph drainage in the bedridden. Massage therapy has been reported to decrease the amount of pain medication needed by patients and to help patients sleep and eat better. Massage may also be used to facilitate the patient's parasympathetic nervous system. As the body is more relaxed, this may aid in the patient's healing process, which may then help speed recovery and reduce the incidence of complications and possible hazards of immobility.

Massage therapy can be utilized in rehabilitation to increase muscle tone, decrease scar tissue, decrease adhesions, and increase soft-tissue health for the reduction of pain and recovery of muscle and joint use.

Some massage therapists in hospitals also treat patients' family members, friends, and significant others to address the stress of being close to someone who is ill or dying. Feeling nurtured and more relaxed can enable family and friends to better care for their ill loved one. Massage therapists also may teach family members and friends to give the patient gentle massage, such as a foot, hand, or back rub. This can help both to alleviate stress in the hospital situation and to nurture the patient, as energy and attention are diverted from worrying and into actively caring for and helping the person who is ill.

Massage therapists may work with hospital staff either in an "on-site" format, giving short 5- to 10-minute chair massages during the work day or by being available to staff members for 1/2 and full-hour massages when off-duty. On-site massages can help decrease staff members' stress levels during their shift, which in turn may allow them to be more attentive, caring, efficient, and focused in their work. Staff members who further take advantage of massage therapy services on their off-hours may report overall decreased stress and increased health. Decreased stress and increased soft-tissue health may contribute to the prevention or minimalization of stress- and work-related problems such as headaches, back strains, carpal tunnel syndrome, and sciatica-like symptoms. This means that massage therapy may be a factor in reducing sick leave and workers' compensation claims.

Some hospital-based massage therapists also treat the general public through an office in the hospital. Massage programs may also offer wellness classes such as self-massage, *t'ai chi*, yoga, and infant massage for parents.

Some massage therapists in hospitals volunteer their services. Some massage programs are based solely on internships, externships, or research projects. Such programs are often conducted in association with a massage therapy school, and the massage therapists involved may volunteer their time, pay for training, or receive a minimal fee.

Some hospital-based massage therapy programs are directed by a paid part- or full-time coordinator (often a massage therapist who is also an R.N.) who coordinates several paid or volunteer massage therapists. Many of the original hospital-based massage therapy programs founded in the 1980s were created as volunteer programs because this was perhaps the easiest way to be accepted into the hospital. However, in the health care reform climate of the 1990s, some volunteer programs were terminated because they were not revenue-generating. Another potential drawback to volunteer programs is that they may be difficult to maintain and develop because people usually cannot afford to volunteer full-time or long-term.

Other massage therapists are paid to work in the hospital. They may work as independent contractors or be hired as employees. They may obtain insurance reimbursement or be paid solely by patients

out-of-pocket. Some massage therapy programs are run in full or in part on funding provided by the hospital. Massage therapists may be paid by the session or by an hourly rate (regardless of whether they are doing massage or paperwork), or they may be hired on salary with benefits. Massage therapy positions range from part- to full-time.

Some massage therapists have their own offices in which to treat in- and outpatients, patients' family and friends, staff, and even the general public. Other massage therapists travel around the hospital with a massage chair to perform on-site massages with staff. Massage therapists may travel from unit to unit treating patients and their attending family members in their beds, chairs, or on massage tables. Massage therapy may be rationed on one area, or just a few units, or may be available throughout the hospital.

Massage therapy techniques and treatment lengths vary based on who is being treated. Acute care patients generally receive more gentle work for shorter periods of time. "Energy work" therapies, such as Reiki and Therapeutic Touch, placing the hands on the body without moving them, and gentle massage of the feet, hands, and scalp including gentle reflexology are some techniques that may be used with patients in acute care. Massage therapists must be trained to understand how approach and technique may vary among patients.

Currently, education and laws governing massage therapy vary widely throughout the country. Therefore, each hospital must create its own standards and guidelines for massage therapists. A hospital considering the creation of a massage therapy program will want to be familiar with state and local laws governing massage therapy, as well as curricula of local massage therapy schools. If there are no state laws governing training requirements for massage therapists, a minimum of 500 hours of training in massage therapy may be considered. To work with staff, patients' family and friends, and the general public, massage therapists should have all the training they would need from a comprehensive massage therapy school. However, massage therapy school basic curricula often do not cover how to work with hospitalized patients. Therefore, massage therapists usually need additional training in this area.

Particularly in the case of inpatients, it is essential that massage therapists know how to work safely around hospital beds and medical equipment, and cautions, indications, and contraindications based on diagnoses, treatments, and medications. Massage therapists may also need further training in pathology, universal precautions, operational protocols, safety standards and guidelines, medical terminology, charting, and working effectively as an interdisciplinary team member.

When initiating a hospital-based massage therapy program for inpatients, it is best to hire massage therapists already knowledgeable in working within medical settings, or to have massage therapists work initially under direct supervision or collaboration with a nurse. Eliciting the assistance of a consultant in hospital-based massage therapy can be an invaluable asset to the success of a hospital massage program.

LAURA KOCH

HUMOR AS A COMPLEMENTARY THERAPY

Humor therapy uses laughter to decrease the effects of stress and pain on the body. While the benefits of humor were acknowl-edged as far back as Biblical times, modern use of humor therapy can be traced to the 1930s, when clowns were used to cheer up children hospitalized with polio. In the 1950s the alternative medicine movement began, and use of humor was subsequently added as it widened to embrace more modalities (Fry, 1994).

How humor affects health may be explained by psychoneuroimmunology (PNI) theory. According to PNI theory, complementary interventions that lead to changes in neurotransmitters, hormones, and immune functioning can subsequently influence health (Solomon, 1987). Because PNI theory acknowledges the holism of healing, it is a useful guide for complementary practitioners (Zeller, McCain, & Swanson, 1996).

According to a recent study of cancer patients (Bennett & Lengecher, in press), 50% of persons surveyed were currently using humor, and an additional 13% stated they would definitely try it. Unfortunately, research data concerning the effect of humor on health are just beginning to emerge. According to Fry (1994), "as with most grassroots movements, there is little laboratory, statistical, analytic, or otherwise scientific evidence to justify the huge degree of enthusiasm for uses of humor in this context."

Humor Research

Laughter, Stress, and Pain Perception

In a series of studies looking at stress and pain, it was found that subjects who laughed before a dental procedure reported less stress afterward (Trice & Price, 1986), elderly persons exposed to humorous videos reported decreased pain and improved mood compared with those exposed to non-humorous videos (Adams & McGuire,

1986), and college students exposed to a humorous tape had increased pain tolerance compared with the control group (Hudak, Dale, Hudak, & DeGood, 1991). Unfortunately, studies of stress hormones have conflicting results. In a study of 20 females, urinary excretion of epinephrine and norepinephrine increased following a humorous film (Levi, 1965). However, a more current study of 10 males found that those exposed to a humorous video had no changes in epinephrine and norepinephrine, while demonstrating decreased stress related cortisol, growth hormone, and dopac levels (Berk, Tan, Fry, Napier, Lee, et al., 1989).

Laughter and Immune Function

Several studies have demonstrated that humor can lead to increased salivary immunoglobulin A (SIgA) (Dillon, Minchoff, & Baker, 1985; Labott, Ahleman, Wolever, & Martin, 1990; Lambert & Lambert, 1995; Lefcourt, Davidson-Katz, & Kueneman, 1990). However, studies using SIgA have been challenged due to assay methodology and the questionable clinical significance of SIgA levels. Natural killer (NK) cell assays give some of the clearest and most replicable results in studies of stress and immune function (Schulz & Schulz, 1992). NK cells are effective against a variety of viruses and tumor cell lines (Levy, Herberman, Lippman, & D'Angelo, 1987). Unfortunately, only three studies of laughter and NK cytotoxicity are available.

In a study of 22 breast cancer patients, it was found that viewing a humorous video did not lead to significant changes in NK numbers or cytotoxicity (Wise, 1989). However, this study had methodological problems and was published in abstract form only. In a controlled study of 10

males, NK cell cytotoxicity was significantly increased following a humorous video (Berk, Tan, Napier, & Evy, 1989). Additional work by this same group has demonstrated that males exposed to a humorous video have a significant increase in serum IgA, interferon, number of activated T cells, and number of NK cells (Berk & Tan, 1995).

In a recent controlled study of 33 women, subjects exposed to a humorous video had significantly decreased stress compared with the distraction group. Mirthful laughter, measured using the Humor Response Scale (HRS), significantly correlated with poststress and with change in NK cytotoxicity for persons in the humor group. Subjects who laughed more (HRS scores over 24) had significantly improved NK activity compared with their baseline values, and as compared with the remaining participants (Bennett, 1997).

Summary

It appears that laughter has the potential to reduce stress and stress hormones, subsequently reducing the effect of stressors on immune function. As low NK activity has been linked to increased incidence of viral infections, this mechanism could explain one link between humor and health. In addition, as low NK activity has been linked to metastases and poorer prognosis in persons with cancer, it is plausible that humor may be a useful complementary therapy in the care of oncology patients.

MARY PAYNE BENNETT

HYPNOSIS APPLIED TO BIRTH

Hypnosis can be very helpful during pregnancy. David Cheek, obstetrician and hypnotherapist, described many uses for hypnosis in his various papers (collected by Ernest Rossi), including treatment for hyperemesis gravidarum (excessive vomiting in early pregnancy), prevention of miscarriage, prevention of premature labor, shortening of labor, turning abnormal presentations of the baby to the normal vertex (head down) presentation, stopping hemorrhage, and restoring stalled labor (uterine inertia) to a normal rate of progress.

The author studied 500 pregnant subjects during their first or second trimesters. Women with high anxiety and stress tended to have more complicated births, as did women who exhibited high levels of fear about birth, a poor sense of themselves as a mother (maternal identity), negative beliefs about birth, and high levels of life stress, depression, or anxiety. The use of hypnosis during pregnancy saved all of these women from having abnormal births. Depression was measured by the Beck Depression Inventory and anxiety was measured by the Taylor Manifest Anxiety Scale.

In another study, the author used hypnosis with 100 pregnant women whose fetuses were in the breech presentation. The estimated gestational age of their fetuses was 37–40 weeks. The treatment group received hypnosis with suggestions for general relaxation with release of fear and anxiety. Hypnosis was offered as a means of reducing overall arousal from fear, anxiety, or the general stresses of life, thereby reducing autonomic arousal and allowing relaxation of the lower uterine segment. The success rate of the experimental group was tested against a comparison group who received standard obstetrical care without the opportunity for hypnosis. Eighty-one percent of the experimental group converted to vertex presentation compared with 48%

of the comparison group. This difference was statistically significant at p levels of less than 0.001.

In a third study, the author used hypnosis with randomly selected women who were being aggressively treated for preterm labor. The hypnosis group was statistically significantly more likely to stop premature labor and to leave the hospital, going on to term, than a comparison group who did not receive hypnosis.

The author has reported 14 cases of hypnosis being used successfully for treating hyperemesis gravidarum during early pregnancy. One of those patients provides an interesting example of how hypnosis can be used. This woman was a psychologist trained in hypnosis. She was certain that her vomiting had no psychological component, but through suggestion she was willing to accept that her vomiting could be resolved by low-dose thyroid medication. During this time, fear of the pain of birth arose and was addressed. Fear of the changes that having a baby would bring for her professional career also emerged and was addressed. Then, when she was given a minuscule dose of thyroid hormone, her symptoms resolved. She continued to claim that no psychological processes had affected her hyperemesis; it was all related to her thyroid status.

The most common use of hypnosis for birth is as birth visualization in preparation for labor. Typically, the author uses a technique in which the subject becomes deeply relaxed for the first 15 minutes of the session. Then she is asked to describe her labor and birth. The author carefully notes areas of distortion and neglect in the woman's description. Hypnosis is then used to create a multisensory, imagined experience of labor. The woman goes through a birth in which the contractions are experienced and the pain of labor is reframed as healthy, intense, and easily handled by the woman. Through this process, the woman who has never had a baby before develops the poise and confidence of a woman who has already given birth.

Hypnosis techniques are (1) making rapport, (2) achieving harmony of communication, (3) use of truisms, (4) use of embedded commands, (5) use of metaphor, (6) use of synesthesia, (7) use of implied causatives, (8) use of storytelling, (9) use of personal self, and (10) use of body language. The full potential benefits of hypnosis for pregnancy and birth remain to be fully discovered and merit further research.

Lewis Mehl-Madrona

HYPNOTHERAPY

Hypnotherapy consists of any therapeutic efforts that use hypnosis to improve a person's health or well-being. Hypnosis itself may involve any approach that guides or teaches a person to become very highly mentally and physically relaxed.

A person may be said to be hypnotized when he or she has achieved a state of mind involving an increased degree of inner focus, shutting out the outside world for the time being. People undergoing a state of hypnosis are then generally able to put their minds to the goals of therapy. They thus allow themselves to be more open to suggestion. (Although hypnosis can be used to aid sleep, hypnotic subjects are *not* asleep as normal sleep is understood.)

Hypnotic suggestions may consist of direct commands, ideas, and mental imagery or visualization. A direct command may involve the suggestion that a person can move an arm or leg that has been injured or in pain and that they've feared to move (despite the fact that the limb is considered "medically able" to function).

A hypnotic idea suggestion may be one in which the subject undergoing hypnotherapy is able to develop ideas for an invention, a composition, giving a speech, or being more assertive with other people. Mental imagery or visualization during hypnotherapy involves subjects "seeing" themselves (as in a dream) accomplishing some goal successfully (e.g., overcoming fear of water by wading in a pool, dumping fattening food in the garbage, eating healthy food, exercising, dancing, driving over a bridge, flying in an airplane, etc.).

Modern hypnotherapy (and competent hypnosis) involves teaching the subject the art of self-hypnosis. Breathing exercises, muscle relaxation exercises, and nightly practice, which may include a hypnotic practice audiotape, are procedures often used in teaching self-hypnosis. Self-hypnosis has the advantage of allowing repeated practice of the skill. With repeated practice, as with any skills, a learning curve is gradually built up. Not only does the subject become more adept at moving the mind to the relaxed-open hypnotic state more easily, but also the targeted goal behavior, such as overcoming chronic pain, giving up a habit, or developing more courage to achieve something, is gradually improved.

"One-shot" (one-session) quick hypnosis is still practiced, as is "stage" hypnosis (Barber, 1969). One shot is disappointing in that the effects are not generally well learned so do not last. Stage hypnosis creates the false impression that hypnotists can make people do silly things against their will. (These subjects are usually pre-screened before a performance.)

The history of hypnosis may well be as old as the discovery of fire. Our human ancestors may well have experienced trance states as they stared into the fire. The experience of sitting calmly and staring into the fire, akin to watching nonviolent TV programs, can be hypnotherapeutic in that the relaxed state alleviates mental and physical stress.

More recent history usually mentions mesmerism (ASCH, 1985), named after the Austrian physician Anton Mesmer (1734–1815). Mesmer's theory of hypnosis was based on his creative notions of the process being due to animal magnetism. Mesmer attempted to mesmerize (hypnotize) the famous American Benjamin Franklin (1706–1790) to help Franklin with his chronic gout and pain. Franklin, however, got no benefit from Mesmer's therapy because he was extremely skeptical and out to prove that Mesmer was a fraud and a quack.

The term "hypnosis" was not used until it was legitimized by James Braid, M.D., in the early 1840s. The American Medical Association finally approved the use of hypnotherapy in 1958.

In addition to the uses already mentioned, hypnotherapy is either the therapy of choice or a helpful additional therapeutic tool in treating anxiety, phobias, depression, alcoholism, eating disorders, chronic pain, memory and concentration, and sexual disorders. Psychological hypnotherapy is not only useful in overcoming habits but also is well established as an alternative therapy to psychoactive "medications." Medical uses for hypnotherapy include anesthesia (more common before chemical anesthetics were developed), control of bleeding, dermatology (e.g., wart removal), burn therapy, and so on.

Hypnotic techniques are often used with other oncological therapies with cancer patients. Many dentists are well trained in hypnotic techniques, using them to reduce fear, for surgery, tongue biting, saliva control, gagging, and general hygiene.

There are hundreds of different hypnotic procedures and many different definitions of hypnosis. Hypnotherapy has an extensive research base throughout the world, ranging from fine-grained studies of brain chemistry and neurological studies to empirical results based on what works under different conditions, techniques, and individual differences (ASCH, 1985; Barber, 1969). Current theory on the hypnotic process is based on the observation that subjects actively call upon their own preexisting imaginative and cognitive skills to produce their own individualistic experiences of hypnotic effects. It is important to realize that all therapists do have a good deal of responsibility to other people. You don't need to be a hypnotist or use hypnosis to influence someone else's actions. Even a casual suggestion given at a certain time may profoundly influence another person's behavior (Hafling, 1974).

W. R. HAFLING

HYPNOTIC PREPARATION FOR SURGERY

Hypnosis has been used as a process to prepare patients for surgery since the 1960s. An effective modality, its use is still not widespread. The theory behind this type of preparation is that the mind influences physiological responses and the patient is, through hypnosis, able to control many physiological responses created within a surgical situation.

Through the hypnotic process, the patient is instructed to participate in his or her own healing process and control blood flow, pain, and other surgical responses. The results are enhanced when hypnosis training of the patient occurs 2 to 3 weeks prior to surgery.

Uses for Hypnotic Surgery Preparation

Hypnosis can be used for any surgical procedure. All hypnosis should be done with a trained and experienced hypnotist, and all medical hypnosis should be done only by referral of the appropriate medical practitioner.

A typical surgical hypnosis session has four parts:

1. The patient presents with a referral from the appropriate medical practitioner. The hypnotist and the patient discuss the surgical procedure.
2. The patient is told how hypnosis works and what hypnosis can and cannot do. The patient is asked if he or she has any questions or concerns regarding the hypnotic process. All questions are answered and concerns addressed before the session proceeds.
3. The patient is asked to get comfortable and the induction begins. Each hypnotist uses his or her own induction and language. In the induction the patient is told that the mind and body work together and that the body can be controlled by positive instructions from the mind.

The patient is guided through a visualization, which includes arriving at the hospital, being taken to the surgical suite, awakening in recovery, returning to the patient's room, leaving the hospital, and experiencing a perfect follow-up office visit. The hypnotist becomes familiar with the patient's procedure and tailors the visualization and posthypnotic suggestions to fit that patient. The purpose of this visualization is to allow the patient to experience a successful rehearsal prior to experiencing the actual surgery.

Posthypnotic suggestions are implanted throughout the session. When creating posthypnotic suggestions, the hypnotist phrases the suggestion in the present (i.e., "All bleeding is minimal," rather than, "All bleeding will be minimal"). Also, all posthypnotic suggestions are phrased in the positive (i.e., "I am comfortable," rather than, "I will not feel pain").

4. Next, the patient is brought out of hypnosis and given a list of posthypnotic suggestions to repeat at home throughout the days prior to surgery.

Posthypnotic Suggestions Throughout the Surgical Process

The patient's list of posthypnotic suggestions is taken to the hospital and read to the patient once the initial sedative has been administered and the patient begins responding to the drug. This sedated state simulates the hypnotic trance. The list of suggestions is taken with the patient and read to the patient through the entire surgical procedure. Ask the transport personnel to read the suggestions to the patient while transporting to the operating room. The list is next given to a nurse or anesthesiologist, who reads the suggestions while in surgery.

Following surgery, the list is given to the recovery room personnel to read to the patient. When the patient returns to his or her room, the suggestions can continue to be read. Using hypnosis in preparation for surgical procedures gives the patient a sense of control that reduces stress levels and healing times.

KATE LEVENSOHN

ICE MASSAGE FOR CONTROL OF LABOR PAIN

Until 25 years ago, little was known about pain, although pain is the most common complaint of clients seeking health care. Pain relief programs have evolved from one of controlling the person's expression of pain to today's widespread programs that explicitly describe pain relief as a top priority in three areas: chronic pain, hospice, and childbirth.

The childbirth education movement makes up one of the largest groups engaged in one of the most prolonged efforts ever made to control pain without drugs. The major components of pain relief taught in this movement are reduction of fear, relaxation techniques, effleurage, breathing techniques, hydrotherapy, and counterstimulation.

Ice Massage for Pain Relief

The early work of Denny-Brown, et al. (1945) showed effective blocking of nerve conduction in sensory fibers at cold temperatures. In 1964, Dr. A. E. Grant advocated massage with ice in the treatment of musculoskeletal pain, naming his technique "cryokinetics."

Dr. C. M. Marshall in 1971 published a study using ice cube massage for the relief of chronic pain of herpes of the eye. Drs. R. Melzack, S. Guite, and A. Gonshor in 1980, and Drs. R. Melzack and K. C. Bentley in 1983, found that intense sensory input produced by ice massage of the web of skin between the thumb and the forefinger of the hand resulted in a 50% reduction in acute dental pain. Drs. Melzack, M. E. Jeans, and J. G. Stratford later demonstrated the efficacy of ice massage in the reduction of low back pain in a comparison test with transcutaneous electrical stimulation (TENS).

Probably the most important factor relating to the studies described above is that they did not eliminate the source of the pain. Melzack and colleagues felt that their work indicated the mode of reduction of pain was due to the engaging of the gate control pain system. In recent years, Melzack's gate control pain theory has come under question in the scientific community. However, real or unproved theory, the techniques of pain relief involving the use of ice massage are effective, noninvasive, and nonpharmaceutical.

Ice Massage for the Control of Labor Pain

Until 1992, there had been no quantitative scientific work looking at ice massage for control of labor pain. A study described in the book *Massage During Pregnancy* (1995) performed ice massage on women in active labor. The web of skin between the thumb and forefinger was massaged using a small ice bag during contractions. The technique was the same as the one used by Melzack and colleagues in their study of dental pain. The anatomical area used for the ice massage is referred to in acupuncture literature as Large Intestine 4 or LI4. Some books refer to this point as *Hoku*.

Although this was a small study, the results were impressive. Eighty-six percent of the women in the study experienced a decrease of pain unpleasantness as well as a decrease in pain intensity. Table 1 shows how the group dropped in rank in describing their memory of pain unpleasantness.

The study was designed to carry out the ice massage for a period of 30 minutes. However, 57 percent of the women in the study felt they received so much relief from the ice massage intervention that they continued with the technique, requesting family members and nursing staff to perform ice massage during each contraction until they were completely dilated and ready to begin pushing. Some participants felt they had more relief on one hand than the other. Thirteen percent of the women in the study felt that the ice massage did not reduce their labor pain.

Steps for Hands-On Ice Massage Technique for Labor Pain

1. Tools needed are crushed ice and a small washcloth.

2. Place a small amount of crushed ice in the center of the washcloth. Twist the cloth around the ice making a miniature ice bag.

3. At the beginning of each contraction, use the ice bag to massage the web of skin between the thumb and the forefinger continuously until the end of the contraction.

4. The pressure of the massage should measure approximately 6 on a scale of 1 (being very light pressure) to 10 (pressure as hard as one can apply).

5. Experiment with massage on opposite hands to find which hand gives the most relief.

6. It is not practical to attempt to continue ice massage once the women reaches the pushing stage. Plus, the act of pushing is pain-relieving.

Note: Ice Massage for the Control of Labor Pain, a research project, was carried out at Dade City Hospital, Dade City, Florida in 1991–92. The research paper was presented June 1992 at the University of Southern Queensland, Toowoomba, Queensland, Australia, as part of Australian-American Nurses Exchange program. It was also presented at a Midwifery Education Seminar at Tampa General Hospital, Tampa, Florida.

BETTE WATERS

TABLE 1   Description of Memory of Pain

Pain level	Before ice	After ice
Excruciating	21.4%	7.1%
Horrible	42.9%	21.4%
Distressing	7.1%	14.3%
Mild	0.0%	14.3%

IMAGERY

Imagery is a natural thought process, using one or more of the five senses and usually associated with emotions. Imagery is how the right brain conceptualizes, and is the bridge between the conscious and subconscious mind. It is simply one way the mind thinks. Just as we all dream, we all use imagery to picture a scene in our mind's eye, recall a pleasant childhood memory, or hear a favorite piece of music being played in our head. This thought process is also active when one imagines a future event that has not happened yet. It would be impossible to be in a creative thought process without using the imagination.

Imagery is as old as man and as new as a fresh thought. For nearly 20,000 years, imagery has been an integral ingredient in healing practices, for it is the link to the spiritual level of healing. All religious beliefs have icons that hold meaning and great power. Ancient and modern indigenous peoples use some form of imagery or symbolism in their rituals. Shamanic healing involves going into the imaginal realm to seek help for someone who is ill and guidance during times of crisis.

Consider the mind-body connection as a conceptual framework. Imagery is the language by which the mind and body communicate. A thought or image is generated in the cerebral cortex and relayed to the limbic system, the emotional center of the brain. Through the nervous system, via neurotransmitters that act as messenger molecules, a message is sent from the brain to a part of the body, activating a physiological response. This is the basis of the exciting body of scientific research called psychoneuroimmunology (PNI), which specifically studies the interconnectedness of the mind, nervous system, and immune function. Through this series of connections, the imagery thought process directly elicits a physical reaction in the body. An example of this is a perceived, not actual, fearful situation, such as a threat of being attacked in a dark alley. This creates an alarm reaction in the body, causing an ele-

vation of heart rate, blood pressure, respiration, a tingling in the nerves, anxiety in the pit of the stomach, sweaty palms, setting into motion the fight/flight response. Another, *pleasurable*, example might be thinking about a sexual fantasy, which causes physical arousal and sensations quite different from the first. Both examples are not actual occurrences yet are very real in the mind and physical body.

Types of Therapeutic Imagery

Therapeutic imagery is taking this natural thought process and directing it to a desired, positive outcome. Guided imagery refers to using the power of the imagination to evoke positive mind-body-emotional responses to enhance innate healing potential. The process is directed by a practitioner or audiotape with scripted suggestions or images. For instance, a client is directed to relax and imagine he or she is going on a healing journey, up a mountaintop, where there is a cave and inside there is a wise shaman who administers a powerful healing medicine. The client then imagines thanking the healer and comes down the mountain back into current time and place. The journey and "imaginary" medicine can have a powerful effect on the body.

Another more personal and spontaneous type of imagery is called interactive guided imagery, or interactive imagery. This method takes the same therapeutic process to an even deeper level by eliciting and interacting with a person's own images. This is the most meaningful and empowering way to use imagery because it taps into one's own inner resources. A case example will help illustrate this. A 49-year-old man, with a classic type A personality, presents with chronic, debilitating tension headaches. The guide assists the client in relaxing and releasing tension in his head and body, which in and of itself is effective stress management. The client then focuses his attention on the area of the headache. The client is asked to bring to mind an image of the headache and describe the first image that arises. Immediately, an image of a volcano about to explode appears. With the assistance of the guide, the client explores information about this image as it relates to his headaches. By understanding the meaning of the volcano, the client learns that he needs to release his accumulated stress in small amounts at the end of each day, so the pressure does not build up and explode. With daily practice, the headaches gradually subside.

Uses and Applications

Although imagery occurs in the mind all the time, the therapeutic imagery process is best facilitated by a relaxation exercise, which sets the stage for the process to unfold. Coined by Herbert Benson (1975), the relaxation response is a psychophysiological state, in which the muscles of the body are released of tension and lactic acid; the heart rate, blood pressure, and respirations are decreased; the brain is in an alpha (alert, yet calm) state; and the parasympathetic nervous system is activated. Relaxation exercises have proven to be effective for hypertension, migraines, stress, pain, ulcers, and anxiety. Coupled with imagery, it is an ideal mind-body event.

The uses of imagery are unlimited. As stated by Martin L. Rossman, codirector of the Academy for Guided Imagery, "It can be used to remember and recreate the past, develop insight into the present, influence physical health and healing, enhance creativity or inspiration, and anticipate possible futures." Imagery is being used in business to create visions of the future and solve current dilemmas. It has been used in sports for quite some time. Studies have shown enhanced performance when imagery rehearsal of the athletic event is combined with physical practice.

In health care, there are a multitude of areas where imagery is highly effective. Guided imagery and interactive guided imagery are being used to reduce anxiety, relieve pain and symptoms, prepare for surgery, procedures, and childbirth, potentiate wound healing, and enhance quality of life. Specific strategies could include working with an image of the problem or disease, inner healing resources such as an inner guide or healer, physiological processes like bone mending, external treatments, medications or chemotherapy, and the desired end state of being healed or of well-being.

Research

There is an increasing body of research that validates the therapeutic effectiveness of imagery. The majority of studies have been conducted with cancer patients. Behavioral interventions such as psychological support, group psychotherapy, and hypnosis, imagery, and relaxation have proven beneficial in persons with cancer (Richardson et al., 1997). Surgery is the other major area where the effects of imagery intervention has been tested. One recent study at Cleveland Clinic revealed that the average length of stay was reduced by 1.5 days, pain medication was decreased by 50%, and bowel function returned to normal 1.2 days sooner.

The imagery process is a valuable healing tool. Within the modality, there are many skills and techniques used by an expert guide.

SUSAN EZRA

See also
   Anxiety/Panic (II)
   Cancer (II)
   Headache (II)
   Mindfulness (IV)
   Psychoneuroimmunology (IV)

IMAGERY, MOVEMENT, AND BREAST CANCER

Alternative and holistic approaches have just begun to take their place in established health care. To do this, they need to be visible, produce results, and be available for the education, training, and healing of health professionals in ongoing health settings. Arts medicine is a new interdisciplinary field that can provide ways in which dance and the healing arts can be integrated into health care settings. In this way, arts medicine can help heal the split between mind and body in modern medicine, heal the healers, and bring the arts as medicine into the community.

To heal is to make whole. This program brings healing through the use of the arts—dance, music, and visual arts—which have been used since ancient times to connect the individual with life's creative energies. Drawing from the Greek concept of preventive medicine, the course on imagery, movement, and breast cancer will use imagery and ritual to promote a harmonious balance between mind, body, and spirit.

The 12-week courses in movement and arts therapy for adults and children are de-signed to teach participants skills to improve their sense of well-being, body image, and verbal and nonverbal communication skills. Participants will be encouraged to develop vision and purpose and to make meaningful changes in their lives.

The movement and imagery group for breast cancer has three parts. The first part sets the intention to heal and establishes the circle of group support. After a check-in surfaces the predominant themes for the day, simple folk dance steps and group warm-ups raise the energy level in the room. The second part amplifies themes and images that emerged from part one through repetition of movement expressions, mirroring and listening in dyads, and drawing the personal healing images on paper. If one of the participants is facing a difficult medical intervention or surgery, the group works with her to develop images or rituals for healing. The third part brings the circle back together to share and reflect on the images. Common themes are fear, archetypal images of the female warrior, body balance and comfort, sensuousness and sexuality, and connectedness.

The objectives of these groups are:

1. Clinical: To provide ongoing groups using dance, ritual, kinesthetic, and visual imagery to work with women with cancer. These groups, would provide support, develop coping strategies, discover meaning, and build sustaining connections in the context of community. The project director would initially teach these groups, but the intention is to train interns and spread the work. Graduates of the program are now leading groups in the community, and we are

investigating the effects of this modality with different ethnic groups.

2. Educational: Continued education and public lectures to doctors, nurses, and interns make the work accessible to the professional community. Training is now taking place with medical students and other health professionals. A videotape of the work was edited and produced by one of the group members as an example of the healing power of creativity.

3. Research: Documentation of this work takes place through rigorous outcome research and training videotapes. Displays and publications of patient art would also increase public awareness. Group participants are planning events for the community, such as leading a movement opening ritual for the annual Race for the Cure during Breast Cancer Awareness month. These events further the healing process by empowering group members to take leadership roles in the community, using the creative skills they learned in the group.

Research

Breast cancer is the major cause of death for women between the ages of 35 and 45. Thirty years ago, breast cancer occurred in 1 in every 20 American women. The rate is now 1 in 9, with a rate of 1 in 8 for the San Francisco Bay area. The diagnosis and treatments may have profoundly disturbing effects on body image, mood, quality of life, and spirituality of these women. Nonverbal and integrative treatment modalities directly address these variables. Because these treatment modalities are noninvasive and potentially cost-cutting, they need to

be researched as complements to traditional medicine. Some studies have investigated the effects of social support groups on quality and length of life (Spiegel et al., 1989; Fawzy et al., 1990). A few studies have looked at the effects of physical movement on breast cancer (Dubbert, 1992). But no published studies have been done on the effects of physical activity and imagery on psycho-social-spiritual variables; therefore, a study done at California Pacific Medical Center in San Francisco from 1995 to 1997 researched the effect of movement therapy on the psycho-social-spiritual adaptation of women to breast cancer.

The treatment modality was Kinaesthetic Imagining, a form of dance/movement therapy which involves a warm-up, development of the themes through movement and art, and group sharing of affect and content. Groups are supportive, encourage connection through rhythm, play, and structured exercises, and are based on group process and led by experienced psychologists/dance therapists. The group meets for 2 hours weekly over a 12-session period. The study used three groups of 12 weeks each. Subjects were recruited from the community through letters, fliers, and an advertisement. Any woman with any stage breast cancer were eligible; minority women were encouraged to attend.

A previous quasi-experimental study was done in 1995 to launch the program and its recruitment drive, pilot the methodology, operationalize the definition of change, and refine the scales and interview questions. Two pilot study groups were completed, starting with 30 subjects, and ending with 20 completed sets (attrition was due to dropouts and/or effects of chemotherapy or radiation). Preliminary data from this study suggest that trends exist in the area of mood and quality of life. In particular, significant trends exist in the fatigue and confusion/bewilderment scales of the POMS. The movement analysis pointed to trends in the concaveness of torsos and restriction in pelvic mobility. Pre- and postinterviews probed more deeply into the women's subjective experience of quality of life, mood, body image, and spirituality. Because the body image scale was not appropriate for women with breast cancer, a content and discourse analysis of the interviews focusing specifically on the area of body image were completed. Using five raters, the resulting data were grouped into categories, and the categories placed into an inventory called the Kinaesthetic Imagery Profile (KIP).

During the second year of the research, the KIP was piloted on three different groups. A more thorough movement analysis using videotapes of the sessions, as well as a range of motion scale administered by a staff physical therapist, supplied behavioral observations of change.

This study therefore combined traditional quantitative psychosocial assessments (MAC, POMS, Jourard Body-Cathexis, Purpose in Life) with an innovative pilot inventory, the KIP based on qualitative analysis from semi-structured interviews. The two unique features of this study are its content (the use of movement on issues of body image and sexuality in women with breast cancer), and its methods (a combination of quantitative and qualitative). Such innovative methods best serve the innovative content and treatment modality and can begin to fill a gap in the literature on the effects of exercise and movement on the treatment of women with breast cancer.

ILENE A. SERLIN

INTERACTIVE GUIDED IMAGERY

Interactive guided imagery (IGI) is an educational and therapeutic approach to mind-body healing, brief psychotherapy, and self-healing developed by Martin L. Rossman, M.D., and David E. Bresler, Ph.D., through their Academy for Guided Imagery in Mill Valley, California. It utilizes imagery as a primary language of the unconscious in an interactive guiding format that encourages the client to become comfortable and proficient in using their unconscious resources for healing.

IGI draws from roots in Jungian therapy, psychosynthesis, Gestalt therapy, mindfulness meditation, Ericksonian hypnosis, and neurolinguistic programming. Both Rossman and Bresler were introduced to the core ideas by Dr. Irving Oyle, a physician doing experimental work in holistic healing in California in the early 1970s. Dr. Oyle was instrumental in synthesizing emerging approaches to healing, including visualization, hypnosis, biofeedback, acupuncture, meditation, and psychoneuroimmunology, into a coherent approach that encouraged patient participation and self-efficacy in healing. This emphasis on patient empowerment through gentle yet effective means continues to be a foundation of IGI.

IGI is based on the premise that there is an innate drive toward healing and wholeness within each of us, and that learning to respectfully attend to and interact with this process allows us to learn from it and support it. Healing is considered as a multidimensional process that moves us toward integrity and that has physical, emotional, mental, and spiritual aspects. While healing on one level may or may not be accompanied by healing on other levels, we value and support any healing that can happen.

The objectives of IGI depend on the objectives of the patient or client. In general, the objective is healing, symptom relief, or improved coping through utilizing the inner resources of the client or patient. IGI has applications in stress reduction, stimulation of natural physical healing processes, development of insight into the meaning of symptoms, creative problem-solving, conflict resolution, and reality-based action planning.

IGI involves using a simple relaxation technique to help clients focus their attention on their unique inner world, then teaches them skills that they can use to be more effective in problem solving, conflict resolution, goal setting, stimulating healing responses in the body, and using their own strengths and resources most effectively.

IGI is used by physicians, psychotherapists, nurses, and other helping professionals to help people with a tremendously wide range of physical and mental health issues. The clinical applications range from common chronic illnesses such as headaches, neck and back pain syndromes, arthritis, allergies, asthma, digestive problems, and reproductive problems, to aspects of life-threatening illnesses such as heart disease, cancer, and AIDS. They also include anxiety disorders, depression,

PTSD, addictions, and sequela of childhood abuse. IGI is also a powerful thought technology for conflict resolution, problem solving, generating creativity, and envisioning and reaching goals, and is useful for personal growth work.

As with any potentially powerful intervention, IGI can pose certain risks when used by poorly trained personnel. There is a possibility of uncovering traumatic insight, or overwhelming affect, and the certified IGI guide is trained and prepared to help prevent this whenever possible and to help work through it should it occur. These risks are rare but real, which is why the Academy for Guided Imagery feels strongly about clear criteria for the awarding of certification to only health professionals with demonstrated competence and high ethical standards.

All guides certified by the Academy subscribe to the high ethical standards articulated in the Code of Ethics of the American Psychological Association, which fully accredits Academy for Guided Imagery training.

A certified IGI guide has taken at least 150 hours of training beyond their graduate and professional licensure requirements, including 52 hours of direct supervision to ensure their mastery of these methods. The guide helps the client learn to use his or her mind to help relieve stress, encourage physical healing, bring about emotional balance, and enhance the quality of daily life.

IGI is most often conducted with the client lightly relaxed and focusing their attention inside. The client is fully aware of the guide's suggestions and questions and is engaged in an active dialogue at all times with the IGI guide. Terminating the work simply requires opening the eyes and returning attention to the outer world. The guide and client work collaboratively, with agreement about their goals and methods.

The Academy for Guided Imagery was founded in 1989 by Martin L. Rossman, M.D., and David E. Bresler, Ph.D. The mission of the Academy is to help people access and utilize the power of the mind/body connection for healing. Objectives include (1) to further understanding of the imagery process in human life and development, with special attention to its uses in the healing professions; (2) to provide systematic, high-quality training and guidance to health professionals who want to use IGI in their practices; (3) to help network this community; and (4) to help the public at large access and utilize their own innate abilities for self-healing.

MARTIN L. ROSSMAN
DAVID E. BRESLER

JIN SHIN DO BODYMIND ACUPRESSURE

Jin Shin Do is a unique synthesis of acupressure theory, Western psychology, and Taoist philosophy, developed by Iona Marsaa Teeguarden, M.T., M.A., L.M.F.CC from the early 1970s to the present. It is modern, yet true to traditional theory and philosophy. Acupuncture/acupressure theory, the most ancient aspect of Jin Shin Do, is said to be at least 5,000 years old. It was developed by Taoist philosophers as a way of maintaining health and promoting longevity. The Jin Shin Do Foundation is a member of the American Oriental Bodywork Therapy Association's Council of Schools and Programs and is approved by

the National Certification Board for Therapeutic Massage and Bodywork as a continuing education provider. Classes are avocational and adjunctive training, offered at both growth centers and massage schools.

Theory Behind Jin Shin Do and Its Uses

Jin Shin Do Bodymind Acupressure is a unique synthesis of: acupuncture theory, Western psychology, and Taoist philosophy. *The Way of the Compassionate Spirit* is a bodywork method that provides many of the beneficial effects of acupuncture by application of firm, gentle, supportive touch rather than needles.

As modern quantum physics and Albert Einstein have demonstrated, all matter is energy. Since the body is a physical entity, it is also basically energy. Biophysical energy, or *qi*, is unformed, subtle, not yet physical, but when organized, it becomes matter: atoms, molecules, cells, tissues, organs. Very simply described, acupuncture theory maps the movement of *qi* through the body along both superficial and internal pathways. Where the pathways of *qi* are open and the instructions for its flow and configuration are intact, the physical body flourishes. Where there are blockages or deficiency of flow, disease develops. The beauty of this system is that one may actually prevent the development of disease by identifying germinal imbalances in the flow of *qi* before they become physical. By working with points, breathing, and visualization to release physical tensions and enhance the flow of *qi*, acupressure can often ameliorate discomfort and enhance the body's own healing potential.

"Acupressure" refers to any technique using finger pressure on the acupuncture points to reduce stress and balance the body energy. At the simplest, a method may address common problems like headache or muscle tension by using points at the site of the symptom. At its most sophisticated, a method will address the root and development of an imbalance, including environmental, emotional, and physiological contributing factors. Jin Shin Do can be a powerful self-help tool and a profound professional modality.

Jin Shin Do is based on the strange flows, energy pathways that provide a short-cut to balancing the body energy. At the basic level, it uses 45 points and simple release examples that anyone can use. The student progresses to learn the 12 meridians (energy pathways), the five elements, and the emotional associations of the meridians and segments, and eventually, over 200 points. Classes teach how to combine these powerful points by pressing one or more "distal points" while a point of tension or "local point" is held. The distal points help to release tense areas more easily, deeply, and pleasurably. At the very least, it can bring about harmonious, deep relaxation and increased awareness of both body and the emotional/mental self.

Acupressurists and acupuncturists work primarily with the model that *qi* follows longitudinal pathways. In fact, the classics describe a "loom" between heaven and earth upon which the body is "woven." Some meridians start at the upraised fingertips and flow toward earth; some start at the toes and flow toward heaven. Jin Shin Do is unique in that it recognizes the influence of horizontal holding patterns in the musculature ("armoring segments") that may interrupt the smooth flow of *qi* across several meridians. Wilhelm Reich pioneered this Western concept of emotional armoring. One can imagine what the mus-

cles of the jaw and back of the neck (the "oral segment") do when one must "hold one's tongue." When the points and flows associated with the tension are held and the awareness directed to the tension through the breath and visualization, one may also contact the distressing feelings held there: anxiety, guilt, anger, resentment. As the *qi* begins to gently flow through the segmental "dams," one can learn to transform, rather than repress, those painful feelings. With supportive touch, this opening to the deep aspects of body mind and spirit is a safe, often pleasurable process.

Taoist philosophy views everything as part of an eternal wholeness. Rather than dividing the world up into good and bad aspects that must be kept or eliminated, it sees the interplay of complementary opposites. Therefore, even healing is not about getting rid of anything, but returning to proper balance. It is not about curing, but about reuniting the pieces of oneself to become whole. It is not the germ alone that causes the disease, but the interaction of the germ and the host. In most cases, where the host is strong, there is peaceful coexistence. So sometimes one must weaken the germ (use antibiotics, proper hygiene), but one must not overlook the host. Certainly today we can thank the war on germs for surviving infancy. This is the benefit of modern medicine. But these invasive procedures like drugs and surgery also tax the host. We can do much to strengthen ourselves so that this intervention is reserved for extreme situations. Jin Shin Do is one way of doing that, through self-care and professional assistance.

Though Jin Shin Do is not to be interpreted as a technique for diagnosing or treating physical or emotional problems or any disease, it can assist the physical and emotional well-being of those in the process of healing and staying well. Jin Shin Do addresses common problems such as neck, shoulder, and back tension/pain, headache (Kroll, 1995), chest problems, menstrual difficulties, pelvic tension, digestive stress, respiratory difficulty (Weisbord, 1997), insomnia, joint problems, creative blocks, muscle spasm, pain, tension, and stress-related difficulties. Among many other applications, it has been used in hospitals by massage therapists and nurses, in classrooms (Teeguarden, 1985) for children with developmental problems, and by physical therapists for people with cerebral palsy. Because it is gentle and is done with the recipient clothed, Jin Shin Do can provide the ease and comfort of safe physical touch in many instances where other types of massage are contraindicated, or where physical or sexual abuse has made touch an issue.

DEBORAH VALENTINE SMITH

See also
Acupuncture and Chinese Medicine (IV)
Hospital-Based Massage Therapy (IV)

JIN SHIN JYUTSU

Jin Shin Jyutsu is an ancient art administered as either a self-help tool or received from a practitioner. Self-help is an important aspect of the practice because it is believed that self-awareness helps maintain balance and harmony and evoke relaxation and peace. Whoever administers the procedure, it is used to help harmonize the flow of life-giving energy throughout the body.

According to the Record of Ancient Things in the Imperial Achieves of Japan (A.D. 712) Jin Shin Jyutsu was practiced in ancient times. Brought to the United States in the 1950s by Mary Burmeister, it was called alternately the Art of Happiness, the Art of Longevity, and the Art of Benevolence. Mary's teacher, Master Jiro Murai, came to call the art Jin Shin Jyutsu, or the Art of the Creator through Man of Knowing and Compassion.

Jin Shin Jyutsu employs 26 safety-energy locks throughout the body. These are found along various pathways through which the universal energy travels. They create and support life and all bodily functions. For many reasons—heredity, character, stress, accidents, tension of daily lifestyle, and so forth—these pathways may become blocked, causing symptoms or illness. By placing the hands (the jumper cables) on these safety energy locks in specific sequences, called flows, they can be unlocked and harmony and balance restored.

To apply Jin Shin Jyutsu, the hands are placed on the clothed body of the client. There is no massage or manipulation involved. The practitioner or client holds the three middle fingers on the lock and waits to feel the rhythmic pulsation in the safety energy indicating that harmony and balance have been restored.

Jin Shin Jyutsu is an art and not merely a technique. It is strongly supported by its underlying philosophy that brings an awareness of self and a connection to the universal energy. By maintaining this, individuals remain in harmony—happy and healthy. When the philosophy is forgotten, the jumper cables recharge internal batteries and restore the proper body functioning.

A Jin Shin Jyutsu session lasts about an hour. The recipient lies face up on a table or any available comfortable surface. The practitioner will "listen" to the pulses, not for diagnosis, but to determine which energy function flows might be utilized to bring the body to its natural state of harmony. The recipient may feel a sense of relaxation and deeper breathing patterns as the energy flow is restored. The immediate effects of the session will continue for eight hours, as the circulation pattern is completed.

DAVID BURMEISTER

KETOGENIC DIET

Seventy percent of children who have a single seizure will never have another. Seventy percent of those who have a second seizure will have their seizures successfully controlled by medication. But if a first medication fails, the chance that a second or third will fail increases (Freeman, Kelly, & Freeman, 1994). Medication can also be combined and seizure control may be attained, but mental alertness and clarity decrease. Learning ability and quality of life diminish as well. One fifth of children with epilepsy cannot be controlled on medication; they either continue to seize or suffer unbearable drug side effects. The primary reference for this article is *The Epilepsy Diet Treatment* by Freeman, Kelly, and Freeman (1994).

What is the Ketogenic Diet?

"The Ketogenic Diet is a rigid, mathematically calculated, doctor-supervised diet" (Freeman et al., 1994). The diet is high fat and low protein and carbohydrate. Three to five times the amount of fat than carbohydrate and protein combined is required. Strict fluid restrictions and calories are also a must. The calories are figured at 75% of the recommended RDA amounts. The liquids allowed are usually 1 cc per calorie. A registered dietician calculates what percentage of calories will come from fat, carbohydrate, and protein. All food must be measured on a gram scale. There is no room for error, the exact prescription must be followed. The carbohydrate content of everything put in the mouth is crucial. This includes medicine, vitamins, and toothpaste. The rigidity of the diet is a crucial part of how it works because the proper ratios will trick the body into thinking it is fasting.

"Fasting has long been recognized as one approach to seizure control" (Freeman et al., 1994, p. 26). Since fasting cannot be a permanent solution, the Ketogenic Diet was developed. The Ketogenic Diet, like fasting, produces acidosis, ketosis, and increased levels of uric acid in the blood and urine. These factors control seizures, however, it is not clearly known how. Initiating the diet requires a period of starvation and fluid restriction. Once 10% of body weight is lost or ketones of 5+ are reached, the diet is started. One third of the total diet is given, then increased over several days to full calculation. Blood sugars, ketones, and specific gravity are monitored continuously. Small amounts of carbohydrates may be given if the child becomes symptomatic. If nausea and vomiting occur with no marked acidosis, 30 cc of orange juice is given and rest encouraged. If nausea and vomiting continues, physicians may consider starting the one-third portion of the diet before the 10% weight loss or 5+ ketones is achieved. Once the full diet is tolerated, urinary ketones and specific gravity are monitored by urinary dipstick, two to three times daily for a month, then about two to three times a week thereafter. Late afternoon shows the highest amount of urinary ketones. If ketosis is significantly reduced, an inquiry should be made. Have the exact calculations been weighed properly on a balanced gram scale? Has the child "cheated"?

Dr. Jay Ellis, a neurologist practicing in Massachusetts, worked with children on the diet at the University of Virginia. He states "noncompliance of children or adults administering the diet incorrectly was the primary factor for failure" (personal communication, August 1995). The extremely small portions and high fat content are difficult to accept as a parent or recipient.

Efficacy

Efficacy of the diet is determined within the first three months. This allows time to adjust calculations and view benefits versus burdens of administering this very involved diet. If the diet is done correctly benefits will appear within this time frame. Complete control can take much longer. The decision to continue is decided after a commitment of three months. It must be noted that the point at which seizures are deemed controlled or better varies from family to family. Each person or family has different definitions of success. This point is needed to determine when a child may end the diet. Once the diet's full benefits have been realized, weaning may begin. A child who is totally controlled for two years may lower his fat to protein and carbohydrate ratio to 3 to 1 for six months, then to 2 to 1 for six months, then to a normal diet. The child who has had no seizures and no medications during the diet has the greatest chance to remain seizure free. The children who have not been completely controlled may continue the diet longer, rather than increasing or adding medications. If a child resumes seizures once off the diet, it can be restarted. The children for whom medication and/or the diet have failed are faced with continued drug trials or surgery.

Aside from the answer "No one knows," a combination of factors are needed to have the diet work. The first factor being ketone bodies. Although they have a sedative, appetite suppressing, and anticonvulsant effect, ketones by themselves do not adequately explain the diet's effectiveness. For example, if large amounts of carbohydrates are eaten, seizures may occur even if urinary ketones are not clearly affected. Ketones present in blood and urine are only one necessary aspect of the diet.

Acidosis is the second factor. Ketone bodies are acids and therefore cause acidosis. Acidosis influences seizure threshold. The body will quickly compensate for the acidosis to readjust its pH, therefore this cannot be a major determinant either. The third factor is dehydration. The limited fluids in the diet may affect the electrolytes, particularly the sodium level. Excess water is known to provoke seizures. Limited fluids, however, cannot take sole credit for the diet's success either. Clearly more research is needed, probably looking at other influences of metabolism on seizure threshold.

Metabolism problems can also be a complication of the diet. Initiating the diet may produce transient hypoglycemia. The diet is also deficient in vitamins and calcium.

Supplements, carbohydrate free, must be taken. Since weight gain is discouraged, growth may slow down but will quickly catch up once the diet is discontinued, usually in 2 years. "Despite the high fat content, the diet does not appear to cause atherosclerosis. Kidney stones can occur, but may be prevented by appropriate fluid intake" (Freeman, Vining, & Pillas, 1991, p. 155). Constipation is also a problem due to the lack of fiber and suppositories are often needed to facilitate a bowel movement. There are no risks associated with the diet if followed correctly. This includes administration of food, medications if indicated and blood tests every four to six weeks. No effects on long-term renal functions have been documented. However, very little research is available. Most studies date back to the 1920s to 1950s.

Conclusion

The Ketogenic Diet has traditionally been used as a last resort when seizures are incapacitating and medication a failure. The diet improves control of seizures in nearly three quarters of the children who try it and eliminates seizures often permanently in half the children who stick to it rigidly (Freeman et al., 1994). "Johns Hopkins Hospital has found 70% of children with intractable seizures who are put on the diet, children who are often retarded or severely brain damaged as well, will have their seizures controlled" (Freeman et al., 1994, p. ix). If the diet is so effective in this extreme population, why is it not used earlier in difficult to control epilepsy? Perhaps John M. Freeman has the answer when he says "If the Ketogenic Diet were a drug, it would probably be the treatment of choice for difficult-to-control epilepsy" (Freeman et al., 1994, p. 4).

Baystate Medical Center in Springfield, Massachusetts, has three children on the diet. Dr. Joseph Donnelly, pediatric neurologist, and Paula Serafino Cross, registered dietician, have been instrumental in making the diet available in our area. Of the three children, two have been removed from the diet. One parent found the diet too intense and the other child had difficulty with Depakote and the diet. The third child is my son who is 12 years old, and not a perfect candidate because of his age. He has been on the diet 5 months and his seizures have been greatly reduced. Baystate, Boston Children's Hospital and others have not had the success Johns Hopkins has experienced. Dr. Donnelly may be onto something when he suggests "The large number of patients at Johns Hopkins plus a careful screening process may be the reason for their greater success" (personal communication, August 1995).

JEANNIE LAUREYNS BELL

See also
Epilepsy (II)

KINESIOLOGY, APPLIED

Applied kinesiology (AK) was devised by a Michigan chiropractor, George J. Goodheart. It is a popular diagnostic and therapeutic system used by many health care practitioners. In 1964, Goodheart reported he could correct a chronic winged scapula by pressing on nodules near the origin and insertion of the involved serratus anterior muscle. This finding led to the origin and insertion treatment, the first method developed in AK. Other diagnostic and therapeutic procedures were developed for neurolymphatic reflexes, neurovascular reflexes, and cerebrospinal fluid flow originally described by Frank Chapman, D.O., Terrence, J. Bennet, D.C., and William G. Sutherland, D.O. Influenced by the writing of Felix Mann, M.D., Goodheart incorporated acupuncture meridian therapy into the AK system. Based on phenomena proposed by L. L. Truscott, D.C., the vertebral challenge method and therapy localization techniques were added.

CAROLYN CHAMBERS CLARK

LIFESTYLE CHANGE

The pursuit of change, altering habits, and replacing behaviors are core components of growth for individuals and humanity. Since the beginning of time, humans have endeavored not only to meet their personal needs but also to improve their existence. This is exemplified in the evolution of the human species. Religion has played an important role in this process as evidenced in religious manuscripts such as the Bible and the Koran. For instance, the Bible not only provides standards and principles that focus on spiritual conduct, but also the early writings addressed health-related behaviors such as dietary *laws* that reduced the transmission of disease.

The countless number of books, programs, and professionals addressing *lifestyle issues* in areas such as health, relationships, parenting, weight loss, self-esteem, spirituality, and addiction demonstrates that many people in society continue in the evolution toward change and growth.

Counseling theories continue to evolve in an attempt to define human behavior and create successful change. Each theory offers a varied perspective with specific therapeutic techniques based on its constructs. However, if someone is seeking professional assistance, the feeling of trust and personal attributes of the helper are often stated to be more significant than the particular theory or techniques used (Okun, 1987).

Psychological factors for successful change have also been identified. Danielson and Wanzel found that exercisers who failed to meet their goals dropped out approximately twice as fast as those exercisers who were more successful. Self-motivation supported by previous successes appears to be a key factor in exercise maintenance.

Similarly, Ornstein and Sobel (1989) found that an optimistic belief in one's ability is a critical feature for successful change, more significant than skills and capacities. Each success, regardless of how small, creates a feeling of confidence and capability that will improve an individual's ability to make and maintain lifestyle changes.

Creating an optimistic belief and experiencing frequent successes are two components necessary for successful change. Treasure mapping is one tool that can help clients clearly define their desires visually and will help them identify with what they want to create (Dzelzkalns, 1991). Once completed, framing the desired change into performance (action) goals rather than outcome goals is a concept for increasing confidence. For example, if an individual would like to lose weight and create a more healthy lifestyle a performance goal of *exercise four times weekly* is more effective than an outcome goal of *losing 10 pounds in 4 weeks*. Individuals have control of their behaviors but not how their body responds to lifestyle changes. By planning and assessing performance goals daily and weekly, success can be evaluated more frequently which is encouraging and improves one's sense of capability.

Finally, critical moment choices is a concept to remember in the process of change. Goal-supporting decisions have to be incorporated into the challenges and complexities of everyday life. This is not always easy. However, regardless of previous choices or misdirected responses, each and every moment offers a new opportunity for success.

KIMBERLY SIBILLE

LIGHT THERAPY

Light therapy is the use of natural or artificial light to promote healing. Sunlight has been used for healing throughout history. Healing temples of light and color existed at Heliopolos in Egypt, as well as in early Greece, China, and India (Gerber, 1996). Hippocrates, the ancient Greek physician, prescribed sunlight for several disorders, sending his clients to recuperate in roofless buildings. In the Middle Ages, red light was used to treat smallpox. Windows of sick rooms and bodies of ill people were wrapped in red sheets (Somerville, 1997).

Bright light has been used to treat seasonal affective disorder (SAD), a form of depression. Full-spectrum light has also been used to treat blood pressure, skin problems, insomnia, premenstrual syndrome, migraines, jet lag, and jaundice in newborns, but it has not undergone rigorous scientific study.

CAROLYN CHAMBERS CLARK

See also
Color Therapy (IV)
Depression (II)

LYMPHATIC MASSAGE

Massage therapy in general exerts a positive impact on the circulation of lymph, but a specialized technique known as manual lymph drainage (MLD) directly stimulates this flow. MLD was created to help assist the lymphatic system perform its crucial function of drainage.

Unlike the blood, lymph does not have a heart to pump it through an extensive and elaborate network of superficial and deep collecting vessels. This transparent or slightly opalescent fluid moves along slowly with the aid of several forces. Within lymphatic ducts themselves, rhythmic contractions of the smooth muscles in the walls help propel the liquid. Outside the system, contractions of voluntary or skeletal muscles during exercise and of intestinal muscles during peristalsis squeeze the lymphatic vessels. Pulsating arteries also provide some massage.

External hands-on stimulation is a boon to increasing the passage of lymph, especially when it stagnates at any of hundreds of lymph nodes located throughout the body. These sites filter lymph and produce lymphocytes, which secrete antibodies to neutralize bacteria. Uninterrupted activity of the lymph nodes is therefore vital to the body's immune system.

The importance of the lymphatic system's drainage process cannot be overstated. Although the total amount of fluid it collects is minor when compared with how much blood is pumped in a day, it is essential to survival. Lymph removes excess fluid, protein, bacteria, viruses, and waste products from the tissues and interstitial spaces. Then it transports them to the blood to be eliminated. When this cleansing is disrupted, the accumulation of lymph causes edema (swelling), congestion, and ultimately pathological conditions. The stagnant fluid can interfere with wound healing and provide a breeding ground for bacteria. If the lymphatic system completely fails to carry out its task, within 24 hours death can result from protein poisoning. While blood capillaries are incapable of reabsorbing larger protein molecules and cell debris, lymphatic ducts have special structures—flap valves—that can open to admit such materials.

The origins of lymphatic massage can be traced to various ancient cultures around the world, but European interest in developing a nonsurgical method to relieve edema was sparked in the late 1800s by a Belgian professor of surgery and two German medical doctors. In 1922, Frederic Millard, a Canadian osteopathic physician, published his findings on the lymphatic system. Ten years later, clinical research conducted by physiotherapists Estrid and Emil Vodder led to the creation of MLD. At the beginning of World War II, the Vodders founded the first MLD Institute in Copenhagen to train therapists. In turn, the Vodders passed on their knowledge to Hildegard and Gunther Wittlinger, who established another school and clinic in Austria in 1972, which is now the leading institute of this method.

In the 1980s, German physician Michael Földi combined MLD with compression therapy, exercises, and skin care into complete decongestive physiotherapy (CDP). More recently, French physician Bruno Chikly innovated lymph drainage therapy (LDT), which is based on traditional drainage methods as well as direct perception of the direction, rhythm, and quality of lymphatic flow. Medical doctors, massage therapists, and physical therapists who trained in MLD in Europe have brought the method and its spinoffs to the United States and Canada. They have set up treatment centers and educational programs, and some have formed the North American Vodder Association of Lymphatic Therapy (NAVALT).

According to Chikly, it took some 30 years for the Vodder method to be taken seriously by Europe's medical profession. Johannes Asdonk, a prominent German physician, worked with 20,000 hospital patients to validate the effectiveness of MLD by measuring efficiency and determining indications and contraindications. His successful research has encouraged medical doctors to routinely prescribe lymphatic drainage to facilitate healing and more comfortable recovery after surgery. The procedure is widely available in European hospitals.

The original Vodder method of MLD includes four basic movements to address both aspects of the lymphatic system—a superficial one that drains the skin and underlying tissues and a deep one that drains the muscles. In working with either area, practitioners are required to use a subtle and precise touch rather than brute strength. In fact, too much pressure can damage the fragile lymphatic vessels and cause the system to stop operating. The fundamental technique is an on-off pulsing pressure, like a smooth pumping action, which has an immediate lulling effect on the autonomic nervous system. Therapists repeat a rhythm of six to seven strokes per minute over an area a square inch or larger until they sense a change in the tissue. They vary the light pressure according to how much distension there is. When dealing with edema in superficial tissues, practitioners move the fluid toward the lymph nodes, which is not the same direction as venous drainage. To drain muscles, they apply the same rhythm but deepen the pressure and move the lymph from the ends of the muscle to the center, following venous drainage. The other three motions—scooping, rotary, and stationary circles—also exert a torquing stretch force on the vessel walls. Both the pumping and stretching techniques massage the lymphatic channels and cause the lymph to flow faster.

Because the light alternating pressure simultaneously stimulates mechanoreceptors in the skin, it inhibits impulses traveling from pain receptors (nociceptors) and thus decreases pain sensations. That allows therapists to work on swelling immediately after an injury. Even if they cannot work directly on the affected area because of severe burns or other conditions, they still can massage the opposite side of the body or near the site of injury and bring about the same results.

Both manual therapists and medical doctors report success with MLD in a variety of conditions: edema due to soft tissue injury (sprains and bruises); localized edema in hands, feet, and face because of insufficient exercise; puffiness in the face following cosmetic or dental surgery; muscular spasms from overuse or chronic tension; and lymphedema following injury, scarring, excision, and/or radiation therapy of the lymph nodes in cancer. Research indicates that lymphatic massage is more effective than mechanized methods or diuretic drugs in controlling lymphedema secondary to radical mastectomy. The technique is also applicable prior to surgery to prepare the patient by draining toxins, stimulating the immune system, and inducing relaxation of the autonomic nervous system. Surgeons find that well-drained tissue is easier to cut.

In addition, MLD plays a role in the treatment of emphysema, migraines, tinnitus, spinal injuries, sinusitis, open ulcers, burns, acne, scars, arthritis, trigeminal neuralgia, and some cerebral disorders. If a pregnant woman receives lymphatic massage before her fifth month, it can help prevent swelling and stretch marks.

Because MLD is a gentle, noninvasive procedure, there are few contraindications. Slight nausea might follow a treatment, but that can be remedied by flushing out the connective tissue and lymph system through greater fluid intake. However, in cases of malignant diseases or acute infections or inflammations, lymphatic massage should not be administered if there is a risk of further spreading through the lymphatic system. This is equally true when there is danger of dislodging a clot or embolism. And last, it is to be avoided in edemic conditions related to congestive heart failure.

MIRKA KNASTER

MAGNET THERAPY

Magnet therapy refers to the use of magnetic fields for therapeutic purposes and has been in existence for over 4,000 years. Our earliest existing written medical record, *The Yellow Emperor's Canon of Internal Medicine*, c. 2000 B.C., describes how lodestones applied to specific skin sites could restore the normal flow of *qi* energy, much like the insertion of acupuncture needles. The *Vedas*, ancient Hindu religious scriptures that also date back several thousand years, similarly mention the treatment of diseases with *ashmana* and *siktavati*, "instruments of stone," which were almost certainly lodestones. The word "lode" is derived from the ancient Teutonic *laithō*, which meant "way" or "course," and is the basis for our verb to lead. "Lodestone," or "leading stone," came from its use as a compass. "Magnet" is believed to stem from *Mágnes líthos*, "stone from Magnesia," a region of Greece rich in magnetic stones, which later became *magneta* in Latin.

Cleopatra allegedly wore a lodestone on her forehead while sleeping to prevent aging, and Tibetan monks placed them on the skulls of novitiates in a particular configuration to improve their minds during training. In medieval times, lodestones were ground up to make powders that could be applied as magnetic salves to promote wound healing or ingested to treat diarrhea and hemorrhage. William Gilbert's 1600 treatise, *De Magnete*, was the first scholarly attempt to explain the nature of magnetism and how it differed from the attractive force of static electricity. Gilbert allegedly used iron magnets to alleviate Queen Elizabeth's arthritic pains. By the middle 1700s, carbon-steel magnets that were stronger and more permanent were being manufactured in Europe, where they were used to treat numerous complaints. Their most passionate proponent, Franz Anton Mesmer, established a popular salon in Paris with all sorts of magnetic paraphernalia, which, fortified by his own "animal magnetism," could allegedly cure any illness.

Magnet mania swept through the U.S. in the 18th and early 19th centuries, promising relief for everything from baldness and menstrual cramps to impotence and cancer. Every conceivable kind of magnetic device, clothing, wearing apparel, and accessory was readily available in Sears & Roebuck and other mail-order catalogues. The current resurgence of interest is due largely to scientific studies showing that modern and more powerful magnets can accelerate healing, reduce inflammation, and provide a safe and extremely cost-effective treatment for various pain syndromes.

Magnetic fields are also created when a current of electricity flows through a coil of conducting wire. Certain electromagnetic devices are approved by the U.S. Food and Drug Administration for the treatment of fractures that have failed to unite normally and have been successful in several hundred thousand patients, including some in which there had been nonunion for 15 or more years. Electromagnetic fields have also been shown to accelerate the healing of soft tissue injuries and ordinary fractures, reduce pain and edema, prevent osteoporosis, improve glaucoma, and relieve arthritic discomfort and disability. Various types of cranial electromagnetic stimulation approaches have provided significant benefits in patients suffering from insomnia, depression, anxiety, substance abuse withdrawal symptoms, far advanced metastatic malignancy, end stage cardiomyopathy, Parkinson's Disease, multiple sclerosis, epilepsy, and other neurodegenerative disorders. A technique known as rapid repetitive transcranial magnetic stimulation has recently been found to be effective in treating severe depression resistant to drug therapy.

The ability of electromagnetic fields to provide so many diverse clinical benefits suggests a *modus operandi* at a very basic level of cellular function. This appears to be confirmed by research studies demonstrating that they alter the dynamics of calcium, potassium, sodium, and other ion transport across cell membranes. These can have profound effects on essential enzyme systems, such as cytochrome oxidase that modulate mitochondrial adenosine triphosphate (ATP) formation, whose high energy phosphate bonds ultimately provide the fuel for every cellular function. All magnetic fields result from the movement of electrons. In an electromagnet, a wire carrying a current of electricity induces a magnetic field. The field from a permanent magnet comes not from electricity, but the spin of electrons in the material itself. Unlike heat, x-rays, sound, light, and other energies, magnetic fields are unique in that they pass freely through bone and other tissues. That is why magnetic resonance imaging is so superior to conventional x-rays in delineating various organs and structures.

It is unlikely that any biological effect can occur unless there is movement within a magnetic field. All of the benefits in the various disorders noted above have been achieved by electromagnetic fields, which are oscillating and therefore always in motion. Similar claims cannot be made for the static fields emanating from permanent magnets. Since motion is a prerequisite, it has been suggested that magnets influence blood or lymph that is moving within their stationary field. Circulation is said to be improved by the generation of local heat, which causes vasodilatation, possibly by influences on iron in the hemoglobin molecule. It is also claimed that a "Hall effect" or "Faraday law" type of activity generates electrical energy in nerves, thus speeding up the transmission of impulses. Some believe that magnetic fields can activate acupuncture points and meridians to improve the flow of *qi* energy in the body, and that they can be as effective as acupuncture for certain disorders. However, none of these frequently repeated explanations have any scientific support. Recent research suggests that the mechanism of action is most likely mediated by influences on ionic transport and binding, similar to that proposed for electromagnetic fields.

Permanent magnets can be constructed of various alloys containing aluminum, nickel, cobalt, or rare earth elements like neodymium, as well as ceramics. Each of these are said to have specific characteristics that provide greater benefits for certain situations. There are also claims about the superiority of different products that apply both positive and negative poles in a checkerboard fashion (Nikken), concentric rings (BIOflex), or negative (North-Pole seeking) only magnets (TecTonic). However, there are few scientific studies to support most of these allegations.

What can be said based upon available research findings, is that rare earth neodymium TecTonic-type magnets are 100 times more powerful than the magnets used early in this century, and are 10 times more powerful than alnico or any other previous product. They have been shown to be capable of providing prompt and potent pain relief for a variety of disorders, including carpal tunnel syndrome and fibromyositis in double blind trials at major university centers. Further objective proof has been demonstrated by the ability of these magnets to reduce postoperative bruising and edema in patients undergoing liposuction procedures, and to increase beta-endorphin levels 45% within an hour or two after application. That these are not placebo effects can be demonstrated by their beneficial effects in infants and widespread use in veterinary medicine to relieve pain and reduce swelling.

Whether all magnets can provide similar rewards is not known. Electromagnetic devices are more flexible with respect to being able to vary the strength and other characteristics of the magnetic fields they deliver, but are much more expensive. In both instances, it seems clear that we have only scratched the surface of the full potential of magnet therapy, and that this exciting modality will be a mainstay of 21st century medicine that promises to replace many pharmaceuticals.

PAUL J. ROSCH

MASSAGE FOR CANCER PATIENTS

Early on in my massage work with oncology patients I massaged a woman with ovarian cancer. In our conversation she mentioned having a friend who was a massage therapist. I asked if her friend came to the hospital to give her massage. "No, she won't because of the cancer"—a story I've heard more than once over the past year. Oncology specialists, however, and those who care for cancer patients are supportive of massage in most instances. In fact, when East-West College students were approved by the hospital medical board to give massage, it was the board's request that the students' trial run be with oncology patients. As of yet there is not a prolific amount of research in this area, but in the studies that do exist, never once does the issue arise of whether massage should be performed. The questions have been, under what conditions and with what patients is massage beneficial?

Studies of patients "living with cancer" were chosen as the focus of this article,

thereby excluding research of hospice patients. Four of the studies were performed with hospitalized patients, the fifth with elderly cancer patients at home. Also, only massage research has been included and not that of other modalities such as Therapeutic Touch or Reiki.

Tope, Hann, and Pinkson (1943) researched the effect of two or more massages on 104 patients over a 4-year period. The subjects were of two types, either general cancer patients (40%) or autologous bone marrow transplant (ABMT) patients (60%). (In ABMT the patient donates her own bone marrow prior to undergoing high doses of chemotherapy.) The massages were administered by a Licensed Practical Nurse, were limited to 30 minutes, and commonly included work on the back, shoulders, neck, and feet. Upon discharge, patients completed a self-report questionnaire. "Relaxation" or "release of muscle tension" was mentioned by 99% of the patients. In addition, 35% commented on improved mood or sense of well-being, 22% mentioned assistance symptom management (control of pain, inflammation, nausea) and 15% felt a decreased sense of isolation. None of the patients made reference to any negative effects of massage.

Tope and colleagues focused on ABMT patients because of the severity of treatment-related symptoms. "ABMT patients generally experience side effects from toxicity and immunosuppression associated with the procedure, such as high fevers, nausea and vomiting, painful skin rashes, and debilitating fatigue, along with other idiosyncratic symptoms." In addition, they remain in the hospital for extended periods of time (at least 3 weeks), and for a portion of that time are unable to leave the protected environment. These factors, along with the ever present potential of mortality, can increase anxiety and depression in these patients. More data will be forthcoming on the topic of massage therapy for postbone marrow transplant distress as this researcher received an NIH grant in 1993 to further her exploration into this area.

Sims (1986) researched the use of slow-stroke back massage on six female patients receiving radiation therapy for breast cancer. Pre- and post-measures were taken with the subjects serving as their own controls. Thirteen symptoms were measured on a 1–5 scale: nausea (frequency and intensity), pain (frequency and intensity), appetite, insomnia, fatigue, bowel pattern, concentration, appearance, breathing, outlook, and cough. Each massage lasted 10 minutes and consisted of slow, gentle, rhythmical strokes using both hands over the back. One group of three patients received massage for 3 consecutive days. The following week they were scheduled for a 10-minute rest for three consecutive days. Group 2 received the massage and the control intervention (10 min. rest) in reverse order. Three of the six subjects reported an improvement in total symptom distress following the 10 min. rest. Five out of six reported a greater improvement in total symptom distress following the massage. Sims analyzed the data from several different angles. However, for the most part the differences between the massage and the 10 min. rest were not statistically significant. The researcher suggested that the small sample size and large number of symptom variables may have contributed to the results. She also comments that individual patient needs were not taken into account, and "the giving of massage within

a research setting may have undermined its true effects."

Ferrell-Torry and Glick (1993) examined the effects of massage on pain perception, anxiety, and relaxation in patients experiencing significant cancer pain. The subjects had a wide variety of cancers—esophageal, rectal, prostate, stomach, and lung, as well as leukemia and mixed nodular lymphoma. Five of the patients had also been diagnosed with metastases to distant sites. Nine males were given 30 min. massages on two consecutive evenings. Massage consisted of effleurage and petrissage to the feet, back, neck, and shoulders plus myofascial TPs located in the upper, middle, and lower trapezius. "Once TPs were located, slow, milking strokes of increasing pressure were utilized along the length of the effected muscle to gradually reduce the pain associated with the TP." Immediately before and after the massage subjects completed self-reports with regard to pain and relaxation. In addition, heart rate (HR), respiratory rate (R), and blood pressure (BP) were taken just before, immediately after, and 10 min. after massage. Subjects' level of pain perception was reduced by an average of 60%, anxiety by 24%, and feelings of relaxation increased by 58%. HR, R, and BP "tended to decrease from baseline, providing further indication of relaxation."

Weinrich and Weinrich (1990) researched the effect of massage on cancer pain. Twenty-eight hospitalized patients (18 men and 10 women) were assigned to a massage or control group. The massage group received a 10-minute Swedish back massage from senior nursing students, while the control group was visited for 10 minutes by the same students. The control was intended to account for the possibility that any effect might be due to the attention the patients were receiving. Immediately before and after the intervention patients rated their pain on a Visual Analogue Scale, the two end points being "no pain" and "pain as bad as it could possibly be." There was no significant difference in pain for males or females in the control group. For males in the massage group there was a significant decrease in pain immediately after the massage. However, for females there was not. The authors note that the men had a high level of self-reported pain prior to the massage, while the women initially had a low level. This led them to wonder if there are differences in how each gender copes with and perceives pain, or if massage has greater social acceptability among one gender than the other.

The final study looks at pain management for elderly cancer patients at home. Rhiner and associates (1993) designed a three-part pain education program funded by a research grant from the American Cancer Society. The program consists of an overview of pain management, pharmacologic management of pain, and nondrug interventions. In the nondrug portion of the educational program the patient had the opportunity to choose from a menu of five nondrug interventions: heat, cold, massage, relaxation/distraction, and imagery. Massage techniques included both hand massage and electric massager/vibration. The two most popular choices of nonpharmacological relief were heat and massage/vibration. Of the 40 patients, 70% selected heat and 63% chose massage/vibration. "Patients most often chose the vibration with heat, especially those patients with hip and leg pain." Perceived effectiveness was rated on a 0 to 4 scale (0, not at all effective to 4, very effective). Heat's effectiveness rating was 3.17, while massage's was 2.76. Interestingly, "distraction" (hu-

morous or musical audio tapes) was rated as the most effective—3.9. Patients were frequently reminded that the purpose of the nondrug methods was to enhance the effectiveness of the pharmacological interventions.

Three general findings have emerged from the research to date. First, massage positively affects symptoms related to cancer or side effects from treatment procedures, such as nausea, fatigue, insomnia, and pain. Second, massage increases relaxation and decreases muscle tension. Third, patients have an increased sense of well-being, with reduction in anxiety and sense of isolation as a result of massage.

Many questions remain unanswered with regard to massage for people living with cancer, such as: (1) Would the effects be greater if the massages were administered by massage therapists rather than nurses who have only minimal massage training? (2) What cumulative effect would daily massages have? (3) Are there gender-related differences regarding the effects of massage on cancer pain? (4) What would be the findings if massage sessions were individually tailored?

What is not in question, however, is the use of light massage for those with a cancer diagnosis. No evidence exists that comfort-oriented massage is deleterious, and what research there is indicates that it is often beneficial. This is not to say we should throw caution to the wind, but neither should we automatically turn away clients, friends, or family with cancer. Consulting with the patient's oncologist is the advisable thing to do before starting any bodywork.

GAYLE MACDONALD

See also
Deep Tissue Therapy (IV)

Esalen Massage (IV)
Hospital-Based Massage Therapy (IV)
Ice Massage for Control of Labor Pain (IV)
Lymphatic Massage (IV)
Newborn Massage (IV)
Pregnancy Massage (IV)
Reflexology (IV)
Russian Massage (IV)
Sports Massage (IV)
Swedish Massage (IV)

MEDITERRANEAN DIET

A typical Mediterranean diet consists of bread, root and green vegetables, fish, fruit, and a large amount of olive oil. Kushi, Lenart, and Willett (1995) pointed out that the consumption of beef, pork, and lamb has traditionally been low in Mediterranean countries and described the benefits of this type of diet. Regular consumption of red meat, part of the typical American diet, has been associated with increased risks of coronary heart disease and colon and other cancers. Possible mechanisms may involve dietary cholesterol, saturated fat, heme iron, and the presence of carcinogens formed in cooking. High consumption of meat also increases urinary calcium losses and may contribute to osteoporotic fractures.

Compared to saturated and partially hydrogenated fats, olive oil reduces low-density lipoprotein (LDL) cholesterol. Although dietary factors may not fully explain the generally good health of Mediterranean populations, available evidence supports the high consumption of fruit and vegetables and whole grains and the low consumption of animal products, saturated and hydrogenated fats, and refined carbohydrates (Kushi et al., 1995).

One study conducted in France (deLorgeril et al., 1994) evaluated the alpha-linolenic, acid-rich diet of 302 people after their first heart attack. The control group consisted of 303 people who ate a regular diet. The Mediterranean group ate fewer fats (saturated, cholesterol, and linoleic acid), and more oleic and alpha-linolenic acids. Results showed increased levels of vitamins C and E in people on the Mediterranean diet. The rate of heart attack was lower for the Mediterranean diet group ($n = 5$) as compared to the control group ($n = 17$). The cardiac death rate was also higher in the control group ($n = 16$) than in the Mediterranean diet group ($n = 3$). The overall death rate was 20 in the normal diet, 8 in the treatment group.

CAROLYN CHAMBERS CLARK

MIDWIFERY

Midwifery is old English for "with woman"; it is a time-honored women's healing art. Although it does not exclude male practitioners, the vast majority of midwives are women. The renaissance of midwifery in the United States in response to the coldness and unsatisfying experiences that were the standard in the late 1960s and early 1970s. Women began to look to one another for defining and meeting their needs.

Midwifery is often defined as woman-centered or consumer-oriented. It is an approach to health care that honors the wisdom of women's bodies: the ability to achieve pregnancy, grow a whole and separate person, labor and birth, to deliver the placenta, to slow down uterine bleeding, and to nourish the infant at the breast. All are taken to be the "normal miracles" of pregnancy. Additionally, the baby is seen as contributing to these processes.

Midwives approach pregnancy with the premise that it is a normal and healthy process that needs support and nurturance. Education (formal or empirical) is based on this ancient knowledge. Direct client care is then infused with skills for self-education and where self-growth is promoted and supported. Most midwives have or supply referrals for clients to access prenatal education (commonly referred to as "Lamaze"). The most ideal education program has material relevant for pre-pregnancy planning or early pregnancy care, along with prepared childbirth methodologies. The best of childbirth education stresses normalcy—how to achieve it, maintain it, and prevent complications. Much emphasis is given to nutrition, exercise, complimentary modalities, communication techniques for clarification between partners, and how and when to initiate emergency services. Complete education includes postpartum concerns as well: initiation of and continued support for breastfeeding, an overview of early parenting issues, including areas of controversy (circumcision, immunizations, prolonged breastfeeding, baby lead weaning), and educational approaches to early childhood development.

In classes as well as in clinical settings, there is a heavy emphasis on informed consent. Midwifery care usually starts out with explanations about who the midwives are and how they were educated. There are two kinds of midwives in the U.S.: direct entry midwife (DEM) or certified professional midwife (CPM), whose training may be formal didactic, apprentice-based, or a combination of both. The other branch of midwifery is composed of nurses who go on for additional training (CNM). As of the date of publication, there are no nurse-midwifery schools that require their students to participate in out-of-hospital birth to gain skills in that area. Most DEM formal programs require at least exposure in a variety of settings so that students gain skills in working with and being comfortable with clients there.

In an ideal community a woman would find midwives offering services for home birth, birth centers, and hospitals, with a corresponding variety of approaches and philosophies. Clients are encouraged to ask many questions about the midwife's training, but more importantly about the philosophy of care and how that will affect them. Women are encouraged to explore all their options, including herbs, chiropractic, massage, aromatherapy, and acupuncture; find their way through pregnancy, their labor, and their births by using a combination of healing or supportive modalities or therapists; and find a midwife that can accommodate those tools that are needed or desired.

The entire pregnancy is one giant adventure in exercising informed consent and can set in motion untold numbers of experiences that lead to confidence building and enhanced self- and couple-esteem. Informed consent is the process of looking at the practitioner, setting, procedure, test, or protocol as a unique experience discussing the advantages and disadvantages, the alternatives, and an acknowledgment of how much time can elapse before a decision must be made. Even in a time-critical situation there still is time to explain what's going on and to obtain the client's cooperation. There is a clear acknowledgment that what is right for one woman is *not* another woman's best choice. One of the biggest compliments that midwives receive is that the client *feels* paid attention to by the very act of being listened to. Consumer-oriented care means that even the most routine procedures are explained and education is provided. Tests are explained before they're obtained and their relevance to the client is reviewed. With this process, there is an understanding that the client is paying for a *service* and that her needs being met are paramount to the exchange.

Midwifery is usually thought of as being the provider for women who are in perfect health and by statistical analysis are expected to have good outcomes (as measured by governments by the number of live babies to pregnancies at births). Historically, though, midwives cared for all women and in most of the world and they continue to care for 75% to 80% of all women, usually with physicians being involved when there is a breakdown of a body system (like diabetes or hypertension) or with a problem in labor.

Most midwives believe in continuity of care, meaning the provider that's most known to the woman follows her through all of her pregnancy and assists at the birth. However, sometimes hospital policies or a physician's protocols will prohibit a midwife from actually being at the birth, so it is important to be specific about the role that the midwife will play throughout her care. For instance, some midwives cannot gain permission to work in a hospital or a physician will not work with her if she wants to be a woman's primary provider.

All midwives are trained to perform the skills necessary to take women from their initial prenatal physical, her labor and birth, her immediate postpartum period, and provide support and continued guid-

ance for breastfeeding. Most midwives provide gynecology or well woman care.

There is ample opportunity for complementary modalities to be used in all phases of pregnancy, labor, in the postpartum and with the newborn. The most commonly applied modalities being massage, chiropractic, and acupuncture. Clients can benefit greatly from these services during pregnancy and/or their births to prevent and treat some of the common problems, e.g., digestive problems, varicose veins, etc., and to help with discomfort and *length* of labors. In a well-integrated plan these modalities can be extremely beneficial and are inexpensive compared with the risks and costs of hospital care.

KARIN KEARNS

MINDFULNESS

Mindfulness is a particular way of paying attention to the present moment. It is one of two major forms of meditation out of the Buddhist traditions in Asia, which are at least 2,500 years old. Mindfulness meditation was developed to help cultivate greater awareness and to help people live fully each moment of their lives, even the painful ones. In the United States, mindfulness is associated with a particular approach to stress management created by Jon Kabat-Zinn.

Mindfulness is sometimes referred to as insight meditation, or *vipassana*. This meditation is begun by focusing attention on one sound or observing the breath. The second part of the process involves allowing the mind to observe any thoughts or feelings that arise and maintaining a nonjudgmental attitude toward whatever occurs, moment by moment. This process allows the meditator to learn about the workings of his or her mind at the present moment and to gain insight into the spending of time and energy. Equal acceptance of the good and bad, pleasant and unpleasant is the goal. The quality of awareness, not the content of the thoughts and feelings, is what is valued. This technique can be practiced in a sitting position or while eating, walking, or doing yoga postures.

Recent History

In 1992, Kabat-Zinn founded the Stress Reduction Clinic at the University of Massachusetts Medical Center. The core training program is an 8-week intensive course to which medical patients with a variety of illnesses and symptoms have been referred. Some have had little or no response to allopathic treatments, and others wish to try a "natural" approach to augment their care.

The training requires a commitment to daily meditative practice. In addition to being offered at the medical center, individually tailored programs have been created for specific groups and presented in prisons, inner city community health centers, and in Spanish as well as English. A training program was instituted to teach health professionals the basic mindfulness meditation techniques and how to teach it to patients.

Uses

The mindfulness meditation program aims to help people mobilize their own inner resources to better understand and care for themselves and complement any medical care they are receiving. The focus is on better coping with the stresses of everyday life, as well as living with a chronic or life-threatening illness. While no promises of symptom relief or illness remission are given, mindfulness meditation, when practiced regularly, can induce deep relaxation, improve symptoms, and help people live more satisfying lives. It is believed that accepting uncomfortable thoughts or feelings is the first step of transforming that reality and one's relationship to it.

Given the positive experience of the University of Massachusetts Medical Center with patients with cardiac and respiratory conditions, human immunodeficiency virus (HIV), diabetes, panic attacks, and other forms of anxiety, it is not yet apparent what kinds of patients or problems cannot benefit from this intensive training. However, high motivation is a critical element because of the daily level of participation required.

JILL STRAWN

MUSIC AND IMAGERY IN HEALING

A modality that affects physiological changes and, at the same time, expands the boundaries of consciousness to allow for new frames of mind sounds a little like magic. In actuality, it is achieved through the combination of two healing agents from the ancient world—music and imagery.

Music and imagery, separately, have been demonstrated as effective agents in managing pain. Achterberg (1985) explains the role of sound in filtering out pain. Auditory tracts passing directly into the reticular activating system of the brain stem coordinate sensory input and alert the cortex to incoming information. Sound traveling through this system activates the

brain and competes for cognitive awareness. Other sensory stimuli, such as pain
and nausea, can be gated out. Achterberg
speaks of images as electrochemical events
that carry messages from the brain to the
body. Thus, combining music and music-
induced imagery in the healing process
provides a powerful synthesis that engages
the whole of a person. Besides the management of physical symptoms, music and mu-
sic-induced imagery are used effectively
in such treatment needs as psychological
factors surrounding chronic or terminal illness; a broad range of mental, emotional,
and relationship problems; assisting individuals through the stages of dying
(Skaggs, 1997); and meeting spiritual and
existential crises.

The Role of Music

Response to music alone is involuntary.
Heart rate, respiratory rate, and other body
rhythms begin to match the rhythm and
tempo of music, in an act of entrainment
where human pulse matches music pulse.
Studies have indicated that music lowers
heart rate and blood pressure and creates
a less stressful, healthier environment.

More than a tool for affecting physiological changes, however, music represents
human emotional processes (Storr, 1992).
As a metaphor for human relationships,
music is in constant motion, tones relating
to tones, questioning and answering in con-
versational style, generating tension and
resolution. It provides diversity, which
keeps interaction vital and engaging, yet
offers the quintessential example of how
unity survives and thrives amidst diversity.
As a complex system of communications,
music is both a reflection of and a model
for universal life patterns (Skaggs, 1997b).

Archetypal patterns inherent in great music
and the symbolic language elicited through
listening provide a bridge between conscious and nonconscious levels of awareness and link personal history to the collec-
tive history of mankind.

Music-Induced Imagery

Music touches at the cellular level and
stimulates responses that go far beyond
mental imagery. As imagery in sound, music is the stimulus that may awaken all of
the senses of perception—visual imagery,
sensations of taste, smell, hearing, and feeling, emotions, and intuition. These responses arise from the depths of the psyche
and are unique to the listener's experience.
Images arising spontaneously in this manner belong authentically to the imager. Images initiated by the reading of someone
else's script tend to be strongly influenced
by the belief system inherent in the script.

A part of any healing process is the activation and strengthening of inner resources. By connecting individuals with
their own image-producing capacity, we
assist them in accessing their true and most
creative nature. With a strong sense of their
own essence, individuals have a resource
that is always available, one that allows a
sense of control over their lives. Images
emerging from such a primary level tend
to "hook" the imager. The ambiguity of
the images prevents their becoming understood with any finality or totality. This elusive nature holds the imager's attention in
an ongoing involvement. Images spawn
more images, serving to maintain a sense
of freshness and excitement. The imager
is not likely to become bored with his or
her healing process or to feel burdened
with the obligation of repeating the same

visualization day after day in a ritualized manner.

The ambiguous, abstract, unfolding nature of music without words provides an open environment for the individual psyche to resonate and respond with its unique language of symbols and images. Healing music may simultaneously stir emotions while containing and supporting them, allowing for the expression of the previously inexpressible. The therapist well trained in the language of symbol and metaphor can assist in the emergence of content from the depths of a person in a manner which offers safety, respect for the experience, and encouragement for growth towards wholeness.

Responsibility in Practice

Since the choice of music influences the sense of safety and the nature of responses, the responsible therapist is trained in the use of music in therapeutic practice. There is music—and there is music. When music is used as medicine, it deserves the same respect that, for example, pharmacology or cardiology commands. The therapist with competent knowledge and experience in the physiological, psychological, and spiritual potentials contained in, or absent from, music can choose music that is isomorphic in function; that is, qualities in the music will match the healing need, whether the need is physiological, emotional, or spiritual in character. When combined with attention to internal responses, this practice is what native Americans might refer to as good medicine.

RUTH SKAGGS

MUSIC THERAPY

Music can be used as a modality to promote change and enhance living for a number of health purposes. Music therapy is a profession that uses music as treatment for rehabilitation, for maintenance of quality of life, and for habitation for persons with physical, intellectual, and emotional disabilities (National Association for Music Therapy, 1997). Music therapists are certified by the Certification Board for Music Therapists.

Music, if analyzed through music theory, is composed of tonal sound intervals and harmonies that are timed in their delivery to designate meaning through rhythm, volume, and the use of lyrics. Theories in music therapy relate to a number of variables, including physiological response to music, emotional response to music (including the impact of memory and earlier life experience), the effect of music on coordination and balance, and cultural influences of music (Music Therapy Program, California State University, 1997).

With children, music therapy is often used in the schools as a vehicle to improve physical coordination, concentration skills, fine motor skills. Music also assists with the acquisition and application of study habits and academic fundamental skills, improving socialization skills, building self-esteem, developing basic life skills, and expanding the quality of life through the enjoyment of music and through creative self-expression.

With adolescents and adults, music can be used therapeutically with those who have behavioral, emotional, or mental problems to assist them to develop new adaptive skills, explore feelings, and resume functioning within society. As a complementary modality, music is often used to decrease stress and anxiety and prevent the development of depression. Audiotaped music is the most often used complementary modality, since it is readily available and consistently reusable. Some audiotapes are researched, such as the Munro Institute hemisync tapes, and may contain hypnotic suggestion through binaural integration (the combination of rhythm and beat delivered asymmetrically and separately to each ear through the use of headphones). The rhythms and beat combined variably with the use of voice-guided imagery focuses specifically on the context of the purpose for use. For example, one of the Munro series of tapes is used in preparation for surgery, during surgery, and following surgery. Each tape varies the prevalence of music over voice or voice over music (Oz, Lemole, Oz, Whitworth, & Lemole, 1996).

Music also is used in the complementary sense when it is used to provide a background for relaxation. The choice of music should be soothing to the person who will listen, so that the time spent in the presence of the music is perceived as pleasurable. The perception of pleasure may be relaxing or stimulating, depending on the intended use. Relaxation promotes reduction in anxiety, whereas enhanced stimulation may help to focus attention. Focused attention can improve concentration and study habits.

ANN BURKHARDT

MUSIC THERAPY RESEARCH

Research in music therapy is diverse and involves many different populations throughout the lifespan and under normal conditions or artificial conditions. It involves all age groups, but is often centered in hospital-based practice. Studies have been done in neonatal intensive care units in hospitals in an effort to mask stimuli and reduce the risk for failure to thrive (Standley & Moore, 1995a). Through earphones, half of the infants studied listened to lullabies and half listened to recordings of their mother's voice for 20-minute intervals over 3 consecutive days. Oxygen saturation levels were measured by pulse oxymetry. During the first day, the infants listening to music had better oxygenation levels than those listening to their mother's voice. During the second and third days, the infants listening to music were fine while they listened, but their oxygenation levels dropped when the music stopped. Overall, the infants who listened to the music had significantly less occurrences of oxymeter alarms than those who listened to their mother's voice.

Music has also been used in cancer treatment settings with both infants and adults (Standley & Moore, 1995b; Sabo & Michael, 1996). The focus of intervention in cancer is often to reduce anxiety and pain, perception of chemotherapy side effects, fear, stress, or grief. The reduction of pain is correlated with decreased dependence on the use of analgesic pain medications. Quality of life may be measured by tools such as the state anxiety scale (Sabo & Michael, 1996) or the locus of control (Standley & Hanser, 1995b). Anxiety has been demonstrated to be significantly less in patients using music during chemotherapy treatment.

Intraoperative and postoperative perception of pain has been measured by the intake of anesthesia during procedures as well as by consumption of analgesic pain medications and the impact on mood, pain, and anxiety or heart-rate variability (Baranson, Zimmerman, & Nieveen, 1995; Byers & Smyth, 1997; Good, 1995; Zimmerman, Nieveen, Baranson, & Schmaderer, 1996). Overall, a generalized physiological relaxation response as measured by heart rate and diminished systolic and diastolic blood pressure have been commonly demonstrated. Concerning the quality-of-life measurers, mood generally improved. However, reduced anxiety has not significantly been demonstrated.

Music has also been used with neurologically impaired populations. Melodic intonation has been used with aphasics to improve decoding of verbal messages when there has been a receptive aphasic component (Popovici, 1995). Music has also been used with patients who have dementia as a stimulator to improve food intake (Ragneskog, Brane, Karlsson, & Kihlgren, 1996). In addition to having greater intake of amounts of food during meals when soothing age and culturally appropriate music were played, patients were noted to have decreased irritability, fear-panic, and depressed moods.

Finally, music has been demonstrated as having an effect on coping ability when well people are under mental or physical duress (Tsenova, 1996). Physically related symptoms of neurosis including sleep disturbance, stress-related cardiovascular symptoms, stomach and muscle pains, irritability, and a sense of emotional imbalance all improved during regulative music therapy sessions.

ANN BURKHARDT

MYOFASCIAL RELEASE

Myofascial release is a specific manual therapy approach to connective tissue dysfunction. It is a therapy that applies prolonged light pressure with specific directions applied to the structural orientation of the fibrous tissue of the skin (Tappan, 1988). This structural orientation of the body was discovered in the mid-1800s by Carl Ritter von Langer, an Austrian anatomist, who discovered natural cleavage lines of the body present in all body areas and visible in only certain sites, such as the palms of the hands (Thomas, 1985). These lines are commonly known as Langer's lines, used today by surgeons who make incisions parallel to the lines to reduce the visible presence of a postsurgical scar. In myofascial release techniques, the hand movements follow a set pattern for tissue manipulation along Langer's lines.

Theory

To further understand myofascial release therapy, it is important to review the general anatomy and physiology of muscle in relationship to fascia. *Myo* comes from the Latin word for "muscle"; *fascia* comes from the Latin word for "a covering or band" (Thomas, 1985). Thus, "myofascia" means "a covering of the muscle." It is commonly known that muscle is a tissue composed of fibers, capable of contracting and relaxing to effect bodily movement. Fascia is a connective fibrous tissue that has ground substance, a viscous liquid that surrounds all cells in the body. It is this tissue fluid that provides an essential medium through which the cellular elements of other tissues are brought into functional relation with blood and lymph (Seeley, Stephens, & Tate, 1995). Thus, fascia has a nutritive function. It also has collagen fibers, long white fibers that create intercellular support responsible for strength, tensile strength, resiliency, and structural integrity. By virtue of its fibroplastic activity, it also aids in the repair of injuries by the decomposition of collagenous fiber/scar tissue.

The functions of fascia are many, with the greatest role being supporting and providing cohesion to the body structures. It supplies restraining mechanisms by the differentiation of retention bands and fibrous pulleys, for example. Fascia also provides fascial planes, pathways for nerves, circulatory, and lymphatic vessels. Deep fascia ensheaths and preserves the characteristic contour of the limbs and promotes the circulation in the veins and lymphatic vessels; the ensheathing layer of deep fascia, as well as intermuscular septa and interosseous membranes, provides additional surface areas for muscular attachment. Superficial fascia allows for storage of fat and provides a surface covering that aids in the conservation of body heat.

In summary, the relationship of muscle to fascia (myofascial) is understood through the properties of each component part, the muscle and the fascia, as shared. General properties and function of myofascia, as a unit, are outlined. The myofascial unit has (1) a rich supply of nerve endings, (2) the ability to contract and to stretch elastically, (3) fascial planes, creating pathways for nervous, circulatory, and lymphatic functions, and (4) the function to support, stabilize, and enhance postural balance of the body, thereby being involved in all aspects of motion (Chaitow, 1988).

The need for the application of myofascial therapy can only be understood within the context of alterations in the myofascial unit, or connective tissue structure, function, and behavior. Sudden or sustained tension or traction of the myofascial unit creates alterations in the tissue itself. Thickening, shortening, calcification, and erosion of the tissue, with resultant distortion in tissue structure and function, interferes with stabilizing and maintaining upright posture, for example. Even the slightest alteration in the normal balance of the various spinal segments, primarily responsible for upright posture, is accompanied by some degree of soft tissue change. Over time, an accumulation of stress and strain produces pain when stagnation of acids and other toxins create chronic passive congestion in a given area. Vasoconstriction and hypoxia of the tissues are associated with changes in the hydrogen ion concentration and calcium and sodium balance in the tissue. In turn, these cellular and tissue changes affect the pain sensors and proprioceptors (Chaitow, 1988). This further predisposes towards dysfunction, pain, and tenderness, especially in the areas of bony attachment, areas of calcification, and in areas where stress forces converge (Chaitow, 1996). Stress forces produce definite stress bands within the myofascial unit, and with sudden stress/trauma on fascial tissue, a burning type of pain ensues (Travell & Simons, 1983). Obviously, myofascial pain is most often the complaint that mobilizes the person to seek the use of manual therapies.

Most of the literature describes myofascial pain in reference to trigger points. A trigger point is a focus of hyperirritability in a tissue that, when compressed, is locally tender and, if sufficiently hypersensitive, gives rise to referred pain and tenderness, and sometimes to referred autonomic phenomena and distortion of proprioception (Travell & Simons, 1983). Myofascial pain is referred from trigger points in specific patterns characteristic of each muscle. It is important to note that manual trigger point zone therapy differs significantly from my-ofascial release therapy. In brief, manual trigger point zone technique localizes and addresses patterns of specific muscle points directly, using deep pressure. Myo-fascial release technique follows Langer's lines and focuses on diffuse areas, using light gentle pressure and stretching.

Application

Previous to utilizing any manual therapy, evaluation of the person's physical, mental, emotional, and spiritual status is most im-portant. It is common knowledge that the integration of these component parts cre-ates balance of body-mind-spirit and pro-motes health of the individual. An imbal-ance of any one of the component parts of the person creates imbalance in health. For example, a person with low self-esteem may exhibit a postural distortion, with a bowing forward of the shoulders. Through simple inspection and observation, valu-able assessment information can be ascer-tained. Inspection and observation are in-valuable tools used to provide data about the whole person. In fact, postural assess-ment provides significant information about the body-mind-spirit holding pat-terns of the person.

Obtaining and utilizing information col-lected from a postural assessment is benefi-cial to determining and planning the course of action taken in a myofascial release ther-apy session. A few important points in-volved in accurate postural assessment are reviewed: (1) observe for correct posture: the head is centered over the pelvis, the face directed forward, and the shoulder gir-dle approximately on the same plane as the pelvis; and (2) observe for poor posture: the head is carried forward, scapulae are held in abduction giving the shoulders a rounded appearance, dorsal curve is in-creased, and chest is flattened (Wadsworth, 1988). Assessment of particular shortened muscles and groups of shortened muscles, also indicating postural distortion, is inte-gral to accurate assessment.

Palpation is another way to successfully diagnose the person's problem. To engage in palpatory diagnosis, run the fingers lightly over the area being checked, taking note of the changes in the skin and tissues below the area. After localizing any changes, deeper structures can be assessed by applying deeper pressure. Touch must be firm and at the same time light, to dis-cern the minute tissue changes. Specific changes noted with palpatory diagnosis are: (1) the skin will feel tense and will be relatively difficult to move or glide over the underlying structures when assessed using lighter pressure; (2) the skin and superficial musculature will demonstrate a tension and immobility indicating fibrotic changes within and below these structures when assessed using deeper pressure; (3) a local-ized increase in temperature may be evi-dent, indicating acute dysfunction, and a localized decrease in temperature may be found in chronic dysfunction due to rela-tive ischemia; (4) tenderness in the area may be experienced (note that this is often misleading as it may indicate local or reflex problems in acute or chronic dysfunction); and (5) edema, found by fullness and con-gestion of the tissue, can be felt in the overlying tissue usually found in acute dys-function. Edema is usually absent in chronic dysfunction as it is replaced by fibrotic changes (Wadsworth, 1988).

Upon discerning information about the areas of tissue distortion, the data are used to indicate the primary focal areas where myofascial release techniques are emphasized. Light, gentle pressure with subtle stretching of the focal and encompassing areas using Langer's lines is employed. This creates friction, generating heat and increasing the temperature and energy level of the tissue. The added energy promotes a more fluid ground substance; the myofascial unit can then be more easily molded. As a result, nutrients and cellular waste conduct their exchange more efficiently. Thus, the buildup of acids as a result of trauma and/or sustained muscle tension or traction lessens and resolves, creating balance within in the myofascial unit. Pain symptoms improve.

Uses for myofascial release therapy extends beyond pain relief. As previously mentioned, fascia has fascial planes that create pathways for nervous, circulatory, and lymphatic functions. Fluids and infectious processes often travel along these planes. Myofascial release therapy facilitates the flow of fluids, contributing to the reduction of the systemic toxic load. Cellular and tissue nutrition is thus enhanced.

Obviously, myofascial release therapy is useful for most people. This therapy remains most effective when body-mind-spirit holding patterns are identified and the person is encouraged to actively engage in measures to correct these patterns. Myofascial release therapy, then, used within the framework of self-responsibility and action to correct identified holding patterns, greatly contributes to body-mind-spirit balance and individual health.

BONNIE T. MACKEY

MYOTHERAPY, BONNIE PRUDDEN

Myotherapy is a method of relaxing muscle spasm, improving circulation, and alleviating pain. To defuse trigger points, pressure is applied to the muscle for several seconds by means of fingers, knuckles, and elbows. The success of this method depends on the use of specific corrective exercise for the freed muscles. The method was developed by Bonnie Prudden in 1976 (Taber's Cyclopedic Dictionary). It is a hands-on, drugless, noninvasive method of relieving muscle-related pain, emphasizes speedy, cost-effective recovery and active patient participation for long-term relief. It relaxes muscles, improves circulation, and alleviates pain throughout the body. It also increases strength, flexibility, coordination, stamina, and energy and improves posture, gait, and sleep patterns. Work and athletic performance are enhanced very quickly and effectively. Although Bonnie Prudden Myotherapy has its origins in the medical discipline of trigger-point injection therapy developed by Janet Travell, M.D., it is noninvasive and very teachable. This has encouraged widespread use by lay individuals.

History

Myotherapy has its origins in work done by Dr. Max Lange in Germany in the mid-1930s. He discovered that there are "tender areas" in muscles, and using a sclerometer he found that those areas were slightly more dense than the surrounding tissue and that they had the ability to throw the muscle into spasm. Also in the 1930s, Dr. Hans Kraus, an Austrian orthopedist, developed Therapeutic Exercise together with Austria's Olympic trainer, Heinz Kowalski. In the 1940s, Dr. Janet Travell began her pioneering experiments in the United States with trigger-point injection therapy followed by muscle-stretching exercise facilitated by muscle-relaxing coolant sprays, ethylchloride and fluorimethane. The two medically valid disciplines complement each other, as trigger-point injections are followed by stretch exercises, which are facilitated by the muscle-related coolant sprays.

In 1976, Bonnie Prudden found that non-invasive pressure to trigger points using fingers, knuckles, or elbows, followed by specific corrective exercises, yielded superior results to those engendered by injection followed by "spray and stretch." In 1978, Desmond Tivy, M.D., a London University graduate and internist, coined the term myotherapy for Bonnie Prudden's discovery. In 1980 and 1985, Bonnie Prudden authored the two books on myotherapy: *Pain Erasure the Bonnie Prudden Way* and *Myotherapy, Bonnie Prudden's Complete Guide to Pain-Free Living*. These two books, with forewords and afterwords by Dr. Tivy, put myotherapy into the able hands of the general public. These books were followed by four others written for different age groups, including chapters on myotherapy specific to those populations.

The Theory

Bonnie Prudden Myotherapy is the noninvasive offshoot of the two medical disciplines, trigger-point injection therapy and therapeutic exercise. Travell holds that injecting procaine and saline into trigger points denies them oxygen and in effect defuses them, allowing painful muscles to relax. Stretch exercises are then used as a coolant spray is applied to the painful area. Prudden discovered that manual pressure applied to trigger points is far less painful, covers much larger muscle areas, and often works more quickly. Specific therapeutic exercises performed immediately following the manual pressure to trigger points erases the pain. A daily program of the same simple exercises makes recovery sure and lasting.

Myotherapy Treatment Session

Treatments typically are consistent from one practitioner to another, since there is only one school of Bonnie Prudden Myotherapy. The first treatment session is 90 minutes and includes the vital history. Subsequent sessions are 60 minutes. Depending on location, fees range from $40 to $150. Objectives are to erase muscle spasm and pain, increase range of motion, and prevent the return of pain by reeducating the muscles with specific exercises designed for each individual problem.

There are typically four components to an initial Bonnie Prudden Myotherapy session. During the history, patients are asked about their birth, past and present occupations, sports activities, accidents, operations, injuries, and the presence of diseases such as multiple sclerosis. Next, the patient is given the medically valid Kraus-Weber test to determine the minimum strength and flexibility of key posture muscles. The myotherapist then locates (based on the history) and erases the trigger points believed to be most directly responsible for the pain, limited range of motion, nerve or circulatory problems, and/or muscle fatigue, weakness, and dysfunction.

The treatment is considered to be a partnership, and the patient is instructed to direct the force of the pressure by letting the therapist know when a trigger point is found and the level of pain on a scale of 1 to 10. The newly relaxed muscles are then passively stretched and the patient is given corrective exercises to do at home.

These keep the muscles free of spasm and are the key to the success of the treatment.

After an initial treatment, patients are usually very relaxed and use words like "looser," "lighter," and "warmer" to describe how they feel. It is normal to note what would seem to be a remarkable reduction of pain and increased flexibility after the first treatment. Patients also report improved sleeping patterns following the reduction of pain. These immediate changes usually hold until the next treatment and become long-term changes especially if the patient faithfully performs the homework exercise and self-help techniques as prescribed.

Benefits, Limitations, Contraindications

Bonnie Prudden Myotherapy is effective whenever pain is muscle-related. Examples are back pain, headaches, sciatica, shoulder and neck pain, repetitive motion injuries such as carpal tunnel syndrome, sports injuries, temporomandibular joint (TMJ) pain, hip, knee, or foot pain, menstrual cramps, and pain associated with disease. While myotherapy does not cure the disease, it does relieve the pain and provide a better climate for recovery.

Myotherapy concentrates solely on functional muscle anatomy and has virtually no side effects other than occasional bruising. Myotherapy almost always works very quickly; the myotherapist usually knows after one treatment whether or not it will be effective. Most patients require fewer than 10 treatments to erase the pain and to learn the corrective exercises and self-help myotherapy necessary to prevent the pain's return.

Pathology must be addressed by the physician prior to embarking on a series of Myotherapy treatments.

Practitioner Evaluation

Certified Bonnie Prudden Myotherapists (CBPMs) train for 1,300 hours (9 months) at the Bonnie Prudden School for Physical Fitness and Myotherapy, the only school of its kind. To maintain certification, 45 hours of update training is required every two years.

BONNIE PRUDDEN
ENID WHITTAKER

NATIVE AMERICAN MEDICINE

Cultures rise and fall. Discovering what is truly traditional amid today's Native American peoples is impossible. Earlier manuscripts from the 18th and 19th centuries provide us with some pre-Christian perspective. Nevertheless, the going is rough in recovering authentic from Christianized practice. Despite this, there are commonalities across most tribes that reflect a unified heritage about which we can reflect and reconstruct. First and foremost, Native Americans grew up within an unshakable faith in healing—that it is possible, that it is a gift from God and the spirits, and that, when it happens, it is miraculous.

Native Americans look to the spiritual world for help with earthly problems. They cry out for help from the spirits with whom they share the earth and sky. Within this context, Native Americans are the original holistic doctors of North America. Native Americans are familiar with herbs; hands-on healing or therapeutic touch; imagery; sacred art; counseling of individuals, families, and extended kinship groups; and, of course, ceremonies. The therapeutic work of Native healers is guided by a kind of diagnosis, usually a narrative tale of the origins of the illness, its growth and development, and its daily life, complete with a prescription for how to overcome the illness implicit in the tale.

How do typical healers work? First they elicit the client's and the family's story of the illness. Healers hear the subtle nuances in voice tone and phrasing, which provide the clues for doors into the story where change can be introduced. Alternative endings are planned for the story in healing. The story reveals the strengths and the weaknesses of the client. Through listening to the story, healers see the spirit of the client and the spirit of the illness. It becomes obvious what plant or animal spirits (medicines) are needed to strengthen the client's spirit. Sometimes this vision inspires sacred art, as in shields or sand paintings. Imagery is sometimes used, through the literal translation for the word is more powerful: "putting them to sleep so that they dream like they're asleep but they're really awake." Through this process, the healer can speak to the illness, learn how it entered the person, who nurtured its growth and development, what it eats to survive, and how healers and clients might best work together to get rid of it. From there it is possible to begin to counsel the patient and the family and to plan a ceremony.

Each tribe has its sacred ceremonies. Sioux ceremonies are becoming increasingly prevalent, achieving almost a pan-Indian status. These ceremonies include the *inipi*, or sweat lodge ceremony; the *hanblecheya*, or vision quest, the sun dance ceremony, the *yuwipi*, or darkness curing ceremony, a rite of passage into adulthood ceremony, to mention the most common. The Dineh people have intricate ceremonies that include sand painting and complex songs and stories. The Cherokee have im-

portant summer and winter solstice ceremonies. The Mojave tribe had a rattlesnake protection ceremony to prevent rattlesnake bites all summer long.

What is common to all these ceremonies is the belief that the prayers of the many are synergistic in the supplication for the one. The candle light of a single person's prayers become the laser light of the group's prayers.

In hearing about Native American medicine, Westerners typically want to be told what techniques work best with which particular illnesses. The assumption behind this question is contrary to the essence of Native American medicine, which would start with the idea of asking who can work best with a particular patient. The personalities of healers and clients must match in some specific ways. Each healer is best with certain kinds of individuals and, for others, cannot do a thing. For example, healers generally do not try to work with clients who have the same psychological ailments as their parents had when the healer was a child. It would be too difficult for them to be as fully present with that client as they should be.

After matching the energy, personality, and style of the healer and the client, then a legitimate question is where to start. Regardless of what techniques the healer is most acquainted with, a diagnosis phase precedes treatment. That diagnosis may be made, for example, in the Dineh tradition, by a hand trembler, who reads the aura of the person and the illness, determining what is wrong (within a particular metaphorical system) and prescribing the proper ceremony or healer. Then it is up to the client to seek out the healer or ceremonial "singer" who can help. Within most Native American traditions (including the Lakota and Cherokee), the healer diagnoses the problem through careful listening and rapport-building. Once the healer understands the problem (again, within one or more of several metaphorical systems), a treatment plan can be constructed, usually a combination of botanical treatments, individual counseling with the healer, family counseling, purification (as in the sweat lodge), healing ceremonies for the family and the community, and sometimes massage therapy, which was particularly well developed among the Cherokee (as well as the Apaches and the native Hawaiians).

It is generally beyond the scope of an afflicted individual to understand what technique will be most helpful to them. We cannot step outside of ourselves far enough to see how to help ourselves. The exception, of course, is the Divine Guidance that clients sometimes receive in dreams or visions, telling them how healing can best be accomplished. For a practitioner, the two modes are easy to distinguish. When a person intellectually reasons out what will help, the healer will usually try this, but always in conjunction with other methods thought to be more helpful. This is because the mind generally cannot rationally solve the problem of illness. On the other hand, when a person comes with an intuitive sense of what will help for which there is no rational argument, the healer is more willing to believe that it will be so. Healers or any health practitioners need to be trustworthy, for whom others can vouch for their integrity and skill. The client must be willing to do what the healer says, unless it seems outrageous or dangerous.

LEWIS MEHL-MADRONA

NEUROMUSCULAR THERAPY

Neuromuscular therapy (NMT) is a form of soft tissue massage therapy that is highly effective in the treatment of most chronic pain syndromes. NMT is a muscle-by-muscle examination of all soft tissues that may be associated with a particular injury or pain syndrome. It is detailed and specific and requires the therapist to have a thorough understanding of anatomy and physiology.

NMT addresses the following six physiological factors that create or intensify pain in the body:

1. Ischemia: Lack of blood and oxygen caused by muscular hypertonicity (spasm).
2. Trigger points: Areas of increased metabolic waste deposits that excite segments of the spinal cord and cause referred pain or sensations to other parts of the body.
3. Nerve entrapment and/or compression: Pressure on nerves by soft tissue (muscle, tendon, ligament, fascia, or skin) or by hard tissue (bone or disk), respectively.
4. Postural distortion: The body's deviation from an anatomically correct position in coronal, sagittal, or horizontal planes.
5. Poor nutrition: The intake of nutrients irritating and stimulating to the central nervous system and insufficient intake of nutrients necessary for cellular metabolism and tissue repair.
6. Emotional well-being: The ability to handle stress.

Neuromuscular therapy originated in the late 1970s from the work of Raymond

Nimmo, D.C., which he called Receptor Tonus Techniques. It also was deeply influenced by trigger point therapy as developed by Janet Travell and David Simons. These techniques have been expanded on and developed into treatment routines by Paul St. John and Judith (Walker) DeLany. A similar form of soft tissue work developed simultaneously in Europe under the influences of Stanley Lief, Boris Chaitow, and Leon Chaitow, under the name neuromuscular technique. Treatment techniques of the two versions are somewhat diverse, although the common links between the two styles appear to be Nimmo's techniques and trigger point applications.

By physically removing the waste products from the muscles, heating fascial casings, and stimulating the pain control (analgesia) system of the brain and spinal cord, application of NMT may affect both fast (sharp) pain signals and slow (burning) pain signals, therefore affecting both acute and chronic pain. Inhibition of pain transmission may be evoked by chemicals, such as enkephalin and serotonin. These chemicals are believed to cause presynaptic inhibition of neurostimulation. Other chemicals in the analgesic system, which resemble opiate-like substances, such as endorphin and dynorphin, may also be released.

In the gate control theory, it is postulated that a modulating gate mechanism exists within the nervous system that screens the transmission of impulses into the cord and assists in the establishment of facilitated segments (reflex arcs). When the secondary stimulation enters the cord, it may override an established reflex arc, which is transmitting the pain signals. Overriding stimulants may include heat, cold, acupuncture, pressure, tactile stimulation, electrical stimulation, vibration, and a number of other possibilities. During the time of the secondary stimulation, the reflex arc is interrupted by the inhibitory gate, possibly by chemical inhibition. If the arc reestablishes itself after the new stimulus is removed, it will usually be lessened and may be completely eliminated. This may be why most forms of therapy, from hydrotherapy to skin counter irritants to TENS units, are effective. It is the theoretical basis of NMT.

NMT has been found highly effective in the treatment of most chronic pain syndromes, including headaches, migraines, back and neck pain, bursitis, shoulder and hip pain, tennis elbow, tendonitis, carpal tunnel syndrome, whiplash, temporomandibular joint dysfunction, sciatica, breathing problems, and pain from auto accidents, work-related injuries, sports and recreational traumas, and repetitive strains. It is also effective in the prevention of injury by eliminating dysfunctional biomechanics, latent trigger points, and existing ischemia, all of which are more prone to injury.

JUDITH WALKER DELANY

NEWBORN MASSAGE

The term "infant massage" is an umbrella for massage with all babies up to the age of walking and includes newborn massage. This includes the full-term healthy newborn and those babies with altered nervous systems caused by prematurity, drug exposure, iatrogenic causes, birth trauma, or trauma incurred in utero. The documented benefits of massaging babies includes increased weight gain, improved elimination, improved sleep-wake states, improved performance on Brazelton neurological functioning scales, improved ability for social interaction, and enhanced bonding or attachment behaviors (Rice, 1977; Field, 1986; White-Traut, & Carrier-Goldman, 1988; Ludington, 1977).

Most infant massage research has been done with the prematurely born infant, and particular guidelines for touching these infants has been established. However, the training for instructors of the actual care givers that was available prior to the Baby's First Massage (BFM) program (Ramsey, 1992) did not differentiate how to touch those babies with more vulnerable nervous systems. There was no program available to meet the needs of new families at the time of birth that was simple enough, and short enough to be easily taught to families, considering their short attention span and the overload of information presented to them.

Conserving Energy

The traditional medical view acknowledges that healing babies need to conserve energy. This is addressed by keeping the newborn swaddled or wrapped during the massage, exposing only the body part being massaged. If a baby hasn't stabilized its body temperature yet, the strokes may be done over clothing. Crying is prevented as much as possible. *Note: two primary patterns of crying are identified: the "I need help" cry and the "Talking" cry. With the talking cry, a baby is able to hold your gaze while crying. Being able to "talk" and be heard is a primal need.* A baby crying the "I need help" cry needs assistance as soon as possible, and should not be "pushed" by continuing giving massage at that time. The abdominal strokes take

into consideration the possible presence of an umbilical cord.

Stroke Patterns

The parasympathetic nervous system (PNS) is targeted for stimulation by particular massage strokes and patterns of stroking (Rice, 1977). The PNS is vegetative and responsible for digestion, absorption, elimination, sleep, healing, growth, and development. This is exactly what the newborn needs. All strokes are cephalo caudal and repeated at least three times. In the BFM program, stroking patterns are incorporated, including the hand positions, the amount of pressure to use, and the number of repetitions to use to obtain the documented effects. However, strokes begin with the legs rather than the head. The International Association of Infant Massage teaches that the legs are much less threatening as an area to begin massaging. Many newborns have experienced birth trauma to the head and shoulders. Other changes to the BFM approach include the elimination of a stroke down and alongside the throat (*BFM is oriented to teaching parents and it feels risky to teach parents to do this stroke as the vagus nerve is close to the surface in this area and bradycardia could be a result from too much pressure on it*), elimination of the stroke over the linea alba in the chest, the addition of two abdominal strokes (the "I Love You" stroke and abdominal reflex stroking), and an opening stretch of the lumbo sacral area that feels like bobbing on an ocean wave.

Time-Out Signals

Time-out signals or disengagement cues (Als, 1986) are respected, and attention is turned to comforting the baby and bringing the baby back to a centered state (or PNS functioning). Als (1986) has thoroughly studied the communication coming out of the nervous system of the very prematurely born, very fragile infant. She presented an extensive list of dramatic autonomic and motor nervous system signals that indicate a baby is becoming very unstable and intervention must be done to calm the baby. If this isn't done with the very fragile baby, neurological damage is a likely consequence. Five or six of these cues commonly seen in the full-term newborn and very frequently seen in the prematurely born. These are arching the back, splaying the fingers, hiccuping and spitting up not related to eating, avoiding the gaze, and inconsolable crying (which is the "I need help" cry taken too far). The primary modes of comforting are related to recreating the womb, such as wrapping tightly, placing the baby in the fetal position, encouraging the baby to suck a finger, a pacifier, or nipple if breastfeeding. These are all forms of "containment" (Als, 1986).

Infant Stability

Newborn massage is appropriate only with the medically stable infant. An easy rule of thumb for stability is if the baby is in an open crib and able to take feedings. There are a few variables in some cases, but this indicates the baby's systems are operating more smoothly. With the prematurely born baby, there are two other guidelines: The baby weighs at least 3 pounds, and it has reached 32 weeks gestation (White-Traut & Carrier-Goldman, 1994). Around 32 weeks gestation, the gag reflex is maturing, and the baby reaches a milestone called "coming out" that means it is more able to interact with the outside world without destabilizing the heart rate, blood pressure, or oxygen saturation. If massage is attempted with babies before they are able to maintain basic homoeostatic mechanisms, we are pushing babies, courting negative consequences, and at a minimum being disrespectful of their needs.

Teachers of infant massage are indebted to the many researchers for their clear and repetitive documentation of the many benefits of infant massage. However, the real power lies in the hands of the parents or care givers. If the only massage a baby receives is with a researcher, then families are not empowered to integrate this into family life. The potential is present for instructors to use a short process (30 minutes long) that teaches a new parent how to identify a talking cry and the "I need help" cry, along with the other time-out signals, several ways to comfort their baby, and 13 simple massage strokes that enhance digestion, absorption, elimination, rest, and healing. Woven throughout this simple interaction is a role modeling of "being present" with the baby. The Scottish have identified this art as "kything" (Savary & Berne, 1988): listening to the baby's ways of communication, listening with their hands as they stoke their baby, staying in the present moment. When a baby presents time-out cues that are respected by the parent, and the parent stops massaging and explores ways to comfort the baby, not only is love being expressed but also the baby is getting a very early opportunity to exercise power over its body.

The BFM program trains and certifies participants as newborn massage instructors to teach new parents how to massage their newborn baby in a respectful, neurologically protective way as soon after birth as possible. It is based on research, and it embodies and intermingles traditional medical views on the needs of a newborn with the more holistic view of massage as a healing art. It supports the basic psychosocial need of all humans to feel welcomed into the family at birth. In all its aspects, the art of listening, being present, or "kything" is subtlety and overtly emphasized.

TERESA KIRKPATRICK RAMSEY

NONDIETING

Nondieting (Tribole & Resch, 1995; Hayes, 1993) consists of making choices about food, exercise, body image, and general self-care that honors pleasure and health without engaging in restrictive dieting, or eating less than one desires or is hungry for. The nondieting movement is gaining more prominence as research continues to confirm that diets simply do not work for most individuals: 90% of all persons trying to lose weight by dieting eventually fail and regain the weight (Foreyt & Goodyrick, 1992).

The "dieter's dilemma," first coined by William Bennett at Harvard University, proceeds as follows: Due to a desire to be thin, eating is restricted; this results in cravings and reduced self-control, which leads to a loss of control and overeating, which in turn leads to regain weight and a need to repeat the cycle (Foreyt & Goodrick, 1992). Example consequences of dieting include a slowed metabolic rate as the body is primed to conserve post-diet calories, feelings of failure, lowered self-esteem, and an eroded sense of trust in oneself regarding food choices. In addition, dieting plays a role in binge-eating, bulimia, and anorexia.

Cultural messages, reinforced by a $30 billion weight-loss industry, equate the absence of body fat with worth, health, and success, especially for girls and women and now increasingly for boys and men. In the media, thin and muscular bodies are portrayed as the ideals. According to Jeanine Cogan of the Office of Public Policy at the American Psychological Association, obesity has been socially constructed as the number-one killer based on the following errors. Research findings on the negative correlates of obesity rather than health benefits of obesity have been selectively reviewed. In addition, key research findings on the potential health risks of weight loss and regain, the important role of genetics in determining body weight, and the inefficacy of restrictive dieting for long-term weight loss are invisible (Cogan, 1997). In this context, dieting continues to be prevalent as Americans, on average, continue to get heavier.

A nondieting approach respects genetic predispositions to a certain body shape or size. It discards externalized rules of dieting and aims to restore trust in inner capabilities to eat flexibly and freely in response to hunger, fullness, satisfaction, and physical feelings. Health at any weight is emphasized rather than weight loss. In general, this involves attending and responding to hunger and other needs (e.g., emotions), being physically active for enjoyment, nurturing rather than disliking the body, and paying attention to how the body feels after various foods are consumed.

Example techniques for a nondieting approach include the following:

- A comprehensive assessment of general health and eating behavior, including eating disorders, personal and family members' weight histories, exercise, and body image. A food diary often is helpful to understand eating patterns.

- Assuming that dieting has failed, exploration of the dieter's dilemma and prior strategies the client has tried, and the benefits and consequences of each strategy.

- Self-monitoring via a food journal. Even though this is a tedious task, a food journal is invaluable for increasing consciousness about what is eaten, the circumstances and feelings before, during, and after eating, and ratings of physical hunger to help assess whether eating is in response to hunger or other reasons. If a person is eating excessively in response to circumstances or to cope with emotions, then awareness of these circumstances or emotions can be increased and alternative strategies for addressing them can be formulated.

- Increasing awareness of hunger signals. Many chronic dieters' physiological hunger signals have faded over time due to being ignored during the dieting process. Hunger sensations can be reestablished by noticing them and by eating at regular intervals.

- Avoiding becoming overhungry due to the tendency for rapid eating or overeating to satisfy extreme hunger. Giving oneself permission to satisfy hunger and permission to eat again when hungry contradicts the external rules of restrictive dieting, which encourage dieters to bypass hunger.

- Allowance of all foods. Once foods are no longer restricted, their power as forbidden foods is decreased. In tandem with freeing food choices, the eater pays attention to what food is wanted, savors food slowly and consciously, and stops when full. Attention is also paid to physical and psychological feelings after eating various foods, which results in consciousness about how eating various foods makes one feel.

- Exercise for pure enjoyment, energy, and vitality, rather than body sculpting or fat- or calorie-burning. Moving one's body is helpful for boosting mood, body image, and overall health.

- Body affirmation, rather than body dissatisfaction: Treat the body with respect. Unhealthy cultural messages that keep a majority of women dissatisfied with their bodies are identified and resisted.

- Encouragement of flexibility with the eating and nondieting process, because the goal of nondieting is self-care rather than achieving perfection.

- Attention to overall needs. For example, cultivating a support system, planning ahead to take care of oneself, and taking time to make eating a conscious, satisfying experience rather than an automatic or stressful experience is encouraged.

The nascent research on the effects of nondieting methods has documented decreased binge eating and increased quality of life and well-being but not weight loss (Goodrick, Poston, Kimball, Reeves, & Foreyt, in press; Polivy & Herman, 1992). The King Medical Group in Salinas, California, reports success with a nondieting approach for regulating blood sugar in diabetes. Tribole and Resch (1995) also summarize research that consistently shows toddlers are natural nondieters who, given free access to food, will balance their nutritional intake over time even though their meal-by-meal intake may be highly variable.

Since the U.S. Dietary Goals no longer recommend ideal body weights, and the National Institutes of Health acknowledge the failure of traditional dieting treatments and instead suggest focusing on health benefits independent of weight loss (Erdman, 1995), nondieting approaches undoubtedly will receive increasing attention for their emphasis on overall well-being rather than weight loss as a primary goal. Due to the complex nature of weight management, obesity, and eating disorders, and the potential for harm to clients of various methods, it is important for professionals to obtain training and supervision or consultation for work with clients in these areas.

MAUREEN M. CORBETT

NUTRITION

Nutrition is the science that studies the various aspects of food acquisition, input, digestion, absorption, metabolism, and excretion, as well as the identification of the needs for specific substances in specific amounts to sustain life, to promote well-being, and to avoid disease. The history of nutritional science tells a fascinating story. At any point in time, that history pinpoints the lack of knowledge or the extent of knowledge available to its researchers. Both laboratory scientists and clinical investigators have contributed to the body of nutritional data. The availability of "space age" technology to quantify nutrient elements in body tissues (extracellular and intracellular) has permitted many therapeutic advances. For example, the presence of an abnormally low level of serum potassium, a potentially life-threatening finding, may be corrected by the rapid administration of intravenous potassium or more slowly by the feeding of a high-potassium food, such as orange juice or banana. The availability of reliable measurements to detect and monitor the low-potassium state permits proper dosing of medication, the proper alteration of diet, and the proper choice of potassium-wasting or potassium-sparing drugs. The same could be said in regard to the measurement of the nutrient glucose and many other substances.

The need for and attainment of scientific precision and quality-control standards for commercial laboratories have been outstanding accomplishments of modern chemical laboratories. Reliable scientific data has permitted rigorous nutritional research, thus providing to the practicing physician a host of biochemical probes to properly evaluate the levels of nutrients in patients whose health is compromised or in those who have health and wish to keep it. As a result, much of the trial and error, guesswork, or unsubstantiated notions that may have abounded have been dispelled. Human tissues commonly examined for their nutritional characteristics include hair (scalp or pubic), red blood cells, white blood cells, plasma or serum, whole blood, urine, and tissue scrapings from the oral mucosa. Nutritional elements of clinical significance are vitamins, minerals, amino acids, organic acids, and accessory nutrients. Note particularly that the ability to grow living cells in vitro permits a functional analysis for nutrients.

Although the overwhelming effect of appropriate laboratory data is positive, one must recognize that nutritional laboratory findings represent only one aspect of a person. Sometimes, laboratory results may need to be interpreted only as a minor character in the drama of health/illness that the patient presents. Sometimes, too, nutritional data can be misleading. When the serum potassium is high, for example, the blood may have been injured in the process of obtaining it from the patient. The resultant breaking apart of the red blood cells (hemolysis) releases potassium to the serum with a factitious result. If the patient truly has a low potassium and the report is abnormally high, a life-threatening condition could be missed. That is only one example of "false," artifactual, or erroneous results. Comprehensive understanding of the patient, the diet, medications, nutrient supplements, symptoms, and lifestyle are requisite to the proper interpretation of nutritional data.

The broad view of nourishment recognizes the nutritional totality provided by pure air, pure water, pure foods, and pure nutrient supplements, love, loving- and therapeutic-touch, judicious exercise, appropriate quality and quantity of REM-adequate sleep, pleasing music and artistic experiences, as well as positive thoughts, nontoxic family members, and friends and coworkers who operate in nontoxic environments. On a practical level, however, the remainder of this discussion shall focus on food, nutritional supplementation, and the gastrointestinal tract.

Food

Foods eaten must be free of contaminating infectious organisms and sufficient in amount to satisfy caloric needs. Fresh, whole foods are always desirable. A wide variety of foods should be eaten so that "the narrow diet" is never embraced unless recommended by a nutritional- or medical professional. A corollary of that is advice to rotate and diversify foods. When one eats according to seasonal patterns that tends to occur, but greater variety than that may be desirable. Usually a moderate intake of individual foods is preferred in quantity and frequency. Unless a specific diet has been prescribed, avoid the monotonous overuse of any individual foods. One shall wish to avoid foods that cannot truly be defined as food. Candy bars could possibly qualify as food, if all other foods are not available, but in ordinary circumstances, candy, sodas, chips, and the like must be considered as not belonging to the category of true food—the sustenance that builds our bodies and maintains them over decades. As a help, one may think of foods as God's foods and man's foods. With certain (but rare) exceptions, natural foods (a potato, for example) will always be preferable to manufactured foods (a potato chip, for example).

Whenever possible, foods should be eaten raw or semiraw. The tiny side salad may be better than none at all, but a plate full of vegetables and a large salad containing four or more vegetables is desirable. Noncarbohydrate vegetables are commonly the most supporting foods for health but the least represented in the diet. Asparagus, kale, broccoli, cabbage, romaine, and tomatoes represent this group. Carbohydrates are best obtained from potatoes, sweet potatoes, winter squash, corn, beans, peas, lentils, and beets. Proteins may be of animal or plant origin. D'Adamo (1996) has compiled a telling case for paying attention to the blood type as a guideline for the relative consumption of meats and carbohydrates. Whole grains or sprouted grains usually are desirable. They may be in the forms of cereals, breads, pastas, and crackers. Brown rice, barley, oats, and buckwheat are first-rate.

The swing away from high fat foods has given rise to an overreliance on grain-based carbohydrates that feeds yeast overgrowth and various bowel dysfunctions. Eating fruit rather than fruit juice complies with nature although the addictive "popping" of cans and bottle tops (usually sodas) has programmed many to expect and rely on liquid rather than the need-to-be chewed solid fruit. Seeds and nuts (and sometimes their butters and milks), when not salted and roasted, are useful foods to supply plant proteins. Sesame, pumpkin, and sunflower seeds enhance vegetables, soups, or cereals but may be eaten—in moderation—alone. Except for certain individuals (most blood-group O persons and certain ones who require meats, milk, or eggs for maintenance of nourishment), the consumption of animal products in most cases has been overdone. The relative ease of their use, their easy satiety effect, and their appealing taste (to many) has driven their overuse. If one contemplates reduction of chicken, turkey, beef, pork, milk, milk products, and eggs, one should do so slowly. Rapid change, unless necessitated by a medical emergency, should never be carried out. Legumes, the bevy of beans and lentils from the plant kingdom, are excellent protein foods that detoxify the body.

Fresh, whole, raw, or semiraw (steamed), organic, locally grown, and seasonal foods are those that place an individual in touch with his or her natural origins. They are the foods that counter disease and promote health. Our present culture assaults that concept for a variety of rea-

sons. Nevertheless, it is the basis of our defense against the toxins of a polluted planet.

Nutritional Supplements

Because the assumption of a desirable diet that runs counter to that of the mainstream culture may be difficult to attain and maintain, and because the best foods available may not possess a full quota of nutrients, and because the toxic, environmental assault upon us is so great, a wide variety of nutritional supplements is commonly needed. If that statement is doubted, one should obtain a blood test to determine lipid peroxides (the measurement of free-radical attack upon our tissues) as well as the total oxidative protection index (top, the measure of our "defensive shield" against oxidative attack). Experience suggests that such an individual shall hasten to alter the diet and/or to add antioxidant protection when his or her results are received. The testing of the individual's specific nutrient-needs can be carried out initially, or an informed judgment can be made by the patient (who has the knowledge of his or her body) and the nutritional physician (who has a body of knowledge) acting in consort as to the desirable number and strengths of supplements that should be used for the individual. Supplements are selected from vitamins, minerals, amino acids, herbs, accessory nutrients, and various food supplements in liquids, powders, or capsule/tablet forms. Phytogreens, for example, may include barley grass, wheat grass, alfalfa, chlorella, or spirulina. A wide variety of vegetable and fruit capsules or tablets is also available. The subject of nutritional supplementation could be covered best only in a series of volumes that has not yet been written.

Gastrointestinal Tract

With every decade of life after 30 or 40 years of age—and progressively more often in younger adults and children—the decay or degeneration of faulty function of the gut increases. The availability of measurements and bacteriological and parasitic assays of the nutritional and toxic components in the gut has shown us the extent of intestinal dysbiosis, "leaky" (hyperpermeable) gut, and colonization by unwanted bacteria and parasites with the elaboration of toxic enzymes and bacterial byproducts that may adversely impact any or all organs or tissues of the body. Why do we so often find an absence or marked reduction of the protective, nutritive friendly bacteria? Consider the frequent use (and overuse) of antibiotics. Consider the fact that the vast majority of animals eaten have antibiotic residues in the meat. Consider that chlorine kills bacteria, and chlorine in drinking water and bath water and most swimming pools has protected us but also affected us all for many years. Let us remember, too, that the friendly bacteria in our intestine are nutritional factories. They manufacture vitamin K, for example, but play a far greater role than that in the total integrity of bowel and body health. Those little bowel critters and the proper medium of gastrointestinal support for them provide the defensive shield against the host of aerobic and anerobic opportunistic pathogens that so earnestly move in to compromise our intestinal (and bodily) health over the passage of years. When one realizes the enormity of that truism, he or she then understands the reason why the best-selling drugs in "developed" countries are those for gastro-intestinal conditions.

RAY C. WUNDERLICH, JR

ORTHOMOLECULAR MEDICINE

Orthomolecular medicine is defined as the provision of the optimum molecular constitution, especially the optimum concentration of substances that are normally present in the body, for the purposes of treating disease and preserving health. The term was coined by Linus Pauling in his 1968 theoretical analysis of megavitamin therapy in psychiatry.

Megavitamin therapy is most closely identified with Abram Hoffer and Humphry Osmond, who in 1954 published the first double blind controlled study in psychiatry, on the treatment of schizophrenia with nicotinic acid and nicotinamide. However, substantial doses of vitamins as therapy for medical and psychiatric conditions had been reported in the 1940s, and even earlier.

In orthomolecular medicine, diseases are assumed to originate from multiple nonspecific causes, congenital and acquired. These causes give rise to biochemical aberrations, the accumulation of which results in symptoms and signs, from which the perception of a disease state follows. Clinically apparent diseases may be described as fuzzy sets of biochemical anomalies. Clearly, it is advantageous for physicians to recognize and to correct patients' small sets of biochemical anomalies at early stage, before expansion of the sets results in recognizable diseases.

In practice, the orthomolecular doctor relies heavily on laboratory testing. In addition to standard clinical chemistries, orthomolecular doctors now employ a wide range of sophisticated laboratory analyses, including those for amino acids, organic acids, vitamins and minerals, functional vitamin status, hormones, immunology, microbiology, and gastrointestinal function. It is to be expected that, as the Human Genome Project progresses, orthomolecular practitioners will increasingly utilize genetic probes to assess the hereditary components of disease.

The orthomolecular model of disease complements and extends the standard medical model, rather than replacing it. As Hoffer wrote (1989): "Nor is orthomolecular treatment a replacement for standard treatment. A proportion of patients will require orthodox treatment, a proportion will do much better on orthomolecular treatment, and the rest will need a skillful blend of both."

Orthomolecular therapy consists in providing optimal amounts of substances normal to the body, by oral or parenteral administration. In the early days of orthomolecular medicine, this usually meant high-dose, single-agent nutrient therapy. However, some ailments require the withholding of normal substances (e.g., the orthomolecular amount of phenylalanine for a phenylketonuric infant approaches zero). Thus, "optimal" is a matter for clinical judgment. Most often, the orthomolecular practitioner employs multiple vital substances—amino acids, enzymes, nonessential nutrients, hormones, vitamins, minerals, and so on—in a therapeutic effort to restore those (or derivative substances) to levels statistically normal for healthy young persons.

The power of the orthomolecular approach is illustrated by its broad relevance.

Hoffer in particular (1989) has outlined orthomolecular strategies for cardiovascular diseases, gastrointestinal disorders, arthritis, neurological diseases, metabolic stress, psychiatry, cancer, and dermatological disorders. Although a full understanding of the aging process remains elusive, orthomolecular medicine offers a rational way to address the multiple cellular and metabolic derangements associated with aging, especially those related to oxidative stress.

Orthomolecular medicine rests on the broad research base of the world's scientific literature in nutrition, metabolism, endocrinology, biochemical genetics, and cell biology. Some of the more clinically relevant literature has been abstracted by Werbach (1996). Clinical studies, reviews, letters, and editorials are published quarterly in *Journal of Orthomolecular Medicine*, edited by Hoffer.

RICHARD P. HUEMER

POLARITY THERAPY

Polarity therapy is a comprehensive health system incorporating bodywork, diet, exercise, and counselling. It is based on the concept of the human energy field, electromagnetic patterns that are expressed in mental, emotional, and physical experience. In polarity therapy, health conditions are viewed as reflection of the condition of the energy field, and therapies are designed to stimulate and balance the field for health benefit.

Polarity has strong links to other holistic health systems. For example, the term "polarity" refers to the universal pulsation of expansion/contraction or attraction/repulsion known as yin and yang in Oriental therapies.

History

Polarity therapy was developed by Randolph Stone (1890–1981), who published his findings in the late 1940s. He chose the word "polarity" to describe the basic nature of the electromagnetic force field of the body. He taught that polarized energy currents precede physical form and are primary factors in well-being. He found that the human energy field is affected by touch, diet, movement, sound, attitudes, relationship, and environmental factors. The scope of polarity practice is very broad, with implications for health professionals in many therapeutic disciplines.

In recent years, polarity has gained increased recognition, partially through the leadership of the American Polarity Therapy Association (APTA), the largest professional organization in the field. APTA has accomplished significant progress since 1987, with the creation of the standards for practice and code of ethics, consensus documents defining the scope and practice of polarity therapy. These documents are the basis for polarity therapy professional certification from APTA.

The Four Dimensions of Energy Anatomy

The caduceus is an ancient egyptian and greek picture of the human energy field. The parts of the symbol show four distinct but interdependent parts of the field. The globe at the top and staff in the center is the core of primary energy found in the craniosacral structures and functions. The intertwining snakes are the three principles of attraction, repulsion, and transitional stillness. The five intersections along the central core are the five elements. The wings represent consciousness, humanity's potential to transcend materialism and reunite with its source.

Polarity therapy asserts that these four underlie the totality of human experience, preceding and determining spirit, mind, feelings, and body. Understanding these four dimensions of the human energy field and their applications is the scope of polarity therapy.

In the polarity model, health is experienced when these systems are functioning normally. Energy flows smoothly without significant blockage or fixation on any level. Disease and pain occur when energy is blocked, fixed, or unbalanced. Blockages occur due to stress and trauma, generally crystallizing from the subtle to the gross levels of the field. Therapy is about finding the blockages, releasing energy to normal flow patterns, and maintaining the energy field in an open, flexible condition.

Bodywork

Polarity therapy is best known for its bodywork. The basic premise of polarity bodywork is that touch affects the human energy field. The body is like a bar magnet, with a positive pole at the top and negative pole at the bottom. Similarly, the hands have a charge, which tends to positive on the right and a negative on the left.

Placing the hands on the body affects energy flow, with one placement stimulating and the reverse placement sedating energy flow. By knowing the major flow patterns and key intersections of any of the four dimensions of the human energy field and by using appropriate hand placements, the practitioner can facilitate profound changes in the body-mind. The conscious intention of the practitioner also affects energy flow. So, instruction on conscious touch, mindfulness, boundaries, and related topics is an important part of polarity therapy training.

Healing is generally seen to come from within the client. The practitioner is a facilitator or helper, not an external curative force. Emphasis is placed on awareness and sensitivity rather than mechanical correction.

Bodywork techniques are based on specific considerations, locations, and therapeutic intentions. For primary energy, techniques center on the craniosacral system. The subtle movements and functions of the cranium, spine, and sacrum are studied. Focus is on the energetic potency and free movement of the cerebrospinal fluid (CSF), the conveyor of the most subtle and powerful energy essence in the body, known as the breath of life or ordering principle. The writings of Stone support and coincide with the teachings of pioneering cranial osteopath William Garner Sutherland in appreciating the significance of the breath of life within CSF.

Basic qualities of yin and yang are studied for the three principles, well described in traditional Ayurvedic and Oriental medical systems. All tissues and functions and all microcosmic and macrocosmic relationships can be understood in terms of charged energy, categorized in polarity as positive, negative, and neutral. These three are in constant dynamic tension with one another, creating the basis for physical manifestation. In physics, this is most clearly seen in the structure of the atom, with proton (positive), electron (negative), and neutron (neutral) in constantly self-adjusting interrelationships with one another. In polarity bodywork, understanding of the three principles is applied in terms of energetic assessment, location and quality of touch, balancing of the nervous systems, and in numerous other ways.

The five elements relate to five stages of density in the form and function of the body. The five elements are also known as five *chakras* (from Sanskrit, meaning "wheel of energy"). From gross to subtle, the five elements are earth (solids), water (liquids), fire (heat), air (gases), and ether (space that contains all others). These functions are associated with specific body areas and specific types of emotional and/or physical problems.

Consciousness is affected by techniques for releasing old trauma and establishing new blueprint-level attitudes and expectations about self and others. Polarity therapy involves both cognitive (becoming more aware of factors affecting consciousness) and noncognitive methods (when energy is released, new behaviors arise spontaneously, without conscious activity).

Other Polarity Techniques

Polarity incorporates diet, exercise, and other dimensions of healing. A vegetarian diet with no meat, fish, fowl, or eggs is recommended, along with a cleansing diet consisting primarily of fresh and cooked vegetables and herbal cleansing practices and formulas.

Stone developed easy stretching posture, or polarity yoga, based on Hatha yoga and the Oriental martial arts. Stone's writing contain wide-ranging references to the full spectrum of human experience, particularly spiritual development.

JOHN CHITTY

PREGNANCY MASSAGE

There are few quantitative data available dealing with massage and any aspect of pregnancy. Studies by Dundee and colleagues (1988) and Hyde (1989) examined acupressure therapy for the reduction of morning sickness of pregnancy. These two studies resulted in the widespread use of acupressure bands for the relief of nausea associated with pregnancy. Kennell and Klaus (1991) initially looked at emotional and social support for women in labor by lay female birth companions at the Social Security Hospital in Guatemala City, Guatemala. The study was repeated at Jefferson Davis Hospital in Houston, Texas. Touch was an important part of the support offered. The simple interventions of these laywomen resulted in shortened labors by several hours. Complications were reduced and the cesarean section rate was decreased. Women's satisfaction relating to the labor experience was greatly enhanced. This work underlies the beginning of today's popular "doula" programs for labor support.

A study by Bette Waters (1995) looked at using ice massage for the control of labor pain. Fields of The Touch Institute at the University of Miami is presently conducting a long-term study looking at the pregnancies and outcomes of pregnant teens who receive regular massage. Some schools of massage in the United States provide information about pregnancy within their curricula. However, this is not widespread, nor is it a part of mandated massage education for licensing.

Massage therapists in private practice teach prenatal massage classes for currently licensed therapists. Courses usually are several days in length and offer either continuing education or some type of certification. There is no state or national certification for prenatal massage specialty. There is a national organization of massage therapists and others interested in pregnancy massage, the National Association of Pregnancy Massage Therapists (NAPMT). The NAPMT publishes a quarterly newsletter and sends membership directories to its members.

Benefits of Prenatal Massage

Our medical system has determined that stress is a major cause of premature birth. The major cause of infant death in the United States is premature birth. Thus, the pregnant woman has more of a need for regular massage because of the known association between increased stress and premature labor.

Stress reduction benefits of massage include increased production of brain endorphins that can last as long as 3 days. Children with chronic asthma show improved lung function and lower levels of the stress hormone cortisol with a 20-minute massage each night.

Tactile stimulation in babies is critical to life. The diagnosis of infants "failure to thrive" is in the medical texts. Infants who receive food, have a clean environment, and are free from disease will waste away and die without human holding, cuddling, and touch. Premature babies who receive several daily massages of 15 minutes show a significant increase in weight gain and neurological development over preemies without massage.

Other benefits of massage of the pregnant woman include reduction of pain and discomfort by releasing stored tension, increased circulation, bringing nutrients to the cells, and helping to flush out metabolic wastes. Therapeutic touch in a safe setting provides the pregnant woman with the important experience of being nurtured.

Contraindications for Pregnancy Massage

Deep venous thrombosis (DVT) in the lower extremity is an absolute contraindication for massage of pregnant women. Up until the 1950s, DVT of the lower extremity was seen mostly in women in the postpartum period. Early ambulating and avoiding bedrest, even in women delivered by cesarean, has resulted in a dramatic decrease of the problem, so much so that now the incidence of DVT is greater in the prenatal period, 1 to 2 in 1,000 pregnancies.

Women who have used oral contraceptives (birth control pills) before becoming pregnant are at greater risk for DVT during pregnancy. This risk group also includes women who work at jobs requiring sitting for long periods of time.

The symptoms of DVT are an abrupt onset of severe pain and edema, heat, and redness of the leg and thigh. Usually, this condition involves most of the deep venous system from the foot to the iliofemoral region.

Massage, especially deep massage, in a client with any degree of DVT can serve to dislodge small blood clots that can travel to the lungs or brain, becoming a life-threatening event.

Massage of the breasts of the pregnant woman is contraindicated. It is well documented in the scientific literature that nipple stimulation causes extended contractions lasting several minutes. These type of contractions do not routinely cause the cervix to begin to open, but long extended periods of the uterus squeezing on the baby can decrease circulation of blood to the baby, decreasing oxygen and food nutrients, resulting in stress.

Clinical Application of Massage in Pregnancy

The anatomical and physiological changes associated with pregnancy are major. However, the traditional massage techniques practiced by massage therapists are safe used on the normal healthy pregnant woman. The most critical clinical element associated with pregnancy massage is the correct body alignment on the massage table.

Traditionally, the supine and prone positions are used for performing massage. The supine position is contraindicated after the woman is 3 months pregnant in order to avoid supine hypotensive syndrome. In the supine position, the enlarged pregnant uterus compresses the venous system that returns blood to the heart from the lower half of the body. Cardiac filling from blood returned via the vena cava slows and causes decreased cardiac output which stress the fetus. Supine hypotensive syndrome also greatly increases blood pressure in the femoral venous system causing severe varicose veins in the pelvis and lower extremities.

The pregnant woman may experience this event as dizziness while lying on her back. Whether she experiences dizziness or not, the event still occurs.

As the pregnant woman's abdomen increases in size and rises from the pelvis to become an abdominal organ, she will find it impossible to lie in the prone position. Table positions such as semisitting or right side and left side lying are the positions of choice. These modifications can be easily accomplished with the use of pillows.

BETTE WATERS

PRENATAL REGRESSION

Since the 1960s, prenatal regression has been used in traditional therapy by practitioners considered alternative. The 1990s have seen an increased use of this process within the mainstream therapeutic community. Originally seen as a religious concept, past-life experiences are now thought to hold keys to current-life issues. Whether or not there are, in fact, past-life experiences and therefore past-life memories cannot be proven; these experiences may simply be metaphors of the mind that the client has created to frame current issues that are now blocking health and well-being.

The theory behind prenatal regression is that each person incarnates into this lifetime carrying memories of unresolved issues from prior experiences. These memories can affect the current life in many ways (i.e., a person may hold pain from old wounds, accidents, and illnesses). In this life, these prior conditions may manifest in pain that medical examination and testing cannot account for. A prenatal regression may reveal a bullet wound in this area. Psychologically, fears and relationship issues may exist (e.g., a person may experience tremendous fear of water that might be psychological residue from a previous lifetime drowning). Relationship issues can be carryovers; these can include repeating the same patterns relationship after relationship. Regression might reveal the same pattern being unresolved in a past lifetime.

Uses for Prenatal Regression

The main purpose for prenatal regression is to assist the client in releasing or reframing old issues that are impeding his or her well-being. Addressing current issues through the modality of prenatal regression allows the client a framework and safe distance to examine issues that may be repressed. A prenatal regression session contains four parts:

1. The client is asked about his or her belief system regarding past lives. If the belief in past lives is inconsistent with the client's belief system, an explanation of metaphors of the mind is given.
2. An explanation of the process is then given to the client, and the client is asked if he or she has any questions or concerns. Questions are answered and concerns addressed before proceeding.
3. Prenatal regression occurs through hypnosis or deep relaxation and should be done only by a qualified hypnotist. The client is asked to get comfortable, and the induction begins. The client is told that these memories are there and accessible. The client is told that once back in the past life, he or she will be asked to answer questions, and the more he or she responds, the more vivid the images or information become.

4. It is further explained that not everyone visualizes to let go of preconceived expectations and to allow the experience. The client is told that rationalizing will bring him or her out of the hypnotic state and rationalizing can be done after the regression. The client is instructed to follow the process describing aloud, whatever he or she is experiencing. The regressionist uses the images the client is describing, being very careful not to ask leading questions.

Again, the purpose of a regression session is moving the client from a state of ill health and concern with his or her issue through releasing the past. This occurs through the reframing process. Each practitioner chooses his or her reframing process based upon the client's needs. The session concludes with dialogue between the client and the regressionist. Whether in fact past lives exist, prenatal regression, done by a skilled regressionist, is a valid process for reframing and releasing issues that are concern to the client.

KATE LEVENSOHN

PROGRESSIVE MUSCLE RELAXATION TRAINING

Progressive muscle relaxation (PMR) training is a simple, straightforward, and effective form of treatment for helping people learn how to relax. It can be used effectively with almost anyone—either as a primary treatment modality or as an adjunct to other medical or psychological interventions. PMR, also known as deep muscle relaxation, was originated by Edmund Jacobson in 1929. Jacobson, a Chicago physician, discovered that by using a prescribed system of tensing and releasing muscles, one could reach deeper levels of relaxation than could be reached by simply sitting still and trying to relax. He developed his system, progressive relaxation, to give people a specific, systematized way to relax the muscles of their body.

Jacobson's work was based on the theory that (1) the body responds to anxiety-provoking thoughts and events by producing muscle tension, as well as other autonomic nervous system responses (this reaction is also known as the "fight or flight response"); (2) this physiological tension, in turn, increases the subjective experience of anxiety; and (3) deep muscle relaxation decreases physiological tension, thereby reducing the subjective experience of anxiety. Jacobson believed that deep muscle relaxation was incompatible with anxiety and was thus effective in interrupting the anxiety cycle.

Jacobson found that by giving patients a straightforward, systematic program for relaxing their muscles completely, they made impressive gains in restoring their health, physically and mentally. He believed that tense muscles made tense minds and that mental relaxation naturally follows physical relaxation. His research, which measured the effectiveness of his progressive relaxation method by measuring the amount of electrical activity in muscle fibers, was conclusive, demonstrating that the method indeed produced profound muscle relaxation.

Over the years, there has been much refinement of Jacobson's method. Instead of the 200 exercises that Jacobson included in his original method, more recent PMR techniques have narrowed this to 15 to 20 exercises, with no loss of clinical effectiveness.

As stated previously, PMR is a systematic program for training people to relax muscles completely. PMR gives patients a simple, straightforward way to relax their bodies (and their minds) deeply and completely. It provides a way to identify particular muscles and muscle groups and to distinguish between sensations of tension and relaxation. Simply stated, PMR helps people increase their awareness of their muscles and their body and thus helps them learn when they are tense. By being able to notice the difference between tension and relaxation, they can then more easily learn how to relax their muscles at will.

In PMR training, people are taught to tense and then release the muscles (or muscle groups) in their bodies. This method is used because research and clinical evidence has shown that after tensing, a muscle will automatically relax more deeply when released. Additionally, it has been found that increased relaxation results from patients' noticing the difference in their muscles between tension and relaxation. Evidence also points to the fact that patients cannot have a feeling of warm well-being in their body and at the same time experience psychological stress. Therefore, teaching patients to produce the deeply relaxed state characteristic of PMR will help them to reduce tension in their bodies and in their minds.

The benefits of PMR are many. PMR relaxes muscles, reduces pulse rate, reduces blood pressure, decreases perspiration, and decreases respiration rate. It has been shown to have excellent results in the treatment of tension headaches, backaches, tightness in the jaw or around the eyes, muscle spasms, high blood pressure, insomnia, and racing thoughts. Additionally, PMR is effective in treating fatigue, irritable bowel syndrome, neck and back pain, stuttering, mild phobias (e.g., fear of flying), fear of public speaking, performance anxiety, test anxiety, athletic performance anxiety, sleep disturbances, anxiety, and depression. PMR also has all the clinical benefits of the relaxation response described by Benson (1975): decreased generalized anxiety; decreased anticipatory anxiety related to phobias; decreased frequency and duration of panic attacks; increased concentration; increased sense of control over moods; increased self esteem; and increased spontaneity and creativity.

People can learn PMR by following a written outline/script, listening to a prerecorded tape, or having someone guide them through the exercises. Initially, it is usually best to have the patient listen to a tape or have someone guide them.

PMR is done by tensing and releasing, in succession, the 15 to 20 different muscle groups of the body. The patient is instructed to tense hard, but not strain, each muscle group for 7 to 10 seconds. While doing this, they might also be instructed to visualize in their mind the muscle group they are tensing. After holding this tension for 7 to 10 seconds the person is instructed to "let go" (i.e., release the tension) abruptly or suddenly and to relax the muscle group for 15 to 20 seconds—letting the muscles go completely limp. While doing this tensing and relaxing, they are also instructed to notice very carefully the feelings of tension and relaxation in the muscles, especially noting the contrast. They may also be instructed to repeat a phrase (such as, "I am relaxing") silently each time they release the tension in a muscle. This tensing/releasing procedure is used in sequence on the 15 to 20 muscle groups of the body. The tensing/relaxing is usually done once with each muscle group but may be repeated two or three times when working with particularly troublesome (tense) areas (e.g., neck and shoulders). Subjects are encouraged to maintain a focus on their muscles and told that if their attention wanders they are simply to bring their attention back to the muscle group.

PMR can be done lying down or in a chair with the head supported. At the beginning of a session, patients are instructed to close their eyes, take several deep breaths, and to begin to relax. They then proceed through the 15 to 20 muscle groups using the tense/relax procedure. It is recommended to do PMR in a quiet location, especially at first, and not to do it right after having eaten. Digestion of food can interfere with one's ability to relax.

PMR should be practiced 20 to 30 minutes per day, and practicing once per day is mandatory to obtain maximum benefit. Once the procedure is well learned, daily practice time can be reduced to 15 to 20 minutes. With practice, people can relax muscle groups more quickly and easily, thus resulting in less practice time. Practicing every day increases the generalization effect of PMR (i.e., that the relaxed feeling experienced during practice will carry over to the rest of the day). Also, with practice, people are able to relax, at least partially, at only a moment's notice. For example, using what is referred to as "creative cuing," people can learn to do PMR while waiting at a stoplight, or while waiting for the elevator. Such cue-controlled relaxation is very effective in reducing tension.

When doing PMR, people are instructed to adopt a passive, detached attitude. What this means is that during their practice time they are to simply do the exercise, without worrying about how well they are doing, how much they are relaxing, or whether they are doing it correctly. They are instructed to simply "let go" and follow instructions. Developing this attitude is very important in the practice and in their lives.

PMR can usually be learned in 1 to 3 weeks if practice is done as recommended. There are no contraindications except where muscles to be tensed and relaxed have been injured. Cramping in feet is also common, especially at first. Care should be exercised in these cases. If someone is on tranquilizer-type medication, PMR may enable a decrease in dosage.

MICHAEL C. MURPHY

PSYCHONEUROIMMUNOLOGY

Physiological and psychosocial theories related to health and disease leave many questions unanswered. Why do people who are exposed to the same stressors or pathogens react differently? What environmental or disease patterns influence individual disease development? How does negativity, stress, and coping contribute to the development and progression of physical illness? Can complementary therapies contribute to decreasing the progression of the disease process? Research in psychoneuroimmunology can provide the answers to these questions.

Ader and Cohen (1981) coined the term "psychoneuroimmunology" (PNI) to describe the interactions between the nervous system and the immune system and the subsequent effects of these interactions upon disease development and progression.

PNI is a rapidly evolving science concerned with the interactions between the central nervous system, neuroendocrine, and the immune systems in response to factors such as feelings, behavior, and other psychosocial influences that may mediate these interactions. The link of behavior to the immune system activity and therefore to health and disease is the concern of psychoneuroimmunology.

PNI goes beyond Cartesian dualism, in which the psychological, neuroendocrine, and immune systems are considered separate entities (Caudell, 1996). PNI developed because research findings contradicted the immune system as an autonomous self-regulating system, which considered the immune processes and part of the organism's psychobiological adaptation to its environment (Ader, 1987; Solomon, 1985).

PNI is concerned with the central nervous system, endocrine system, and immune system interaction, which can further be subdivided by examining the effects of personality, stress, emotions, and coping on infections and cancer, other resistive diseases, and allergic and autoimmune disease (Solomon, 1987). PNI operates with the similar premise of the indivisibility of the mind and body, such as psychosomatic medicine or psychophysiology. It is different, however, in that PNI emphasizes the hypothesis that the immune system can serve to mediate the effects of psychosocial factors on pathophysiological states, and the understanding of these relationships has important clinical implications (Ader, 1987).

PNI as an emerging paradigm, or framework, originated by the development of a multifactorial model developed by Engel (1962), which included stress, coping, and disease formation. This was further enhanced by Solomon and Moos (1964) and Solomon (1985, 1987) to include stress on the immune system in disease formation. PNI has been described as an excellent paradigm to examine the stress response, where physiologically the stress response causes an activation of the neuroendocrine system, which leads to increased cortisol production and suppression of the immune system (Munck & Guyre, 1991).

The psychoneuroimmune network is the complex network of cells that communicate with one another by the release and uptake of a myriad of antibodies, mediators called cytokines, and other molecules (Balkwill & Burke, 1989). The neuroendocrine system is the link between the CNS and the immune system (Camera & Danao, 1989). Neurons and lymphocytes share most of the properties of the parenchymal cell targets of hormones (receptors, coupling mechanism in cell membranes), identical second messengers, and identical systems for the activation or inhibition of the genome. The immune system is an intricate part of a complex neuroimmune network and the challenge is to discover how the network affects of health and disease.

PNI theory acknowledges the relationship between psychological being, wellness, and illness. A clear link between the psyche and immunological changes has yet to be demonstrated, although the emerging field of PNI is providing scientific evidence to support the mind-body connection. Current links between psychosocial factors and behavior such as anxiety, chronic hostility, depression, loss of loved ones, and coping and the immune system are being explored in research (Kiecolt-Glaser & Glaser, 1988; Fawsey et al., 1990; Irwin, Daniels, Bloom, Smith, & Weiner,

1987). This research is examining these behaviors and stressors on specific aspects of the immune system such as T-lymphocytes and natural killer cells. PNI provides a holistic and an interdisciplinary approach to examine the pathophysiological processes involved in disease and provides an opportunity to examine behavioral interventions that can used to influence ones' health and reaction to disease.

Research related to PNI has centered on three broad areas: (1) behavioral studies; (2) studies on the anatomical connections between the nervous, endocrine, and immune systems; and (3) studies on the physiological and biochemical mechanisms that mediate this communication (Institute of Medicine, 1989). In the past 15 years, researchers in PNI have examined the effects of stress on the immune system in animals and humans. In addition, they have begun to examine the effects of behavioral interventions on immune function and concepts related to stress, quality of life, mood states, and depression. Behavioral interventions including relaxation, guided imagery, and support groups improve the immune response (Fawzy et al., 1990; Fawzy & Fawzy, 1994; Spiegel et al., 1989). Although some studies show that behavioral interventions are not universally effective, they are well received by most patients, are cost-effective, and cause no adverse events (Redd, 1994).

Redefining concepts and beliefs related to the immune system and disease could expand our knowledge of the psychoneuroimmune network. Rather than looking at the immune system as a defense system that protects the body from conquering invaders, Booth (1990) suggests that the immune systems could be viewed as an extension of the brain, supporting the body's relationship to the environment, with the immune system acting as a molecular sense organ.

This conceptual analysis can affect the way we see disease. Through this new model, disease would no longer be seen as an unnatural state that had to be conquered; it would be considered a source of the dynamic process of existence, providing an opportunity for transformation, adaptation, and evolution (Booth, 1990). In this model, disease is promoted by disconnection, and health is promoted through the optimal connectiveness or coherence of persons with their environment. The theory of PNI and the psychoneuroimmune network can be useful to guide research and practice in the use of complementary or alternative therapies.

CECILE A. LENGACHER

PSYCHONEUROIMMUNOLOGY RESEARCH

Research on the enhancement and stabilization of the immune system during stressful life events is important to demonstrate in the new field of psychoneuroimmunology (PNI). Many research studies have been conducted on the effects of stress on the suppression of the immune system, but relatively few have focused on how to enhance the immune system. This study describes an accurate and precise procedure to measure the lymphocytes in the immune response and suggests that hypnosis may be an effective technique to stabilize the immune system during stressful life events.

Research Methods

Twenty-eight subjects were included in the study, 22 females and six males. Both the experimental group and the wait list control group had 11 females and three males. The average age of the subjects in the wait list control group was 31.43, with a range of 22 to 49. The average age of the experimental subjects was 33.07, with a range of 23 to 50.

Subjects were randomly assigned to one of two groups: an experimental group that received self-hypnosis training, and a wait list control group. Each group had blood samples drawn for determination of total lymphocyte number, total T-cell levels, helper T-cell levels, suppressor T-cell levels, natural killer T-cell levels, and B-cell levels. The blood samples were drawn 3 weeks apart for both groups and assessed using six monoclonal antibodies that detect antigens on human lymphocytes. The monoclonal antibody test for lymphocytes contains a monoclonal antibody linked to a fluorescent dye. This conjugate specifically binds to lymphocytes, which can be detected when the dye is excited by light from a fluorescence-activated cell sorter (FACS). The FACS analysis involves hitting a thin stream of the cell suspension with a laser beam and then utilizing light detectors to collect the scattered light. Fluorescently labeled cells can be quantified accurately by this method of analysis.

Four individual self-hypnosis training sessions were conducted for each experimental subject over a 3-week period. The sessions covered: (1) the definition, misconceptions, and applications of self-hypnosis; (2) self-hypnosis training; (3) research findings in immunology; (4) biochemical details of the immune response; and (5) direct and indirect suggestions for increased self-confidence and improved immune response.

Results and Discussion

The results of this study suggest that self-hypnosis training may alter immune system functioning. Control subjects experienced a significant decline in their total T-lymphocyte levels. These subjects also experienced a significant drop in their T-helper cells. These results are consistent with the literature reports that psychosocial factors that stress an individual's adaptive capacity are associated with alterations of specific immune functions that tend to suppress the immune system. The research by Kiecolt-Glaser and coworkers showed that medical students had significantly lower percentages of helper T-lymphocytes during stressful exam periods and a significant decline in natural T-killer cell activity.

The experimental subjects who received the self-hypnosis training did not experience a significant decline in their mean level of total T-lymphocytes. Also, the subjects who received the self-hypnosis training did not have a significant decrease in their T-helper cells. This demonstrates that the self-hypnosis training prevented the significant decline in the immune system that graduate students typically experience. The students who received self-hypnosis training were significantly different from the control group in the change in level of total T-lymphocytes, helper T-cells, total number of lymphocytes, natural killer T-cells, and suppressor T-lymphocytes. This suggests that psychological intervention in the form of self-hypnosis may prevent the significant decline in the level of immune cells in graduate students as they progress into the semester.

The belief that psychological states and life circumstances have an effect on the health of an individual has been a repeated theme in medical theory. However, experimental attempts to study the impact of such effects on health did not occur until the recent beginning of the PNI field. Research has consistently found decreased immune function in patients experiencing severe depression and in individuals who experience stressful life events. However, relatively few have been able to demonstrate biochemically a stabilization or enhancement in the immune system. This control study describes a state of the art procedure to measure the lymphocytes in the immune response and suggests that hypnosis may be an effective technique to stabilize the immune system during stressful life events.

BEREE R. DARBY

QI GONG

Qi Gong, or *Qigong* (pronounced "chee-gong"), is the cultivation of *qi*. *Qi*, or *chi*, is the term used in Chinese medicine to denote the body's vital energy. *Qi Gong* dates back thousands of years. The modern practice of ritual breathing, exercise, and meditation flows from Buddhist, Taoist, and Confucian philosophies.

The practice can take many forms, from fairly vigorous exercises or spontaneous movement to slow, flowing movements, and still, standing postures. There are standing, sitting, lying, and walking postures. The difference between Qi Gong and aerobic exercise is the attention paid to *qi*. The aim is to open the body, clear the channels, and allow the *qi* to flow smoothly, while strengthening the body's ability to build and conserve energy. Some Qi Gong masters claim to emit external *qi*, and transmit energy from themselves to another person for healing purposes.

Qi Gong is a way of life, to be practiced daily. It is believed to boost circulation and enhance overall wellness. Although it is used for specific ailments ranging from allergies to asthma, diabetes, liver disorders, high blood pressure, and even cancer, it is most properly a wellness maintenance procedure.

CAROLYN CHAMBERS CLARK

QUANTUM MEDICINE AND MICROWAVE RESONANCE THERAPY

Sergei Sitko, Ph.D., is Merit Scientist of the Ukraine, a nuclear physicist who has received recognition from Belgium and from an international panel of scientists, include a Nobel laureate physicist. In 1982, Dr. Sitko began his investigations of quantum medicine, the quantum physics of the living system, and microwave resonance therapy, introduced 12 years earlier and used to treat 200,000 patients.

With a staff of 200, including many university physicists and medical specialists, Sitko developed the principles of quantum medicine's five major principles:

1. The electromagnetic frame of the human body, which consists of quantum fluxes in the microwave field from cells and organs. These resonances range from 52 to 78 GHz.
2. The resonance frequencies flow in channels from internal organs to the tips of fingers and toes and are reflected from bone to skin back to the organs, producing vectorgrams of microwave energy. At a quantum level, it may be similar to cardiac body mapping.

3. The reflective skin points, in disease, become tender and may show impedance and other electrical characteristic changes.
4. In various diseases, the amplitude of the intrinsic (eigen) frequencies is interrupted.
5. Application of a deficient frequency at very low levels of power is capable of restoring the amplitude and assisting the body in restoring homeostasis.

The fifth principle is a derivative of quantum synergetic theory: the susceptibility of a system to external influences approaches infinity at the phase transition point.

The most basic research has been done in cultures of *E. coli*, where it has been demonstrated that DNA compacting occurs at microwave power intensities only 10^{-1} levels above background or at 10^{-11} watts/cm^2. This affects growth but is reversible and at all power levels up to 100 microwatts/cm^2 microwave resonance therapy (MRT) is capable of causing damage.

As a quantum principle, the resonance effect has no intensity threshold, so that a nanowatt may be as effective as a microwatt.

MRT has been used clinically with 200,000 patients with extensive laboratory documentation of clinical improvement in a variety of patients. The greatest effect of MRT appears to be improvement in immune function as well as in pain. After the Chernobyl nuclear incident, only 60 miles from Kiev, many immunological defects have been seen. Numerous clinical studies have been done at the Ukraine Endocrinology Institute (120 endocrinologists), the Orthopedic Institute, and the Cardiology

Institute (400 cardiologists), as well as at other hospitals.

Published articles, some in peer-reviewed international journals in English, German, or Spanish, were provided to Americans. A number of patients were observed during various stages of MRT therapy (usually in courses of 10 days, 20 to 30 minutes per day). Some current laboratory studies, with personal microscopy observations, confirmed the reports of enzymatic improvement.

Pain improvement in peptic ulcers, rheumatoid and osteoarthritis, and phantom limb were particularly prominent. The American team was encouraged to participate in the treatment. An engineer verified the electronic competency and validity of the equipment, as specified. It appears that MRT, beginning now to be tested at 17 centers in the U.S., offers significant potential for pain management.

C. NORMAN SHEALY

REFLEXOLOGY

Reflexology is a science that deals with the principle that there are reflex areas in the feet and hands that correspond to all of the glands, organs, and parts of the body (see Figure 1). Reflexology is a unique method of using the thumb and fingers to apply specific pressures to these reflex points. Foot and hand reflexology includes, but is not limited to, (1) relieving stress and tension; (2) improving blood supply and promoting the unblocking of nerve impulses; and (3) helping nature achieve homeostasis.

As a reflexologist works each reflex, it triggers a release of stress and tension in

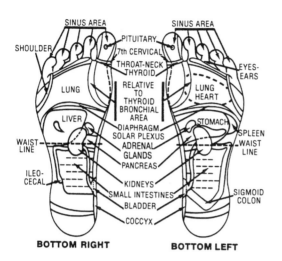

SINUS AREA   SINUS AREA

SHOULDER   PITUITARY
            7th CERVICAL
            THROAT-NECK   EYES-
            THYROID   EARS
    LUNG   RELATIVE   LUNG
            TO   HEART
            THYROID
            BRONCHIAL
    LIVER   AREA   STOMACH
            DIAPHRAGM
WAIST   SOLAR PLEXUS   SPLEEN
LINE   ADRENAL   WAIST
            GLANDS   LINE
            PANCREAS
ILEO-
CECAL   KIDNEYS
            SMALL INTESTINES   SIGMOID
            BLADDER   COLON
            COCCYX

BOTTOM RIGHT   BOTTOM LEFT

FIGURE 1   Reflex areas of the feet. Copyright © 1980 International Institute of Reflexology.

the corresponding area or body zone, as well as an overall relaxation response. The release of tension unblocks nerve impulses and improves the blood supply to all parts of the body. Because reflexology works from the inside, it also has a balancing effect on each gland, organ, and body region. Clients typically express relief from tension and pain along with a greater feeling of well-being and increased energy. Exactly how this works is still under debate. Ray Wunderlich, Jr. offers one explanation: "The fact that there are 7,200 nerve endings in each foot may explain why we feel so much better when our feet are treated. Nerve endings in the feet have extensive interconnections through the spinal cord and brain with all areas of the body. The feet are the ideal site from which to release tension and enhance health." A strong advocate of reflexology, Wunderlich suggested that "therapists who are certified in reflexology provide a practical

method of whole body therapy which results in greater returns for clients and therapists alike."

Differences Between Reflexology and Massage

While both massage and reflexology involve the use of the hands to administer treatment, they have fundamental differences. Massage is the systematic and scientific manipulation of the soft tissues of the body. Reflexology is the application of specific pressures to reflex points in the feet and hands. Massage treatments benefit the muscles or connective tissue, which are the direct recipients of the manipulation, while reflexology benefits the contact treatment sites (feet or hands) only incidentally. The primary benefits of reflexology result from the generalized relaxation of the entire body as well as from the balancing effect it has on specific organs, glands, zones, or body regions.

Origins of Reflexology

We know some form of reflexology was practiced by ancient Egyptians, judging by inscriptions and drawings found in a physician's tomb dating back to 2300 B.C. Eunice Ingham stated in her books (1938, 1951) that the credits for the origin of reflexology in Europe and the United States must go to Dr. William H. Fitzgerald (1917), who discovered the Chinese method of zone therapy, which we know today as reflexology. Additionally, pioneering efforts of Joe S. Riley and his wife in the field of zone therapy were instrumental in introducing Ingham to this alternative health care modality. She attributed her knowledge and the inception of the original Ingham method as a direct result of the knowledge of zone therapy imparted to her by Dr. Riley and his wife.

As an early proponent of what was to become reflexology, Fitzgerald—an eye, ear, nose, and throat specialist—wrote the book *Zone Therapy* (1917) and used a form of reflexology to anesthetize areas of the body before surgery. Fitzgerald's discovery of the Chinese method of zone therapy opened up the path for further development of this discovery of 10 zones of the body and the location of each particular organ in the body corresponding to one or more of these zones. Fitzgerald recognized Riley for the use of his zone markings chart to inform the world of their collaborative findings.

Reflexology in its current form was researched and developed by Eunice Ingham in *Stories the Feet Can Tell* (1938). That book was followed by the sequel, *Stories the Feet Have Told* (1951). From the early 1930s until shortly before her death in 1974, Ingham traveled around the country practicing and teaching her original Ingham method of reflexology to individuals, groups, and medical schools. She is considered throughout the world as the pioneer and developer of reflexology as it is known today and was succeeded by her nephew, Dwight Byers, who carries on her work today teaching throughout the world. *Better Health with Foot Reflexology* (Byers, 1983) has been published in nine languages. This book is a practical guide which includes the introduction to every anatomical system of the body and a step-by-step guide in applying the tenets of reflexology. Every section is fully illustrated to assist in the practical application of techniques.

The stated opinions among reflexologists, alternative healers in other modalities, and physicians who have experienced and now endorse reflexology is that the study of reflexology enhances one's understanding of the workings of the body, and its practice enhances the health of those who receive it. Andrew Weil and Julian Whitaker have used reflexology as an integral part of their treatment and recommend it as an alternative healthcare treatment.

Stress reduction and treating the mind and the body as a single entity can have a significant impact on the prevention and management of disease. There is growing evidence that emotions can influence resistance and immunity to infection, even to cancer. There have been several studies documenting the fact that positive approaches and outlooks by both doctor and patient can have a beneficial effect on a variety of disorders.

DWIGHT C. BYERS

REFLEXOLOGY: RESEARCH AND USES

Reflexology is the physical act of applying pressure techniques to the feet and hands in an orderly pattern. While simple in concept, reflexology has garnered supporters throughout history and around the world today. Artifacts of past work on the feet reflect health systems created in ancient Egypt, India, China, and Japan (Kunz & Kunz, 1993). Reflexology professional associations in 35 countries reflect the interest today (www.reflexology.org).

Reflexologists and several government agencies in Denmark cooperated with consumers to study and find positive effects of reflexology work on headaches. When reflexology services were provided to workers, one Danish company found that the workers missed fewer days due to illness and saved the company $30,000 a year (Eriksen, 1995).

Research has given a clue to the exact nature of what happens when reflexology technique is applied. Kunz and Kunz (1987) found that reflexology work applied to paralysis by spinal cord injury produced specific results. Limbs moved in as if taking a step and internal organs responded with growling or perspiration. They theorized that it resulted from communication between the extremities of the body and internal organs, through a process called autonomic-somatic integration. One recent Chinese study (Liang, 1996) found reflexology to 93.63% effective in an analysis of 8,096 clinical cases. The study found reflexology to be significantly effective in 50% of the cases for 26 diseases. Chinese theories vary but all revolve around an idea of stimulus-response, applying pressure in a particular pattern and obtaining a particular response.

Uses of Reflexology

Pressure technique is applied to specific areas to achieve a specific effect and the overall hand or foot to achieve an overall effect such as relaxation. Different methods for applying pressure have been developed. Practitioner techniques are applied by hand, using the flats of the fingers and inner edge of the thumbs. The advantage of practitioner-applied technique as opposed to self-applied technique is that a skilled practitioner can target stressed areas and create an enhanced sense of relaxation. The advantage of self-help techniques is

that pressure techniques can be applied frequently almost anytime and anywhere. Self-help techniques include applying pressure by self-applied hand techniques and tools. Tools include a golf ball for rolling or a smooth rock for standing.

When considering how long and how frequently to apply reflexology techniques, think in terms of any exercise program. Frequency, duration, and focus play a role in getting results. A successful self-help program includes application of technique for 5 minutes, 4 times a day. After 2 weeks, evaluate the results. To improve results, apply the technique more frequently or consider applying pressure to further reflex areas.

When seeking a reflexology service provider, ask questions. Look for an individual who has completed a course of study in reflexology and who has experience as a reflexology practitioner. Try a brief session. Evaluate the reflexologist's technique application for comfort level. Consider the level of relaxation after the session. After work on one foot, ask permission to get up and move around. Consider how the one foot feels as opposed to the other.

Use of reflexology techniques for health benefits has expanded beyond individual's efforts and will continue to grow. Workers at a Shiseido cosmetics factory in Japan, for example, voted to install a reflexology walking path for health improvement rather than a typical gym.

KEVIN AND BARBARA KUNZ

REIKI

Reiki is a form of touch therapy or healing that began in Tibet and spread to India, China, Japan, and the United States. Reiki, or "universal life force energy," is derived from *ki*, the Japanese word for "energy." The term is similar to the Chinese *qi* or *chi*, the Indian *prana*, the Hawaiian *mana*, and the Native American *orenda*.

Reiki is a way of applying the life force energy to relieve pain and speed the healing process, as well as to regenerate, revitalize, and calm. It differs from touch therapy in its use of formal physical positions applied over the *chakras*, or body energy centers.

Reiki is taught in a series of steps, or degrees. The first degree opens the learner to the ability to channel energy and teaches the healing positions. The second teaches distance healing processes. The third teaches the ability to open or attune others.

The healer never tires because she receives energy through the crown of the head and allows it to flow through her body and into her hands. The energy then flows through her hands and is directed to the areas of pain in the person being touched. The thumb and fingers are always held close together to link energy. A meditation asking for openness to heal is used, and the healer may enter a meditative state to focus on the areas that need to be healed. Then the healer holds her hands for 5 minutes over each of three head positions (eyes, sides and back of head), nine body positions (throat, chest, solar plexus, pelvis, and pubic region), and several optional positions (knees, feet, and back).

Treatments are completed with the body fully clothed. In cases of acute illness or accidents, Reiki is used directly over the pain area. If an area cannot be touched, the practitioner holds the hands above the spot, though not touching the person. Reiki is believed to ease trauma, reduce stress and pain, keep tissue damage to a minimum, and prevent or lessen swelling, blistering, and bleeding. Practitioners believe that the treatments help the body to regenerate itself.

CAROLYN CHAMBERS CLARK

REIKI: HISTORY AND THEORY

Reiki is a system of natural healing involving intentional touch by the practitioner with a receptive client. The Japanese word *Reiki* means "universal life force energy." It is the traditional laying on of hands that has been used for over 3,000 years. The practice was renewed and named in the 1800s by Mikao Usui.

There are three levels or "degrees" of Reiki healers in the traditional Usui system. The first degree teaches the practitioner to do a basic treatment on others and to use self-healing techniques. The second degree increases the intensity of the healing energy and introduces three symbols for use in traditional healing sessions and healing at a distance. The third degree is the Reiki master. A final symbol is given in the traditional system, and the master is empowered to initiate others and teach classes. There are specific hand placements on the body during a healing session. A healing session usually lasts 45 minutes to 1 hour.

Other schools of Reiki have been developed within the last 20 years. Additional symbols and levels have been added to the traditional system. Many of the symbols are ancient Tibetian in origin.

History/Theory

Usui, the president of Doshisha University in Japan, was challenged by his students to explain how Christ was able to heal. His journey took him all over the world and back to writings in the ancient Sanskrit language as well as his own meditation practice for the answers. He began to treat others and teach throughout Japan. Before his death around the turn of the century, he gave responsibility for the Reiki lineage to a trusted colleague, Chujiro Hayashi, who founded the first Reiki clinic in Tokyo. Hawaya Takata was initiated as a Reiki master in the late 1930s and brought the practice to the United States.

Reiki is said to work by transference of universal energy to the recipient through the Reiki practitioner. The philosophy is that the practitioner takes Reiki energy into their bodies through the crown *chakra*, where it passes through their bodies and out of their hands. It is therefore not energy that originates with the practitioner. It is said to also bring healing to the practitioner as it passes through to the recipient.

Principles of Reiki are:

- Just for today I will live the attitude of gratitude.
- Just for today I will not worry.
- Just for today I will not anger.
- Just for today I will do my work honestly.
- Just for today I will show love and respect for everyone.

Uses

Reiki is a complementary practice that can be used alone or in combination with any Western medical technique in a variety of settings. Recipients and providers report a subjective increase in well-being. The relaxation response is initiated, placing the person in a balanced state for healing to occur. The hand placement in a Reiki treat-

ment covers major human organs. Each recipient is said to draw energy to areas of need and/or deficiency to promote balance and rejuvenation of the human energy system within the body. Reiki is said to accelerate the process of psychotherapy and reduce anxiety. The subjective experience of pain has been reported to be reduced.

Reiki energy may be delivered by a single practitioner or by the use of self-healing techniques. Healing circles where individuals take turns giving and receiving Reiki energy is a common practice.

Research Base

There has been little traditional research on Reiki as its use by Western medical systems is only beginning to be explored. Descriptive studies have shown an increase in the electromagnetic energy field of the healer and the recipient during a Reiki treatment. Illustrations of this phenomena have been illustrated using Kirlian photography. Like traditions of energy healing have allowed measurement of brain activity in both the sender and the recipient through electro-encephalography. Results have illustrated a consistent decrease in the levels of anxiety and increase in levels of calmness. Numbers and effectiveness of natural killer cells in the immune system have shown to increase with regular use of the practices.

LINDA HEIN

RELIGIOUS SCIENCE PRACTITIONERS

Religious Science is part of the uniquely American religious movement known as New Thought (Anderson & Whitehouse,

1995). The roots of New Thought lie in the teachings and philosophies of Phineas Parkhurst Quimby, Emma Curtis Hopkins, Ralph Waldo Emerson, and Thomas Troward. One of the basic beliefs of New Thought is that the power of God is within us and available to us at all times. Implicit in this is that what happens to us is more a function of our own internal thought processes and beliefs than external factors.

Dr. Ernest Holmes (1887–1960), founder of Religious Science, combined Eastern and Western philosophies, science, and religion in his book *Science of Mind* (1938). Holmes's book has become the textbook for Religious Science and its practitioners.

The central theme of Religious Science is that there is a direct and unfailing cause and effect connection between one's thoughts and beliefs and the conditions that are manifested in one's life. Those who have completed three years of study, an internship, and have submitted documentation regarding successful applications of science of mind principles are licensed as practitioners. Practitioners are professionals who work with clients to effect healings of all types, including healing of physical conditions. Practitioners are trained to listen to a client and detect the negative mental images that the client has embraced. The practitioner then denies that this negative mental equivalent has any power, replacing it with a positive affirmation.

The practitioner uses affirmative prayer, which is referred to in Religious Science as a spiritual mind treatment. It is a specific five-step process. The first step is the recognition that there is but one God power. The second step, unification, acknowledges that each of us is a manifestation of God—that God is an in-dwelling presence in every human being no matter what the outward appearances may be. It is in this step that the practitioner enters into a spiritual oneness with God and the client. The third step of spiritual mind treatment is the process of making the desired positive affirmation. In this step, the present tense is always used as if the results have already been accomplished. The practitioner sees beyond the temporary physical conditions of the patient to the spiritual self, which is always perfect, complete, and whole. This process of outpicturing the desired result in mind is the cause that creates the effect of changing conditions including, but not limited to physical healing. The fourth step is thanksgiving, and the fifth and final step is release, believing in God's infinite power and allowing that process to occur. This process of stating and believing completely in an outcome is the essence of spiritual mind treatment. It is not unlike the process of physical faith healing successfully utilized in other religious groups. It transcends just physical healings, however, because it is believed in Religious Science that spiritual mind treatment works in all areas of life at all levels—physical, spiritual, and emotional.

While there are a multitude of documented, anecdotal instances of Religious Science principles being successful in physical healings, there are no controlled studies regarding the efficacy of spiritual mind treatment that meet academic research criteria. The primary thrust of Religious Science is to live the principles on a daily basis. It is believed that the proof of the teaching lies in individual application and demonstration of results.

There are currently 650 active licensed Religious Science practitioners in Religious Science International (RSI). They are all listed in *Creative Thought*, a monthly magazine published by RSI.

LINTON I. HARRIS

RITUAL AS A CREATIVE HEALING EXPERIENCE

Ritual is the archetypal response of human beings to the mysteries of life. All cultures develop ritual behaviors around deeply meaningful, emotional experiences such as birth, puberty, marriage, illness, and death. The purpose of ritual is to enable a person to regain a sense of participation, control, and integration during a challenging or threatening time of their life. Ritual not only commemorates change but also provides a symbolic vehicle to move us through change.

There are two types of ritual: prescribed and creative. Prescribed rituals occur in such forms as religious ceremony, funeral traditions, behavior at family gatherings, and cultural holiday customs. These ritualistic behaviors are constant over time, and their very constancy is comforting and re-affirming of values.

Like prescribed rituals, creative rituals also mark life's passages or assist with journeys of growth and change. Unlike prescribed rituals, they are creative, intuitive acts, even though they often follow a set format. The images and symbology of creative ritual attract the attention of the senses and the unconscious—the nonreasoning aspect of our total self. In bypassing the logical mind, creative ritual engages the artistic mind and the power of the unconscious, producing a shift in consciousness, which allows growth and integration of the challenging situation.

Creative rituals are emerging as a way to address the meaning of an illness and return some control and wholeness to the client. They have a positive impact on illness behaviors and on the way individuals feel about themselves. Healing rituals can be performed in private or with any number of participants. While the rituals themselves are varied and creative, most follow a format:

1. Definition of intention: The purpose of the ritual is defined. This drives the rest of the ritual, so the purpose must be clear.
2. Preparation: This is the period of time leading up to the actual ritual and helps move the individual into a more creative, spontaneous, open state of mind. It may include a time of introspection, meditation, prayer or fasting, securing and preparing "props," and deciding upon and securing a ritual space.
3. Creation of sacred space: Sacred space sets the time and place of the ritual apart from ordinary reality. A room in the client's home or the practitioner's office can be transformed into sacred space by intent and by props. A quiet spot outdoors is calming and establishes a connection with nature. In creating sacred space, one generally invites beneficial influences into the space. For some, this may be religious in nature. It may include invoking the energy of ancestors, of symbolic beings (archetypal god or goddess forms), of saints or angels, or one of the many names or manifestations of a supreme deity. The highly personal and spiritual nature of preparation for ritual and cre-

ating sacred space often leads to an altered state of consciousness—a sense of the holy that allows personal transformation and shifts in perception to occur during the ritual.

4. State the intent of the ritual aloud in sacred space.

5. Body of the ritual: Using creativity, decide beforehand what will be done symbolically to accomplish the intention. Symbols, colors, symbolic actions, active imagery, song, chants, music, drumming, candles, or anything else that attracts the creative mind can be used. The body of the ritual is the means by which perceptions of reality are transformed while in a sacred space in an altered state of consciousness (meditative or prayerful state). This might include imagery, meditation or prayer, or even charging an object with the intention to create a talisman (a physical link or reminder of an act in one's body-mind-spirit's creative will). The body of the ritual is the outward, physical form that acts as the focal point or vehicle for the inner will. During this time, energy is raised and directed with imagination, desire, and will toward the purpose.

6. Grounding: The energy that has been raised is directed toward the purpose. Any excess energy is given to the earth, where it is transformed. This is often done simply by laying the hands on the ground with intention. Grounding reestablishes a connection with the earth plane, providing a centering and stabilizing aspect.

7. Closing sacred space and reentering earth time. The participants give

thanks and know that the work is done.

Healing rituals can be used in all aspects of healing the mind-body-spirit, and regardless of the stated purpose, they always affect the whole person (mind-body-spirit). A ritual can mark the beginning of a change in lifestyle and support a change in attitude that will facilitate healing. It can mark the beginning of a course of medical treatment. It can commemorate the beginning or the end of a life. Rituals can help (on a deeply unconscious and symbolic level) to release guilt or lay to rest old relationships, earlier woundings, and other emotional challenges. Some examples of healing rituals are using colored candles to represent oneself and another person, moving the candles closer each day, symbolically indicating a desire to grow closer. Tying knots in a cord can symbolize the intention to establish new behaviors. Cutting a cord can indicate a severing (of a relationship or of old behaviors). Writing a letter to another, and then ceremoniously burning it, tying it to a helium-filled balloon, or casting it in moving waters often eases unresolved issues in a former relationship.

When shared, rituals also establish a very close personal human bond with another. Ritual demands full attention and presence, and this focus extends to others present. Creating and performing a ritual for another person is a gift of love and healing. Being present at a ritual for another is a strong declaration of support and a witness for healing.

Our society has made tremendous technological advances in the last 60 years but has largely ignored the lived experience of illness. As recognition of the personal meanings of illness increases, practitioners will continue to incorporate more holistic ways of healing, focusing more on the transformative journey, not just the prescribed treatment. Ways of supporting people as they go through their healing journey will be sought, with participation through ritual in the mysteries of life.

KATHLEEN S. FASNACHT

ROLFING: STRUCTURAL INTEGRATION

Rolfing is a manual therapy comprising the holistic philosophy, science, and art of integrating the structural, functional, and energetic patterns of the human body in gravity. Rolfing explores and introduces change to these patterns by systematically lengthening and repositioning the body's connective tissue in a highly detailed, principles-based series of sessions which can facilitate transformation on many levels. Ida P. Rolf (1896–1979) originally defined and named her work "structural integration" to set her revolutionary approach apart from other systems of manual manipulation that treated the body symptom by symptom instead of as an "integrated" whole. Rolf's unique vision was that health, well-being, and even freedom to evolve are dependent on the ability to adapt to gravity. The original, nongeneric "brand name" of structural integration is rolfing. The extent to which rolfing values and explores gravity's impact on human structure is the hallmark of the work and distinguishes it from all other types of manual therapy.

The most common misconception about rolfing is that it is a gratuitously painful process. It's not. Rolfers are trained to sensitively uncover patterns of holding and shortening in the body that may or may not be experienced, subjectively, as painful. The rate of change, specificity of intention, and finesse of the rolfer, appropriate boundaries and communication as well as the client's history, are key determinants.

History

Ida Rolf was born in 1896 in the Bronx, New York, and earned her undergraduate degree in science from Barnard College in 1916. In 1920, she received her doctorate in biological chemistry from Columbia University's College of Physicians and Surgeons. Rolf then went to work as a research scientist at the Rockefeller Institute, an opportunity that was unique for a woman at the time. In addition to her traditional academic pursuits, Rolf was very interested in more unorthodox healing modalities, such as yoga, homeopathy, and osteopathy. These interests were reinforced by her extensive travel, reading, and intrepid desire to solve her own family health problems including scoliosis, arthritis, and prediabetes. Rolf possessed an amazing ability to understand intuitively, had a genius-level I.Q., and through trial and error combined her knowledge of science and physical manipulation to create not only a pioneering method of somatic therapy but also a truly original inquiry into the human experience.

During the 1950s, after 25 years of developing her revolutionary work, Rolf presented structural integration in the United States, Great Britain, and Canada, primarily to osteopaths and chiropractors. Rolf had much respect for A. T. Still, the founder of osteopathy. Rolf was concerned that her work was myopically seen by some as an ancillary technique to "fix" specific problems and would be diluted if merely observed and coopted in a smorgasbord-like manner. Rolfing structural integration entered an arena of greater recognition in the late 1960s, when Rolf visited the Esalen Institute in Big Sur, California. Esalen was the epicenter of the nascent human potential movement and was an experiential potpourri of many of the most current therapies and thought forms. It was here that rolfing developed the reputation as a desirably intense and cathartic form of process and release. Fritz Perls, the director of Esalen and the founder of Gestalt therapy, was convinced that Rolf had saved his life by healing his severe angina attacks.

The eponym "rolfing" reputedly was coined at Esalen. It was while she was at Esalen that Rolf was persuaded, reportedly by Perls, to establish a school so that her remarkable work would not die with her.

Rolf felt at home at Esalen and continued to practice and teach there until 1972, when she and her small group of teachers established the Rolf Institute in Boulder, Colorado. The Rolf Institute of Structural Integration remains the only school that certifies rolfers and advanced rolfers, although there have emerged several other schools of structural integration emanating out of her work.

Theory

Rolfing is based on the insight that our bodies are not soft machines made of parts but are unified seamless wholes capable of adapting their forms to an ever-changing environment, gravitation being the principle component. Modern physics no longer describes gravity as a force that pulls downward but as a multidimensional activity that relates all bodies and acts in continually curving motions. Structural integration is an expression of ongoing, multidimensional, and multisystem interactions that are possible only because of the presence of the organizing action of gravity. The unending influence of this force, along with normal developmental events and the random traumatic events of life, affect how we are shaped. All adaptations in human shape occur primarily as alterations in connective tissue structures, primarily fascia. These ubiquitous structures bind muscle fibers together, attach muscle to bone, and surround and invest the bones, organs, nerves, and blood vessels themselves. Fascia shortens and thickens in response to trauma and habitual movement patterns in gravity. Rolfing attempts to alter this process by systematically and sensitively freeing fascial adhesions, restoring joint mobility, and calling for appropriate movement from the client. The proactive nature of the work is another distinguishing feature. From the rolfing perspective, if the whole body is not properly prepared to receive the effects of local manipulations, either the change will not be maintained or strain will show up in other areas.

Uses

We must deal with gravity like other material structures. Whether from poor posture, injury, illness, or emotional distress, a misaligned or "random" body is at war with gravity. We experience this war as stress, depleted energy, and pain. In studies, rolfing has shown to significantly reduce chronic stress, enhance neurological functioning, improve spinal biomechanics, and create more economical and refined patterns of movement. The effectiveness of rolfing is determined by the client's capacity to incorporate new proprioceptive and sensory information arising from rolfing-induced changes. These changes can include shifts in position, stature, and emotional states, along with increased potentials for order, expression, and experience. People from all walks of life seek rolfing not only as a way to ease pain and chronic stress but also as a way to improve performance in their professions and daily activities. Rolf was not only concerned with easing the pain and stresses of human life but also was profoundly interested in creating a system that could transform the whole person at every level.

CHRISTOPHER AMODEO

THE RUBENFELD SYNERGY METHOD

Rubenfeld synergy is a body-centered psychotherapy with strong elements of psychophysical reeducation. Using gentle touch together with active listening, verbal dialogue, imagery, movement, and metaphor, the Rubenfeld synergy method facilitates self-healing and integration on all levels—physical, mental, emotional, and spiritual.

Rubenfeld synergy is based on the beliefs that (1) body, mind, emotions, and spirit are integrally related and that change in one brings about change in the others; (2) we all have an innate wisdom and a capacity for self-healing; (3) the body tells the truth; and (4) ultimate responsibility for change rests with the client. The work is about moving away from habit and toward conscious choice.

Feelings and beliefs that develop early in life or from traumatic situations later on exert strong, often unconscious, influence on our lives today. These feelings and beliefs may be responsible for physical pain or dysfunction, disease, low self-esteem, tension, confusion, depression, troubled relationships, and many other conditions that affect the quality of life. Through the Rubenfeld synergist's use of light touch and in the safety provided by the synergist's nonjudgmental attitude, clients are assisted in bringing these feelings and beliefs from the body and the hidden recesses of the psyche into conscious awareness. From this awareness and with the caring support of the synergist, the client can discover the origins of these underlying beliefs and feelings, experience them from a new perspective, and explore more positive alternatives. Many clients then choose to let go of old, self-defeating patterns and replace them with patterns that are more life-affirming.

What distinguishes Rubenfeld synergy and makes it such a powerful therapy is the multilevel communication that develops between synergist and client through the simultaneous use of gentle touch and talk. Touch helps the synergist create the safety and trust that are essential for the client to allow repressed feelings and painful memories to surface so that they can be released. With gentle hands and subtle movements, the synergist directly senses what is happening with the client. Feeling the pulsations of energy around certain words or issues, the synergist can sense where the energy is blocked and by bringing the client's awareness to the area help the client release tensions and holding patterns. Touch, along with gentle verbal probes, directs the client's awareness to moment-to-moment bodily sensations and emotional states.

Metaphor, visualization, and inner dialogue help clients connect what is happening in the body to what is happening in their lives, thus revealing their underlying belief systems and feelings. To give an example: In response to a general question, a client reports that she is noticing a lump in her throat. The synergist asks her to give the lump a voice and let it tell her what it's doing there. The lump says that it's there to keep her from saying things she shouldn't. The synergist develops this by asking the client what she might say and to whom if the lump weren't there to restrain her. This leads to things she would like to say to her current boss but doesn't out of fear. Then the realization comes that these are things she really wanted to say to her father as a child, but couldn't. So she had unknowingly repressed her feelings and projected them onto other people. With this awareness, she is able to recognize that her feelings about her boss's behavior are inappropriate to the current situation, and she begins to alter them. In that session and future sessions, she works through the issues with her father and is able to let go of feelings and beliefs that interfere with living the life she wants.

A typical Rubenfeld synergy session lasts about 50 minutes and takes place with the client fully clothed and lying on a padded table or sitting in a chair. Since Rubenfeld synergy is designed to facilitate personal growth and change, it is an ongoing therapy, most often done on a weekly basis and continuing for as long as needed. Although the work is most often done with individuals in private sessions, an individual's session can also be witnessed by a supportive group.

Because Rubenfeld synergy is a gentle, noninvasive therapy that respects the uniqueness of each individual and puts the client in charge of finding his or her own wisdom and healing, it is appropriate for all but the most seriously disturbed.

Benefits

Rubenfeld synergy facilitates the changes people want in their lives; these changes will vary depending on the person. Some of the benefits enjoyed include relief of stress and tension, greater self-esteem, resolution of painful issues and experiences, recovery from physical and/or emotional trauma, inner peace and calm, increased ease of movement, greater inner capacity for self-healing, and increased body-mind awareness and acceptance.

Origin and Founder

The Rubenfeld synergy method was developed in the 1960s by Ilana Rubenfeld, an early pioneer in the field of body-centered psychotherapy. As is so often the case, this unique work developed out of her own journey in search of healing.

A student at Julliard School of Music in the early 1950s, Rubenfeld developed a painful back spasm from her practice as a conductor. When doctors were unable to provide anything but temporary relief, she went to a teacher of the Alexander technique, who helped her learn how to use her body without stressing it. The lessons, in which her teacher touched and guided her gently, elicited many emotions. To deal with all the feelings that were surfacing, Rubenfeld was advised to see a psychoanalyst. However, to her distress, she was unable to reproduce those deep emotions when talking with the analyst. For several years, Rubenfeld went back and forth between the two—one who talked but would not touch and one who touched but would not talk.

From this experience, Rubenfeld came to the realization that neither touch nor talk was sufficient by itself; they needed to happen simultaneously. She went on to become a teacher of the Alexander technique and later studied with Moshe Feldenkrais, the creator of the Feldenkrais method. Both these approaches emphasize the mind-body connection and work in subtle ways to reeducate the body for optimal functioning, movement, and ease.

While the Alexander technique and the Feldenkrais method were the beginning points in the development of Rubenfeld synergy, Gestalt therapy provided much of its theoretical basis. Some of the similarities include emphasis on body awareness, focus on the present experience, and dialogues with one's own body and with people who are not present. Rubenfeld's years of study with Fritz and Laura Perls, cofounders of Gestalt therapy, and her work with several other gifted therapists brought psychotherapeutic understanding and technique into her work. The fourth major influence in the development of Rubenfeld synergy was hypnotherapy as taught by the renowned psychotherapist, Milton Errickson.

In its fully developed form, Rubenfeld synergy is a unique system that is far more than the sum of its parts; it is a synergistic blend. Rubenfeld continues to develop and refine the system as she teaches and lectures around the world and directs the training program at the Rubenfeld Center in New York. The Rubenfeld synergy training program, begun in 1977, is currently a 1,600-hour program that meets six times a year for 4 years. Students attend three week-long modules and three weekends annually. Conducted by Ilana Rubenfeld and her faculty, it is the only source of training and certification of Rubenfeld synergists.

JEANNE REOCK

RUSSIAN MASSAGE

Russian massage is a form of massage that is based on the physiology of a dysfunction instead of focusing on the anatomical structure as the primary guideline for treatment. The techniques are based on the belief that the body is its best healer and that massage can teach the body how to help itself. Therefore, the major goal of each massage is to introduce the body to the solution that it lacks and to produce the effects that the body will use to correct an existing problem. Often, pharmaceutical drugs have been replaced with these massage techniques.

Massage influences the body by means of mechanical stimulations provided to the tissues by the techniques of effleurage (stroking), friction (rubbing), petrissage (kneading), and vibration. The great variety of strokes used in Russian massage allows for varying degrees of influence from very light to very deep. The techniques that influence the tissues stimulate the mechanoreceptors, also called tactile receptors, with which the body converts the energy of mechanical stimulation (including touch) into specific activity of the nervous system, the signals that transmit information to the nerve centers.

History/Theory

Use of massage as a form of medicine dates back thousands of years. However, massage was not studied or used scientifically in Russia until 1860, when M. Y. Mudrov used massage and movement to treat illnesses. The treatment methodologies used by Russian massage therapists were further developed by Soviet physicians to solve post–World War II problems because few affordable pharmaceutical solutions were available. While the Western world busily developed pharmaceutical drugs, the USSR put hundreds of physiatrists (MDs with a Ph.D. in physical therapy) to work finding benefits of natural means of healing. Massage became one of the major forms of treatment in traditional Russian medicine. Through extensive research, physiatrists set out to determine how each stroke affects the body in general and each system in particular.

Russian doctors took the same principles on which medication works in the body of an ill individual and set to match the healing process with the use of massage. To use massage as a form of medicine, physicians had to know what massage does not only to a healthy individual but also to people with different dysfunctions. Various strokes were found to have different effects on the body. Although the names of the Russian massage techniques appear to resemble traditional Swedish massage, they vary greatly in terms of performance and in their effects on the body.

For example, effleurage can increase the amount of leukocytes and erythrocytes in the blood, as well as relieve pain and slow down an irritated central nervous system. Friction can increase the heating of tissues, and therefore improve local arterial circulation up to 140 times (Kunidev, 1979). Russian massage developed a form of petrissage that can reverse the atrophy process in muscles and can, therefore, be used as a tool to grow muscle tissue. Russian

vibrational techniques done in specific frequencies can relax, stimulate, or even anesthetize an area.

Movements of massage are perceived by the body as stimuli of tactile reception. Massage stimulates the mechanoreceptors of the skin, which sends a signal via the afferent nerves causing the feeling of touch, pressure, or vibration. The intensity of the tactile stimulation and its amount are caused by the strength of the massage motion. The stronger the stimulation, the greater the electrical potential because of the greater number of impulses sent to the nervous system. The higher the speed with which the stimulation is given to the skin, the greater the feeling of pressure. This principle will allow a substitution of speed for depth, especially useful when deep touch is not tolerable.

All of the movements of massage work on the basis of reflexes. Russian physiologists such as I. M. Sechenov, N. E. Vedensky, A. A. Uxtomsky, and I. P. Pavlov (Belaya, 1983) found that the major function of massage is based on neurohumoral and neuroendocrine reflective action, which is regulated by the higher centers of the central nervous system. By influencing the body with a methodical (i.e., properly formulated for a particular individual with a particular condition) dosage of massage movements, a chain of adaptive reactions is formed. For example, massage normalizes blood pressure, which means that with similar techniques, a person with high blood pressure will have it lowered, and a person with low blood pressure will have it increased.

Uses

In Russian clinics, physicians addressing multiple dysfunctions realized that the type of dysfunction decides the type of massage that should be given. Russian massage can be used to treat neurological, cardiovascular, dermatological, intestinal, musculoskeletal, postsurgical, and various internal dysfunctions. As Russian massage follows the standard medical model, proper diagnosis and referral from a physician are necessary for treatment. Russian massage is not indicated for most acute conditions; however, it can be used to resolve edema and other immediate posttraumatic cases.

Some of the conditions that can be treated with Russian massage include bursitis, rotator cuff injury, headaches, occipital nerve irritation, trigeminal neuralgia, ulnar neuritis, cervical and thoracic scoliosis, carpal tunnel syndrome, arthritis, plantar faciatis, tendinitis, meniscus tears, sciatic radiculitis, hip strains and sprains, herniated discs, lower back strain, fibromyalgia, chronic gastritis, chronic colitis, atherosclerosis, hypertension, hypotension, and lateral and medial epicondylitis.

ZHENYA KURASHOVA WINE

SHEALY BACK PAIN MANAGEMENT PROGRAM

In 1971, an active behavioral modification program for chronic pain was instituted at the Pain Rehabilitation Center in La Crosse, Wisconsin, based on the work of Dr. Wilbert Fordyce at the University of Washington in Seattle (Fordyce, 1968). Beginning in 1966, he used the concept of behavioral modification or operant conditioning. Working with a maximum of four individuals at a time, he treated 100 for chronic pain, selecting only 25% of those sent to him. Participants were conditioned to avoid pain posturing or behavior and

were weaned from all pain or mood-altering drugs. Over a 2-month in-hospital program, at a 1966 cost of $5,000, 60% improved markedly. Six months later, 40% of the men and 33% of the women remained improved. Considering that all of them had been failures of conventional medicine, the results were impressive.

In 1972, Fordyce reported an average per person prior expense of $50,000. His program, at that time, cost $5,000. He estimated that society would break even if only 10% of the participants in his program returned to work. If one takes into account the income produced by those who return to work, even less than 10% work-return success would produce a break-even point for society.

At the Pain Rehabilitation Center, 90% of the applicants had failed back pain syndrome with an average of 6 or more unsuccessful back operations. Virtually all were iatrogenically addicted to opioids and benzodiazepine tranquilizers. A majority had significant pretreatment stress illness such as hypertension, diabetes, peptic ulcer, etc. They were withdrawn from all mood and pain altering drugs and kept out of bed at least 12 hours per day. Working with 24 to 40 patients at a time, caregivers routinely assigned patients all the following treatments: slapping/pounding massage 4 times per day; ice rubdowns 4 times per day; vigorous mechanical massage by a nurse 4 times per day; whirlpool 30 minutes daily; swimming pool exercises for 1 hour per day, 5 days per week; massage by a massage therapist 2 times per week; specified other exercise regimens, including walking hall laps starting with 10 and adding 1 daily, and guided limbering exercise by a physical therapist; application of Electreat 1 hour 4 times per day (this was the only electrical stimulator available for pain control at that time); acupuncture 2 times per week; 30 minutes of autogenic training 2 times per day; and temperature, EMG, or EEG biofeedback training 1 hour per day.

Patients continued in the program for 4 weeks. They were discharged home with recommendations to them and their home physician for continuing physical exercise, relaxation/autogenic training, and no drugs.

At the end of the first year, 400 patients had been treated with an average hospital stay of 30 days at an average cost of $3,200. Seventy percent were markedly improved over admission as measured by them on a five-point pain profile: intensity of pain, percent of time pain is present, affect of pain on physical activity, affect of pain on mood, and drug consumption.

Of the 94% of 800 patients who eventually completed the program, 600 were followed for 2 years, and 200 were followed for 6 months. Results reveal that 35% of those patients returned to work; 90% were off all drugs except aspirin or acetaminophen; 70% were improved 50% to 100% measured on pain intensity, percent of time in pain and in physical activity; 30% who did not improve greatly almost invariably did not practice the techniques taught (as reported by them); 5% had a facet rhizotomy, the procedure for denervating the facet joints of selected vertebrae, done with a percutaneous approach under local anesthesia; 25% continued the use of TENS (transcutaneous electrical nerve stimulation) for at least 6 months ("TENS" is the term applied to use of the Electreat and its more modern adaptations); pain intensity was reduced over an average of 70% as measured by patients; the percent of time pain was present was reduced an average of 65% as measured by patients; mood was

improved in 90% of patients as measured by them; less than 5% had additional surgical procedures after treatment; drug expenses after therapy were reduced 85%; hospitalization after therapy was reduced 90%; total medical expenses were reduced after therapy 80% to 85%; and cost of treatment ranged from $4,000 to $5,500.

In 1974, the self-regulation training was intensified, keeping participants in the hospital only 3 weeks, the last 3 days doing 8 hours per day of guided autogenic training, visualization, relaxation exercise, and hypnotherapy. The results: 85% of patients improved 50% to 100% over all aspects of the pain profile. Six months later, 72% remained improved. Three years later, 70% remained improved (as measured by their pain profile).

In August of 1974, the program was converted to a 12-day outpatient format, continuing the most important treatments: TENS, acupuncture, an adapted form of self-regulation training called Biogenics, massage, physical exercise, trigger point nerve blocks, facet nerve blocks, and psychological counseling.

This has been the foundation of work for the subsequent 23 years. The Pain Rehabilitation Center evolved into the Shealy Institute. In the last 3 years, the American Academy of Pain Management has consistently found, as an outside independent agency, that the treatment of back pain at the Shealy Institute has been the most successful and most cost-effective in the United States. For those patients who enter the 12 day, 80 hour treatment program, costs average about $5,500. The cost success index is 60% below the national average.

Recently, in response to the need to consolidate and improve further the cost/success index, based on completed studies, the following protocol was used.

The Shealy Protocol for Back Pain

Treatment

A. Initial management of all currently consumed analgesic medications and substances (caffeine, alcohol, tobacco, and street drugs).
  1. Decrease by 10% per day from initially determined dosage.
  2. Start Bromelain 1,000 mg tid 1/2 hour after meals.
B. Learn to use the visual analogue scale (VAS) for pain measurement at the first appointment with the physician and then continue to complete VASs at all subsequent appointments.
C. Use a TENS unit during all waking hours (electrode placement taught by facility MD or RN).
D. Receive a daily pre-DRS (computerized traction device) vibratory massage or myofascial release using vacuum/inferential current treatment for 30 minutes with heat application to the lower back for 20 sessions.
E. Receive distraction/decompression for 30 minutes on the DRS using 1/2 of the body weight plus 10 pounds for 20 sessions.
F. After DRS, place a Polar Pack on the lower back for 30 minutes.
G. After 1 week (5 DRS sessions), any participants with clinical and diagnostic imaging findings of ruptured intervertebral disc who are not 50% improved receive 1 mg/d IV Colchicine and 2 g magnesium/B6 IV for 5 days, then are orally maintained on 0.6 mg/d for 6 months.
H. After the second week of the program (10 DRS sessions), if improved 50%, learn the Shealy exercise program. For those not yet improved 50%, reassess patients with repeat physical examination.
I. For those not 50% better after 10 DRS sessions, consider:
  1. Percutaneous electrical nerve stimulation (PENS) to be done by the facility physician.
  2. Referral to anesthesiologist or neurosurgeon for facet nerve blocks.
  3. Trigger point injections with Sarapin by facility physician.
J. After 20 DRS sessions, or significant improvement of symptoms from multimodality approaches, have an exit physical examination with the facility physician. An aftercare plan will be established calling for the use of the Polar Packs, TENS, exercise, relaxation training, use of any substances, pacing techniques, and proper utilization of body mechanics and posture for daily activities.
K. Return 1 month after treatment for evaluation by the facility physician.

If these fail, then consider facet nerve blocks.

Outcome: Eighty-five percent of patients with acute/subacute ruptured discs and 75% of patients with chronic back pain due to facet arthrosis are markedly improved after 4 weeks.

C. NORMAN SHEALY

SHIATSU

Shiatsu is a relatively recent form of manipulative body therapy coming into recognition around 1920 in Japan. The term came into being as Japanese *anma* and massage therapists tried to avoid government regulations limiting their practice. The three legally recognized forms of manipulative therapy in Japan now are *anma* (the Japanese version of Chinese medicine, diagnosis, and treatment that includes manipulation and pressure), Western massage, and shiatsu. Shiatsu combines techniques of *anma*, accupressure, stretching, and Western massage; the experience of it can vary from practitioner to practitioner, from the almost meditative to highly energetic and deep.

As in all such therapies, finding the most effective treatment for each patient requires keeping an open mind and having a knowledge of the receptivity of the individual patient. Arguments that arise among the various schools of manipulative therapy as to their effectiveness or superiority over others prove relatively nothing. Like other forms of massage, shiatsu enhances lymphatic and blood circulation, can ease tension and muscle aches, and depending upon the technique and intent can calm or invigorate the recipient. Shiatsu can also be more extensive than a massage treatment.

The official definition of shiatsu from the Japanese Ministry of Health and Welfare is that "shiatsu therapy is a form of manipulation administered by the thumbs, fingers, and palms, without the use of any instrument, mechanical or otherwise, to apply pressure to the human skin, correct internal malfunctioning, promote and maintain health, and treat specific diseases." Japanese therapists themselves do not make strict distinctions among the various pressure techniques, although certain specific routines will be named after their originators. In general, the therapist desires

to help the patient achieve wellness and wholeness beyond an hour session for relaxation. Simply put, shiatsu is like acupuncture without needles.

Although the specific techniques are not that difficult for massage therapists to learn, the real difference between the amateur or home remedy treatment and the professional is in the understanding of the theory of the *tsubo*, the energy centers or points, and of diagnosis. Oriental medical theory is quite different from Western theory, and much of the appeal of therapies such as shiatsu is due to its "preventive" nature. Oriental diagnosis and medicine involves sympathy and compassion for the patient's unique condition, and small details or idiosyncrasies often dismissed by Western medicine are many times significant to the Oriental practitioner.

Western medicine has not scientifically proven the existence of meridian lines, the lines of energy that Oriental medicine uses, and upon which the theory of *tsubo* is based. The treatment of the points and meridians unblocks the various flows of energy in the body by contacting these lines and points and stimulating them in various ways. Blocked energies are believed to be the prodrome of disease conditions. Nevertheless, Chinese medicine and its derivatives have a long history of use and effectiveness despite the West's lack of understanding of the mechanisms in play.

Meridians and points may be *kyo* or *jitsu*, meaning roughly flabby or hard, and may be treated by toning or sedating. Depending on the meridian and its condition, one may describe specific psychological and physical details such as being prone to obesity, having dry nasal passages, constipation, yawning, or a tendency to worry over details as well as proneness to serious organ malfunctions. The meridian conditions can describe thousands of other diagnostic symptoms; thus, a professional and well-trained shiatsu practitioner might treat many forms of illness other than muscle aches and pains. There is also self-shiatsu so that individuals can treat themselves at home; this can further empower the patient to take an active part in health maintenance and disease prevention. Common ailments such as headache, tendonitis, periodic cramps, or back aches may well be relieved without medications using relatively simple shiatsu techniques.

Unlike many other forms of massage, shiatsu does not use oils to lubricate the skin. Many of the techniques are relatively stationary and may be performed through loose clothing. Using pressure and stretches, the natural balance of the body is restored and energy returns to parts of the body where it is lacking. One session of any therapy is not likely to reverse a problem that has taken years to develop, however. Shiatsu may be done on a massage table, seated in a chair, or on a futon on the floor.

As with any manipulative body therapy, patients should be aware of their own comfort levels. Does one bruise easily? Is getting up and down from the floor an issue? Is the patient willing to follow a regime that may be foreign to Western habits of eating, exercise, and philosophy, or is he or she just curious as to what a shiatsu session might feel like? Any concern should always be discussed with a therapist prior to initiating any treatment.

There are no miraculous cures even with the most advanced Western medical technology, and to expect that health maintenance or the recovery from illness and injury is other than a process that takes time

and attention could lead to dissatisfaction with alternative and complementary forms of healing.

LESLIE AGUILLARD

SPIRITUALITY AND PSYCHOTHERAPY

Do spirituality and religion belong in psychotherapy? Should the therapist wait for the patient to bring up religion? Or does the therapist deal with it directly, as simply another aspect of the client that requires exploration? Is spirituality a given part of religion, and visa versa? Or is spirituality more, the unqualifiable essence of mental and emotional life? Is the therapist remiss in omitting it from the client's history?

While issues in spirituality and religion can be found in both the general psychology and nursing literature, much of the writing in this area is to be found in the marriage and family therapy literature and in the literature on addictive behaviors. Little of the literature is based on research.

Stander et al. (1994) discuss the integration of family therapy, religion, and spirituality. They note that separation of church and state has evolved into avoidance of religious topics in secular settings. This avoidance can be seen in therapist education that seldom discusses the meaning of religion in the lives of clients. Yet, the authors believe, spiritual values are often the unifying force within a family and should be addressed.

An interesting article that attempts to reframe 12-step programs using a cognitive-behavioral framework discusses the notion of spirituality as empowerment. Ann Bristow-Braitman (1995) views spirituality in the context of a 12-step program as the force that fosters connectedness to the self and others. This leads to both self-efficacy, as a giver and a taker of support, and to responsibility for the self and others. Both self-efficacy and responsibility are empowering. Although admitting to powerlessness while under the influence of a chemical, the substance abuser is empowered with the reframed thought that she or he is powerful enough to handle life's problems in another way (i.e., without chemicals).

Robert Turner et al. (1995) wrote about their drive to make the religious and spiritual dimensions of culture a part of a more culturally sensitive diagnostic classification system. In their article, they discuss the assessment of religious/spiritual problems and how to differentiate between these problems and psychopathology. They make a particular effort to discuss specific types of spiritual problems documented in the literature. Special attention is given to problems occurring with hospitalized psychiatric patients and seriously ill medical patients.

Koenig, Larson, and Matthews (1996) directly address the issue of using religion in the psychotherapy of older adults. They strongly advocate the use of religious interventions in the treatment of religious older patients. Such interventions might consist of Biblical references to support aspects of the psychological treatment or to give comfort in the face of inevitable death. The authors suggest that, at a minimum, a religious history should be taken with all older patients. Furthermore, the therapist's religious beliefs or nonbeliefs are not as important as the therapist's validation of this aspect of the patient's life. Nonreligious therapists can effectively use religious interventions in supportive therapy. When religion is used more actively in therapy,

a match between the patient's and the therapist's beliefs becomes important. Koenig, Larson, and Matthews give various examples of the use of religious interventions in psychodynamic and cognitive-behavioral therapy. A Judeo-Christian religious reference point is used throughout the article.

In the research literature, Shafranske and Malony (1990) surveyed 409 clinical psychologists on their religious and spiritual orientations and their practice of psychotherapy. More than half of the sample held some sort of religious belief and affiliated, to some extent, with organized religion. However, the degree of actual involvement with organized religion was low. Psychologists who held some sort of religious belief were more inclined to approach this aspect of clients' lives than were those without belief. While most of the respondents maintained that psychologists had the skills and knowledge to work on religious issues with their clients, few felt personally able to do so.

Propst, et al. (1992) published a study that compared the effectiveness of religiously oriented cognitive-behavioral therapy (RCBT) and standard cognitive-behavioral therapy (CBT) for symptom reduction in clinically depressed, highly religious individuals. Fifty-nine subjects were randomly assigned to either an experimental or a control group. Control groups consisted of a pastoral counseling group and a wait list group. The therapists in the experimental groups (RCBT, CBT) were equally divided between those who held personal religious beliefs and those who didn't. Both the pastoral counseling group and the religious cognitive-behavioral group reported lower posttreatment depression at 3-month and 2-year follow-up than did the other groups.

A more recent study surveyed the usage of spiritual interventions among Mormon psychotherapists (N = 215). Richards and Potts (1995) found that, as a group, Mormon therapists use spiritual interventions sparingly. When interventions are used, they tend to be centered in the therapist (e.g., silent prayer before or during a session). Many therapists voiced ethical concerns about the use of other spiritual interventions, citing as major concerns the possibility of dual relationships with Mormon clients and the possibility of imposing religious beliefs on non-Morman clients. The authors concluded with a recommendation that therapist education incorporate the religious/spiritual domain as part of standard curriculum.

In summary, while the clinical literature contains numerous writings on the spiritual and religious aspects of therapy, the research literature has lagged behind. While research is moving toward the spirit as a valid subject of inquiry, the questions posited above have not been answered. Certainly, addressing this area in therapy requires sensitivity. Certainly, it requires a foundation of basic religious and spiritual knowledge. Beyond this, it requires an openness to new experience. More importantly, it requires an intellectual and spiritual curiosity. It requires that unqualifiable essence of mental and emotional life—spirituality.

MARIE LOUISE BERNARDO

SPIRITUAL/RELIGIOUS APPROACHES

Complementary health practices of spiritual and religious origins are as old as mankind, arising from a premise that it is possible to link with a suprahuman source of meaning and that the source may be drawn upon for growth, comfort, or healing. In contrast to spirituality, religion concerns acceptance of a specific set of beliefs, that is, a creed concerning the nature of that source. Religion also implies some organized group that worships in accord with the specified set of beliefs. Spirituality is a more global and more individualized concept. Dossey and Guzzetta (1995) define spirituality as involving unfolding mystery, inner strengths, and harmonious interconnectedness—with self, others, higher powers, and environment. Some authors see religion as one subcategory of spirituality.

Two distinct approaches to therapeutics may be differentiated, regardless of whether one is discussing religion or spirituality, the first in which one attempts to apply normal human means of comforting and consoling, and the second in which direct interventions into the health state are intended.

Normal Comforting and Consoling

Normal acts of comforting and consoling are applied in both spiritual and religious contexts and typically invoke rituals with which the client is familiar, such as (on the part of the religious) reading of sacred literature, performing religious rituals (sometimes requiring a special authority figure), reciting religious cants or prayers, or providing religious objects of comfort. Such measures, when requested by the client and drawing on the client's beliefs, evoke meaning and comfort. Effective use of such measures requires knowledge of the client's cultural and religious background and the ability to act within that context. Specter (1996) provides a useful guide to the demands of diverse cultures and religions.

Spiritual aspects of comforting and consoling come closer to practices normally labeled as sensitive human understanding. Donley, for example, gives three therapeutic approaches to relieving suffering: (1) accompaniment, (2) giving meaning, and (3) action. Accompaniment (or presence) implies simply being with the suffering client. A search for the meaning of suffering may occur within a religious or a spiritual context. The recommended action is that of relieving suffering, and this may involve diverse measures, spiritual, psychological, physiological, or biochemical to name a few.

Direct Intervention

Attempts at direct intervention in the client's condition call for a more active involvement with the source, however identified. In the case of some traditional religions, that source may be termed God; in other spiritual and religious traditions, labels range from the Tao, the Light, the Source, an Intelligent Energy, to the Shared Universal Soul Within. Different persons perceive the relationship with that power to occur in different ways, from being a child of God to reaching one's spiritual center within.

In each case, an attempt is made to reach that source by some imagery (reaching up, reaching down, reaching within) and combining that effort at connection with intentionality (to heal, to relieve pain, to allay fear). The first step in these therapeutic approaches is that of making contact with the higher power. Prayer typifies this in religion. Meditation or centering (reaching a deep concentrated point of focus within) serves a similar function in some spiritual approaches.

The second step invokes the healing power/presence. Depending on the set of involved beliefs, this may involve asking the higher power to channel its power through the petitioner, or, alternately, it may be seen as putting oneself in a state in which the power (often seen as universal energy) may be channeled through one's hands. The notion of power as movement of energy is valid for many schools (e.g., Reiki, core energetics). Additionally, some religious groups see the higher source acting directly rather than through an intermediary human agent.

The third step is that of intentionality toward a specific person to be assisted. Here, for example, the religious person may ask that the perceived source directly intervene through petitionary prayer, or, alternately ask that the source act through the petitioner via a laying on of hands. Similarly, the spiritual person often channels energy to an intended client, typically through the hands via touch. Also, in some systems, it is believed that energy can be channeled merely by intention, over space, without touch.

Such energy movement (often termed "therapeutic touch") and laying on of hands may be perceived as drawing on similar powers. Also, such universal energy may be employed in the absence of either religious or spiritual intentions. Krieger (1981), for example, sees the use of therapeutic touch as based on research findings, not faith or belief.

Research into spiritual and religious approaches is conducted from several perspectives. Much of the research involves surveys of how many practitioners and patients use or want a spiritual/religious component to their care (King & Bushwick, 1994). Many of the physician-initiated studies attempt to associate spirituality with improved medical outcomes (Mathews, 1997). Some of the scholarly work builds models to explain the effectiveness of these religious/spiritual therapeutics. Slater (1995a, 1995b), for example, builds an interesting metaphor to explain how energic alternate therapies might work, while Dossey (1995) proposes a physiological model.

BARBARA STEVENS BARNUM

SPORTS MASSAGE

The Eastern bloc countries developed most sports massage techniques as their athletes pushed the limits of training to excel in competition. Ways were needed to help the body recuperate faster. The effectiveness of sports massage on athletes was tested also in Sweden on cyclists, and it was found that the quadriceps muscles were 11% stronger after a brief massage compared with a 10-minute rest. We have only to recall Olympic games early in the 20th century to know these athletes won the medals. Thus sports massage came to the Western world. Does it work? The year the New York Giants started using sports massage was the same year they went to the Super Bowl and won.

Sports massage therapists generally have more training in kinesiology, the science of movement, but like other forms of massage, the techniques are not fundamentally different, and it is still the increased circulation that speeds the healing and recovery time. The intense activity especially in competitive sports creates small traumas in the muscle tissue and swelling. Massage helps to reduce it. Sports massage may be given pre- and/or postevent. Massage preevent is said to help prevent injury; for example, extra time is spent on tendons and ligaments, which are tissues without blood supply so they tend to warm up more slowly. The massage prepares these tissues for the stress of the event, and then they are less likely to be injured. Postevent massage reduces soreness and cramping and helps retain flexibility.

Like myotherapy and deep tissue massage, sports massage also searches out trigger points to treat and will use other familiar techniques such as compression and cross fiber friction strokes. Sports massage may focus more specifically on certain areas of the athlete's body, such as the legs in cyclists or the arms and shoulders in tennis players. Although sports massage "feels" good, the prime focus is not a dreamy meditative experience as in some other massage forms. Sports massage has a mission, and the athletes tend to view it as part of a serious training program. Therefore, it tends to be focused on a certain area of the body and specialized to the performance demands of the athlete. However, some competitors have spoken of receiving several 2-hour sports massages between heavy workouts during a single day. Many sports teams have their own massage therapists traveling with them, and more often sports massage therapists are to be found at the end of long cycling and other amateur events as well. Exercise clubs and spas often have massage therapists on staff, although these may not all be trained specifically in sports massage. Swedish massage itself, for example, is relaxing and also comparable to a 3- or 4-mile walk.

For the noncompeting athlete, a sports massage therapist can give valuable instructions for self-care of sore shins, aching knees and feet, and other transient strains and how to avoid them in the future.

The cautions of when not to massage are no different for sports massage than any other, and some of the more general cautions would not even be considered because athletes are generally in good condition and not suffering from debilitating disease processes. Sports massage is contraindicated when pitting edema is present (for nonpitting edema and other swollen limbs massage is acceptable above the swelling and in the direction of the heart); if a person has high blood pressure or gastric or duodenal ulcers, the abdominal area needs to be avoided; if a person has cancer, TB, a high fever, or malignant or infectious conditions that could spread through the body, massage should also be avoided (in cancer patients when the spread of disease is not a consideration, light massage for comfort is not contraindicated); with blood vessel problems such as varicose veins, phlebitis, and even diabetes, massage therapists need to avoid the legs so as not to possibly break the vessels or dislodge a blood clot, which could have serious repercussions such as aneurysm or stroke; broken bones, cysts, breaks in the skin, and even bruises should be given a wide berth by massage therapists (for example, rubbing no closer than five or six inches from the injured area). It is also a good idea to avoid sports massage for subjects on pain medication, as these could mask pain and inadvertently have massage be too deep for tolerance or have trouble spots be missed by the therapist.

LESLIE AGUILLARD

SWEDISH MASSAGE

Massage has existed for thousands of years. Practitioners around the world administer assorted manipulations to the soft tissues of the body to help restore normal function as well as to maintain health and well-being. Although they primarily use their hands, they also may work with their forearms, elbows, or feet. The various movements directly and indirectly affect the body's systems—musculoskeletal, nervous, circulatory, digestive, and others. By both stimulating and relaxing them, the techniques assist the body to heal itself.

The practice of Swedish massage, as it is known in contemporary times, began in the ancient world. Greek, Roman, and Arabic physicians, such as Celsus, Galen, and Avicenna, recommended massage for everything from insomnia and indigestion to paralysis and gynecological problems, and for sports regimens. Their medical treatises influenced treatment protocols as late as the Renaissance. Hippocrates (ca. 460–ca. 377 B.C.), the father of Western medicine, is still quoted today on the importance of massage. In *On Articulations*, he wrote, "The physician must be experienced in many things, and among others, in friction. Friction can bind a joint that is too loose and loosen a joint that is too rigid."

As discoveries were made about human anatomy and physiology, including circulation of the blood by William Harvey in 1628, interest was revived in the therapeutic benefits of massage. Several physicians developed integrated systems of massage and exercise. The Swedish approach did not appear until 1813, when Per Henrik Ling (1776–1839) established the Royal Gymnastic Central Institute in Stockholm. His Swedish Movement Cure or Swedish Medical Gymnastics was a synthesis of earlier systems, including, some say, Eastern healing arts he supposedly learned in China. As Ling's ideas spread throughout Europe, they inspired others to spread the work. So-called Swedish massage became a remedial science. Many physicians in the United States wrote prolifically on its history, applications, treatment cases, and experiments regarding its physiology, and they prescribed it widely.

The classic Swedish massage consists of five procedures: effleurage, or stroking; petrissage, or kneading; friction, or rubbing; tapotement, or percussion; and vibration. Each one is executed differently, feels different to the receiver, and is employed for different reasons at different points during a session. Skilled practitioners work with great sensitivity of touch rather than a mechanical routine, for appropriate physical contact can be an important form of nonverbal communication with a powerful healing effect.

Effleurage involves smooth, long, and flowing strokes that can be performed with palms, finger pads, or forearms. When repeated rhythmically, they can feel like water gliding and rippling over the body. Because stroking soothes muscles and nerves, it can induce sleep and decrease pain. More firmly done in the direction of the heart, it stimulates circulation of blood and lymph. As fresh blood enters the tissues, more oxygen and other nutrients become available, while waste products are removed. Effleurage warms up and prepares the tissues for the other techniques.

Short and rapid percussive movements include hacking (with the outside edge of the hand), tapping (with fingertips), cupping or clapping (with cupped palms, fingers held close together), pummeling or beating (with loose or tight fists), and plucking (picking up or loosely pinching small patches of tissue between the thumb and forefinger). Tapotement is administered for a few seconds only to the fleshy areas of the body for its stimulating or toning effect. When applied to the upper back and chest, it can break up congestion

in the lungs. However, if prolonged, percussion can lead to overstimulation and exhaustion of nerves and muscles.

Friction is a series of circular, linear, or transverse strokes made with the thumb, fingertips, palm, or heel of the hand. With sufficient pressure, this form of rubbing can reach and spread muscle fibers and free muscles from adhesions and scar tissue developed after an injury. It also is useful in loosening joints and tendons.

In kneading, the practitioner lifts muscle away from bone and then squeezes, presses, and rolls it. By using both hands or thumbs alternately, it is possible to provide a continuous milking-like motion that flushes the tissue of fluids and metabolic by-products. This reduces edema and decongests muscles. For dancers and athletes, petrissage can be invigorating before performance and cleansing afterward to prevent soreness and stiffness.

To effect vibration, practitioners use one hand or fingertips to create a rapid trembling, shaking sensation. This technique stimulates nerves and relaxes tight muscles. When applied to the abdomen, it can activate the digestive organs.

In addition to these five movements, range of motion is often incorporated to help mobilize joints through rotation, flexion, and extension. This passive form of exercise along with massage can help keep unused muscles from atrophying and provide needed stimulation to all of the body's systems in nonambulatory patients.

Many hundreds of articles in medical journals of North America, Europe, and the former Soviet Union have documented the physiological and psychological benefits of massage. The Touch Research Institute at the University of Miami School of Medicine alone has conducted dozens of clinical trials demonstrating its broad versatility in helping to facilitate growth, attentiveness, and learning, alleviate pain, improve immune function, ameliorate stress, heal psychiatric problems, and overcome addiction.

For example, premature infants who receive daily massage gain more weight, leave the hospital sooner, and score better on development scales than unmassaged babies. Cocaine-exposed preterm infants also improve significantly, with fewer postnatal complications and stress behaviors. HIV patients experience a decrease in anxiety, stress, and cortisol levels with a corresponding increase in serotonin and natural killer cells, which are known to ward off cancer and viral cells. For women in labor, massage reduces pain and the need for medication, speeds up the progression of labor, minimizes the hospital stay, and lessens the possibility of postpartum depression. In the case of fibromyalgia, massage abates pain, improves sleep patterns, and diminishes levels of fatigue, anxiety, depression, and cortisol. Massage is known to trigger the body's innate ability to control pain naturally by stimulating the production of endorphins, opiate-like neuropeptides.

Other trials indicate that smokers who learn self-massage crave less intensely, smoke fewer cigarettes, and, in some cases, completely give them up. Following massage treatments, women suffering from premenstrual syndrome have less anxiety, pain, and water retention, and show improved mood. Child and adolescent psychiatric patients sleep better, exhibit less depression, have lower anxiety and stress hormone levels but higher body image scores, and make clinical progress. Depressed teenage mothers and adolescent girls with bulimia and anorexia display similar results.

Still other studies focus on migraine headaches, back pain, coma and spinal cord injuries, carpal tunnel syndrome, irritable bowel syndrome, cystic fibrosis, arthritis, hypertension, multiple sclerosis, depression, cerebral palsy, Down's syndrome, eczema and psoriasis, burns, diabetes, autism, posttraumatic stress disorder, ADHD, and more.

Because deep pressure, rubbing, and manipulation may aggravate certain conditions, massage is sometimes contraindicated. A highly trained massage therapist knows what to avoid entirely, when to modify pressure, how to work around rather than directly on the difficulty, and when to consult with a physician. Caution is advised in the following: broken bones, fractures, dislocations, or severe sprains; acute infection or inflammation; injury, abrasion, or disease of the skin; hemorrhaging; large hernias; cancerous tumors; torn ligaments, tendons, or muscles; cardiovascular conditions; advanced diabetes; osteoporosis; frostbite; kidney disease; and hypertension.

MIRKA KNASTER

See also
   AIDS/HIV (II)
   Anxiety/Panic (II)
   Depression (II)
   Eating Disorders (II)
   Fibromyalgia (II)
   Pain (II)
   Pregnancy (II)
   Premenstrual Syndrome (PMS) (II)

T'AI CHI

T'ai chi is a series of slow gentle movements designed to enhance mind and body function usually practiced outdoors. *T'ai chi* is a moving meditation, with each move having symbolic meaning. Since so many Chinese people practice *t'ai chi* every morning, it is believed to be the most widely practiced exercise in the world. All that is required to practice *t'ai chi* is within the student. There is no need for spoken word or music, just silence and space. Because of its gentle nature, *t'ai chi* is accessible to people of all ages. Practice of *t'ai chi* leads to both physical and mental well-being. The movements improve awareness of different body parts while having positive effects on the cardiovascular, skeletal, muscular, and nervous systems. Its tranquil nature also reduces stress and stress-related conditions.

Another health promoting aspect of *t'ai chi* is its ability to build internal strength through enhanced circulation of *qi*, the immaterial force of all living objects. This vital life force can become blocked, resulting in illness. *Qi* is expressed through the principles of yin and yang, the two polar forces that are opposing, yet complementary, and present in all living organism. *T'ai chi* works to keep the yin and yang energies balanced with the body, with a goal of achieving health and quality of life.

Several research studies have demonstrated the usefulness of *t'ai chi*. Jin (1992) assigned 48 male and 48 female *t'ai chi* practitioners to four treatment groups: *t'ai chi*, brisk walking, meditation, and neutral reading. Heart rate, blood pressure, and urinary catecholamine changes were similar to walking at a speed of 6km/hr and superior to neutral reading in the reduction of state anxiety and the enhancement of vigor. Since the subjects' high expectations could account for some gains, the researcher recommended further assessment. Province et al. (1995) used a preplanned

meta-analysis of seven frailty and injuries: Cooperative Studies of Intervention Techniques independent, randomized, controlled clinical trials that assessed the reduction of falls and frailty in elderly persons. All included an exercise component for 10 to 36 weeks with a 2- to 4-year follow-up. Participants ranged from 100 to 1,323 per study with a minimum age of 60. One of the exercise components was *t'ai chi*. They concluded that exercise, including *t'ai chi*, reduced the risk of falls.

Wolfson et al. (1996) evaluated the effects of *t'ai chi* and computerized balance training on frailty and falls. Two hundred persons aged 70 and older living in the community comprised the sample. Fear of falling responses and intrusiveness responses were reduced after the *t'ai chi* intervention compared with the balance training intervention. After adjusting for fall risk factors, *t'ai chi* was found to reduce the risk of multiple falls by 47.5%.

Wolf et al. (1997) explored whether *t'ai chi* or an educational computerized balance training group would affect the ability to minimize postural sway of 72 relatively inactive older people. *T'ai chi* was most helpful in promoting confidence about falls, but not in enhancing postural stability.

Lai et al. (1995) found that practicing *t'ai chi Chuan* regularly may delay the decline of cardiorespiratory function in older individuals. The researchers suggested that *t'ai chi* be prescribed as an aerobic exercise for older adults.

In 1991, Kirsteins and colleagues tested joint tenderness, joint swelling, time to walk 50 feet, hand-grip strength, and a written functional assessment for 11 people diagnosed with rheumatoid arthritis and compared them with a control group. They found *t'ai chi* safe for those with rheumatoid arthritis and suggested it be used as an alternative for their exercise therapy and become part of their rehabilitation program.

SANDRA VAN DE WEERD

THERAPEUTIC TOUCH: DEFINITION, HISTORY, AND THEORY

Therapeutic touch is a contemporary interpretation of several ancient healing practices that is an intentionally directed process of energy exchange during which the practitioner uses the hands as a focus to facilitate healing.

There are several key words in this definition, which comes from the Nurse Healers-Professional Associates (NH-PA). The predominant "ancient healing practices" referred to in therapeutic touch is the laying on of hands. However, therapeutic touch does not have a religious base. Therapeutic touch is a conscious, intentional act of compassion. Healing is used to mean strengthening one's connection with an inner sense of peace to facilitate wholeness of the body-mind.

Intention is of paramount importance with therapeutic touch. Thoughts are used with compassion in a goal-directed manner. The intention of connecting with the universal healing field is primary, coupled with the intent to help. The "hands" are the antennae to assess the energy field, and the mind makes sense of the sensations felt, colored by individual interpretations of reality. To facilitate gives the impression of assistance and support. The practitioner comforts with therapeutic touch; however, clients heal themselves.

The emphasis in therapeutic touch is on centering. The practitioner maintains the centered state throughout the therapeutic touch process. It is this ability to go within oneself and connect with what Dora Kunz, cofounder of therapeutic touch, calls the inner self, as well as connect with what is greater than ourselves, through nature, that allows the healing to happen with therapeutic touch. NH-PA (1992) defines centering as "bringing the body, mind and emotions to a quiet, focused state of consciousness." The other aspects of the Therapeutic Touch process that occur simultaneously with the advanced practitioner, are assessing, rebalancing and reassessment.

NH-PA defines assessment as "using the hands to determine the nature of the dynamic energy field. Sensory cues are intuitive as well as cognitive and vary for each practitioner." While the hands are the tools used to gather the information from the dynamic energy field, interpreting cues 2 to 6 inches from the body, it is the mind's interpretation of that information that determines the actions to assist the client in a therapeutic manner. The intention while assessing is to focus one's sensitivity in the subtle cues that the dynamic energy field radiates. These energetic cues may be interpreted through intuition, kinesthetic, auditory, or the visual sensory systems. Assessment is one of the skills within the therapeutic touch process that only develops over time and is one of the reasons that therapeutic touch is considered a discipline. Consistent practice 6 months to 1 year are necessary, according to NH-PA guidelines, to develop beginning skills. Practitioners with many years of consistent practice develop an unshakable confidence in the meaning of particular cues within themselves, as well as the cues perceived through the hands. The perception of a gentle symmetrical warmth is a common kinesthetic interpretation of the normal dynamic energy field. Most practitioners can easily develop the ability to notice temperature differentials when assessing the energy field.

The rebalancing aspect of therapeutic touch is defined by NH-PA as "facilitating the symmetrical and rhythmical flow of energy through the field by projecting, directing, and modulating energy based on the assessment, thereby assisting to reestablish the order in the system." It is necessary to mobilize the innate rhythm of the field when it is sluggish. This ensures that the dynamic field is open and communicating with its surrounding environment before instilling additional energy into the system. Therefore, the intent during the rebalancing aspect of therapeutic touch is to facilitate the wholeness and flow within the system. The client will spontaneously draw the energy through the practitioner, the centered instrument of peace, as necessary, into the areas of need. Simply be alert to when this flow is occurring and maintain a centered state of consciousness. Each intervention during the therapeutic touch process is based on the continuous reassessment of the energy field.

The final aspect of Therapeutic Touch is reassessment. NH-PA defines reassessment as "using professional, informed, and intuitive judgment to determine when to end a session." It is an ongoing process, it drives responses, intention, and knowledgeable interaction with the dynamic energy field. When the reassessment reveals the balanced, symmetrical, and rhythmical order within the system, there is no more repatterning necessary.

History

While observing the Hungarian healer named Estebany, as well as other renowned healers, Dora Kunz and Dolores Krieger were led to join, as an unlikely pair of healers, to start the therapeutic touch movement in 1972.

Dora Kunz, a natural healer, withstood criticism from other healers that ordinary people could not help heal. It was through Kunz's observations in the early 1970s that she realized that the ability to assist healing, in a manner such as the laying on of hands, was a natural human potential. Kunz invited anyone interested in learning about healing to a gathering at a theosophical encampment in Craryville, New York, in the summer of 1972. Krieger took this opportunity to bring her graduate students and engage in this learning activity as a group process. This is where the formal beginnings of therapeutic touch unfolded, in a tranquil natural setting known as Pumpkin Hollow Farm.

Krieger is responsible for naming the healing process "therapeutic touch." The name is a misnomer of sorts, because therapeutic touch does not require any physical touching.

Theory

Some of the theoretical frameworks that support therapeutic touch are: (1) science of unitary human beings developed by Martha Rogers; (2) human energy field model developed by Dora Kunz; (3) relativity and quantum field theory; and (4) psychoneuroimmunology.

Fundamental to the science of unitary human beings is the idea that all living systems are energy fields, integral with the environmental energy field. Within this conceptual system, nursing is viewed as the study of unitary and indivisible human and environmental fields. The NH-PA has identified four basic assumptions of therapeutic touch. The first assumption is that "people are open, complex, and pandimensional energy systems." This comes directly from the four fundamental precepts that Rogers's theory is based upon: first, that unitary human beings are energy fields and have a corresponding, adjoining, environmental energy field; second, these energy fields are open and infinite; third, these fields are identified by patterns that are continuously changing and becoming more complex and diverse; fourth, these fields are pandimensional or nonlinear and so are not limited by the characteristics of space or time. These precepts are reflected within the three general principles of homeodynamics. The principle of resonancy refers to the pattern of wave frequencies that are always changing within the energy field patterns of a person and the environment. The principle of helicy recognizes the continuously innovative, yet unpredictable propensity for diversity among the human and environmental energy field patterns. The last principle of integrality identifies the mutual and simultaneous human field and environmental field interaction that is always occurring.

Kunz's hypothesis of a human energy field model is congruent in many respects with the science of unitary human beings. It supports the first assumption of therapeutic touch, as well as two additional assumptions. According to NH-PA, the second assumption of therapeutic touch is that "in a state of health, life energy flows freely through the organism in a balanced, symmetrical manner." The third assumption of therapeutic touch is that healing is an in-trinsic movement toward order that occurs in living organisms and can be facilitated by practitioners. Life energy follows the intent to heal. This latter assumption emphasizes that therapeutic touch is a natural human potential. According to Kunz, the four interpenetrating human energy fields are in addition to the electromagnetic fields that surround all living matter. These four fields are the vital, emotional, mental, and intuitional fields.

The vital field is closely associated with the physical body. Each organ in the body actually has a corresponding energetic rhythm within this vital field, which usually extends 1 to 6 inches from the body. The emotional field is made up of feelings and has an elastic quality that allows it to be projected 18 to 48 inches from the body. When strong emotions are combined with thought and intention, this field can be projected 10 to 15 feet. The mental field is actually the personification of thinking and includes visual images, perceptions, and ideas. The intuitional field represents order, creativity, and compassion and is the source of healing. This intuitive or universal healing field, which permeates the whole universe, is what the practitioner makes the intent to connect with during the centering process.

Because therapeutic touch is an energetic intervention, it follows that the relativity and quantum field theories would provide additional frameworks of support. Einstein's relativity theory identifies energy as dynamic and recognizes that mass or matter is nothing but a form of energy. The idea that space and time are intimately connected and form a four-dimensional continuum called space time is a hallmark of relativity theory. When quantum field theory is combined with relativity theory, it describes the force fields of subatomic particles. The paradoxical nature of the world of subatomic particles reveals a basic oneness of the universe, while at the same time embracing the continuous change and rhythm inherent in individual particles. Another key component of quantum field theory is that consciousness is considered an essential feature. It is well recognized that the observer affects the observed during experimental situations.

The relatively new field of psychoneuroimmunology also supports the practice of therapeutic touch. Developments in this field indicate the reciprocal relationship among the nervous, endocrine, and immune systems of the body. The term "body-mind" emphasizes the intimate connection between the body and mind that occurs while communicating using the same peptide system throughout the body. This field substantiates how neuropeptides, as molecules of emotion, are able to move throughout the brain and body forming an intimate information system. New peptides made up of amino acids are continuing to be discovered that unlock the mystery of this communication. Psychoneuroimmunology indirectly supports the fourth and final basic assumption of therapeutic touch identified by the NH-PA, "that human beings are capable of both transformation and transcendence." The intimate connection of the mind and emotions allows individuals to adapt to a different way of looking at beliefs and attitudes. If one chooses to bring awareness to the motives of one's behavior and take the action to change, healing can occur.

BARBARA DENISON

See also
Centering: The Path to Healing Presence (IV)
Psychoneuroimmunology (IV)

THERAPEUTIC TOUCH: USES, RESEARCH, AND STANDARDS FOR PRACTICE

Therapeutic touch has a wide range of usefulness because of its soothing effect. One way this is accomplished is by stimulation of the body's parasympathetic branch of the autonomic nervous system (Krieger, 1993). Often this effect can be elicited within 3 to 5 minutes. Often pain can be diminished or even eliminated. The deep relaxation response that results from a therapeutic touch intervention allows for awareness of the body-mind connection. Extreme peace of mind permeates one's being when this unity is experienced. Calming of any anxiety is possible—for example, the anxiety surrounding a medical diagnosis, upcoming surgery, or lack of control associated with hospitalization.

As with any nursing or medical intervention, the client has the right to decline the intervention or treatment. The frequency and duration of a therapeutic touch session varies according to the assessment, which includes a holistic assessment, whenever possible. Usually 10 to 20 minutes is sufficient, allowing 5 to 10 minutes to rest afterward. Acute conditions may require more frequent and shorter interventions, while chronic conditions need regular consistent interventions over a period of time.

One way to categorize illness or conditions that can benefit from therapeutic touch, as demonstrated by anecdotal evidence from therapeutic touch practitioners, includes: (1) psychosomatic illnesses; (2) postoperative paralytic ileus; (3) circulatory disorders; (4) musculoskeletal problems; and (5) problems associated with impaired functioning of the immune system.

There are several factors that contribute to the individual responses to therapeutic touch. It really can't be predicted how therapeutic touch may help a client because the outcome is not in the practitioner's hands. The relationship among the client's values in general, belief in the intervention, and the ability to relax all contribute to the response. Synchronicity also is a key—if the timing is right and the person is receptive, a change may occur. It is possible, however, for a client to be skeptical of the intervention and still benefit from relief of the symptoms of pain or anxiety to some degree. For lasting effects, demonstrated by shifts in attitudes or changes in perceptions as well as physical responses, it is usually necessary for the client to recognize patterns in thinking and feeling that are not healthy. Such acknowledgment opens the door for the potential of healing.

Research

A biochemist (Grad, 1961 & 1963) at McGill University conducted a series of double blind experiments using the renowned healer, Oskar Estebany. The wounded mice and damaged barley seeds in Estebany's treatment group demonstrated a significantly accelerated healing process compared with control groups under similar conditions. An enzymologist (Smith, 1972) also worked with Estebany in double blind experiments using the enzyme trypsin. The activity of trypsin was significantly stimulated by Estebany's treatment compared with control groups in both its natural state and after being damaged by ultraviolet radiation.

The results of these studies, coupled with a study of Eastern literature and primitive cultures, led Krieger to hypothesize that hemoglobin would be a sensitive indicator of energy exchange. The similarity in function and chemical structure of hemoglobin and chlorophyll, and the fact that both are dependent on enzyme activity, contributed to her decision to use hemoglobin as the dependent variable in her studies. The initial pilot study involved Estebany as the healer (Krieger, 1972). The results showed significant increased mean hemoglobin scores in the clients treated with the laying on of hands. This pilot study was replicated as a full-scale study (Krieger, 1973 & 1976), controlling for additional intervening variables, because of the criticism surrounding the original research quality. Each replicated study supported that therapeutic touch increased mean hemoglobin values in the recipients.

Krieger then replicated the original laying on of hands studies with an important difference (Krieger, 1975). Registered nurses were substituted in the role of healer, who had learned the intervention from Dora Kunz or Dolores Krieger. The results still showed a significant increase in posttest mean hemoglobin values in the group treated by therapeutic touch. While critics reported that it was nothing more than the placebo effect, studies began to be developed that attempted to control for this effect. These studies supported the beneficial effect that therapeutic touch had in clinical situations. Although the exact mechanism of how therapeutic touch worked could not be specifically demonstrated, it was evident by the mounting support from the clinical studies that it was able to effect, at the very least, the relaxation response to decrease state trait anxiety as perceived by the recipients of this healing process. The theories supporting therapeutic touch as an energy exchange remain hypothetical in the Western scientific community.

Early studies provided support that therapeutic touch significantly reduced state trait anxiety (Heidt, 1981; Quinn, 1982). Both studies involved cardiovascular hospitalized clients. Heidt's study divided 90 clients into three groups. One group received casual touch by a nurse taking pulses, one group received no touch, one group received therapeutic touch. Each intervention lasted only 5 minutes, and the group receiving therapeutic touch showed a significantly larger decrease in anxiety compared with the other groups. Quinn replicated Heidt's study, using 60 similar clients. Again the intervention only lasted 5 minutes; however, a mimic intervention was designed. This control group consisted of nurses who had no knowledge of therapeutic touch and performed the hand gestures while mentally counting backward by 7 from 100. According to the Spielberger State-Trait Anxiety Scale, the same measurement scale used in Heidt's study, the group receiving therapeutic touch demonstrated significant decrease in the anxiety scores.

In relation to research studying therapeutic touch and pain, there are three studies to mention. A study that evaluated tension headache pain treated with therapeutic touch (Keller, 1986) on 60 volunteers showed, with a reliable tool to measure pain, that 90% of the experimental group receiving therapeutic touch interventions had a significant decrease in the headache pain compared with the mimic group. A study that reexamined the effect of therapeutic touch on acute abdominal or pelvic pain in 159 postoperative clients (Meehan, 1993) demonstrated the potentiation effect of therapeutic touch when used with analgesia. One group received therapeutic touch and PRN pain agent, one group re-

ceived mimic therapeutic touch and PRN pain agent, and one group received routine nursing care. The experimental group received seven therapeutic touch interventions and waited a significantly longer time before requesting more medication compared with the mimic group. A study on the effect of therapeutic touch and clients experiencing burns (Clark, 1997) that involved 99 clients evaluated whether therapeutic touch would decrease pain and anxiety. It was a single blinded randomized clinical trial. This study showed significant decrease in pain and anxiety in the group receiving therapeutic touch according to the McGill Pain Questionnaire Pain Rating Index and Number of Words Chosen and the Visual Analogue Scale for Anxiety. There was also effect on T-cells in 10 subjects in the therapeutic touch group showing a lower total CD8 + lymphocyte concentration.

Research on the effects on wound healing in deltoid dermal wounds and therapeutic touch (Wirth, 1990 & 1993) demonstrated significantly faster wound healing in the experimental therapeutic touch group. These were well-developed, double blind studies that controlled for the placebo effect. The control group received no treatment. In the first study, 16 consecutive daily interventions of 5-minute duration were given. The wounds were 10 times smaller in the experimental group on day 8 and on day 16, 13 of the 23 treated subject's wounds were totally healed. None of the wounds in the control group had closed completely. The replicated study evaluated wound reepitheliazation on days 5 and 10. The experimental group had five unhealed wounds on day 5 compared with 12 in the control group. The experimental group had two unhealed wounds on day 10 compared with eight in the control group.

A pilot study (Quinn, 1993) with grieving individuals indicated the area of immune response and therapeutic touch needed further research. An expert practitioner of therapeutic touch was shown to have almost half the percentage of suppressor T-cells as the individual treated. The recipients all demonstrated decreased percentages of suppressor T-cells following a course of seven therapeutic touch treatments over 10 days. No definitive conclusions can be made based on this pilot data.

A recent pilot study (Olson, 1997) on medical and nursing students with documented stress prior to taking professional board examinations was funded by the Office of Alternative Medicine. The experimental group received three therapeutic touch interventions the week prior to exams, while the control group received none. The results demonstrated a change in the humoral immunity component reflected by significant differences in levels of immunoglobulins IgA, IgG, and IgM. There was also change in the anticipated direction in cell mediated immunity as measured by CD4. While not enough to be significant, a subsequent similar study demonstrated the significant change in the CD4 level. One purpose of this study was to develop a model that could be used to study a variety of stress-reduction interventions to determine efficacy of their use in individuals who are stressed.

There are multiple dissertation abstracts studying the effect of therapeutic touch. One study (Garrard, 1995) looked at the effect of therapeutic touch on stress reduction and immune function in persons with AIDS. Results showed significant difference in the CD4 counts indicating increased lymphocyte subset pattern. In addition, an increase in coping skills was reflected by a significant difference in response on the Coping Resource Inventory for Stress tool.

Another pilot study (Robinson, 1995) investigating the effects of therapeutic touch on grief demonstrated the experimental therapeutic touch group showed a greater decrease over time in social isolation, loss of control, and somatization. There were more frequent reported favorable effects on their grief by the therapeutic touch group.

A pilot study (Woods, 1996) studying the effect of therapeutic touch on disruptive behaviors of individuals with dementia of the Alzheimer type showed a significant decrease in three of the six behaviors monitored. There was a decrease in the frequency and intensity of the searching and wandering, vocalization, and manual manipulation behaviors.

There is a growing number of qualitative research studies on therapeutic touch that consider the effect on the practitioner as well as the client when involved in the healing process. A qualitative study (Heidt, 1990) revealed that therapeutic touch is a healing interaction significantly affecting both the practitioner and the client. The core variable that linked the experiences of both was described by the term "opening." In the process of giving and receiving therapeutic touch, nurses and clients described their experiences as an "opening intent," "opening communication," and "opening sensitivity." Both the practitioner and client described what seemed to be a transfer of energy taking place on a physical as well as a psychological level during the healing interaction. Another phenomenological study about the experience of receiving therapeutic touch (Samarel, 1992) showed that it was perceived as a fulfilling, multidimensional experience that facilitated personal growth.

Additional basic research would be useful to influence the traditional medical establishment's decision to accept therapeutic touch. However, the substantial clinical research, at the very least, adequately supports the use of therapeutic touch as a comfort, relaxation intervention.

Standards/Criteria

The NH-PA has established guidelines and curricula for teaching therapeutic touch at the beginning, intermediate, and advanced levels. Teachers of therapeutic touch must meet established guidelines and criteria to be referred to as a recognized and qualified therapeutic touch teacher. This peer review process is the closest thing to a certification process that exists for therapeutic touch teachers.

There is currently no certification process for therapeutic touch practitioners. The NH-PA proclaims that the interior process involved in the healing act makes it difficult to contain it to any form of certification. The professional nursing license, for those that practice therapeutic touch who are nurses, is the credential that is necessary. The NH-PA has developed standards of therapeutic touch practitioners and recommended scope of practice for therapeutic touch. In addition, the recommended guidelines suggested by NH-PA for therapeutic touch workshop attendance and consistent therapeutic touch practice ensures the practitioner is providing safe and knowledgeable therapeutic touch.

Therapeutic touch can be practiced by nurses once they have completed an opti-

mum of a 12- or a minimum of a 6-hour program by recognized therapeutic touch teachers. NH-PA can recommend qualified therapeutic touch teachers from among its membership. NH-PA can also refer therapeutic touch practitioners without endorsement because it is the responsibility of the consumer to evaluate the efficacy of the practitioner.

A minimum guideline of consistent practice averaging two times a week is recommended for a therapeutic touch practitioner. The cost of the intervention varies by regional area, practitioner's values and experience, and whether other healing modalities are integrated into the session. Therapeutic touch does integrate with established complementary and traditional interventions. If assessment indicates benefit in combining interventions with therapeutic touch, it needs to be with clarity of intention, awareness, and permission by the client and use of each modality within its original discipline.

There are many other disciplines besides nursing that practice therapeutic touch, as well as non-health care professionals and members of the public. Each discipline is responsible for developing its own standards of care for therapeutic touch.

BARBARA DENISON

THERAPEUTIC TOUCH IN THE HOSPITAL SETTING

Therapeutic touch was initially taught by nurses, to nurses and many consumers have had their first experience with therapeutic touch in the hospital setting. However, the provision of therapeutic touch has generally been happenstance (i.e., if one was fortunate enough to have a nurse that practiced therapeutic touch, then one received treatment). In the past several years, as complementary adjunctive treatments are requested more by consumers, nurses at many hospitals have been working to develop provider systems to identify hospitalized individuals who could benefit from therapeutic touch and deliver the service in a coordinated manner.

The provision of therapeutic touch in a hospital setting is a grassroots movement, usually generated by a small group of staff aware of the benefits of this intervention. The development of an institutional therapeutic touch program is a natural result of living the therapeutic touch lifestyle. By practicing therapeutic touch three to five times a week, the practitioner's life changes in a direction of self-growth and increased awareness of both an inner micro flow of energy and an outer macro energy flow. An inner knowing of what one must do in one's life emerges along with the strength and intuition to proceed. By initially focusing on the individual practice of therapeutic touch with clients or colleagues, a natural progression of comfort and expertise occurs. Natural curiosity and positive results lead colleagues to inquire more about the therapeutic touch process and how they might obtain training. Word spreads quickly among both staff and patients, and soon requests for treatments start coming in.

Working with administration is another exercise in the therapeutic touch lifestyle of speaking one's truth, which can be a bit scary at times. However, with a strong background of positive clinical results, high patient satisfaction, and current research, therapeutic touch providers are finding it easier to gain the ear of administration.

Building support for the development of a therapeutic touch program in a hospital takes personal time and commitment. Offering inservices and providing education at a lecture series can introduce other health care providers to the benefits of therapeutic touch. Demonstrations at the educational sessions are invaluable in providing personal experience of the effects of therapeutic touch. In building the therapeutic touch program at one medical center, classes were offered through the Education Department in beginning level therapeutic touch. This process has spread knowledge and respect throughout the hospital, as well as given staff the tools needed to begin practice.

Therapeutic touch is also a staff morale builder. Encouraging staff to provide treatments to each other for stress, headaches, and so on strengthens sharing and caring behaviors toward one another. Early research on the effects of therapeutic touch on practitioners indicates an improved immune response for both practitioners and clients (Quinn & Strelkauskas, 1993). Anecdotal reports from colleagues providing therapeutic touch in hospital settings indicate that the "mood" of an entire unit seems to be calmer and more focused when therapeutic touch is being integrated into care. This translates into fewer patients turning on call lights, fewer somatic complaints (that may really be calls for individual acknowledgment and reassurance), and fewer employee sick days. Many therapeutic touch practitioners believe burnout can be prevented by staff caring for each other and creating an environment that replenishes the caregiver.

Introducing therapeutic touch in a hospital setting involves risk taking and nonattachment to ego. Many administrators may allow therapeutic touch on a trial or limited basis but not allocate resources to deliver the intervention in a coordinated manner. It takes a strong commitment to the therapeutic touch lifestyle to trust in the therapeutic touch process and not force one's will into the situation. Just as therapeutic touch works on many levels in a gradually healing way, so the development of a therapeutic touch program occurs on many levels, often seeming to move itself along. Therapeutic touch involves a new model of working with others, a model with relationship, compassion, attention, and intention at its core, rather than mechanistically performed tasks focused on pathology or organ systems. As a holistic modality, therapeutic touch often evokes a sense of the sacred; patients and providers both routinely comment on the spiritual aspect of therapeutic touch practice, which goes beyond religious dogma and touches a very personal spirituality many never knew they had. Therapeutic touch practitioner and author Janet Quinn (1992) names this aspect of practice "holding sacred space." Several hospital chaplains have recognized therapeutic touch as a healing practice that is appropriately offered by their volunteer visitors, providing a ministering to spirit as well as to the body.

The practice of therapeutic touch in a hospital setting can be found throughout the hospital. At one facility, a large VA Medical Center, therapeutic touch is practiced on acute wards for pain control, anxiety, and insomnia. The pain clinic physician refers patients to the therapeutic touch clinic (an outpatient clinic). In the extended care/long-term care inpatient program, therapeutic touch is used in wound care, pain control, anxiety, emotional pain, and insomnia. The hospice unit has integrated therapeutic touch into its daily comfort care for clients and their families. Other hospitals have found the benefits of using therapeutic touch in the perioperative period reflected in a reduction of stress and improved pain control.

As a nursing intervention, the provision of therapeutic touch does not need a doctor's order. Consults to providers are usually nurse-to-nurse, although physicians who have seen the benefit of therapeutic touch also send in consultation requests. For new consults, providers can attach an educational handout to their consultation report providing an explanation of the intervention. Therapeutic touch providers also are aware they are educators and provide on-the-spot inservices to curious staff. Explanations to staff physicians are tailored to their approach to medicine. Most physicians are aware of the research documenting the effects of stress on the physical body and accept therapeutic touch as a means of stress reduction. Other physicians, embracing the ideas of holistic health, have been extremely supportive and encouraging to the practitioners.

In a holistic environment, healing is everyone's responsibility. In therapeutic touch classes, staff nurses, physicians, psychologists, psychiatrists, social workers, nurses aides, nurse educators, nurse practitioners, laboratory and imaging personnel, secretarial staff, and hospital volunteers have been taught the procedure. Support has come from these disciplines, as well as from the medical library, which has ordered several books and a videotape series on therapeutic touch. In establishing a program in a hospital, it is important to realize that allies can be found everywhere and any and all services can help smooth the way for the development of a therapeutic touch program.

KATHLEEN S. FASNACHT

THERAPEUTIC WRITING AND IMMUNE FUNCTION

When individuals undergo traumatic or difficult events in their lives, the overwhelming majority of them will turn to another to tell them about it. It seems to be a natural inclination. And while many can bemoan heavy traffic or an overbearing boss without hesitation, there is no easy time to talk about a history of rape or a regretted affair. The keeping of such secrets is both psychologically and physically taxing, placing a chronic, low-level stress on the body. The inhibition of emotionally charged information is associated with markedly higher sympathetic nervous system activity, intrusive thoughts, cognitive vigilance, changes in immune function markers, and increased illness rates (Pennebaker, 1989; Petrie et al., 1995). The obvious question, then, is how can individuals confront these issues without risking the social repercussions of making troublesome topics public? Disclosure through writing offers a kind of analog to psychotherapy, a private means of reducing the stress of emotional memories.

Research Basis of Written Disclosure

The contemporary version of this type of stress-relieving practice was developed and investigated by James W. Pennebaker in the early 1980s. Having witnessed the physiological and psychological effects of criminal confessions, Pennebaker reasoned that many individuals with no criminal history nevertheless might have aspects or events in their personal histories that would be difficult to discuss with others. These issues, in turn, might take a toll on physical health. Quite possibly, then, individuals who *wrote* about traumatic events or upsetting issues might experience health improvements without the social risks (such as judgment, awkwardness, or recrimination) associated with confiding in another.

To test the hypothesis, Pennebaker and colleagues recruited the participation of 80 college undergraduates in an investigation of the health effects of writing exercises. One group was asked to write about their "deepest thoughts and feelings surrounding the most upsetting event or issue you have ever faced." The control group was asked to write about a trivial, nonemotional topic. A third group was asked to write about only their feelings surrounding the topic. In the 3-month follow-up period, the group that expressed both their thoughts and feelings about emotional topics made significantly fewer health center visits for illness than the other groups (Pennebaker, 1989). Pennebaker and others began to search for possible mediating mechanisms, such as autonomic nervous system measures and immune function markers, that would explain the health impact of putting stress into words.

Pennebaker teamed up with two leading researchers in PNI, Janice Kiecolt-Glaser and her husband Ronald Glaser of Ohio State University, to attempt to identify the immune system repercussions of emotional disclosure. Students again were asked to write about either upsetting events or trivial topics and were asked for blood samples before and after writing. Those who wrote about upsetting topics showed better proliferative responses to a number of antigenic challenges than did those who wrote about emotionally neutral topics (Pennebaker, Kiecolt-Glaser, & Glaser, 1988). Finally, in an effort to improve the methodology, a later study was conducted to assess the impact of disclosure on *in vivo* measures of immune function, specifically, response to a hepatitis B vaccination series. Again, emotionally relevant writing subjects showed higher responses to the series than did controls (Petrie, Booth, Pennebaker, Davison, & Thomas, 1995). Furthermore, disclosure of emotional topics issued in dramatic reductions in skin conductance levels, one measure of sympathetic nervous system arousal associated particularly with the stress of inhibiting information. These and similar findings (e.g., Esterling, Antoni, Fletcher, Margulies, & Schneiderman, 1994) pointed to writing as a potent means of relieving the stress of one's personal past in a way that enhances physical health and functioning.

Scope and Nature of Disclosure

Written disclosure exercises should not be confused with the popular conceptualization of journaling. The exercises that issued in reduced nervous system arousal and enhanced health were emotionally engrossing, complete, repeated engagements with painful episodes of subjects' lives. Instructions to subjects were roughly as follows: "For the next 20 minutes, I want you to write about the most upsetting event or issue you have ever faced. Don't worry about grammar, spelling, punctuation, or anything else, just let go and explore your feelings about this difficult time. If you run out of things to write about, just continue writing until the time is up."

In most cases, subjects were asked to continue writing about the same topic for 3 or 4 consecutive days. Related studies have found that reexposure to an upsetting event issues in reduced arousal associated with that event. Writing about upsetting experiences repeatedly, then, encourages a cognitive restructuring of the memory. This cognitive restructuring seems to have several important results. First, the memories elicit less nervous system arousal over time, suggesting that the event's impact on physiology is changed in the process. Second, subjects report that, despite the distressing nature of the exercise, they find it a valuable way to find meaning and hope in even the most difficult of circumstances. Finally, the repetition and restructuring seem to diminish the implicit social barrier that exists when one wants to discuss important topics but can't.

Uses for Disclosure Exercises

Writing about traumatic events for brief periods over consecutive days is a potentially powerful therapeutic tool that takes advantage of individuals' natural tendency to talk about emotional events and to search for meaning in their lives. Samples of HIV+ patients, laid-off executives, college students, and arthritis patients have participated in formal studies of disclosure that have yielded beneficial effects. The advantages of disclosure exercises include low cost, freedom of setting, self-selected topics, and value to participants. Disadvantages would include emotional distress that might accompany the disclosure process, the possibility of lack of benefits, and poor ability to control "dosage"—that is, some individuals have real issues and memories to work through, while others are not engaged by such an exercise.

Disclosure through writing differs from many other complementary health practices in that it is a general, not a specific, prescription. As a health practice, though, it is of sound value. People who are faced with chronic or life-threatening illnesses are confronted with many psychological challenges that go beyond their choice of treatment options. They want to process and understand the role of the illness in their lives. Through writing they can develop conceptions of the cause and the impact, expectations about their own role in disease course, and visions about how their lives might differ in the future. Moreover, the writing exercises are a valuable means of self-expression for individuals whose styles of practices are shunned by their surrounding social network. Minorities, homosexuals, alcoholics, and other marginalized groups may reduce the sense of barrier between themselves and their surroundings by making sense of their lives through writing. Finally, a number of popular authors have asserted that writing in general is a tool for self-discovery and expression that is essential to the unfoldment of one's optimal work (Goldberg, 1986). Even for those whose immune systems are compromised beyond repair, writing offers a practice that heals in the absence of a cure.

KATHRYN P. DAVISON

TOUCH THERAPY RESEARCH

Touch therapy, or massage therapy, is defined as manipulation of body tissues by the hands for wellness and the reduction of stress and pain. Its therapeutic effects derive from its impact on the muscular, nervous, and circulatory systems. Massage therapy sessions usually combine several techniques, including Swedish massage (stroking and kneading), shiatsu (pressure points), and neuromuscular massage (deep pressure). Oils are typically used and aromatic essences are often added for an additional effect. The sessions also feature soft backup music, usually classical or new age music.

The practice of massage has been in the world before recorded time. The word "massage" can be found in many classic texts, including the Bible and the Ayurveda. Hippocrates, as early as 400 B.C., talked about the necessity of physicians being experienced in the art of rubbing. Ancient records from China and somewhat later from Japan refer to massage therapy, and it was also widely used by other early cultures, including Arabs, Egyptians, Indians, Greeks, and Romans. During the Renaissance, massage spread throughout Europe, and Swedish massage was developed early in the 19th century.

Based on existing research, fibromyalgia clients who receive massage therapy are expected to show improved mood state and affect and decreased anxiety and stress hormone levels (salivary cortisol) (Sunshine et al., 1996). These changes have been highly significant based on observations of the client, self-reports by the client, and saliva assays for cortisol. In addition, whenever EEG is recorded, changes occur in the direction of heightened alertness. Longer-term changes also measured in research have typically been evaluated after 46 weeks of treatment. These changes invariably include a decrease in depression, improved sleep patterns, lower stress (as measured by urinary cortisol, norepinephrine, and epinephrine levels), and enhanced immune function (an increase in natural killer cells) (Ironson et al., 1996). Changes have also been noted on clinical measures that are specific to different conditions or considered by clinicians to be gold standards for those conditions. For example, increases have been noted in pulmonary functions including peak air flow for children with asthma, and decreased blood glucose levels have been reported for children with diabetes following 1 month of massage. Another example is a significant increase in weight gain in premature infants given 10 days of massage (Field et al., 1986). These changes are unique to these conditions and would not be expected to occur generally across medical conditions.

Although the primary indications have been for wellness and stress and pain reduction, there are many other ways in which massage therapy is clinically useful, including the following: (1) pain reduction during painful procedures such as childbirth labor and massage therapy prior to debridement for burn patients; (2) pain reduction in chronic pain conditions such as fibromyalgia, premenstrual syndrome, lower back pain, and migraine headaches; (3) the alleviation of depression and anxiety, for example in bulimia, anorexia, and chronic fatigue; (4) stress reduction, including job stress and separation stress; (5) immune disorders including HIV where there is an increase of natural killer cells, which are the front line of the immune system and ward off viral cells and cancer cells and for the autoimmune conditions already mentioned including diabetes and asthma.

Although some therapists have warned of contraindications for massage, there is virtually no research supporting therapists' concerns about these contraindications, including (1) infectious or contagious skin conditions, (2) high fever, (3) scar tissue, (4) varicose veins, and (5) tumors.

Many massage therapists are located in private clinics in the community, or they have treatment rooms in their own homes. They can also be found in spas, workout clubs, hair salons, hotels, airports, and even at car washes in some cities. Finally, they can be hired to come to your own home with a portable table or a portable chair. Unfortunately, although massage therapy used to be routinely practiced in hospitals (as recently as the 1950s), it is rarely seen in hospitals today. The costs are relatively low ($1 per minute is the going rate) and the therapy has been shown to be cost-effective. For example, $4.7 million per year could be saved in medical costs if all premature infants were massaged. That figure derives from 470,000 infants who are born prematurely each year being massaged and discharged 6 days early, at a hospital cost savings of $10,000 per infant. Similarly, using senior citizen volunteers as therapists for infants has been cost-effective and has resulted in lower stress hormones and fewer trips to the doctors' office following 1 month of the therapists' massaging the infants. Similar cost-effective figures are likely to emerge for other conditions since they too benefit significantly from the stress-reduction effects of massage therapy. The therapy lowers stress hormones (cortisol), which in turn enhances immune function resulting in less illness and greater wellness.

TIFFANY FIELD

TRAGER APPROACH

As a young man, Milton Trager spontaneously discovered a way to relieve muscle soreness and joint pain. It began as an intuitive approach that focused on the mind and body connection. As he refined this approach, he affirmed the intuitive aspect and diminished the importance of technique. The Trager approach to psychophysical integration evolved over Trager's lifetime to include a hands-on mode and a movement awareness mode.

His desire to understand more about the mind and body connections led Trager to study medicine. After he became a physician, he applied this approach to many chronic and acute conditions with much success. Other individuals became interested in learning this approach. In conveying the mind-set an individual must achieve to be effective in applying this approach, Trager accentuated the importance of a subtle mental connection between the client and the practitioner. He called this connection "hook-up." While he acknowledged that the physical application was important, he stressed it was the mind of the client that did the work. According to Trager, "In order to make changes in the body we have to reach the mind and to reach the mind we go through the body."

In 1980, The Trager Institute for Psychophysical Integration opened in Mill Valley, California. It is a nonprofit educational corporation that serves to protect the registered names of *Trager* and *Mentastics*, the movement awareness mode. Information dissemination, training, and certification of Trager practitioners are also provided. Individuals who provide the Trager approach to the public must be current members and licensees of the institute.

Description

A hands-on session begins with hook-up, a contemplative mental state that allows connection with the subtle energy forces surrounding and within the body. The touch is light and noninvasive, involving a sequence of gentle rocking and rhythmic movements. This encourages a deepening state of relaxation, a lengthening of the musculature, and a sense of freedom of movement. During this positive subtle communication with the central nervous system, information about the range of movement minus stress or pain is presented. A usual session lasts about 75 minutes. It is concluded with a short Mentastics session. This assists the client in developing an awareness of the fundamental ability to access and affect sensory input through movement.

"Mentastics" is a word coined by Trager from the words "mental" and "gymnastics." It is a series of flowing movements that assist the client in recalling the feeling of movement experienced during the hands-on session. Visualization and imagery are used to encourage expansive movements that become lighter and freer through repetition. It provides a self-directed way to repattern the restricted movements that have created discomfort and pain. The aim is to allow these movements to happen effortlessly. Clients are encouraged to continue these series of movements at home or in a Mentastics class.

Application

The Trager approach has been used to assist individuals with neurological disorders. As an adjunct therapy in the treatment of cerebral palsy, muscular dystrophy, Parkinson's Disease, and others, the effect is an increase in the range of motion. In the treatment of chronic spinal pain associated with surgery or trauma, there is reduction of pain and increased mobility.

As a complementary practice in the treatment of many other medical and psychological disorders, the Trager approach has proven effective in enhancing the mobility of the client and reducing the emotional triggers that often accompany them. The subtlety of the work bypasses the client's initial resistance and allows a sensory-motor new message to be patterned.

Theories

There are several theories applicable in the understanding of how the Trager approach works. Theories relating to the sensory-motor feedback loop; to the reflex response; to biochemical processes; and those concerning the role of neurotransmitters in affecting mood all interact to explain the mind-body connection. It is this connection that is addressed by bodywork in general and by the Trager approach in a soft, effortless manner.

ROBERTA CIROCCO
REGINA KUJAWSKI

TRANSCENDENTAL MEDITATION

The transcendental meditation (TM) program is a simple mental technique practiced 20 minutes in the morning and evening. It works by allowing the mind to relax and experience the least excited state of consciousness, pure consciousness (PC). Wallace has referred to this silent state as a fourth major state of consciousness, an addition to the commonly known states of waking, dreaming, and sleeping, because of the profound psychological and physiological differences between these states. The simplest way to understand the state of PC is to connect it with the other known states of consciousness. The descriptions from sleep and dreaming are from normative data, and the data on TM and waking are from research on the TM program. Based on this data, PC is a low-arousal, high-consciousness state.

PC has been described in religious and philosophical literature for centuries throughout the world as a "state of knowing" or a "state of grace." Plato discussed PC in his classic text, The Republic. TM comes from an ancient tradition that is thousands of years old, and according to Maharishi Mahesh Yogi, the teacher who brought this knowledge to the world, it is timeless and transcends culture because it has its basis in the very functioning of life itself. Travis has shown that pure consciousness occurs in everyone several times a day for a few seconds at the transition point between waking and sleeping, and sleeping and dreaming. It also occurs naturally in individuals with very pure nervous systems. Normally, when an individual is awake, he or she is focusing attention outward through the senses. In TM, a sound with a known positive effect, a mantra, is used to allow awareness to turn inward and focus on itself. PC is described as a state where consciousness experiences its own essential nature.

During the practice of TM, the mind settles down into a silent state, and the body's internal repair mechanisms are turned on to repair the body in a manner similar to what occurs in deep sleep. This is how the physiological benefits of the TM program occur.

Scientific Research on Transcendental Meditation

The TM technique has been tested in over 500 scientific studies at more than 200 in-

TABLE 1   Comparison of Four States of Consciousness on Various Psychophysiological Characteristics

	DEEP SLEEP	DREAMING	WAKING	PC
EEG Pattern	In stage 2, 12–14 Hz spindles and K complexes. In stage 3 & 4 at least 50% delta waves.	Stage 1 REM: Low voltage desynchronized sawtooth waves. Stage 2, 12–14 Hz spindles and K complexes.	Primarily beta, in activity, Eyes closed is low voltage mixed frequency and/or alpha (9–11 Hz—eyes closed).	Predominance of high amplitude alpha and theta with synchronous alpha, theta, and beta spindles occurring.
Subject reports	No awareness	Illusory awareness	Awareness of percepts, thoughts.	Aware of silence in thought and mind
Breath Pattern	Steady, shallow	Erratic and highly variable.	Changes according to the activity.	Very light with virtual suspensions observed in some people.
Heart rate	Lowest level in circadian cycle.	Usually slight increase above sleep. Erratic.	Variable	↓ significantly
Plasma cortisol	↓ Slightly	Slight ↓	Baseline	↓ significantly
Plasma lactate	Unknown	Unknown	Baseline	↓ significantly
Plasma prolactin	Increases gradually	↑ gradually	Baseline	↑ significantly
Plasma phenylalanine	↓ slightly	↓ slightly	Baseline	↑ significantly
Plasma TSH	Unchanged	Unchanged	Baseline	↓ significantly
Seroton	During night sleep cycle it peaks	Increases REM sleep parallels increase serotonergic activity	Relaxed state associated with increased serotonergic activity	Higher than during relaxed waking.
Blood flow to the brain	Unchanged	Acute ↑ during REM sleep.	Baseline	Redistribution of blood flow away from abdomin toward the brain.

Compiled from data in Wallace, R. K. (1986), *Neurophysiology of Enlightenment* (Fairfield, IA: MIU Press) and in Alexander, C. N., Cranson, R. W., Boyer, R. W., & Orme-Johnson, D. W. (1987), Transcendental consciousness: a fourth state of consciousness beyond sleep, dreaming, and waking. In J. Gackenbach (ed.), *Sleep and Dreams: A Sourcebook* (New York: Garland Publishing, Inc., 282–315).

dependent research institutions in 30 countries. One reason why the TM technique has been so thoroughly researched is that it is systematically taught by highly qualified teachers. It also produces dramatic and easy to reproduce results.

TM is a powerful proof of mind-body connection theories and it is easy to research. TM improves both mental and physical health by connecting the mind with its essential innermost nature, the field of pure consciousness, the source of

TABLE 2   Summary of Major Areas of Research on Transcendental Meditation

	AREA RESEARCHED	RESULT
Mental Health	Increased intelligence	Students at MIU increased significantly in intelligence over a 2-year period, compared to control subjects from another Iowa university.
	Increased creativity	Torrance Tests of Creative Thinking measured figural and verbal creativity in matched control and experimental group and the TM group improved significantly.
	Improved moral behavior and advanced ego development	Erickson's and Lovinger's Developmental Scales showed that very long term meditators scored at levels significantly above the mean for the general population.
	Decreased anxiety, improved self-esteem	375 studies were reviewed in a meta-analysis and showed that the TM program was significantly more effective in producing improvements in self-esteem and decreases in anxiety than other techniques for self-development.
	Decreased psychological ill health	Review of Swedish National Health Board Records showed the incidence of admission to psychiatric care units was approximately 150–200 times less for meditators than for the general population.
Substance Abuse and Crime	Decreased use of alcohol, cigarettes, and addictive drugs	A statistical meta-analysis of 198 independent treatment outcomes indicated that TM produced a significantly larger reduction in tobacco, alcohol, and illicit drug use, from 51%–89% over an 18–22 month period.
	Decreased criminal behavior	A nationwide prison project in Senegal Africa, indicated a Reduced National Recidivism Rate-over 70% decrease in prison return rates.
Physical Health	Decrease Blood Pressure	Over a 3-month interval, systolic and diastolic blood pressure dropped by 10.6 and 5.9 mm Hg, respectively, in the TM group, and 4.0 and 2.1. mm Hg in the PMR group, with virtually no change in the usual care group.
	Decrease Blood Cholesterol	In a random assignment study, initial serum levels of both groups were the same TM decreased to 225 ± 9.4 mg/100ml compared to their own baseline Controls remained at baseline with 259 ± 8.9 mg/100ml.
	Increases in DHEAS	LT meditators had the same level of DHEAS in their blood as an individual five to ten years younger.
	Increased in the life expectancy	LT meditators were 5 years were physiologically 12 years younger than their chronological age.
	Decreased Medical Care Utilization	Medical care utilization decreased 50% for meditators compared to a matched control group.

(continued)

TABLE 2   (*continued*)

	AREA RESEARCHED	RESULT
Sociological Health	Improvements in family life	Taylor Johnson Temperament Analysis Benefits for Married Couples found that many of the major characteristics needed for stable marriages such as the ability to be understanding increased with long term TM.
Maharishi Effect	Decrease in violence in a society	Time series analysis was used to compare the intensity of the war in Lebanon before and after the arrival of a group of meditators. War deaths fell 55% and war injuries 38% during the time of the assembly and returned to their previous levels after the group left.

Compiled from data in Chalmers, R., Clements, G., Schenkluhn, H., & Weinless, M. (Eds.), *Scientific Research on Maharishi's Transcendental Meditation Collected Papers Vol 1-5* (MERU Press: Switzerland) and on line at URL http://www.tm.org (Scientific Research on Transcendental Meditation).

thought, the source of life, energy and vitality in an individual.

SUSAN VEGORS

VEGETARIANISM

Krajcovicova-Kudlackova and colleagues (1994) studied 183 vegetarians. Their aim was to judge the state of health and nutrition of this population. Participants ranged in age from 19 to 60 years—102 were between 19 and 39 years, and 81 were older. They had maintained a vegetarian food consumption regime for an average of 4.2 years. One third of the men and one half of the women ate milk products (lacto-vegetarians), the rest ate milk products and eggs (lacto-ovo-vegetarians). The group was compared to 160 nonvegetarians of similar age groupings. Vegetarians showed more favorable lipid parameters, including low values of cholesterol, triglycerids, LDL-cholesterol, and atherogenic index.

Additional favorable factors included the absence of obesity and a higher level of antisclerotic active substances in the blood. Vitamin C and E were significantly higher in the vegetarian population than in the nonvegetarian population; both play an important role in the process of atherogenesis and cancer.

Key, Rhorogood, Appleby, and Burr (1996) examined the dietary habits and mortality in 11,000 vegetarians and health-conscious people in a 17-year follow-up study in the United Kingdom. In the study, 4,336 men and 6,435 women were recruited through health food shops, vegetarian societies, and magazines. The main outcome measures were mortality ratios from ischemic heart disease, cerebrovascular disease, and all malignant neoplasms, lung cancer, colorectal cancer, and breast cancer.

The results included the following: (1) 2,064 of the participants (19%) smoked, (2) 4,627 (43%) were vegetarian, (3) 6,699

(62%) ate whole-wheat bread daily, (4) 2,948 (27%) ate bran cereals daily, (5) 4,091 (38%) ate nuts or dried fruit daily, (6) 8,304 (77%) ate fresh fruit daily, and (7) 4,105 (38%) ate raw salad daily. The cohort had a mortality of half that of the general population. For vegetarians, after adjusting for smoking, a significant reduction in mortality was associated with eating fresh fruit, especially for ischemic heart disease heart disease, cerebrovascular disease, and all causes combined. Conversely, smoking was associated with an increased risk of death from all malignant neoplasms, and diet did not protect those participants.

CAROLYN CHAMBERS CLARK

See also
Antioxidants and Free Radicals (III)
Cancer (II)
Heart and Blood Vessel Conditions (II)

YOGA

"Yoga" in Sanskrit means union of the different aspects of the individual. There are several branches of yoga, each designed to help the individual achieve health, strength, wisdom, and success. *Hatha yoga*, developed by ancient Vedic scholars, brings optimal physical conditioning to the body through a series of postures and breathing techniques. It is an ancient time-proven system that eases muscle strain, promotes physical strength, and vitality, revitalizes mental capacities, and balances one's emotional state. What modern science refers to as biofeedback and psychonueroimmunotherapy is actually yoga.

The original practitioners of *hatha* yoga wanted to meditate for long periods of time to achieve spiritual advancement. A healthy physical body enabled them to sit in meditative stillness for extended periods of time. A disease-free state also enhanced deeper meditations. Today, we are able to benefit from their findings to combat stress and overcome the health challenges that result from poor lifestyles.

In this country, *hatha* yoga has been associated with back care and breathing exercises. *Hatha* yoga postures, when done properly, focus on skeletal alignment, creating space in the body for the organs to function efficiently. By creating length in the spine, the practitioner enables the central nervous system to effectively operate. All of the postures are linked with the breath which is a manifestation of *prana*. *Prana* is the Sanskrit term for life force, or particle of energy. When the breath is flowing freely, the *prana* is flowing as well. When the body's energy is blocked in any way, it can lead to a state of disease. By doing a program of *hatha* yoga, the body and the body's energies are freed and can be utilized for health and vitality for the practitioner.

Yogic body postures make up the majority of *hatha* yoga. The exercises have muscular and structural benefits, in addition to a dynamic healing effect on the internal organs and body chemistry. *Hatha* yoga has been found to help blood pressure, depression, and osteoporosis and to aid in menopausal discomfort. It has been used in India and in different parts of the world for thousands of years as a modality for the prevention of disease and as rehabilitation therapy for those suffering from physical discomfort due to injury.

Each posture was inspired by the natural surroundings of ancient India: tree pose, cobra pose, etc. When the pose is pronounced in Sanskrit, it always ends with the word *asana*. *Asana* means calm, steady state or seat, meaning the practitioner is ideally doing each posture in a state of relaxed activity and active relaxation. *Asana* also implies that each posture is a prelude to the ultimate goal of *hatha* yoga, which is being comfortable and healthy in a seated pose for meditation.

The postures can be simple or complex; each participant is urged to avoid pain and to practice at his or her own level. The student begins slowly, progressing at his or her own pace. As the body becomes attuned to the postures, one moves on to more complex poses. Benefits are achieved through sincere intent and effort. Home practice is encouraged and many aspects of the practices can be done without a teacher, however, a qualified instructor is recommended, especially if there are health issues that need to be addressed.

SHIVAN S. SARNA

Part V

Contributor Directory

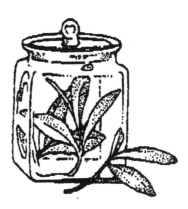

Leslie Aguillard, RN
Reiki Master, CMNT
Classical Homeopathic Practitioner
P.O. Box 40435
Denver, CO 80204

Christopher Amodeo
234 E. 17th Street
Costa Mesa, CA 92627

Hans A. Baer, PhD
Professor
Department of Sociology and Anthro-
  pology
University of Arkansas at Little Rock
University and 28th Street
Little Rock, AR 72204

Barbara Stevens Barnum, RN, PhD,
  FAAN
Columbia University School of Nursing
630 West 168th Street
New York, NY 10032

Mary Payne Bennett RN, DNSc
Assistant Professor
Indiana State University School of
  Nursing
Corner of 8th and Chestnut St.
Terre Haute, IN 47809

Marie Louise Bernardo, RN, MSN, PhD
Licensed Psychologist and Registered
  Nurse
23 Sherman Street
Fairfield, CT 06430

Andy Bernay-Roman, RN, MS, LMT,
  CCHT, National Certified Counselor
718 Buoy Road
North Palm Beach, FL 33408

Tacey Ann Boucher, BA
Program Evaluation Resource Center
Minneapolis Medical Research Founda-
  tion
914 S. 8th Street, Suite D917
Minneapolis, MN 55404

David E. Bresler, PhD, LAc
Co-Founder and Co-Director
Academy for Guided Imagery
10780 Santa Monica Blvd. #290
Los Angeles, CA 90025

Mary Anne Bright, RN, CS, EdD
Associate Professor
School of Nursing
University of Massachusetts, Amherst
Arnold House
Amherst, MA 01003

Carolyn M. Brown, RPh, PhD
Assistant Professor
Pharmacy Practice and Administration
  Division
College of Pharmacy
The University of Texas at Austin
Austin, TX 78712

Ann Burkhardt, MA, OTR/L, BCN
Assistant Director of Occupational
  Therapy
Columbia-Presbyterian Medical Center
Milstein Hospital Bldg.
177 Fort Washington Avenue
New York, NY 10032

David Burmeister
8719 E. San Alberto
Scottsdale, AZ 85258

Dwight C. Byers, President
International Institute of Reflexology
5650 1st Avenue North
P.O. Box 12642
St. Petersburg, FL 33733-2642

Ronald L. Caplan, PhD
Assistant Professor of Public Health
Division of Professional Studies
Richard Stockton College
Jim Leeds Road
Pomona, NJ 08240-0195

Susan E. Cayleff, PhD
Professor and Chair
Department of Women's Studies
San Diego State University
San Diego, CA 92182

Stephen E. Chagnon, RN, LMT
Carpal Tunnel Seminars
110 Glen St.
Glens Falls, NY 12801

John Chitty, RPP
President, American Polarity Therapy As-
  sociation
Director, Polarity Center of Colorado
2888 Bluff Street #149
Boulder, CO 80301

Chung-Kwang Chou, PhD
Department of Radiation Research
City of Hope National Medical Center
1500 East Duarte Road
Duarte, CA 91010-3000

Roberta Cirocco, ARNP CS
3690 Inverrary Drive #1Y
Lauderhill, FL 33319

Carolyn Chambers Clark, EdD, RN,
  ARNP, FAAN, HNC
Founder
The Wellness Institute
3451 Central Avenue
St. Petersburg, FL 33713 and
Doctoral Faculty
Walden University
Phone: (727) 322-0841
Email: cccwellness@earthlink.net

Michael H. Cohen, JD, MBA, MFA
Associate Professor of Law
Specializes in Health Care Law
Chapman University School of Law
1240 S. State College Blvd., Suite 200
Anaheim, CA 92806

Maureen M. Corbett, PhD
Independent Practice
143 13th Avenue North
St. Petersburg, FL 33701 and
University of South Florida/New College
  Counseling and Wellness Center
Sarasota, FL

Beree R. Darby, PhD
Counseling Psychologist
Student Health Care Center
College of Medicine
University of Florida
2531 N.W. 41st St., Suite C
Gainesville, FL 32606

Kathryn P. Davison, PhD
Department of Psychology
Southern Methodist University
Suite 300 Hyer Hall
Dallas, TX 75275

Judith (Walker) DeLany, LMT
Director
NMT Center
900 14th Avenue North
St. Petersburg, FL 33705

Barbara L. Denison, RN, BSN
Education Trustee, NH-PA, Inc.
Therapeutic Touch Practitioner
Coordinator Complementary Healing Ser-
  vices at Via Christi Regional Medical
  Center in Wichita, KS
6609 S. Spencer Road
Newton, KS 67114

Margo A. Drohan, MSN, RNCS, PNP
HC 65 Box 37
Great Barrington, MA 01230

Leslie Ellis, MRC, PhD, CRC
Director of the Fibromyalgia Management Program in St. Petersburg, Florida
P.O. Box 9300
Treasure Island, FL 33740

Susan Ezra, RN
80 Taylor Drive
Fairfax, CA 94930

Kathleen (Kat) S. Fasnacht, MA, MSN, ARNP-C
Bay Pines Veterans Affairs Medical Center
1226 Magnolia Drive
Clearwater, FL 33756

Tiffany Field, PhD
Director, Touch Research Institute
University of Miami School of Medicine
Department of Pediatrics (D-820)
P.O. Box 016820
Miami, FL 33101

Suzanne E. Foster, RN
Biofeedback Therapist
Bay Area Psychological Services
721 11th Street North
St. Petersburg, FL 33705

Judith Gammonley, RN, CS, EdD
Educational Consultant
Pinellas Animal Foundation
Seminole, FL and
Adjunct Instructor
St. Petersburg Jr. College
St. Petersburg, FL
2486 Saddlewood Lane
Palm Harbor, FL 34685

Wilbert M. Gesler, PhD
Professor
Department of Geography
University of North Carolina at Chapel Hill
Chapel Hill, NC 27599-3220

Norman Gevitz, PhD
Professor and Chair
Department of Social Medicine
Ohio University College of Osteopathic Medicine
Athens, OH 45701

Rena J. Gordon, PhD
Research Lecturer in Family and Community Medicine
University of Arizona College of Medicine and Visiting Professor
Arizona State University East
13660 East Columbine Drive
Scottsdale, AZ 85259

W. R. Hafling, PhD
Licensed Professional Psychologist
Diplomate, Board Certified, Forensic Medicine
Bay Area Psychological Services
721 11th St. N.
St. Petersburg, FL 33705

Pamela L. Hamilton, EdD
Bay Area Psychological Services
721 11th Street
St. Petersburg, FL 33705

Carl A. Hammerschlag, MD
Psychiatrist, Author, Speaker
3104 East Camelback Road, Suite 614
Phoenix, AZ 85016

Linton I. (Chip) Harris, BEE, MBA, RScP
147 Windward Dr.
Osprey, FL 34229

Mary E. Hazzard, PhD, FAAN, AM, BSN
Professor of Nursing
Department of Health and Human Services
National University
11255 North Torrey Pines Rd.
La Jolla, CA 92037

Linda Hein, RN, MSN, CHTP
Reiki Master
2006 Main Street
Vancouver, WA 98660

Lourdes Heber
Professor
College of Nursing
University of Saskatchewan
107 Wiggins Road
Saskatoon, Saskatchewan
Canada S7N 5E5

Joseph Heller
406 Berry St.
Mt. Shasta, CA 96067

Carl O. Helvie, RN, DrPH
Professor
School of Nursing
Old Dominion University
Norfolk, VA 23529-0500

Rita Holl, RN, PhD
11200 N. Sharpend Road
Albany, IN 47320

Richard P. Huemer, MD
Medik Research, Inc.
P.O. Box 24
Brush Prairie, WA 98606
and
Hull Eye Center
1739 West Avenue J
Lancaster, CA 93534

Kathleen M. Iwanowski, RN
Our Space to Create
100 E. Tarpon Avenue—Suite 5
Tarpon Springs, FL 34689

Karin Kearns, LM
Executive Director
The Delphi Center, Inc.
702 West Adalee Street
Tampa, FL 33603

Rodger Kessler, PhD
Clinical Psychologist
Mountain Affiliates in Psychology, P.C.
P.O. Box 424
Mountain Road
Stowe, VT 05672-0424

Thomas J. Kiresuk, PhD
Program Evaluation Resource Center
Minneapolis Medical Research Foundation
914 S. 8th Street, Suite D917
Minneapolis, MN 55404

Evan W. Kligman, MD
Private Practice
Family Practice and Geriatrics
Cienega Health and Healing
1845 West Orange Grove Rd., Suite 109
Tucson, AZ 85704

Mirka Knaster, MA, LMT
P.O. Box 7464
Asheville, NC 28802

Laura Koch, CMT
Hospital-Based Massage Network
#5 Old Town Square, Suite 205
Fort Collins, CO 80524

Allen M. Kratz, BSc, MSc, PharmD
HVS Laboratories, Inc.
P.O. Box 8243
Naples, FL 33941

Regina Kujawski
Licensed Massage Therapist
Certified Trager Practitioner
Introductory Trager Workshop Leader
Private Practice
9523 Boca River Circle
Boca Raton, FL 33434

Kevin and Barbara Kunz
Co-Directors of Reflexology Research
Co-Editors of *Reflexions*
P.O. Box 35820, Stn. D
Albuquerque, NM 87176

Zhenya Kurashova Wine
Physiotherapist
President of Kurashova Institute for Stud-
ies in Physical Medicine
P.O. Box 6246
Rock Island, IL 61204

Jeannie Laureyns Bell, RN
195 Eleanor Road
Pittfield, MA 01201

Cecile A. Lengacher, RN, PhD
Professor
University of South Florida
College of Nursing
Health Sciences Center
12901 Bruce B. Downs Blvd., MDC 22
Tampa, FL 33612-4766

Kate Levensohn, PhD
Regressionist/Hypnotist
1820 Bryan Ave.
Winter Park, FL 32789

Pamela Lewis, RN, CFT
Certified Feldenkrais Teacher
1430 Willamette #526
Eugene, OR 97401

Lurrae Lupone, MEd
InnerSpace Feng Shui
Box 220
Madison, CT 06443

Frederic Luskin, PhD
Research Fellow
The Complementary and Alternative
Medicine Program at Stanford Univer-
sity
and
Director
Stanford Forgiveness Project
730 Welch Road
Palo Alto, CA 94304-1583

Gayle MacDonald
4327 NE Mallory Avenue
Portland, OR 97211

Bonnie T. Mackey, MSN, ARNP, CMT
Mackey Health Institute, Inc.
6800 S.W. 45 Lane #1
Miami, FL 33155

David McMillan, MA
Edgar Cayce Foundation
Association for Research and Enlighten-
ment
67th St. and Atlantic Ave.
Virginia Beach, VA 23451

Steve Meeker, Dipl. L.Ac.
Director
Hollywood Clinic
1804 NE 25th
Portland, OR 97212

Lewis Mehl-Madrona, MD, PhD
Medical Director and Faculty, Internal
  Medicine and Family Practice Residen-
  cies
University of Pittsburgh Medical
  Center—Shadyside
5230 Centre Avenue, SON Bldg., Rm
  216
Pittsburgh, PA 15232

Allan R. Meyers, PhD
School of Public Health
Boston University School of Medicine
715 Albany Street, T-W349
Boston, MA 02118

Marc S. Micozzi, MD, PhD
Executive Director
The College of Physicians of Philadel-
  phia
Philadelphia, PA 19103-3097

Richard B. Miles
President
Health Frontiers Professional Network
6876 Pinehaven Road
Oakland, CA 94611

James D. Moran
Belchertown Wellness Center
21 Everett Avenue
Belchertown, MA 01007

Michael C. Murphy, PhD
Clinical Associate Professor
University of Florida
301 Peabody
Gainesville, FL 32611

Alan Rice Osborn, PhD
Instructor
Department of Geography

University of Oregon
4023-L Donald Street
Eugene, OR 97405-3966

Idelle Packer, MS, PT, CTAT
27A Fairfield Road
Greenwich, CT 06830

Joseph E. Pizzorno, Jr., ND
President
Bastyr University
14500 Juanita Drive NE
Bothell, WA 98011

Bonnie Prudden
Bonnie Prudden School for Physical Fitness and Myotherapy
7800 E. Speedway
Tucson, AZ 85710

Teresa Kirkpatrick Ramsey, RN, BSN,
  LMT
P.O. Box 2027
Spring, TX 77383

Daniel Redwood, DC
1645 Laskin Road, Suite 103
Virginia Beach, VA 23451

Ru-long Ren, MD
Department of Radiation Research
City of Hope National Medical Center
1500 East Duarte Road
Duarte, CA 91010-3000

Jeanne Reock
Certified Rubenfeld Synergist
President, The National Association of
  Rubenfeld Synergists
7 Kendall Road
Kendall Park, NJ 08824

Paul J. Rosch, MD, FACP
President
The American Institute of Stress
124 Park Avenue
Yonkers, NY 10703 and
Clinical Professor of Medicine and Psy-
chiatry
New York Medical College
1901 1st Avenue
New York, NY 10029

Martin Rossman, MD
AGI POB 2070
Mill Valley, CA 94942

David M. Sale, JD, LLM
P.O. Box 1615
Annapolis, MD 21404

Shivan S. Sarna
Owner and Instructor
Shivan's Yoga Studio
P.O. Box 25366
Sarasota, FL 34277

Ruth Scaggs, B.Mus, MA
SouthEastern Institute of Guided Imagery and Music
2801 Bufird Hiway #225
Atlanta, GA 30329

Dona Schneider, PhD, MPH
Associate Professor
Department of Urban Studies and Com-
munity Health
Rutgers, The State University of New
Jersey
33 Livingston Avenue
New Brunswick, NJ 08901-1958

G. N. Schrauzer, PhD
Department of Chemistry/Biochemistry
University of California, San Diego
Grillman Dr. and La Jolla Village Dr.
La Jolla, CA 92093

Donna Schwontkowski, DC, MS
4848 South Highland Drive
Suite 215
Salt Lake City, UT 84117

Ilene A. Serlin, PhD, ADTR
Professor of Psychology
Saybrook Institute
450 Pacific Ave.
San Francisco, CA 94133

Laura Servid, OTR/L
Aston-Patterning Practitioner
P.O. Box 3568
Incline Village, NV 89450-3568

Steve Shapiro, PhD
Member, Board of Directors
Multiple Sclerosis Association of
America
103 Saxony Drive
Mt. Laurel, NJ 08054

C. Norman Shealy, MD, PhD
Founder, Shealy Institute for Comprehen-
sive Health Care
Founding President, American Holistic
Medical Association
Research and Clinical Professor of Psy-
chology, Forest Institute of Profes-
sional Psychology
1328 East Evergreen Street
Springfield, MO 65803-4400

Kimberly Sibille, MA, LMHC
Licensed Mental Health Counselor
Certified Health/Fitness Instructor
P.O. Box 582
Safety Harbor, FL 34695

Howard D. Silverman, MD, MS
Chief Medical Officer
American Centers for Health and Medi-
cine
5055 North 32nd Street, Suite 200
Phoenix, AZ 85018

Gail Silverstein, DPA
Vice President of Health Plans
Maricopa Integrated Health Systems
2516 E. University
Phoenix, AZ 85034

Deborah Valentine Smith, BA, LMT
P.O. Box 402
W. Stockbridge, MA 01266

Jill Strawn, EdD, RN, CS
Assistant Professor
Graduate Program in Holistic Nursing
College of New Rochelle
New Rochelle, NY 10805

Deborah A. Sullivan, PhD
Associate Professor
Department of Sociology
Arizona State University
Tempe, AZ 85287-2101

Ann Gill Taylor, MS, EdD, RN, FAAN
Betty Norman Norris Professor of Nurs-
  ing and Director
Center for the Study of Complementary
  and Alternative Therapies
McLeod Hall
15th & Lane Street
University of Virginia
Charlottesville, VA 22903-3395

Nancy J. Terry, M.ED, ADTR
456 49th Street North
St. Petersburg, FL 33710

Valentin and Luminita Tureanu
Street Oltet No. 4
2200 Brasov, Romania

Dana Ullman, MPH
Director
Homeopathic Educational Services
2124 Kittredge St.
Berkeley, CA 94704

John E. Upledger, DO, OMM
President
The Upledger Institute, Inc.
11211 Prosperity Farms Rd. D325
Palm Beach Gardens, FL 33410

Sandra van de Weerd
Tai Chi Instructor
Taoist Tai Chi Society
731 31st Avenue N #2
St. Petersburg, FL 33704

Susan Vegors, EITC, PhD
59 Drake
Pocatello, ID 83201

Bette Waters, ARNP, RN, CNM, SANE
P.O. Box 878
Mesilla, NM 88046

Enid Whittaker
Bonnie Prudden School for Physical Fitness and Myotherapy
7800 E. Speedway
Tucson, AZ 85710

James C. Whorton
Professor
Department of Medical History and
  Ethics
School of Medicine
University of Washington
Box 357120
Seattle, WA 98195

Jacquelyn J. Wilson, MD
Consultant in Homeopathy
Diplomate American Board of Family
  Practice
Diplomate American Board of Homeo-
  therapeutics
Member of the Homeopathic Pharmaco-
  poeia Convention of the United States
536 Brotherton Road
Escondido, CA 92025-6454

Paul Root Wolpe, PhD
Center for Bioethics and Department of
  Sociology
University of Pennsylvania
3401 Market St., Suite 320
Philadelphia, PA 19104

Ray C. Wunderlich, Jr., MD
1152 94th Ave. N.
St. Petersburg, FL 33702

Kenneth Zwolski, RN, EdD
Associate Professor
College of New Rochelle School of
  Nursing
81 Bleeker St.
Lake Peekskill, NY 10537

Part VI

Resource Directory

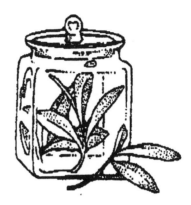

Academy for Guided Imagery. P.O. Box 2070, Mill Valley, CA 94942. Phone: (800) 726-2070. Fax: (415) 389-9342.

Accreditation Commission for Schools and Colleges of Acupuncture and Oriental Medicine. 8403 Colesville Rd., Suite 370, Silver Spring, MD 20910. Phone: (301) 608-9680. Fax: (301) 608-9676.

Alexander Technique International, Inc. 1692 Massachusetts Ave., Cambridge, MA 02138. Phone: (617) 497-2242. Fax: (617) 876-2709.

American Academy of Medical Acupuncture. 5820 Wilshire Blvd., Suite 500, Los Angeles, CA 90036. Phone: (213) 937-5514. Fax: (213) 937-0959.

American Academy of Osteopathy. 3500 DePauw Blvd., Suite 1080, Indianapolis, IN 46268-1136. Phone: (317) 879-1881.

American Academy of Reflexology. 606 E. Magnolia Blvd., Suite B, Burbank, CA 91501. Phone: (818) 841-7741.

American Apitherapy Society. P.O. Box 54. Hartland Four Corners, VT 05049. Phone: (802) 436-2708. Fax: (802) 436-2827.

American Association of Acupuncture and Oriental Medicine. 433 Front St., Catasaugua, PA 18032. Phone: (610) 266-1433. Fax: (610) 264-2768.

American Association of Naturopathic Physicians. 2366 Eastlake Ave, Suite E, Seattle, WA 98102. Phone: (206) 323-7610. Fax: (206) 323-7612.

American Association of Oriental Medicine. 433 Front Street, Catasuqua, PA 18032. Phone: (610) 433-2448. Fax: (610) 264-2768. Email: AAOM1@aol.com Web site: http://www.aaom.org

American Chiropractic Association. 1701 Clarendon Blvd., Arlington, VA 22209. Phone: (703) 276-8800. Email: americhiro@aol.com

American Chronic Pain Association. P.O. Box 850, Rocklin, CA 95788. Phone: (916) 632-0922.

American Council of Hypnotist Examiners. 312 Riverdale Dr., Glendale, CA 91204. Phone: (818) 242-5378.

American Dance Therapy Association. 2000 Century Plaza, Suite 108, Columbia, MD 21044-3263. Phone: (410) 997-4040.

American Herbalist Guild. P.O. Box 746555, Arvada, CO 80006. Phone: (303) 423-8800. Web site: http://www.health.net/pan/pa/herbalmedicine/ahg/index.html

American Holistic Nurses Association. P.O. Box 2130, Flagstaff, AZ 86003-2130. Web site: http://www.ahna.org

American Horticultural Therapy Association. 362A Christoperher Avenue, Gathersburg, MD 20879. Phone: (301) 948-3010.

American Institute of Homeopathy. 1585 Glencoe, Denver, CO 80220. Phone: (303) 898-5477.

American Institute for Mental Imagery. 351 E. 84th Street, Suite 10D, New York, NY 10028.

American Institute of Vedic Studies. P.O. Box 8357, Santa Fe, NM 87504-8357. Phone: (505) 983-9385.

American Massage Therapy Association. 820 Davis St., Suite 100, Evanston, IL 60201. Phone: (708) 864-0123. Fax: (708) 864-1178.

American Oriental Bodywork Therapy Association. 6801 Jericho Turnpike, Syosset, NY 11791. Phone: (516) 364-5533.

American Osteopathic Association. 142 East Ontario St., Chicago, IL 60611. Phone: (312) 280-5800.

American Polarity Therapy Association. 2888 Bluff St., No. 149, Boulder, CO 80301. Phone: (303) 545-2080. Fax: (303) 545-2161.

American School of Ayurvedic Sciences. 10025 N.E. 4th, Bellevue, WA 98004. Phone: (206) 453-8022. Fax: (206) 451-2670.

American Society of Clinical Hypnosis. 2200 East Devon Ave., Suite 291, Des Plaines, IL 60018. Phone: (708) 297-3317. Fax: (708) 297-7309.

American Yoga Association. 513 South Orange Avenue. Sarasota, FL 34236-7598. Phone: (800) 226-5859. Email: AmYogaAssn@aol.com

Associated Bodywork and Massage Professionals. 28677 Buffalo Park Rd., Evergreen, CO 80439. Phone: (303) 674-8478.

Association for Applied Psychophysiology and Biofeedback. 10200 West 44th Avenue, Suite 304, Wheat Ridge, CO 80033-2840. Phone: (800) 477-8892. Fax: (303) 422-8894.

Association for Network Chiropractic. 444 North Main St., Longmont, CO 80501. Phone: (303) 678-8101.

Aston-Patterning. P.O. Box 3568, Incline Village, NV 89450-3568. Phone: (702) 831-8228. Fax: (702) 831-9855.

Ayurveda Holistic Center of New York. 82A Bayville Ave., Bayville, NY 11709. Phone/Fax: (516) 628-8200.

Ayurvedic Institute. P.O. Box 23445, Albuquerque, NM 87192-1445. Phone: (505) 291-9698. Fax: (505) 294-7572.

Bastyr University of Natural Health Sciences. 144 N.E. 54th Street, Seattle, WA 98105. Phone: (206) 523-9585. Fax: (206) 527-4763.

Bonnie Prudden Institute for Physical Fitness and Myotherapy Pain Erasure Clinic. 7800 E. Speedway, Tucson, AZ 85710. Phone: (602) 529-3979 or (800) 221-4634.

Biofeedback Certification Institute of America. 10200 W. 44th Ave., Suite 304, Wheatridge, CO 80033. Phone: (303) 420-2902.

Canadian Naturopathic Association. P.O. Box 4520, Station C, Calgary, Alberta T2T 5N3. Phone: (403) 244-4487.

Cancer Support and Education Center. 1035 Pine Street, Menlo Park, CA 94025. Phone: (415) 327-6166. Fax: (415) 327-2018.

Center for Mind/Body Medicine. P.O. Box 1048, La Jolla, CA 92038. Phone: (619) 794-2440.

Center for Attitudinal Healing. 33 Buchanan, Sausalito, CA 94965. Phone: (415) 331-6161.

College of Maharishi Ayur-Ved, Maharishi International University. 1000 4th St., DB-1155, Fairfield, IA 52557-1155. Phone: (515) 472-7000. Fax: (375) 472-1189.

Council of Colleges of Acupuncture and Oriental Medicine. 1010 Wayne Avenue, Suite 1270, Silver Spring, MD 20910. Phone: (301) 608-9175. Fax: (301) 608-9576.

Council for Homeopathic Certification. P.O. Box 157, Corte Madera, CA 94976.

Council on Homeopathic Education. 801 N. Fairfax, No. 306, Alexandria, VA 22314. Phone: (703) 548-7790.

Council on Naturopathic Medical Education. P.O. Box 11426, Eugene, OR 97440-3626. Phone: (503) 484-6028.

Cranial Academy. 3500 DePauw Blvd., Indianapolis, IN 46268. Phone: (317) 879-0713.

Emory University Alternative Medicine (MedWeb) web site: http://www.Gen. Emory.edu/medweb/medweb. altmed.html

Feldenkrais Guild. P.O. Box 489, Albany, OR 97321-0143. Phone: (800) 775-2118.

Flower Essence Society. P.O. Box 459, Nevada City, CA 95959. Phone: (800) 736-9222

Foundation for Homeopathic Education and Research. 2124 Kittredge Avenue, Berkeley, CA 94704. Phone: (510) 649-8930.

Health Frontiers Professional Network, 6876 Pinehaven Road, Oakland, CA 94611. Phone: (510) 655-9951. Fax: (510) 654-6699. Email: rbmihpn@ aol.com

Hellerwork, Inc. 406 Berry St., Mt. Shasta, CA 96067. Phone: (800) 392-3900. Fax: (916) 926-6839. Email: hwork@snowcrest.net

Herb Research Foundation. 1007 Pearl Street, Suite 200, Boulder, CO 80302. Phone: (303) 449-2265.

Homeopathic Academy of Naturopathic Physicians. P.O. Box 69565, Portland, OR 97201. Phone: (503) 795-0579.

Homeopathic Educational Services. 21224 Kittredge St., Berkeley, CA 94704. Phone: (510) 649-0294.

Indic Traditions of Healthcare Dharma Hinduja Indic Research Center, Columbia University. Mail Code 3367, 1102 International Affairs Building, New York, NY 10027. Phone: (212) 854-5300. Fax: (212) 854-2802. Email: dhirc@columbia.edu

Insight Meditation Society. Pleasant St., Barre, MA 01005. Phone: (508) 355-4378.

Insight Meditation West. P.O. Box 909, Woodacre, CA 94973. Phone: (415) 488-0164.

Institute for Music, Health, and Education. 3010 Hennepin Avenue South, No. 269, Minneapolis, MN 55408. Phone: (800) 490-4968. Email: imhemn@pressenter.com

Institute of Noetic Sciences. 475 Gate Five Road, Suite 300, Sausalito, CA 94965. Phone: (415) 331-5650. Fax: (415) 331-5673.

Institute of Transpersonal Psychology. 744 San Antonio Road, Palo Alto, CA 94303. Phone: (415) 493-4430. Fax: (415) 493-6835.

Institute for Frontier Science. 7711-D McCallum Street, Philadelphia, PA 19118. Email: 101471.1777@compuserve.com

Integrative Medicine Resources on the Internet. Web site: http://www.HealthWWWeb.com

Interactive BodyMind Information System (IBIS). Web site: http://www.Integrative-Medicine.com

Interfaith Health Program. The Carter Center, One Copenhill, Atlanta, GA 30307. Phone: (404) 614-3757. Fax: (404) 420-5158.

International Association of Infant Massage. 5660 Clinton St., Suite No. 2, Elma, NY 14059. Phone: (800) 248-5432.

International Association of Yoga Therapists. 20 Sunnyside Avenue, Suite A243, Mill Valley, CA 94941. Phone: (415) 868-1147. Email: IAYT@yoga-net.com

International Chiropractic Association. 1110 N. Glebe Rd., Suite 1000, Arlington, VA 22201. Phone: (800) 423-4690.

International Foundation for Homeopathy. 2366 Eastlake Ave. E, Suite 325, Seattle, WA 98102. Phone: (206) 304-8230.

International Institute of Reflexology. 5650 First Avenue North, P.O. Box 12641, St. Petersburg, FL 33733. Phone: (813) 343-4811.

International Massage Association. 3000 Connecticut Ave., NW, Suite 102, Washington, DC 20008. Phone: (202) 387-6555. Fax: (800) 776-NAMT.

International Society for the Study of Subtle Energies and Energy Medicine. 356 Goldco Circle, Golden, CO 80403-1347. Phone: (303) 278-2228. Email: 74040.1273@compuserve.com Web site: http://www.vitalenergy.com/issseem/index.html

Jin Shin Do Foundation for BodyMind Acupressure. 366 California Ave., Suite 16, Palo Alto, CA 94306. Phone: (415) 328-1811.

Jin Shin Jyutsu, Inc. 8719 E. San Alberto, Scottsdale, AZ 85258. Phone: (602) 998-9331.

Milton H. Erickson Foundation. 306 North 24th Street, Phoenix, AZ 85016. Phone: (602) 956-6196. Fax: (602) 956-0519.

Mind/Body Medical Institute. Deaconess Hospital, 1 Deaconess Road, Boston, MA 02215.

National Acupuncture and Oriental Medicine Alliance. 14637 Starr Road, S.E., Olalla, WA 98359. Phone: (206) 851-6896. Fax: (206) 851-6883.

National Acupuncture Detoxification Association (Addictive and Mental Disorders). P.O. Box 1927, Vancouver, WA 98668-1927. Phone/Fax: (360) 260-8620. Email: NADAclear@aol.com

National Association for Holistic Aromatherapy. P.O. Box 17622, Boulder, CO 80308-7622. Phone: (800) 566-6735.

National Association for Music Therapy. 8455 Colesville Road, Suite 1000, Silver Spring, MD 20910. Phone: (301) 589-3300. Email: info@namt.com

National Association of Nurse Massage Therapists. P.O. Box 1268, Osprey, FL 34229. Phone: (813) 966-6288. Fax: (813) 918-0522.

National Association of Pregnancy Massage Therapists. P.O. Box 81453, Atlanta, GA 30341. Phone: (404) 633-7731.

National Association of Trigger Point Myotherapists. 2600 S. Parker Rd., Suite 1-214, Aurora, CA 80014.

National Center for Complementary and Alternative Medicine (NCCAM), NCCAM Clearinghouse, P.O. Box 8218, Silver Spring, MD 20907. Phone: (888) 644-6226. Fax: (301) 495-4957. Web site: http://www.altmed.od. nih.gov/nccam

National Center for Homeopathy. 801 N. Fairfax St., No. 306, Alexandria, VA 22314. Phone: (703) 548-7790.

National Certification Board for Therapeutic Massage and Bodywork. 8201 Greensboro Drive, Suite 300, McLean, VA 22102. Phone: (703) 610-9015. Fax: (703) 610-9005 or (800) 296-0664.

National College of Naturopathic Medicine. 11231 S.E. Market Street, Portland, OR 97216. Phone: (503) 255-4860.

National Commission for Certification of Acupuncturists. 1424 16th St. N.W., Suite 501, Washington, DC 20036. Phone: (202) 232-1404. Fax: (202) 462-6157.

National Certification Commission for Acupuncture and Oriental Medicine. P.O. Box 97075, Washington, DC 20090-7075. Phone: (202) 232-1404. Fax: (202) 462-6157.

National Institute of Craniosacral Studies, Inc. 7827 N. Armenia Ave., Tampa, FL 33604-3806. Phone: (813) 935-0583. Fax: (813) 933-6355.

Neuromuscular Therapy Center. 900 14th Ave. N., St. Petersburg, FL 33705. Phone: (813) 821-7167.

North American Society of Homeopaths. 10700 Old County Road 15, No. 350, Minneapolis, MN 55441. Phone: (612) 593-9458.

North American Society of Teachers of the Alexander Technique. P.O. Box 112484, Tacoma, WA 98411-2484. Phone: (800) 473-0620. Email: nastat@ix.netcom.com

Nurse Healers Professional Associates, Inc. 1211 Locust Street, Philadelphia, PA 19107. Phone: (215) 545-8079. Fax: (215) 545-8107. Email: 73764.123@compuserve.com

Pacific Institute of Aromatherapy. P.O. Box 6723, San Rafael, CA 94903. Phone: (415) 479-9121. Fax (415) 479-0119.

Qigong Institute East West Academy of Healing Arts. 450 Sutter Place, Suite 2104, San Francisco, CA 94108. Phone: (415) 788-2227. Fax: (415) 788-2242.

Reflexology Research. P.O. Box 35820, Station D, Albuquerque, NM 87176. Phone: (505) 344-9392.

Reiki Alliance. P.O. Box 41, Cataldo, ID 83810-1041. Phone: (208) 682-3535.

Reiki Outreach International. P.O. Box 609, Fair Oaks, CA 95628. Phone: (916) 863-1500. Fax: (916) 863-6464.

Rolf Institute of Structural Integration. 205 Canyon Blvd., Boulder, CO 80302. Phone: (800) 530-8875.

Rosen Method Professional Association. 2550 Shattuck Ave., Box 49, Berkeley, CA 94704. Phone: (510) 644-4166.

Rubenfeld Synergy Center. 115 Waverly Place, New York, NY 10011. (212) 254-5100. Fax: (212) 254-1174.

School for Body-Mind Centering. 189 Pondview Dr., Amherst, MA 01002. Phone: (413) 256-8615. Fax: (413) 256-8239.

Society for Light Treatment and Biological Rhythms. 10200 West 44th Avenue, Suite 304, Wheat Ridge, CO 80033-2840. Phone: (303) 424-3697. Email: sltbr@resourcenter.com

Society of Ortho-Bionomy International. P.O. Box 1974-70, Berkeley, CA 94701. Phone: (800) 743-4890.

Society for the Study of Neuronal Regulation. 4600 Post Oak Place, Suite 301, Houston, TX 77027. Phone: (713) 552-0091. Fax: (713) 552-0752. Email: ssnr@primenet.com

Soma Institute of Neuromuscular Integration. 730 Klink St., Buckley, WA 98321. Phone: (360) 829-1025.

Sound Healers Association. P.O. Box 2240, Boulder, CO 80306. Phone: (303) 443-8181.

Southeastern Institute for Music-Centered Psychotherapy. 2801 Buford Highway, Suite 225, Atlanta, GA 30329. Phone: (404) 633-8224.

Southwest School of Botanical Medicine (Bisbee, AZ)
Web site: http://www.chili.rt66.com/hrbmoore/HOMEPAGE/HomePage.html

Sports Massage Training Institute. 2156 Newport Blvd., Costa Mesa, CA 92627. Phone: (714) 642-0735.

Taoist T'ai Chi Society of U.S.A. 1060 Bannock Street, Denver, CO 80204. Phone: (303) 623-5163. Fax: (303) 623-7908.

Trager Institute. 33 Millwood St., Mill Valley, CA 94941. Phone: (415) 388-2688. Fax: (415) 388-2710.

Upledger Institute, Inc. 11211 Prosperity Farms Rd., Palm Beach Gardens, FL 33410. Phone: (800) 233-5880.

Vedic Sciences Institute. P.O. Box 2537, Jupiter, FL 33468-2537. Phone: (407) 745-2164.

Wellness Community. 2716 Ocean Park Blvd., Suite 1040, Santa Monica, CA 90405. Phone: (310) 314-2555.

Wellness Resources. 3451 Central Avenue. St. Petersburg, FL 33713. Phone: (727) 322-0841. Email: cccwellness@earthlink.net Web: http://home.earthlink.net/~cccwellness

World Federation of Chiropractic. 78 Glencairn Avenue, Toronto, Ontario M4R 1M8. Phone: (416) 484-9978. Fax: (416) 484-9665.

Yoga International. Himalayan Institute, RD 1, Box 88, Honesdale, PA 18431.

Yog-Ayu. 237000 Edmonds Way, Edmonds, WA 98026. Phone: (206) 542-3528.

Zero Balancing Association. P.O. Box 1727, Capitola, CA 95010. Phone: (408) 476-0665.

REFERENCES

ABC on mercury-poisoning from dental amalgam fillings. (1997). Stockholm: Swedish Association of Dental Mercury Patients.

Abbott, R. D., Curb, J. D., Rodriguez, B. L., Sharp, D. S., Burshfield, C. M., Yano, K. (1996). Effect of dietary calcium and milk consumption on risk of thromboembolic stroke in older middle-aged men: The Honolulu Heart Program. *Stroke*, *27*(5), 813–818.

Abraham, A., Brooks, B., & Eylath, U. (1992). The effects of chromium supplementation on serum glucose and lipids in patients with and without non-insulin-dependent diabetes. *Metabolism, 41*, 768–771.

Abraham, I. L., Neundorfer, M. M., & Currie, L. J. (1992). Effects of group interventions on cognition and depression in nursing home residents. *Nursing Research*, *41*(4), 196–202.

Academy of Psychosomatic Medicine. (1996). Mental disorders in general on medical practices. *Behavioral Health Tomorrow*, *5*(5), 55–62.

Acanda Roque, M. C., Gonzales Valente, A., & Fialio Sanza, A. (1990). Psychogeriatrics and psychoballet. *Rev Cubana Enferm*, *6*(2), 198–204.

Access to Medical Treatment Act, H.R. 2019, 104th Cong., 1st Sess.; S. 1035, 104th Cong., 1st Sess. (1995). The bill has been reintroduced as H.R. 746, 105th Cong., 1st Sess. (Feb. 13, 1997); and S. 578, 105th Cong., 1st Sess. (Apr. 18, 1997).

Accredited surgical facilities offer protection for patients. (1993). *Plastic Surgery News*, *5*(5), 1+.

Achterberg, H., et al. (1994). *Rituals of healing: Using imagery for health and wellness*. New York: Bantam Books.

Achterberg, J. (1985). *Imagery in healing, shamanism in modern medicine*. Boston & London: New Science Library.

Ack, M., Norman, M. E., & Schmitt, B. D. (1984). A conservative approach to enuresis. *Patient Care*, *28*(1), 54–81.

Acute Low Back Problems Guideline Panel. (1994, December). Acute low back problems in adults. Clinical practice guideline no 14 (AHCPR Pub. No. 95-0642). Rockville, MD: Agency for Health Care Policy and Research, Public Health Service, U.S. Department of Health and Human Services.

Acute Pain Management Guideline Panel. (1992, February). Acute pain management: Operative or medical procedures and trauma. Clinical practice guideline no 1 (AHCPR Pub. No. 92-0032). Rockville, MD: Agency for Health Care Policy and Research, Public Health Service, U.S. Department of Health and Human Services.

Adams, E., & McGuire, F. (1986). Is laughter the best medicine? A study of the effects of humor on perceived pain and affect. Special Issue: Therapeutic activities with the impaired elderly. *Activities, Adaptation and Aging*, *8*(3–4), 157–175.

Ader, R. (1987). Clinical implications of psychoneuroimmunology: Commentary. *Developmental and Behavioral Pediatrics*, *8*(6), 357–358.

Ader, R., & Cohen, N. (1981). Conditioned immunopharmacologic responses. In R. Ader (Ed.), *Psychoneuroimmunology* (pp. 6–38). New York: Academic Press.

Ader, R., & Cohen, N. (1982). Behaviorally conditioned immunosuppression and murine systemic lupus erythematosis. *Science*, *214*, 1534–1536.

Ader, R., Felten, D., & Cohen, N. (Eds.). (1991). *Psychoneuroimmunology* 2nd edition. New York: Academic Press.

Adler, A. J., & Holub, B. J. (1997). Effect of garlic and fish-oil supplementation on serum lipid and lipoprotein concentrations in hypercholesterolemic men. *American Journal of Clinical Nutrition*, *65*(2), 445–450.

Adlercreutz, H., & Mazur, W. (1997). Phyto-oestrogens and Western disease. *Ann Med*, *29*(2), 95–120.

Agency for Health Care Policy and Research. (1994). *Acute low back problems in adults* (Clinical Practice Guideline No. 14). Washington, DC: U.S. Government Printing Office.

Agte, V., Chiplonkar, S., Joshi, N., & Paknikar, K. (1994). Apparent absorption of copper and zinc from composite vegetarian diets in young Indian men. *Annals of Nutrition and Metabolism*, *38*(1), 13–19.

Alabaster, O., Tang, Z., & Shivapurkar, N. (1997). Dietary fiber and the chemopreventive modulation of colon carcinogenesis. *Mutation Research*, *350*(1), 185–197.

Aldori, W. H., Giovannucci, E. L., Rimm, E. G., et al. (1994). Association between dietary fiber, sources of fiber, other nutrients, and the diagnosis of symptomatic diverticular disease. *American Journal of Clinical Nutrition*, *60*(5), 757–764.

Aldori, W. H., Giovannucci, E. L., Stampfer, M. J., Rimm, E. B., Wing, A. L., & Willett, W. C. (1997). Prospective study of diet and the risk of duodenal ulcer in men. *American Journal of Epidemiology*, *145*(1), 42–50.

Alexander, F. M. (1996). *The use of the self*. New York: E. P. Dutton.

Allen, J. J., & Schnyer, R. N. (1994). *An acupuncture treatment study for unipolar depression*. http://www.altmed.od.nih.gov/oam/cgi-bin/research/search_simple.cgi

Allen, V. (1997). Childhood cancer on the rise. EPA Conference, September 15, Washington, D.C.

Aloisi, P., Marrelli, A., & Porto, C. (1997). Visual evoked potentials and serum magnesium levels in juvenile migraine patients. *Headache*, *37*(6), 383–385.

Alon, R. (1990). *Mindful spontaneity*. New York: Avery Publishing Group, Inc.

Alpert, J. E., & Fava, M. (1997). *Nutrition and depression: The role of folate* [Online]. Available: http://www.medscape.com [April 1997].

Als, H. (1986). The high risk neonate: Developmental therapy perspectives. *Physical and Occupational Therapy in Pediatrics*, *6*, 3–55.

American Academy of Orthopaedic Surgeons. (1995). News Release. 222 S. Prospect Avenue, Park Ridge IL 60068. (800) 346-2267.

American Academy of Pediatrics Committee on Nutrition. (1985). Use of oral fluid therapy and post treatment feeding following enteritis in children in a developed country. *Pediatrics*, *75*, 358–361.

American Association of Health Plans. (1996). *State penetration rates*. Washington, DC: Author.

American Association of Retired Persons (AARP). (1995). *A profile of older Americans*. Washington, DC: AARP Program Resources.

American College of Sports Medicine Position Stand. (1994). Exercise for patients with coronary artery disease. *Med Sci Sports Exerc*, *26*(3), i–v.

American Dietetic Association. (1994). American dietetic association issues position on functional foods. American Dietetic Association News Release, November 16, 1994, Chicago, Illinois.

American Heart Association (AHA). (1996). *Heart and stroke facts: Statistics supplement*. Author.

American Institute for Cancer Research. (1997). *Healthy flavors of the world: Asia*. Washington, DC: Author.

American Psychiatric Association. (1994). *Diagnostic and statistical manual of mental disorders* (4th ed., pp. 394–403). Washington, DC: Author.

Anderson, C. A., & Whitehouse, D. G. (1995). *New thought*. New York: The Crossroads Publishing Company.

Anderson, J. E. (1983). *Grant's atlas of anatomy*, 8th edition. Baltimore: Williams & Wilkins.

Anderson, J. W., Johnstone, B. M., & Cook-Newell, M. E. (1995). Meta-analysis of the effects of soy protein intake on serum lipids. *New England Journal of Medicine*, *333*, 276–282.

Anderson, M. (1979). *Colour healing: Chromotherapy and how it works*. New York: Samuel Weiser, Inc.

Anderson, M. (1996, March). Larry Dossey, MD is finding common ground between alternative and conventional medicine. *Natural Foods Merchandiser*, *17*(3), 48–52.

Anderson, R. (1993). Chromium and its role in lean body mass and weight reduction. *Nutr Rep, 11*(41), 46, 48.

Anderson, R. A. (1997). Chromium as an essential nutrient for humans. *Regul Toxicol Pharmacol, 26*(1), S35–S41.

Anderson, R. A., Cheng, N., Bryden, N. A., Polansky, M. M., Cheng, N., Chi, J., & Feng, J. (1997). Elevated intakes of supplemental chromium improve glucose and insulin variables in individuals with type 2 diabetes. *Diabetes, 46*(11), 1786–1791.

Anderson, R., Meeker, W. C., Wirick, B. E., et al. (1992). A meta-analysis of clinical trials of spinal manipulation. *Journal Manipulative Physiol Ther, 15*, 181–194.

Andreas, C., & Andreas, S. (1989). *Heart of the mind*. Moab, UT: Real People Press.

Andrews, B. (1997). Bodily shame in relation to abuse in childhood and bulimia: A preliminary investigation. *British Journal of Clinical Psychology, 36*(Part 1), 41–49.

Andrews, L. B. (1996). *The Shadow Health Care System: Regulation of Alternative Health Care Providers*, 32 Houston L. Rev. 1273.

Angell, M. (1985). Disease as a reflection of the psyche. *New England Journal of Medicine, 312*, 1570–1572.

Ankri, S., Miron, T., Rabinkov, A., Wilcheck, M., & Mirelman, D. (1997). Allicin from garlic strongly inhibits cysteine proteinases and cytopathic effects of *Entamoeba histolytica. Antimicrob Agents Chemother, 41*(10), 2286–2288.

Appel, L. J., Moore, T. J., Obarzanek, E., Vollmer, W. M., Svetkey, L. P., et al. (1997). *New England Journal of Medicine, 336*(16), 1117–1124.

Appels, A., Bar, F., Lasker, J., et al. (1997). The effect of a psychological intervention program on the risk of a new coronary event after angioplasty: A feasibility study. *Journal of Psychosomatic Research, 43*(2), 209–217.

Arase, Y., Ikeda, K., Murashima, N., et al. (1997). The long-term efficacy of glycyrrhizin in chronic hepatitis C patients. *Cancer, 79*(8), 1494–1500.

Arena, J. G., Bruno, G. M., Hannah, S. L., & Meador, K. J. (1995). A comparison of frontal electromyographic biofeedback training, trapezius electromyographic biofeedback training, and progressive muscle relaxation therapy in the treatment of tension headache. *Headache, 35*(7), 411–419.

Aruin, L. I. (1997). Helicobacter pylori infection is carcinogenic for humans. *Arkh Patol, 59*(3), 74–78.

Ashizawa, K., Sugane, A., & Gunji, T. (1990). Breast form changes resulting from a certain brassiere. *Journal of Human Ergology, 19*(1), 53–62.

Ashley, B. (1988, October 31). It's never too late to feel fit. *Marin Independent Journal.*

Ashton, C., Jr., Whitworth, G. C., Seldomridge, J. A., et al. (1997). Self-hypnosis reduces anxiety following coronary artery bypass surgery: A prospective, randomized trial. *Journal of Cardiovascular Surgery, 38*(1), 69–75.

Astin, J. A. (1997). Stress reduction through mindfulness meditation: Effects on psychological symptomatology, sense of control, and spiritual experiences. *Psychother Psychosom, 66*(2), 97–106.

Aston, J. (1991). Your ideal body. *Physical Therapy Today, 14*(2), 30.

Aston, J., & Low, J. (1991, Fall). Your three-dimensional body—The Aston system of body usage, movement, and fitness. *Physical Therapy Today, 12*, 14–16, 18, 20–22, 24.

Aston, J., & Miller, B. (1993). A new approach to the dynamics of posture. *Physical Therapy Today, 16*(3), 47–53.

Aston, J., Molnar, M. A., & Krier, L. (1992). In your best shape with gravity's assistance. *Physical Therapy Today, 15*(3), 50–59.

Auguet, M., De Feudis, V., Clostre, F., & Deghenghi, R. (1982). Effects of an extract of Ginkgo biloba on rabbit isolated aorta. *Gen Pharmac, 13*, 225.

Augusti, K. T. (1996). Therapeutic values of onion (*Allium cepa L.*) and garlic (*Allium sativum L.*). *Indian Journal Exp Biol, 34*(7), 634–640.

Auteroche, B., Navailh, P., Maronnaud, P., & Mullens, E. (1986). *Acupuncture en gynécologie et obstétrique*. Paris: Maloine.

Avorn, J., Monane, M., Gurwitz, J. H., Glynn, R. J., Choodnovskiy, I., & Lipsitz, L. A. (1994). Reduction of bacteriuria and pyuria after ingestion of cranberry juice. *Journal of the American Medical Association, 271*(10), 751–754.

Azar, B. (1996). Intrusive thoughts proven to undermine our health. *APA Monitor, 27*(10), 34.

Azen, S. P., Qian, D., Mack, W. J., Sevanian, A., Selzer, R. H., Liu, C. R., Liu, C. H., & Hodis, H. N. (1996). Effect of supplementary antioxidant vitamin intake on carotid arterial wall intima-media thickness in a controlled clinical trial of cholesterol lowering. *Circulation, 94,* 2369–2372.

Badam, L. (1997). In vitro antiviral activity of indigenous glycyrrhizin, licorice and glycyrrhizic acid (Sigma) on Japanese encephalitis virus. *Journal Communicable Diseases, 29*(2), 91–99.

Baer, H. A. (1982). Toward a systematic typology of black folk healers. *Phylon, 43,* 327–343.

Baer, H. A. (1989). The American dominative medical system as a reflection of social relations in the larger society. *Social Science and Medicine, 28,* 1103–1112.

Baer, L. D., & Good, C. M., Jr. (1998). The power of the state. In R. J. Gordon, B. Nienstedt, & W. M. Gesler (Eds.), *Alternative therapies: Exploring options in health care* (pp. 45–66). New York: Springer Publishing Company.

Bagga, D., Capone, S., Wang, H., et al. (1997). Dietary modulation of Omega-3/Omega-6 polyunsaturated fatty acid ratios in patients with breast cancer. *Journal of the National Cancer Institute, 89*(15), 1123–1131.

Bahr, F. (1978). *Introduction to scientific acupuncture.* Kalamazoo, MI: The German Academy for Auricular Medicine.

Baker, M. E. (1994). Licorice and enzymes other than 11 beta-hydroxysteroid dehydrogenase: An evolutionary perspective. *Steroids, 59*(2), 136–141.

Balch, J. F., & Balch, P. A. (1997). *Prescription for nutritional healing* (2nd ed.). Garden City Park: Avery.

Baldwin, C. (1994). *Calling the circle: The first and future culture.* Newberg, OR: Swan, Raven & Co., S. (1991).

Baldwin, R. (1986). *Special delivery.* Berkeley: Celestial Arts.

Balkwill, F. R., & Burke, F. (1989). The cytokine network. *Immunology Today, 10,* 299–304.

Ballaban-Gil, K., et al. (1996). Ketogenic diet and treatment of intractible epilepsy in adults. *Eppilepsia, 37*(5), 92.

Baltes, P. B. (1993). The aging mind: Potential and limits. *Gerontologist, 33*(5), 580–594.

Bandura, A. (1982). Self-efficacy mechanism in human agency. *American Psychologist, 37,* 122–147.

Bang, H. O., Dyerberg, J., & Sinclair, H. M. (1980). The composition of Eskimo food in north western Greenland. *American Journal of Clinical Nutrition, 33,* 2657–2661.

Barlow, W. (1990). Use and disease. In W. Barlow, *The Alexander technique* (pp. 92–124). Rochester, VT: Healing Arts Press.

Baranson, S., Zimmerman, L., & Nieveen, J. (1995). The effects of music interventions on anxiety in the patient after coronary artery bypass grafting. *Heart and Lung: Journal of Critical Care, 24*(2), 124–132.

Barber, T. X. (1969). *Hypnosis, A Scientific Approach.* New York: Litton Educational Publishing, Van Nostrand Reinhold.

Barber, T. X., Spanos, N. P., & Chaves, J. F. (1974, 1979). *Hypnotism, Imagination, and Human Potentialities.* Pergamon General Psychology series. New York: Pergamon Press.

Barden, M. (1987). Body odyssey: Exploring Bodywork techniques. *Shape, 12*(8), 90–93, 142, 144, 146, 149–151.

Barnes, F. S. (1995). Typical electric and magnetic field exposures at power-line frequencies and their coupling to biological systems. In M. Blank (Ed.), *Electro-magnetic fields, biological interactions and mechanisms* (pp. 37–55). Washington, DC: American Chemical Society.

Barnes, S., Sfakianos, J., Coward, L., & Kirk, M. (1996). Soy isoflavonoids and cancer prevention. Underlying biochemical and pharmacological issues. *Adv Exp Med Biol, 401,* 87–100.

Barnett, L., & Chambers, M. (1996). *Reiki - energy medicine.* Rochester, VT: Healing Arts Press.

Barrett, M. (1994). Potential role of ascorbic acid and beta-carotene in the prevention of preterm rupture of fetal membranes. *Int Journal Vit Ntr Res, 64,* 192–197.

Baschetti, R. (1995). Chronic fatigue syndrome and licorice. *New Zealand Medical Journal, 157.*

Basmajian, J. V. (Ed.). (1989). *Biofeedback: Principles and practice for clinicians* (3rd ed.). Baltimore: Williams & Wilkins.

Basset, S. W., & Lake, B. M. (1958). Use of cold applications in management of spasticity: Report of three cases. *Physical Therapy Review, 3–8,* 333.

Basso, A., Dalla, P. L., Erle, G., et al. (1994). Licorice emeliorates postural hypotension caused by diabetic autonomic neuropathy. *Diabetes Care, 17*(11), 1356.

Bastian, H. (1993). Personal beliefs and alternative childbirth choices: A survey of 552 women who planned to give birth at home. *Birth, 20,* 186–192.

Bastien, J. W. (1992). *Drum and stethoscope: Integrating ethnomedicine and biomedicine in Bolivia.* Salt Lake City, UT: University of Utah Press.

Bauer, R. (1996). Echinacea drugs—effects and active ingredients. *Z Arztl Forthild (Jena), 90*(2), 111–115.

Bauer, U. (1984). 6-month double-blind randomised clinical trial of Ginkgo biloba extract versus placebo in two parallel groups in patients suffering from peripheral arterial insufficiency. *Arzneimittelforschung, 34*(6), 716–720.

Beal, M. F., & Matthews, R. T. (1997). Coenzyme Q10 in the central nervous system and its potential usefulness in the treatment of neurodegenerative diseases. *Mol Aspecgts Med*(Suppl. 18), S169–S179.

Bear, M., Dwyer, J. W., Benveneste, D., et al. (1997). Home-based management of urinary incontinence: A pilot study with both frail and independent elders. *Journal of Wound Ostomy Continence Nursing, 24*(3), 163–171.

Beauchemin, K. M., & Hays, P. (1997). Phototherapy is a useful adjunct in the treatment of depressed in-patients. *Acta Psychiatr Scand, 95*(5), 424–427.

Beck, A. T. (1976). *Cognitive therapy and the emotional disorders.* New York: International Universities Press.

Beck, A., & Katcher, A. (1996). *Between pets and people.* West Lafayette, IN: Purdue University.

Becker, V. H. (1982). Against snakebites and influenza: Use and components of *Echinacea augustifolia* and *purpurea. Deutsche Apotheker Zeitung, 122*(45), 2020–2023.

Beijing, Shanghai, and Nanjing Colleges of Traditional Chinese Medicine, The Acupuncture Institute of the Academy of Traditional Chinese Medicine. (Compilers). (1980). *Essentials of Chinese acupuncture.* Beijing: Foreign Languages Press.

Bekyarova, G., Yankova, T., & Galunska, B. (1996). Increased antioxidant capacity, suppression of free radical damage anderthryocyte aggrerability after combined application of alpha-tocopherol and FC-43 perfluocarbon emulsion in early postburn period in rats. *Artif Cells Blood Substit Immobil Biotechnol, 24*(6), 629–641.

Belaya, N. A. (1983). *Manual of therapeutic massage.*

Bellavite, P., & Signorni, A. (1995). *Homeopathy: A frontier in medical science.* Berkeley, CA: North Atlantic Books.

Belluomini, J., Litt, R. C., Lee, K. A., & Katz, M. (1994). Acupressure for nausea and vomiting of pregnancy: A randomized, blinded study. *Obstet Gynecol, 84*(2), 245–248.

Bemporad, J. R. (1996). Self-starvation through the ages: Reflections on the pre-history of anorexia nervosa. *International Journal of Eating Disorders, 19*(3), 217–237.

Bender, M. L. (1971). *A study of the relationships between persistent immaturity of the symmetric tonic neck reflex and learning disabilities in children.* Unpublished doctoral dissertation, Purdue University, West Lafayette, IN.

Bender, R., Eastop, J., & Keller, M. J. (1994). Retreat: A different approach to team building. *Medsurg Nursing, 3,* 135–138.

Bendix, A. F., Bendix, T., Lund, C., Kirkbak, S., & Ostenfeld, S. (1997). Comparison of three intensive programs for chronic low back pain patients: A prospective, randomized, observer-blinded study with one-year follow-up. *Scand Journal of Rehabil Med, 29*(2), 81–89.

Bennett, M. (1997). The effect of mirthful laughter on stress and natural killer cell cytotoxicity. *Dissertation Abstracts International.* Chicago: Rush-Presbyterian-St. Lukes Medical Center.

Bennett, M., & Lengecher, C. Design and Testing of the Complementary Therapy Rating Scale. *Alternative Health Practitioner, 4*(3): 179–198.

Benson, H. (1975). *The relaxation response.* New York: Avon Books.

Benson, H. (1996). *Timeless healing.* New York: Simon & Schuster.

Benson, J. (1975). *The relaxation response.* New York: William Morrow.

Bentsen, H., Lindgarde, F., & Manthorpe, R. (1997). The effect of dynamic strength back exercise and/or a home training program in 57-

year-old women with chronic low back pain. Results of a prospective randomized study with a 3-year follow-up period. *Spine*, *22*(13), 1494–1500.

Benvenuti, S. (1988). Putting new life into old bodies. *The Ark*, *16*(9).

Berger, B. G., & Owen, D. R. (1992). Mood alteration with yoga and swimming: Aerobic exercise may not be necessary. *Percpt Motor Skills*, *75*(3, Pt. 2), 1331–1343.

Berger, M. M. (1995). Role of trace elements and vitamins in perioperative nutrition. *Ann Fr Anesth Reanim*, *14*(Suppl. 2), 82–94.

Berggren-Thomas, P., & Griggs, M. J. (1995, March). Spirituality in aging: Spiritual need or spiritual journey? *Journal of Gerontological Nursing*, *21*(3), 5–10.

Berglund, F. (1995). *150 Years of Dental Amalgam*. Orlando, FL: Bio-Probe.

Berjeron-Oliver, S., & Oliver, B. *Working without pain*. Chico, CA: The Pacific Institute of the Alexander Technique.

Berk, L., & Tan, S. (1995). Eustress of mirthful laughter modulates the immune system lymphokine interferon-gama. *Annals of Behavioral Medicine Supplement, Proceedings of the Society of Behavioral Medicine's Sixteenth Annual Scientific Sessions*, *17*, C064.

Berk, L., Tan, S., Fry, W., Napier, B., Lee, J., Hubbard, R., Lewis, J., & Eby, W. (1989). Neuroendocrine and stress hormone changes during mirthful laughter. *American Journal of the Medical Sciences*, *298*, 391–396.

Berk, L., Tan, S., Napier, B., & Evy, W. (1989). Eustress of mirthful laughter modifies natural killer cell activity. *Clinical Research*, *37*, 115A.

Berkeley Holistic Health Center. (1978). *The Holistic Health Handbook*. Berkeley, CA: And/Or Press.

Berkow, R., & Fletcher, A. J. (1992). *The Merck Manual of Diagnosis and Therapy*. Rahway, NJ: Merck Research Laboratories.

Berman, B. M., Hartnoll, S. M., Singh, B. B., & Singh, B. K. (1997, July). Homoeopathy and the U.S. primary care physician. *British Homoeopathic Journal*, *86*, 131–138.

Bernard, R. J., Inkeles, S., & Jung, F. (1994). Diet and exercise in the treatment of NIDDM: The need for early emphasis. *Diabetes Care*, *17*, 1354.

Bernstein, J. E., et al. (1989). Topical capsaicin treatment of chronic posttherapeutic neuralgia. *Journal Am Acad Dermatol*, *21*, 265–270.

Bernstein, L., Henderson, B. E., Hanisch, R., Sullivan-Halley, J., & Ross, R. K. (1994). Physical exercise and reduced risk of breast cancer in young women. *Journal of the National Cancer Institute*, *86*, 1403–1408.

Beverley, L., & Travis, I. (1992). Constipation: Are natural laxatives better? *Journal Gerontol Nsg*, *18*, 6.

Bezerra, J., Stathos, T., Duncan, B., & Gaines, J. (1992). Treatment of infants with acute diarrhea: What's recommended and what's practiced. *Pediatrics*, *90*, 1–4.

Bigos, S., Bowyer, O., Braen, G., et al. (December 1994). Acute lower back problems in adults. Clinical Practice Guideline, Quick Reference Guide Number 14. Rockville, MD: U.S. Department of Health and Human Services, Public Health Service, Agency for Health Care Policy and Research, AHCPR Pub. No. 95-0643.

Bilger, B. (1997). Nature's pharmacy. Hippocrates (November): 20–27.

Birk, T. J. (1995). The use of massage therapy in HIV-l patients. Office of Alternative Medicine Research Grant Results. http://www.altmed.od.nih.gov/oam/cig-bin/research/search_simple.cgi

Birlouez-Aragon, I., Ravelontseheno, Villate-Cathelineau, B., et al. (1993). Disturbed galactose metabolism in elderly and diabetic humans is associated with cataract formation.

Blalock, J. E., & Smith, E. M. (1985). The immune system: Our mobile brain? *Immunology Today*, *6*, 115–117.

Blank, M. (1997). *Electromagnetic Fields: Biological Interactions and Mechanisms*. Washington: American Chemical Society.

Blot, W. J., Li, J., Taylor, P. R., Guo, W., Dawsey, S., Wang, G., Yang, C. S., et al. (1993). Nutrition intervention trials in Linxian, China: Supplementation with specific vitamin/mineral combinations, cancer incidence, and disease-specific mortality in the general population. *Journal of the National Cancer Institute*, *85*(18), 1483–1492.

Blumenthal, M., Goldberg, A., Gruenwald, J., Hall, T., Riggins, C. W., Rister, R. S. (Eds.), Klein, S., Rister, R. S. (Trans.). (1998). *German Com-*

mission E Monographs: Therapeutic Monographs on Medicinal Plants for Human Use. Austin, TX: American Botanical Council.

Blumsohn, A., Herrington, K., Hannon, R., et al. (1994). The effect of calcium supplementation on the circadian rhythm of bone resorption. *Endocrinology and Metabolism, 79,* 730–735.

Bo, K., & Talseth, T. (1996). Long-term effect of pelvic floor muscle exercise 5 years after cessation of organized training. *Obstetrics and Gynecology, 87*(2), 261–265.

Bohmer, D., & Ambrus, P. (1992). Behandlung von Sportverletzungen mit Traumeel-Salbe Kontrollierte Doppelblind-Studie. *Biologische Medizin, 21,* 260–268.

Boik, J. (1996). *Cancer and natural medicine* (pp. 99–102, 161–168, 177–198). Princeton, MN: Oregon Medical Press.

Boissevain, M. D., & Mc Cain, G. A. (1991). Towards an integrated understanding of fibromyalgia syndrome. I: Medical and pathophysiological aspects. *Pain, 44,* 227–238.

Boline, P., Kasak, K., Bronfort, G., Nelson, C., & Anderson, A. V. (1995). Spinal manipulation vs. amitriptyline for the treatment of chronic tension-type headaches: A randomized clinical trial. *Journal Manipulative Physiol Ther, 18*(3), 148–154.

Bollumar, F., Olsen, J., Rebagliato, M., & Bistanti, L. (1997). Caffeine intake and delayed conception: A European multicenter study on infertility and subfecundity. European Study Group on Infertility and Subfecundity. *American Journal of Epidemiology, 145*(4), 324–334.

Boniface, R., & Robert, A. M. (1996). Effect of anthocyanins on human connective tissue metabolism in the human. *Klin Monatsbl Augenheilkd, 209*(6), 368–372.

Bonis, P. A., & Norton, R. A. (1996). Irritable bowel syndrome. *American Family Physician, 53,* 1229.

Bonjour, J. P., Schurch, M. A., & Rizzoli, R. (1996). Nutritional aspects of hip fractures. *Bone, 18*(Suppl. 3), 139S–144S.

Bonne, O. B., Gur, E., & Berry, E. M. (1995). Hyperphosphatemia: An objective marker for bulimia nervosa? *Comprehensive Psychiatry, 36*(3), 236–240.

Booth, R. J. (1990). The psychoneuroimmune network: Expanding our understanding of immu-

nity and disease. *New Zealand Medical Journal, 103*(893), 314–316.

Booth, R. J., & Ashbridge, K. (1993). A fresh look at the relationship between the psyche and the immune system: Teleological coherence and harmony of purpose. *Advances, 9,* 4–23.

Bortz, W. M. (1989). Redefining human aging. *Journal of the American Geriatrics Society, 37,* 1092–1096.

Borysenko, J. (1987). *Minding the body, mending the mind.* New York: Bantam Books.

Borysenko, J. (1989). Removing barriers to the peaceful core. In R. Carlson & B. Shield (Eds.), *Healers on healing* (pp. 198–196). Los Angeles: Jeremy P. Tarcher.

Boscaro, M., & Armanini, D. (1994). Licorice ameliorates postural hypotension caused by diabetic autonomic neuropathy. *Diabetes Care, 17*(11), 1356.

Bossy, J., Guevin, F., & Yasui, H. (1990). *Nosologie traditionnelle chinoise et acupuncture* (pp. 156–158). Paris: Masson.

Boucher, T. A., & Kiresuk, T. J. (in press). Alternative therapies. In A. Graham & T. Schutlz (Eds.), *Principles of addiction medicine* 2nd ed.

Bouldin, A. S., Smith, M. C., Garner, D. D., Szeinbach, S. L., Frate, D. A., & Croom, E. M. (1997, March). *Herbal medicine in community pharmacy practice.* Paper presented at the meeting of the American Pharmaceutical Association, Los Angeles, CA.

Bourdiol, R. (1982). *Elements of auriculotherapy.* Moulins-les-Metz, France: Maisonnueve.

Bourgoin, B. P., Evans, D. R., Cornett, J. R., et al. (1993). Lead content in 70 brands of dietary calcium supplements. *American Journal of Public Health, 83,* 1155–1160.

Bourne, E. J. (1990). *The anxiety and phobia workbook.* Oakland: New Harbinger Publications.

Bouskela, E., Cyrino, F. Z., & Marcelon, G. (1994). Possible mechanisms for the inhibitory effect of *Ruscus* extract on increased microvascular permeability induced by histamine in hamster cheek pouch. *Journal Cardiovascular Pharmacology, 24*(2), 281–285.

Bowman, A. J., Clayton, R. H., Murray, A., Reed, J. W., Subhan, M. M., & Ford, G. A. (1997). Effects of aerobic exercise training and yoga on the baroreflex in healthy elderly persons. *Euro-*

pean Journal of Clinical Investigation, 27(5), 443–449.

Boyce, M. L., Robergs, R. A., Roldan, C., Foster, A., Montner, P., Stark, D., & Nelson, C. (1997). Exercise training by individuals with predialysis renal failure: Cardiorespiratory endurance, hypertension, and renal function. *American Journal of Kidney Diseases, 30*(2), 180–192.

Bradley, L. A. (1989). Cognitive-behavioral therapy for primary fibromyalgia. *Journal of Rheumatology, 16*(Suppl.), 131–136.

Brady, K. (1995). Prevalence, consequences and costs of tobacco, drug, and alcohol use in the United States. Training about alcohol and substance abuse for all primary care physicians. Proceedings of a conference sponsored by the Josiah Macy, Jr. Foundation. October 2–5. 1994 (in Circa, C. M. (Ed.)), Phoenix, AZ.

Braeckman, J. (1994). The extract of *Serenoa repens* in the treatment of benign prostatic hyperplasia: A multicenter open study. *Curr Ther Res, 55*, 776–785.

Braith, R. (1996). Moderate exercise, angiotensin II, aldosterone and vasopressin. Reported at the November 11th annual meeting of the American Heart Association, New Orleans.

Brancati, F., & Kao, L. (1997). Low magnesium levels may predict type II diabetes in Caucasians. Presented at the Annual meeting of the American Diabetes Association, June.

Branch, L. G., et al. (1994). Urinary incontinence: What many don't know. *Journal of the American Geriatrics Society, 42*, 1257.

Breithaupt-Grogler, K., Ling, M., Boudoulas, H., & Belz, G. G. (1997). Protective effect of chronic garlic intake on elastic properties of aorta in the elderly. *Circulation, 96*(8), 2649–2655.

Bremness, L. (1994). *Herbs.* New York and London: Dorling Kindersley.

Brennan, B. A. (1987). *Hands of light: A guide to healing through the human energy field.* New York: Bantam Books.

Brennan, M. J., Duncan, W. E., Wartofsky, L., et al. (1991). In vitro dissolution of calcium carbonate preparations. *Calcified Tissue International, 49*, 308–312.

Briere, J., Woo, R., McRae, B., Foltz, J., & Sitzman, R. (1997). Lifetime victimization history, demographics, and clinical status in female psychiatric emergency room patients. *Journal of Nervous Mental Disease, 185*(2), 95–101.

Briggs, L., & Joyce, P. R. (1997). What determines post-traumatic stress disorder symptomatology for survivors of childhood sexual abuse? *Child Abuse Negl, 21*(6), 575–581.

Brigham, D. D. (1994). *Imagery for Getting Well.* New York: Norton & Co.

Bristow-Braitman, A. (1995). Addiction recovery: 12-step programs and cognitive-behavioral psychology. *Journal of Counseling and Development, 73*, 414–418.

Britton, J., Pavord, I., Richards, K., Wisnewski, A., Knox, A., Lewis, S., Tattersfield, A., & Weiss, S. (1995). Dietary antioxidant vitamin intake and lung function in the general population. *American Journal of Respiratory and Critical Care Medicine, 151*, 1383–1387.

Britton, J., Pavord, I., Richards, K., Wisniewski, A., Knox, A., Lewis, S., Tattersfield, A., & Weiss, S. (1994). Dietary magnesium, lung function, wheezing, and airway hyperreactivity in a random adult population. *Lancet, 344*(8919), 357–362.

Broadman, J. (1958). A review of the foreign literature on bee venom for the treatment of all rheumatism. *General Practice.*

Brodsky, M. A., et al. (1994). Magnesium therapy in new-onset atrial fibrillation. *American Journal of Cardiology, 73*, 1227–1229.

Brody, L. (1993). Axling: A new spin on fitness. *Shape, 12*(8), 80–84.

Brooks, A., Thomas, S., & Droppleman, P. (1996). From frustration to red fury: A description of work-related anger in male registered nurses. *Nursing Forum, 31*(3), 4–15.

Brown, E. R. (1979). *Rockefeller's medicine men.* Berkeley, CA: University of California Press.

Brown, G. K., Beck, A. T., Newman, C. F., Beck, J. S., & Tran, G. Q. (1997). A comparison of focused and standard cognitive therapy for panic disorder. *Journal Anxiety Disord, 11*(3), 329–345.

Brown, R. K., McBurney, A., Lunec, J., & Kelly, F. J. (1995). Oxidative damage to DNA in patients with cystic fibrosis. *Free Radical Biology and Medicine, 18*(4), 801–806.

Brownley, K. A., Light, K. C., & Anderson, N. B. (1996). Social support and hostility interact to influence clinic, work, and home blood pressure in black and white men and women. *Psychophysiology*, *33*(4), 434–445.

Bruder, G. E., Steward, J. W., Mercier, M. A., et al. (1997). Outcome of cognitive-behavioral therapy for depression: Relation to hemispheric dominance for verbal processing. *Journal of Abnormal Psychology*, *106*(1), 138–144.

Bruyere, R. L. (1994). *Wheels of light*. New York: Simon & Schuster.

Buchan, W. (1769). *Domestic medicine*. Edinburgh: Balfour, Auld and Smellie.

Buchbauer, G., Jirovetz, L., Jager, W., et al. (1991). Aromatherapy: Evidence for sedative effects of the essential oil of lavender after inhalation. *Z Naturforsch*, *46*(11–12), 1067–1072.

Bucher, H. C., Guyatt, G. H., Cooke, R. J., Hatala, R., Cook, D. J., Lang, J. D., & Hunt, D. (1996). Effect of calcium supplementation on pregnancy-induced hypertension and preeclampsia. A meta-analysis of randomized controlled trials. *Journal of the American Medical Association*, *275*(14), 1113–1117.

Buchner, D. M., Cress, M. E., de Lateur, B. J., et al. (1997). A comparison of the effects of three types of endurance training on balance and other fall risk factors in older adults. *Aging (Milano)*, *9*(1–2), 112–119.

Buck, G. M., Sever, L. E., Batt, R. E., & Mendola, P. (1997). Lifestyle factors and female infertility. *Epidemiology*, *8*(4), 435–441.

Burckhardt, C. S., Mannerkorpi, K., Hedenberg, L., et al. (1994). A randomized, controlled clinical trial of education and physical training for women with fibromyalgia. *Journal of Rheumatology*, *21*, 714–720.

Burke, S. O., Kauffman, E., Costella, E. A., & Dillon, M. C. (1991). Hazardous secrets and reluctantly taking charge: Parenting a child with repeated hospitalizations. *Image: Journal of Nursing Scholarship*, *23*, 39–45.

Burns, K., Cunningham, N., White-Traut, R., Silvestri, J., & Nelson, M. (1994). Infant stimulation modification of an intervention based on physiologic and behavioral cues. *JOGNN*, *9*, 581–589.

Burros, M. (1997, December 15). U.S. weighs rules on organic foods. *Arizona Republic*, pp. A1, A8.

Burroughs, S. (1993). *Healing for the age of enlightenment: Balanced nutrition, vita flex, color therapy*. Auburn, CA: Burroughs Books.

Burton, A. K., Symonds, T. L., Zinzen, E., Tillotson, K. M., Caboor, D., et al. (1997). Is ergonomic intervention alone sufficient to limit musculoskeletal problems in nurses? *Occup Med*, *47*(1), 25–32.

Byers, D. C. (1983). *Better health with foot reflexology*. Saint Petersburg, FL: Ingham Publishing, Inc.

Byers, J. F., & Smyth, K. A. (1997). Effect of a music intervention on noise annoyance, heart rate, and blood pressure in cardiac surgery patients. *Am Journal Crit Care*, *6*(3), 183–191.

Caan, B., Duncan, D., Hiatt, R., et al. (1993). Association between alcoholic and caffeinated beverages and premenstrual syndrome. *Journal Reprod Med*, *38*(8), 630–636.

Caihn, K. (1983). Mental and emotional aspects of long distance running. *Psychosomatics*, *24*(2), 133–151.

Calvert, R. (1988, October–November). Exclusive interview, Judith Aston, developer of Aston-Patterning Bodywork. *Massage Magazine*, *16*, 12–13, 15, 17–19.

Camera, E., & Danao, T. (1989). The brain the immune system: A psychosomatic network. *Psychosomatics*, *30*(2), 140–146.

Cameron, J. (1992). *The artist's way: A spiritual path to higher creativity*. New York: Putnam.

Cameron, J. (1996). *The vein of gold: A journey to your creative heart*. New York: Putnam.

Cannon, W. (1939). *The wisdom of the body*. New York: W. W. Norton.

Cano Cuenca, B., Marco Algarra, J., Perez del Valle, B., & Pellicer Pascual, F. J. (1995). The effect of Ginkgo biloba on cochleovestibulary pathology of vascular origin. *An Otorrinolaringol Ibero Am*, *22*(6), 619–629.

Caplan, D. (1987). *Back trouble*. Gainsville, FL: Triad Publishing.

Caplan, R. L. (1984) Chiropractic. In J. W. Salmon (Ed.), *Alternative medicines: Popular and policy perspectives* (pp. 80–113). New York: Tavistock Publications.

Caplan, R. L. (1996, January–February). Managed health care: Reorganization without reform. *Dollars and Sense*, pp. 42–43.

Cappelli, R., Nicora, M., & Di Perri, T. (1988). Use of extract of *Ruscus aculeatus* in venous disease in the lower limbs. *Drugs Exp Clin Res*, *14*(4), 277–283.

Caprio, F. *Better health self hypnosis*. Prentice Hall.

The capsaicin study group. (1992). Effect of treatment with capsaicin on daily activities of patients with painful diabetic neuropathy. *Diabetes Care, 15*, 139–165.

Carey, O. J., Cookson, J. B., Britton, J., & Tattersfield, A. E. (1996). The effect of lifestyle on wheeze, atrophy and bronchial hyperreactivity in Asian and white children. *American Journal of Respiratory and Critical Care Medicine, 154*(2) part 1, 537–540.

Carey, O. J., Locke, C., & Cookson, J. B. (1993). Effect of alterations of dietary sodium on the severity of asthma in men. *Thorax, 48*(7), 714–718.

Carlston, M., Stuart, M. R., & Jonas, W. (1997). Alternative medicine instruction in medical schools and family practice residency programs. *Family Medicine, 29*(8), 559–562.

Carter, C. M., Urbanowicz, M., Hemsley, R., et al. (1993). Effects of a few food diet in attention deficit disorder. *Arch Dis Child, 69*(5), 564–568.

Cassidy, J. D., Lopes, A. A., & Yong-Hing, K. (1992). The immediate effect of manipulation versus mobilization on pain and range of motion in the cervical spine: A randomized controlled trial. *Journal Manipulative Physiol Ther, 15*(9), 570–575.

Caudell, K. (1996). Psychoneuroimmunology and innovative behavioral interventions in patients with leukemia. *Oncology Nursing Forum, 23*(3), 493–502.

Cayleff, S. E. (1992). *Wash and be healed: The water-cure movement and women's health*. Philadelphia: Temple University Press.

Cellini, L., Di Campli, E., Masulli, M., et al. (1996). Inhibition of Helicobacter pylori by garlic extract (*Allium sativum*). *FEME Immunol Med Microbiol, 13*(4), 273–277.

Cerda, J. (1996). Florida nutrition research advocates cholesterol-lowering foods instead of drugs. Press Release, University of Florida, Health Science Center, PO Box 100253, Gainesville FL 32610-0253.

Ceremuzynski, L., Chamiec, T., & Herbaczynski-Cedre, K. (1997). Effect of supplemental oral L-arginine on exercise capacity in patients with stable angina pectoris. *American Journal of Cardiology, 80*(3), 331–333.

Chai, J., Guo, Z., & Sheng, Z. (1995). Protective effects of vitamin E on impaired neutrophil phagocytic function in patients with severe burn. *Chung Hua Cheng Hsing Shao Shang Wai Ko Tsa Chih, 11*(1), 32–35.

Chaitow, L. (1988). *Soft-tissue manipulation: A practitioners guide to the diagnosis and treatment of soft tissue dysfunction and reflex activity*. Rochester, VT: Healing Arts Press.

Chaitow, L. (1996). *Modern neuromuscular techniques*. New York: Churchill Livingstone Publishers.

Chaitow, L. (1996). *Positional release techniques*. New York: Churchill Livingstone.

Chakalis, E., & Lowe, G. (1992). Positive effects of subliminal stimulation on memory. *Percept Motor Skills, 74*(3, Pt. 1), 956–958.

Chalmers, K., Thomson, K., & Degner, L. F. (1996). Information, support and communication needs of women with a family history of breast cancer. *Cancer Nursing, 19*(3), 204–213.

Chang, S., & Risch, H. A. (1997). Perineal talc exposure and risk of ovarian carcinoma. *Cancer, 79*(12), 2396–2401.

Changing your mind about your body. (1980, August). *Los Gatos Magazine*, 6–9.

Chappell, L. T., & Jason, M. (1996). EDTA chelation therapy in the treatment of vascular disease. *Journal of Cardiovascular Nursing, 10*, 78–86.

Chappell, L. T., & Stahl, J. P. (1993). The correlation between EDTA chelation therapy and improvement in cardiovascular function: A meta-analysis. *Journal of the Advancement in Medicine, 6*, 139–160.

Chappell, T. (1995). *Questions from the heart, Answers to 100 questions about chelation therapy, a safe alternative to bypass surgery*. Charlottesville, VA: Hampton Roads Publishing.

Charlesworth, E. A., & Nathan, R. G. (1982). *Stress management: A comprehensive guide to wellness*. New York: Ballantine Books.

The Charlie Foundation. (Producer). (1994). An introduction to the Ketogenic Diet. [Videotape]. Santa Monica, CA: Author.

The Charlie Foundation. (Producer). (1995). A primer in calculating and administering the Ketogenic Diet: A dietitian and nurses point of view. [Videotape]. Santa Monica, CA: Author.

Chasean-Taber, L., Selhub, J., Rosenberg, et al. (1996). A prospective study of folate and vitamin B6 and risk of myocardial infarction in U.S. physicians. *Journal of the American College of Nutrition, 15*(2), 136–143.

Chemtob, C. M., Novaco, R. W., Hamada, R. S., & Gross, D. M. (1997). Cognitive-behavioral treatment for severe anger in posttraumatic stress disorder. *Journal of Consulting and Clinical Psychology, 65*(1), 184–189.

Chen, W., & Zuoxu, L. (1994). Treating osteoarthritis of the knee joint by traditional Chinese medicine. *Journal of Traditional Chinese Medicine, 14*(4), 279–282.

Cheung, N. (1995). Looking at dietary effects on weight loss and diarrhea in HIV seropositive patients: a pilot project. *Nutrition and Health, 19*(3), 201–202.

Chikly, B., and A. (1997). Applications of pre- and post-surgical lymph drainage therapy. *Massage and Bodywork* (summer/fall), 64–67.

Chin, R. M. (1992). *The Energy Within, the Science Behind Every Oriental Therapy from Acupuncture to Yoga*. New York: Paragon House.

Chiou, W. F., Shum, A. Y., Liao, J. F., & Chen, C. F. (1997). Studies of cellular mechanisms underlying the vasorelaxant effects of rutaecarpine, a bioactive component extracted from an herbal drug. *Journal of Cardiovascular Pharmacology, 29*(4), 490–498.

Chitty & Muller. (1990). *Energy exercise*. Boulder, CO: Polarity Press.

Choe, M. A., & Heber, L. (1997). Dance/movement: Listen to the music. *Sigma Theta Tau International Reflections*, 2nd quarter, 17.

Chou, C. K. (1995). Radiofrequency hyperthermia for cancer therapy. In *CRC Biomedical Engineering Handbook* (pp. 1424–1430). CRC Press, Florida.

Chou, C. K., McDougall, J. A., Ahn, C., & Vora, N. (1997). Electrochemical treatment of mouse and rat fibrosarcomas with direct current. *Bioelectromagnetics, 18*, 14–24.

Chou, J. (Sept. 1986). A biological investigation of succussed serial microdilutions. *Journal Amer Inst Homeop*, Vol 79, No. 3, 100–105.

Christensen, A. J., & Smith, T. W. (1993). Cynical hostility and cardiovascular reactivity during self-disclosure. *Psychosomatic Medicine, 55*(2), 193–202.

Christensen, J. H., Ejlersen, E., Jessen, T., et al. (1995). Fatty acids and ventricular extrasystoles in patients with ventricular tachyarrhythmias. *Nutrition Research, 15*, 1–8.

Christensen, L. (1993). Effects of eating behavior on mood: A review of the literature. *International Journal of Eating Disorders, 14*, 171–183.

Christensen, L., & Burrows, R. (1990). Dietary treatment of depression. *Behavior Therapy, 21*, 183–194.

Christensen, L., & Redig, C. (1993). Effect of meal composition on mood. *Behavioral Neuroscience, 107*, 346–353.

Chuong, C. J., & Dawson, E. G. (1994). Zinc and copper levels in premenstrual syndrome. *Fertility and Sterility, 62*(2), 313–320.

Cichewicz, R. H. J., & Thorpe, P. A. (1996). The antimicrobial properties of chile peppers (Capsicum species) and their uses in Mayan medicine. *Journal of Ethnopharmacology, 52*(2), 61–70.

Cichoke, A. J. (1997). Are you a victim of syndrome X? *Health Counselor, 5*(5), 33–35.

Claire, T. (1995). Rubenfeld Synergy® Method: Touch Therapy Meets Talk Therapy. In *Bodywork*. New York: William Morrow and Company, 149–165.

Clark, A. J., Turner, J., Gauthier, D., & Williams, M. (1997). *The Effect of Therapeutic Touch on Pain and Anxiety in Burn Patients*. Manuscript submitted for publication.

Clark, C. C. (1996). *Wellness Practitioner, Second Edition*. New York: Springer.

Clauw, D. J. (1994). The pathogenesis of chronic pain and fatigue syndromes, with special reference to fibromyalgia. *Medical Hypotheses*, 369–368.

Clawson, G. A. (1996). Protease inhibitors and carcinogenesis: A review. *Cancer Investigation, 14*(6), 597–608.

Cleveland, C. S. III (1997). Vertebral subluxation. In D. Redwood (Ed.), *Contemporary chiropractic* (pp. 38–44). New York: Churchill Livingstone.

Cline, A. D. (1993). *Stress fractures in female Army recruits: Implications of exercise, calcium intake, and bone density*. Dissertation Abstracts International, Colorado State University. Volume: 54-06, Section B, 3002.

Coates, T. J., McKusick, L., Keno, R., & Stites, D. P. (1989). Stress reduction training changed number of sexual partners but not immune function in men with HIV. *American Journal of Public Health*, *79*, 885–886.

Cockerham, W. C. (1998). *Medical sociology*. Upper Saddle River, NJ: Prentice Hall.

Coetzer, H., Claassen, N., van Papendorp, D. H., & Kruger, M. C. (1994). Calcium transport by isolated brush border and basolateral membrane vesicles: Role of essential fatty acid supplements. *Prostaglandins Leukotrienes and Essential Fatty Acids*, *50*(5), 257–266.

Cogan, J. C. (1997, August). Feminist challenge to psychology's approach to obesity and eating disorders. Paper presented at the annual convention of the American Psychological Association, Chicago, IL.

Coghill, G. E. (1941). The educational methods of F. Matthias Alexander. In F. M. Alexander, *The universal constant in living* (pp. xxi–xxxiii). New York: E. P. Dutton.

Cohen, M. H. (1995). *A Fixed Star in Health Care Reform: The Emerging Paradigm of Holistic Healing*, 27 Ariz. State L. J. 79.

Cohen, M. H. (1996). *Holistic Health Care: Including Alternative and Complementary Medicine in Insurance and Regulatory Schemes*, 38 Ariz. L. Rev. 83.

Cohen, M. H. (1998). *Complementary and Alternative Medicine: Legal Boundaries and Regulatory Perspectives*. Baltimore: Johns Hopkins University Press.

Cohen, M., Mezoff, A., Laney, W., Bezerra, J., Beane, B., & Drazner, D. (1995). Use of a single solution for oral rehydration and maintenance therapy in infants with diarrhea and mild to moderate dehydration. *Pediatrics*, *95*, 639–645.

Cohen, S., Doyle, W. J., Skoner, D. P., et al. (1997). Social ties and susceptibility to the common cold. *Journal of the American Medical Association*, *277*(24), 1940–1944.

Cohen, S., Tyrell, D., & Smith, A. (1991). Psychological stress and susceptibility to the common cold. *New England Journal of Medicine*, *325*, 606–912.

Collins, J. A., & Rice, V. H. (1997). Effects of relaxation intervention in phase II cardiac rehabilitation. *Heart Lung*, *26*(1), 31–44.

Colt, H. G. (1996, September). See me, feel me, touch me, heal me. *Life*, pp. 35–40, 42, 46–47, 50.

Combest, W. L., & Nemecz, G. (1997). Herbal remedies in the pharmacy. *U.S. Pharmacist*, *22*(7), 50, 52, 55–56, 59.

Connors, M. E., Johnson, C. L., & Stuckey, M. K. (1984). Treatment of bulimia with brief psychoeducational group therapy. *American Journal of Psychiatry*, *141*(12), 1512–1516.

Cook, J. (1985, December). Body Ease. *Self Magazine*, 146.

Cook, P. (1973). *The relationship of Bender facilitating exercises to ocular control and to achievement test scores*. Ph.D. dissertation, Purdue University.

Cooney, N. L., Litt, M. D., Morse, P. A., Bauer, L. O., & Gaupp, L. (1997). Alcohol cue reactivity, negative-mood reactivity and relapse in treated alcohol men. *Journal of Abnormal Psychology*, *106*(2), 243–250.

Cooper, P. J., Coker, S., & Fleming, C. (1996). An evaluation of the efficacy of supervised cognitive behavioral self-help bulimia nervosa. *Journal of Psychosomatic Research*, *40*(3), 281–287.

Cooper, R. A., & Stoflet, S. J. (1996, Fall). The education and practice of alternative medicine clinicians (DataWatch). *Health Affairs*, pp. 226–238.

Cordell, G. A., & Arajuo, O. E. (1993). Capsaicin: Identification, nomenclature and pharmacotherapy. *Ann Pharmacother*, *27*, 330–332.

Corey, G. (1991). *Theory and practice of counseling and psychotherapy*. Pacific Grove, CA: Brooks/Cole.

Cornell, J. (1994). *Mandala: Luminous symbols for healing*. Wheaton, IL: Quest Books.

Cornwell, D. A. (1994). The role of lavender oil in relieving perineal discomfort following childbirth; a blind randomized clinical trial. *Journal Adv Nurs*, *19*, 89–96.

Coulehan, J. L. (1985). Chiropractic and the clinical art. *Social Science and Medicine*, *21*(4), 383–390.

Coulter, H. (1975). *Divided legacy: The conflict between homeopathy and the American Medical Association*. Berkeley, CA: North Atlantic Books.

Cowley, G., King, P., Hager, M., & Rosenberg, D. (1995, June 26). Going mainstream. *Newsweek*, pp. 56–57.

Cowrie, J. B., & Roebuck, J. (1975). *An ethnography of a chiropractic clinic.* New York: The Free Press.

CQ Researcher, 7(6), 121–144. (1997, February 14). Washington, DC: Congressional Quarterly.

Craig, W. J. (1997). Phytochemicals: Guardians of our health. *Journal Am Diet Assoc, 97*(Suppl. 10), S199–S204.

Cranton, E. (Ed.). (1989). *A textbook on EDTA chelation therapy,* special issue of *Journal of Advancement in Medicine, 2*(1, 2).

Cranton, E. (Ed.). (1994). *Bypassing bypass: The new technique of chelation therapy, a non-surgical treatment for improving circulation and slowing the aging process.* Trout Dale, VA: Medex Publishers.

Crawford, H. (1995). *Chronic pain and hypnosis.* http://www.altmed.od.nih.gov/oam/cgi-bin/research/seach_simple.cgi

Crawford, J. G. (1996). Alzheimer's disease risk factors as related to cerebral blood flow. *Medical Hypotheses, 46*(4), 367–377.

Crawford, R. D. (1995). Proposed role for a combination of citric acid and ascorbic acid in the production of dietary iron overload: A fundamental cause of disease. *Biochemistry and Molecular Medicine, 54*(1), 1–11.

Crits-Cristoph, P., & Singer, J. L. (1981). Imagery in cognitive-behavior therapy: Research and application. *Clinical Psychology Review, 1,* 19–32.

Csikszentimihalyi, M. (1996). *Creativity.* New York: Harper Collins.

Culliton, P. D., Boucher, T. A., & Bullock, M. L. (in press). Complementary/alternative therapies in the treatment of alcohol and other addictions. In J. Spencer & J. Jacobs (Eds.), *Complementary medicine: An integrated approach.* Philadelphia: Mosby-Yearbook, Inc.

Culliton, P. D., Boucher, T. A., & Carlson, G. A. (1997). Substance misuse and alternative medicine. In A. Watkins (Ed)., *The physician's handbook of mind-body medicine.* London: Churchill-Livingston.

Culliton, P., & Kiresuk, T. (1996). Overview of substance abuse acupuncture treatment research. *Journal of Alternative and Complementary Medicine, 2*(1), 149–159.

Cummings, S. R., Nevitt, M. C., Browner, W. S., et al. (1995). Risk factors for hip fracture in white women. *New England Journal of Medicine, 332*(12), 767–773.

Cunningham, MacDonald, Gant, Deep Venous Thrombosis, WILLIAMS OBSTETRICS, Twentieth Edition, Appleton & Lange, Prentice Hall, 1997; 1112–1117.

Cunningham, MacDonald, Gant, Supine Hypotensive Syndrome, WILLIAMS OBSTETRICS, Twentieth Edition, Appleton & Lange, Prentice Hall, 1997; 210.

Curhan, G. C., Willett, W. C., Rimm, E. G., Spiegelman, D., & Stampfer, M. J. (1996). Prospective study of beverage use and the risk of kidney stones. *American Journal of Epidemiology, 143*(3), 240–247.

Curhan, G. C., Willett, W. C., Speizer, F. E., Spiegelman, D., & Stampfer, M. J. (1997). Comparison of dietary calcium with supplemental calcium and other nutrients as factors affecting the risk for kidney stones in women. *Annals of Internal Medicine, 126*(7), 553–555.

Curhan, G. C., Willett, W. C., Rimme, E., & Stampfer, M. J. (1993). A prospective study of dietary calcium and other nutrients and the risk of symptomatic kidney stones. *New England Journal of Medicine, 328,* 833–838.

Curtis, K. M., Savitz, D. A., & Arbuckle, T. E. (1997). Effects of cigarette smoking, caffeine consumption, and alcohol intake on fecundability.

Cushman, K. (1995). *Midwife's apprentice.* New York: HarperCollins.

D'Adamo, P. J., with Whitney, C. (1996). *Eat right for your type.* New York: G. P. Putnam's Sons.

Dale, A., & Cornwell, S. (1994). The role of lavender oil in relieving perineal discomfort following childbirth: A blind randomized clinical trial. *Journal of Advanced Nursing, 19*(1), 89–96.

Dalery, K., Lussier-Cacan, S., Selhub, J., et al. (1995). Homocysteine and coronary artery disease in French Canadian subjects: Relation with vitamins B12, B6, pyridoxal phosphate, and folate. *American Journal of Cardiology, 75*(16), 1107–1111.

Daly, D. (1995). Alternative medicine courses taught at U.S. medical schools: An ongoing list. *Journal of Alternative and Complementary Medicine, 1,* 293–295.

Daly, M. E., Vale, C., Walker, M., et al. (1997). Dietary carbohydrates and insulin sensitivity: A review of the evidence and clinical implications. *American Journal of Clinical Nutrition, 66*(5), 1072–1085.

Dane, J. R. (1996). Hypnosis for pain and neuromuscular rehabilitation with multiple sclerosis: Case summary, literature review and analysis of outcomes. *International Journal of Clinical and Experimental Hypnosis, 44*(3), 208–231.

Dane, J., & Kessler, R. (1994). Self regulation techniques: and adjunction therapy for pain. In J. Hamill & J. Rowlinson (Eds.), *Handbook of critical care pain management* (pp. 239–250). New York: McGraw Hill.

Darius, I., & Leverett, A. (1995). Magnetic canceling technology and Kamma RPS. Techology White Paper, Connectware, Inc. Richardson, TX 75081.

Dart, R. (1959). An anatomist's tribute to F. Matthais Alexander. In *Skill and poise.* Urbanna, IL: NASTAT Books.

Dashwood, R., & Guo, D. (1995). Protective properties of chlorophylls against the covalent binding of heterocyclic amines to DNA in vitro and in vivo. *Princess Takamatsu Symp, 23,* 181–189.

Dashwood, R., Yamane, S., & Larsen, R. (1996). Study of the forces of stabilizing complexes between chlorophylls and heterocyclic amine mutagnes. *Environ Mol Mutagen, 27*(3), 211–218.

Daughtry, C. (1997). UF study reveals loss in sensory perception may not be linked to aging. Press Release, September 12, University of Florida, Health Science Center Communications, Gainesville, FL 32610-0253. (352) 392-2621.

Daugird, A., & Spencer, D. (1996). Physician reactions to the health care revolution: A grief model approach. *Archives of Family Medicine, 5*(9), 497–500.

Davidson, J. R., Morrison, R. M., Shore, J., et al. (1997). Homeopathic treatment of depression and anxiety. *Alternative Therapies in Health and Medicine, 3*(1), 46–49.

Davidson, P. (1991). *Chronic muscle pain syndrome.* New York: Berkley Books.

Davies, S., McLaren, H. J., Hunnisett, A., & Howard, M. (1997). Age-related decreases in chromium levels in 51,665 hair, sweat, and serum samples from 40,872 patients—implications for the prevention of cardiovascular disease and type II diabetes mellitus. *Metabolism, 46*(5), 469–473.

Daviglus, M. L., Stamler, J., Orencia, A. J., Dyer, A. R., Liu, K., Greenland, P., Walsh, M. K., Morris, D., & Shekelle, R. B. (1997). Fish consumption and the 30-year risk of fatal myocardial infarction. *New England Journal of Medicine, 336,* 1046–1053.

Davilla, G. W. (1994). Urinary incontinence: Which treatments help? *Postgraduate Medicine, 96,* 103.

Davis, E. (1992). *Heart and hands: A midwife's guide to pregnancy and birth.* Berkeley: Celestial Arts.

Davis, F. A. (1970). Axonal conduction studies based on some considerations of temperature effects in multiple sclerosis. *Electroencephalog Clin Neorophysiol, 28,* 281–286.

Davis, K. (1994). Press Release, International Asociation of Fitness Professionals, September 6, 1994, 6190 Cornerstone Court East, Suite 204, San Diego, CA 92121-3773.

Davis, L. E., Shen, J., & Royer, R. E. (1994). In vitro synergism of concentrated allium sativum extract and amphotericin B against Cryptococcus neoformans. *Planta Medica, 60*(6), 546–549.

Davis, M. D., Eshelman, E. R., & McKay, M. (1982). *The relaxation and stress reduction workbook* (2nd ed.). Oakland: New Harbinger Publications.

Davison, B. J., & Degner, L. F. (1997). Empowerment of men newly diagnosed with prostate cancer. *Cancer Nursing, 29*(3), 187–196.

Davydova., O. B., Tupitsyna, I., Bendarzhevskaia, A. K., et al. (1994). Submerged hydromassage as a method for the rehabilitation of myocardial infarct patients at the polyclinic stage. *Voprosy Kurortologii, Fizioterapii i Lechebnoi Fizicheskoi Kultury, 6,* 3–6.

Dawson-Hughes, B., Harris, S. S., Krall, E. A., et al. (1997). Effective calcium and vitamin D supplementation in men and women 65 years of age or older. *New England Journal of Medicine, 337*(10), 670–676.

De Angelis, T. (1996, July). Exercise gives a lift to psychotherapy. *Monitor,* American Psychological Association, p. 24.

de Lone, T. (1996). Creative movement for women at risk of cardiac disease. *Alternative Health Practitioner, 2*(2), 121–122.

de Rijk, M. C., Breteler, M. M., den Breeijen, J. H., Launer, L. J., Grobbee, D. E., Van der Meche, F. G., & Hoffman, A. (1997). Dietary antioxidants and Parkinson's disease: The Rotterdam Study. *Archives of Neurology, 54*(6), 762–765.

De Witt, P. M. (1993). The birth business. *American Demographics, 15,* 44–49.

DeAlcantra, P. (1997). *Indirect procedures: A musician's guide to the Alexander Technique.* Oxford, England: Oxford University Press.

DeAngelis, T. (1994). Report of the American Psychological Association's Conference: Psychological and behavioral factors in women's health—creating an agenda for the 21st century, May 11–14, Washington DC. *APA Monitor, 26*(7), 50.

Declair, V. (1997). The usefulness of topical application of essential fatty acids (EFA) to prevent pressure ulcers. *Ostomy Wound Management, 43*(5), 48–52.

DeGood, D. (1995). *Effect of massage therapy on post-surgical outcomes.* http://www.altmed.od. nih.gov/oam.cgi-bin/research/search_simple. cgi

deGroot, A. C., & Frosch, P. J. (1997). Adverse reactions to fragrances: A clinical review. *Contact Dermatitis, 36*(2), 57–86.

Dehpour, A. R., Zolfaghari, M. E., Samadian, T., & Vahedi, Y. (1994). The protective effect of liquorice components and their derivatives against gastric ulcer induced by aspirin in rats. *Journal Pharm Pharmacol, 46*(2), 148–149.

deLorgeril, M., Renaud, S., Mamelle, N., et al. (1994). Mediterranean alpha-linolenic acid-rich diet in secondary prevention of coronary heart disease. *Lancet, 343,* 1454–1459.

Delta Society. (1992). *Handbook for animal-assisted activities and animal-assisted therapy.* Renton, WA.

Dennison, B. A. (1997). Fruit juice consumption by infants and children: A review. *Journal of the American College of Nutrition, 15*(Suppl. 5), 4S–11S.

Dennison, B. A., Rockwell, H. L., & Baker, S. L. (1997). Excess fruit juice consumption by preschool-aged children is associated with short stature and obesity. *Pediatrics, 99*(1), 15–22.

Denny-Brown, D., Adams, R. D., Brenner, C., et al. (1945). The Pathology of Injury to Nerve Induced by Cold. *Journal of Neuropathology and Experimental Neurology, 4,* 305–323.

DePompei, P. M., Whitford, K. M., & Beam, P. H. (1994). One institution's effort to implement family-centered care. *Pediatric Nursing, 20,* 119–121, 132–133.

DerMarderosian, A. H. (1996). Understanding homeopathy. *Journal of the American Pharmaceutical Association,* NS36(5), 317–321.

DerMarderosian, A. H., & Kratz, A. M. (1997). Alternative healthcare. In A. R. Gennaro (Ed.), *Remington: The science and practice of pharmacy* (pp. 829–840). Easton, PA: Mack Publishing.

Deroc, D. (1991). *Les troubles sexuels chez la femme et médecine traditionnelle chinoise.* Séminaire: Actualites 1991—Acupuncture et gynécologie obstétrique, C.H.R.U. de Nimes.

Dewey, J. (1919). Introductory word. In F. M. Alexander, *Man's supreme inheritance.* New York: E. P. Dutton.

Diamond, H., & Diamond, M. *Living health.* New York: Warner.

Diaz, M. N., Frei, B., Vita, J. A., & Keaney, J. F. (1997). Antioxidants and atherosclerotic heart disease. *New England Journal of Medicine, 337*(6), 408–416.

Diehm, C., Trampisch, H. J., Lange, S., & Schmidt, C. (1996). Comparison of leg compression stocking and oral horse-chestnut seed extract therapy in patients with chronic venous insufficiency. *Lancet, 347*(8997), 292–294.

Dienstsrey, H. *Where the mind meets the body.* New York: Harper Collins.

Diet offers hope to children with epilepsy. (1997). *Advance for Nurse Practitioners,* 35–40, 66.

Dillon, K., Minchoff, B., & Baker, K. (1985). Positive emotional states and enhancement of the immune system. *International Journal of Psychiatric Medicine, 15,* 13–18.

Dirschl, D. R., Henderson, R. C., & Oakley, W. S. Jr. (1995). Correlation of bone mineral density in elderly patients with hip fractures. *Journal of Orthopaedic Trauma, 9*(6), 470–475.

Dishong, A. (1994). Florida scientists introduce new pectin-rich food powder to help prevent clogged arteries. *Health Science, 3.*

DNA repair works its way to the top. (1994). *Science, 266,* 1926.

Doblin, B. H., & Klamen, D. L. (1997). The ability of first-year medical students to correctly identify and directly respond to patients' observed behaviors. *Acad Med, 72*(7), 631–634.

Dobson, K. S. (1988). *Handbook of cognitive-behavioral therapies.* New York: Guilford.

Doeksen, G. A., Miller, D. A., & Howe, E. (1988). A model to evaluate whether a community can support a physician. *Journal of Medical Education, 63,* 515–521.

Dohn, N. E. (1994). Building stronger bones through weight training can help prevent osteoporosis. Press Release, University of Florida, Health Science Center Communications, PO Box 100253, Gainesville, 32610.

Dohn, N. E. (1996, February 15). Review of fiber research separates fact from fiction. News Release, Health Science Center Communications. University of Florida, Gainesville.

Dohn, N. E. (1996). Lifting weights shown to reverse effects of osteoporosis in heart transplant patients. Press Release, University of Florida, Health Science Center Communications, PO Box 100253, Gainesville, 32610.

Dolk, H., Shaddick, G., Walls, P., et al. (1997). Cancer incidence near radio and television transmitters in Great Britain. I. Sutton Coldfield transmitter. *American Journal of Epidemiology, 145*(1), 1–9.

Domar, A. D., Sebel, M. M., & Benson, H. (1990). The mind/body program for infertility: A new behavioral treatment approach for women with infertility. *Fertil Steril, 53*(2), 246–249.

Domar, A. D., & Dreher, H. (1996). *Healing Mind, Healthy Woman: Using the Mind-Body Connection to Manage Stress and Take Control of Your Life.* New York: Henry Holt.

Dossey, B. M. (1995). The psychophysiology of bodymind healing. In B. M. Dossey, L. Keegan, C. E. Guzzetta, & L. G. Kolkmeier, *Holistic nursing: A handbook for practice* (2nd ed.) (pp. 87–111). Gaithersburg, MD: Aspen Publishers.

Dossey, B. M., & Guzzetta, C. E. (1995). Holistic nursing practice. In B. M. Dossey, L. Keegan, C. E. Guzzetta, & L. G. Kolkmeier, *Holistic nursing: A handbook for practice* (2nd ed.) (pp. 1–24). Gaithersburg, MD: Aspen Publishers.

Dossey, B. M., Keegan, L., Guzzetta, C. E., & Kolkmeier, L. G. (1995). *Holistic nursing: A handbook for practice* (2nd ed.). Gaithersburg, MD: Aspen.

Dow, I., Tracey, M., Villar, A., Coggon, D., Margettes, B. M., Campbell, M. J., & Holgate, S. T. (1996). Does dietary intake of vitamins C and E influence lung function in older people? *American Journal of Respiratory and Critical Care Medicine, 154*(5), 1401–1404.

Dox, I. G., Melloni, B. J., & Eisner, G. M. (1993). *The HarperCollins Illustrated Medical Dictionary.* New York: HarperPerennial.

Doyle, T. J., Zheng, W., Cerhan, J. R., et al. (1997). The association of drinking water source and chlorination by-products with cancer incidence among postmenopausal women in Iowa: A prospective cohort study. *American Journal of Public Health, 87*(7), 1168–1176.

Drabaek, H., Petersen, J. R., Winberg, N., et al. (1996). The effect of *Ginkgo biloba* extract in patients with intermittent claudication. *Ugeskrift for Laeger, 158*(27), 3928, 3931.

Drury, N., & Drury, S. (1989). *Bach Flower Remedies. The illustrated dictionary of natural health.* New York: Sterling.

Drury, S., & N. (1989). *The Illustrated Dictionary of Natural Health.* New York: Sterling.

Dubbert, P. M. (1992). Exercise in behavioral medicine. *Journal of Consulting and Clinical Psychology, 60,* 613–618.

Dubovsky, S. L. (1997). *Mind-body deceptions: The psychodynamics of everyday life.* New York: W. W. Norton & Company, Inc.

Duke, J., & Vazquez, R. (1994). *Amazonian ethnobotanical dictionary.* Boca Raton, FL: CRC Press.

Dundee, J. W., et al. (1988, August). P6 Acupressure Reduces Morning Sickness. *Journal of the Royal Society of Medicine,* pp. 456–457.

Dunn, F. (1976). Traditional Asian medicine and cosmopolitan medicine as adaptive systems. In C. Leslie (Ed.), *Asian medical systems: A comparative study* (pp. 133–158). Berkeley, CA: University of California Press.

Dunn, S. C., Sleep, J., & Collett, D. (1995). Sensing and improving: An experimental study to evaluate the use of aromatherapy, massage and periods of rest in an intensive care unit. *Journal of Advanced Nursing, 21*(1), 34–40.

Dunstan, D. W., Mori, T., Puddey, I. B., et al. (1997). The independent and combined effects of aerobic exercise and dietary fish intake on serum lipids and glycemic control in NIDDM. A randomized controlled study. *Diabetes Care, 20*(6), 913–921.

Dworkin, B. M., Rosenthal, W. S., Wormser, G. P., Weiss, L., Nunez, M., Coline, C., & Herp, A. (1988). Abnormalities in blood selenium and glutathione peroxidase in patients with acquired immunodeficiency syndrome and AIDS-related complex. *Biological Trace Element Research, 20*, 86–96.

Dychtwald, K. *Bodymind.*

Dyerberg, J., & Bang, H. O. (1979). Haemostatic function and platelet polyunsaturated fatty acids in Eskimos. *Lancet, 2*, 433–435.

Dykman, K. D., Tone, C. M., & Dykman, R. A. (1997). Analysis of retrospective survey on the effects of nutritional supplements on chronic fatigue syndrome and/or fibromyalgia. *Journal of the American Nursing Association*, Supplement 1, 28–31.

Dzelzkalns, L. (1991, April). Treasure mapping. *Shape.*

Eadie, B. *Embraced by the light.* Gold Leaf Press.

Editors of Prevention Magazine. (1997). *New choices in natural healing for women.* Emmaus, PA: Rodale Press.

Edwards, S. (1989). *Breaking the sound barriers of dis-ease.* Unpublished manuscript.

Edwards, S. (1993). *Signature sound: Techniques and technology.* Athens, OH: Forum I Workshop.

Edwards, S. (1994). *Signature sound: Research and results.* Athens, OH: Forum II Workshop.

Edwards, S. (1995). *The first annual spring conference Bio-Acoustics: The Medicine of the Future.* Glouster, OH.

Eiker, D., & Sapphire, Ed. (1995). *Keep simple ceremonies.* Portland, ME: Astarte Shell Press.

Eisenberg, D. M. (1997). Advising patients who seek alternative medical therapies. *Annals of Internal Medicine, 127*(1), 61–69.

Eisenberg, D. M., Kessler, R. C., Foster, C., Norlock, F. E., Calkins, D. R., & Delbanco, T. L. (1993). Unconventional medicine in the United States: Prevalence, costs and patterns of use. *New England Journal of Medicine, 328*, 246–252.

Elder, J. (1997, July 31). Women take health care seriously, want more respect from doctors. *Arizona Republic*, p. HL4.

Elling, R. H. (1981). Political economy, cultural hegemony, and mixes of traditional and modern medicine. *Social Science and Medicine, 15A*, 89–99.

Ellis, A. (1984). Is the unified interaction approach to a cognitive-behavior modification a reinvention of the wheel? *Clinical Psychology Review, 4*, 215–217.

Ellis, A. (1987). The impossibility of achieving consistently good mental health. *American Psychologist, 42*, 364–375.

Emerich, M. (1996, June). Industry growth: 22.6%. *Natural Foods Merchandiser, 17*(6), 1, 22.

Engel, G. (1962). *Psychological development in health and disease.* Philadelphia: Saunders.

Eos, N. (1995). *Reiki and medicine.* Grass Lake, Michigan: Nancy Eos, MD.

Erdman, C. K. (1995). *Nothing to lose: A guide to sane living in a larger body.* New York: HarperCollins.

Eriksen, L. (1995). A Close Up View of Company Reflexology. Danish Reflexology Association Committee Report of February 1995, Copenhagen, Danish Reflexology Association.

Erikson, E. (1959). Identity and the life cycle. *Psychological Issues* (Vol. 1, No. 1). New York: International Universities Press.

Ermalinski, R., Hanson, P. G., Lubin, B., Thorby, J. I., & Nahormek, P. A. (1997). Impact of a body-mind treatment component on alcoholic inpatients. *Journal Psychosoc Nurs Mental Health Serv, 35*(7), 39–45.

Ernst, E. (1996). *Complementary medicine: An objective appraisal.* Oxford: Butterworth-Heinemann.

Eslinger, P. (1995). *Music therapy and brain injury* (Funded study, Office of Alternative Medicine, National Institutes of Health). Abstract available: http://www.altmed.od.nih.gov/oam/cgi-bin/research/search_simple.cgi

Esterling, B. A., Antoni, M. H., Fletcher, M. A., Margulies, S., & Schneiderman, N. (1994). Emotional disclosure through writing or speaking modulates latent Epstein-Barr virus reactivation. *Journal of Consulting and Clinical Psychology, 62*, 130–140.

Estok, P. J., & Rudy, E. B. (1996). The relationship between eating disorders and running in women. *Res Nurs Health, 19*(5), 377–387.

Everson, S. A., Goldberg, D. E., Kaplan, G. A., et al. (1996). Hopelessness and risk of mortality and incidence of myocardial infarction and cancer. *Psychosomatic Medicine, 58,* 113–121.

Faccinetti, F., Borella, P., Sances, G., et al. (1991). Oral magnesium successfully relieves premenstrual mood changes. *Obstetrics and Gynecology, 78*(2), 177–181.

Facino, R. M., Carini, M., Stefani, R., Aldini, G., & Saibene, L. (1995). Anti-elastase and anti-hyaluronidase activities of saponins and sapongenins from Hedera helix, Aesculus hippocastanum, and Ruscus aculeatus: Factors contributing to their efficacy in the treatment of venous insufficiency. *Archives of Pharmacy, 328*(10), 720–724.

Facino, R. M., et al. (1994). Free radical scavenging action and anti-enzyme activities of procyanidines from Fitis vinifera. A mechanism for their capillary protective action. *Arzneim Forsch, 44,* 592–60l.

Fackelmann, K. A. (1992). Hints of a chlorine-cancer connection. *Science News, 142,* 23.

Fairweather-Tait, S., & Pier, Z. (1991). The effect of tea on iron and aluminum metabolism. *British Journal of Nutrition, 65,* 61–68.

Fan, C. F., Tanhui, E., Joshi, S., Trivedi, S., Hong, Y., & Shevde, K. (1997). Acupressure treatment for prevention of postoperative nausea and vomiting. *Anesthesia and Analgesia, 84*(4), 821–825.

Fang, Z. (1982). The honeybee and human health. *NAAS Proc, 5,* 18.

Farkas, C., & leRiche, W. (1987). Effect of tea and coffee consumption on non-haem iron absorption. *British Journal of Nutrition, 65,* 161–163.

Fawcett, J., Sidney, J., Riley-Lawless, K., & Hanson, J. J. (1996). An exploratory study of the relationship between alternative therapies, functional status, and symptom severity among people with multiple sclerosis. *Journal Holistic Nursing, 14*(2), 115–129.

Fawzi, W. W., Herrera, M. G., Willett, W. C., Nestel, P., el Amin, A., Lipsitz, S., & Mohamed, K. A. (1994). Dietary vitamin A intake and the risk of mortality among children. *American Journal of Clinical Nutrition, 59*(2), 401–408.

Fawzy, I. F., Kemeny, M. E., Fawzy, N. W., Elashoff, R., Morton, D., Cousins, N., & Fahey, J. I. (1990). A structured psychiatric intervention for cancer patients: Changes over time in immunological measures. *Archives of General Psychiatry, 47,* 729–735.

Fawzy, I. F., & Fawzy, N. W. (1994). Psychoeducational interventions and health outcomes. In R. Glaser & J. Kiecolt-Glaser (Eds.), *Handbook of human stress and immunity* (pp. 365–402). San Diego: Academic Press.

Fehily, A. M., Burr, M. L., Phillips, K. M., & Deadman, N. M. (1983). The effect of fatty fish on plasma lipid and lipoprotein concentrations. *American Journal of Clinical Nutrition, 38,* 349–351.

The Feldenkrais Guild of North America. (1996). The Feldenkrais Method an overview—video recording. Albany, OR: Author.

Feldenkrais, M. (1972). *Awareness through movement.* Harper and Row: New York Hagerstown San Francisco London.

Feldenkrais, M. (1985). *The potent self.* Harper and Row: San Francisco Cambridge Hagerstown New York Philadelphia London Mexico City Sao Paulo Singapore Syndey.

Felhendler, D., & Lisander, B. (1996). Pressure on acupoints decreases postoperative pain. *Clinical Journal of Pain, 12*(4), 326–329.

Ferrannini, E., Natali, A., Capaldo, B., et al. (1997). Insulin resistance, hyperinsulinemia, and blood pressure: Role of age and obesity, European Group for the Study of Insulin Resistance. *Hypertension, 30*(5), 1144–1149.

Ferrara-Love, R., Sekeres, L., & Bircher, N. G. (1996). Nonpharmacologic treatment of postoperative nausea. *Journal of Perianesthesia Nursing, 11*(6), 3778–3783.

Ferrell, B. A., Josephson, K. R., Pollan, A. M., Loy, S., & Ferrell, B. R. A randomized trial of walking versus physical methods for chronic pain management. *Aging (Milano), 9*(1–2), 99–105.

Ferrell-Torry, A. T., & Glick, O. J. (1993). The use of therapeutic massage as a nursing intervention to modify anxiety and the perception of cancer pain. *Cancer Nursing, 16,* 93–100.

Fick, K. M. (1993). The influence of an animal on social interactions of nursing home residents in a group setting. *American Journal of Occupational Therapy, 47*(6), 529–534.

Field, T. (1986). Tactile/kinesthetic stimulation effects on preterm infants. *Pediatrics, 77,* 5.

Field, T. (1990). Massage alters growth and cate-cholamine production in preterm newborns. *Advances in Touch*, Key Biscayne, FL, Johnson and Johnson Round Table #14.

Field, T. (1995). *Massage effects on development-immune function of HIV-exposed* infants. Office of Alternative Medicine Research Grant Results. http://altmed.od.nih.gov/oam/cgi-bin/research/search_simple.cgi.

Field, T. (1995). The benefits of infant massage on growth and development. *Pediatric Basics* Gerber Products Company, Winter, (71).

Field, T. M., et al. (1987). Massage of preterm newborns to improve growth and development. *Pediatric Nurse*, *13*, 385–387.

Field, T. M., Grizzle, N., Scafidi, F., et al. (1996). Massage and relaxation therapies' effects on de-pressed adolescent mothers. *Adolescence*, *31*(124), 903–911.

Field, T., Quintino, O., Henteleff, T., et al. (1997). Job stress reduction therapies. *Altern Ther Health Med*, *3*(4), 54–56.

Field, T., Schanberg, S. M., Scafidi, F., Bauer, C. R., Vega-Lahr, N., Garcia, R., Nystrom, J., & Kuhn, C. M. (1986). Tactile/kinesthetic stimula-tion effects on preterm neonates. *Pediatrics*, *77*(5), 654–658.

Fischer-Rizzi, S. (1990). *Complete aromatherapy handbook: Essential oils for radiant health*. New York: Sterling.

Fishbein, M. (Ed.). (1935). *Modern home medical adviser*. New York: Doubleday, Doran.

Fisher, K. (1988). Early experiences of a multidisci-plinary pain management programme. *Holistic Medicine*, *3*, 47–56.

Fisher, P., & Ward, A. (1994, July 9). Complemen-tary medicine in Europe. *British Medical Jour-nal*, *309*, 107–110.

Fitzgerald, W. (1917). *Zone Therapy*. Columbus, OH: I. W. Long Publishing.

Fleet, J. C. (1994). New support for a folk remedy: Cranberry juice reduces bacteriuria and pyuria in elderly women. *Nutrition Reviews*, *5*(2), 168–170.

Fleming, J., Mullen, P., & Bammer, G. (1997). A study of potential risk factors for sexual abuse in childhood. *Child Abuse Negl*, *21*(1), 49–58.

Fleming, L., et al. (1994). Parkinson's disease and brain levels of organochlorine pesticides. *Annals of Neurology*, *36*, 100–103.

Fleming, T. (Ed.). (1998). *Physicians' Desk Refer-ence for Herbal Medicines*. Montvale, NJ: Medi-cal Economics.

Fletcher, N. (1970). *The chemical physics of ice*. Cambridge University Press, fig 5.4.

Flowers, B. (1993). Interview with Dr. Candace Pert. *Bill Moyer's healing and the mind*. New York: Doubleday.

Fluge, T., Richter, J., Fabel, H., et al. (1994). Long-term effects of breathing exercises and yoga in patients with bronchial asthma. *Pneumologie*, *48*(7), 484–490.

Flynn, M. A., Irvin, W., & Krause, G. (1994). The effect of folate and cobalamin on osteoarthritic hands. *Journal of the American College of Nutri-tion*, *13*(4), 351–356.

Földi, M., and E. (1993). *Lymphoedema Methods of Treatment and Control*. Portland, OR: Medicina Biologica, 1993.

Food, Drug, and Cosmetic Act, Pub. L. No. 75-717, 52 *Stat.* 2040 (1938), as amended, 21 *U.S.C.* §§ 301 et seq.; Drug Amendments of 1962 (Kef-auver-Harris Amendments), Pub. L. No. 87-781, 76 *Stat.* 780 (1962), codified at 21 *U.S.C.* § 355.

Ford, C. W. (1994). *Compassionate touch*. New York: Parkside.

Fordyce, W., Fowler, R., & DeLateur, B. (1968). An application of behavior modification tech-nique to a problem of chronic pain. *Behavior Research and Therapy*, *6*, 105–107.

Foreyt, J. P., & Goodrick, G. K. (1992). *Living without dieting: A revolutionary guide for every-one who wants to lose weight*. New York: War-ner Books.

Forster, K. A. (1950). Forty years of experience with bee venom therapy. *Che Med*.

42 *U.S.C.* § 1320a-7a(a)(1)(E).

Fotherby, M. D., & Potter, J. F. (1997). Long-term potassium supplementaiton lowers blood pressure in elderly hypertensive subjects. *Int Journal Clin Pract*, *51*(4), 219–222.

Foxman, B., Geiger, A. M., Palin, K., Gillespie, B., & Koopman, J. S. (1995). First-time urinary tract infection and sexual behavior. *Epidemiol-ogy*, *6*(2), 162–168.

Franceschi, S., Bidoli, E., La Vecchia, C., et al. (1996). Tomatoes and risk of digestive-tract can-cers. *International Journal of Cancer*, *59*(2), 181–184.

Franceschi, S., Favero, A., La Vecchia, et al. (1995). Influence of food groups and food diversity on breast cancer risk in Italy. *International Journal of Cancer, 63*(6), 785–789.

Frangolias, D., & Rhodes, E. (1995). Maximal and ventilatory threshold responses to treadmill and water immersion running. *Medicine and Sci in Sports and Exer, 27*(7), 1007–1013.

Frankenburg, W. K., Goldstein, A., & Camp, B. (1971). The revised Denver Developmental Screening Test: Its accuracy as a screening instrument. *Journal of Pediatrics, 79*, 988–995.

Franklin, N. (1984, Spring). Bodywork. *Self Care,* pp. 35–37, 53–56.

Fraser, G. E., Lindsted, K. D., & Beeson, W. L. (1995). Effect of risk factor values on lifetime risk of and age at first coronary event. The Adventist Health Study. *American Journal of Epidemiology, 142*(7), 746–758.

Freeman, J. M., Kelly, M., & Freeman, J. B. (1994). *The epilepsy diet treatment.* New York: Demos Publications.

Freeman, J. M., Vining, E. P. G., & Pillas, D. J. (1991). *Seizures and epilepsy in childhood: A guide for parents.* Baltimore: Johns Hopkins University Press.

Freeston, M. H., Ladouceur, R., Gagnon, F., et al. (1997). Cognitive-behavioral treatment of obsessive thoughts: A controlled study. *Journal of Consulting and Clinical Psychology, 65*(3), 405–413.

Freudenheim, J. L., Marshall, J. R., Vena, J. E., et al. (1996). Premenopausal breast cancer risk and intake of vegetables, fruits, and related nutrients. *Journal of the National Cancer Institute, 88*(6), 340–348.

Friedman, R., & Benson, H. (1997). Spirituality and medicine. *Mind/Body Medicine, 2*(1), 1–2.

Friedman, R., Sobel, D., Myers, D., et al. (1996, Fall). Behavioral medicine, clinical health psychology and cost offset. Medical Cost Offset. pp. 25–48.

Friel, J., Andrews, W., Matthew, J., et al. (1993). Zinc supplementation in very-low-birth-weight infants. *Journal Ped Gastr, 17*, 97–104.

Friese, K. H., Kruse, S., & Moeller, H. (1996). Acute otitis media in children. Comparison between conventional and homeopathic therapy. *HNO, 44*(8), 462–466.

Frozena, C. (1997). Multiple sclerosis. *American Journal of Nursing, 97*(11), 48.

Fry, R. P., Beard, R. W., Crips, A. H., & McGuigan, S. (1997). Sociopsychological factors in women with chronic pelvic pain with and without pelvic venous congestion. *Journal of Psychosomatic Research, 41*(1), 71–85.

Fry, W. (1994). The biology of humor. *Humor: International Journal of Humor Research, 7*(2), 111–126.

Frymann, V. M. (1966). Relation of disturbances of craniosacral mechanisms to symptomatology of the newborn: A study of 1,250 infants. *JAOA, 65*, 1059.

Fuller, C. J., Chandalia, M., Garg, A., Grundy, S. M., & Jialal, I. (1996). RRR-alpha-tocopheryl acetate supplementation at pharmacologic dose decreases low-density lipoproprotein oxidative susceptibility but not protein glycation in patients with diabetes mellitus. *American Journal of Clinical Nutrition, 63*(5), 753–759.

Furacciolo, G., Chirelli, L., Scita, F., et al. (1987). EMG-biofeedback training in fibromyalgia syndrome. *Journal of Rheumatology, 14*, 820–825.

Furhman, B., Buch, S., Vaya, J., Belinky, P. A., et al. (1997). Licorice extract and its major polyphenol glabridin protect low-density lipo-protein against lipid peroxidation: In vitro and ex vivo studies in humans and in atherosclerotic apolipoprotein E-deficient mice. *American Journal of Clinical Nutrition, 66*(2), 267–275.

Gabbay, F. H., Krantz, D. S., Kop, W. J., et al. (1996). Triggers of myocardial ischemia during daily life in patients with coronary artery disease: Physical and mental activities, anger and smoking. *Journal of the American College of Cardiology, 27*(3), 585–592.

Gagne, D., & Toye, R. C. (1994). The effects of therapeutic touch and relaxation therapy in reducing anxiety. *Archives of Psychiatric Nursing, 8*(3), 184–189.

Galbraith, L. K., Kaiser, S., Mahoney, D., Moore-Harris, L., Polman, I., Ross, L., Vaughn, G., & Willenbrink, D. (1992). An overnight retreat to facilitate coping with stress. *Pediatric Nursing, 18*, 372–374.

Galibois, I., Desrosiers, T., Guevin, N., Lavigne, C., & Jacques, H. (1994). Effects of dietary fibre mixtures on glucose and lipid metabolism and on mineral absorption in the rat. *Annals of Nutrition and Metabolism, 38*(4), 203–211.

Gallai, V., et al. (1994). Magnesium content of mono-nuclear blood cells in migraine patients. *Headache, 34,* 160–165.

Galland, L. D., Baker, S. M., & McLellan, R. K. (1986). Magnesium deficiency in the pathogenesis of mitral valve prolapse. *Magnesium, 5,* 165–174.

Gammonley, J., Howie, A., Kirwin, S., Zapf, S., Frye, J., Freeman, G., & Stuart-Russell, R. (1996). *Animal-assisted therapy in the health care professions.* Renton, WA: Delta Society.

Gantes, M., Kirchhoff, K. T., Work, B. A., Jr. (1985, Nov-Dec). Breast massage to obtain Contraction Stress Test. *Journal of Nursing Research, 34*(6), pp. 338–341.

Gao, L. (1991). Study on the adequate dosage of vitamin A in the prevention and treatment of postburn visceral injury. *Chung Hua I Hsueh Tsa Chih (Taipei), 71*(4), 199–201.

Garfinkle, M. S., Schumacher, H. R. Jr., Husain, A., Levy, M., & Reshetar, R. A. (1994). Evaluation of a yoga based regimen for treatment of osteoarthritis of the hands. *Journal of Rheumatology, 21*(12), 2341–2342.

Garg, A., Bonanome, S. A., Grundy, S., et al. (1988). Comparison of a high-carbohydrate diet with a high-monosaturated diet in patients with non-insulin-dependent diabetes mellitus. *New England Journal of Medicine, 319,* 829–934.

Garnefski, N., & Diekstra, R. F. (1997). Child sexual abuse and emotional and behavioral problems in adolescence: Gender differences. *Journal of the American Academy of Child and Adolescent Psychiatry, 36*(3), 323–329.

Garrard, C. T. (1995). *The Effect of Therapeutic Touch on Stress Reduction and Immune Function in Persons with AIDS.* (Doctoral dissertation, University of Alabama at Birmingham.)

Garrett, J. T. (1997). *Cherokee medicine.* Sante Fe, NM: Bear and Company.

Garrison, R., & Somer, E. (1995). Chromium, cobalt, copper, fluoride, selenium, zinc and cobalt. *The Nutrition Desk Reference* (3rd ed.). New Canaan, CT: Keats Publishing, Inc., p. 217.

Gebhardt, R. (1997). Antioxidative and protective properties of extracts from leaves of the artichoke (*Cynara scolymus L.*) against hydroperoxide-induced oxidative stress in cultured rat hypa-

tocytes. *Toxicology and Applied Pharmacology, 144*(2), 279–286.

Gelb, M. (1994). *Body learning.* New York: Henry Holt & Co.

Gelfand, D. M., Teti, D., Seiner, S. A., & Jameson, P. B. (1996). Helping mothers fight depression: Evaluation of a home-based intervention program for depressed mothers and their infants. *Journal of Clin Child Psychol, 25,* 406–422.

Gerard, L. (1997). Group learning behavior modification and exercise for women with urinary incontinence. *Urological Nursing, 17*(1), 17–22.

Gerber, R. (1988). *Vibrational medicine.* Santa Fe, NM: Bear & Co.

Gerber, R. (1996). *Vibrational medicine.* Santa Fe, NM: Bear & Co.

Gerson, S. (1993). *Ayurveda: The ancient Indian healing art.* Rockport, MA: Element Inc.

Gerster, H. (1997). The potential role of lycopene for human health. *Journal of the American College of Nutrition, 16*(2), 109–126.

Gesler, W. M. (1988). The place of chiropractors in health care delivery: A case study of North Carolina. *Social Science and Medicine, 26*(8), 785–792.

Gessner, B., Voelp, A., & Klasser, M. (1985). Study of the longterm action of a *Ginkgo biloba* extract on vigilance and mental performance as determined by means of quantitative pharmaco-EEG and psychometric measurements. *Arzneimittel-Forschung, 35*(9), 1459–1465.

Gevitz, N. (1991). *The D.O.s: Osteopathic medicine in America.* Baltimore, MD: Johns Hopkins University Press.

Gevitz, N. (Ed.). (1988). *Other healers: Unorthodox medicine in America.* Baltimore, MD: Johns Hopkins University Press.

Gibson, R. (1991). Trace element deficiencies in humans. *Canadian Medical Association Journal, 145,* 231.

Gillman, M. W., Belanger, A., D'Agostino, R. B., Ellison, R. C., & Posner, B. M. (1994). Protective effect of calcium intake on development of hypertension. Presented at the 34th Annual Conference on Cardiovascular Disease Epidemiology and Prevention, March 16 and 17, Hyatt Regency Westshore, Tampa, Florida, p. 10.

Gillman, M. W., Cupples, L. A., Gagnon, D., et al. (1995). Protective effect of fruits and vegetables on development of stroke in men. *Journal of the*

American Medical Association, 273(14), 1113–1117.

Gillman, M. W., Hood, M. Y., Moore, L. L., Singer, M. R., Uyen-Sa, N., & Andon, M. B. (1994). Effect of calcium supplementaiton on blood pressure in inner-city children. Presented at the 34th Annual Conference on Cardiovascular Disease Epidemiology and Prevention, March 16 and 17, Hyatt Regency Westshore, Tampa, Florida, p. 10.

Gillum, M. E., Mussolino, & Ingram, D. D. (1996). Physical activity and stroke incidence in women and men: The NHANES I Epidemiologic Follow-up Study. *American Journal of Epidemiology, 143*, 860–869.

Gin, R. H., & Green, B. N. (1997). George Goodheart, J., D.C., and a history of applied kinesiology. *Journal Manipulative Physiol Ther, 20*(5), 331–337.

Giovannucci, E., Ascherio, A., Rimm, E. G., et al. (1995). Intake of carotenoids and retinol in relation to risk of prostate cancer. *Journal of the National Cancer Institute, 87*(23), 1767–1776.

Giovannucci, E., Rimme, E. B., Stampfer, M. J., Colditz, G., & Willett, W. C. (1992). Relationship of diet to risk of colorectal adenoma in men. *J Natl Cancer Inst, 84*(2), 91–98.

Giovannucci, E., Rimme, E. G., Colditz, G. A., et al. (1993). A prospective study of dietary fat and risk of prostate cancer. *Journal of the National Cancer Institute, 85*, 1571–1579.

Girodon, F., Blache, D., Monget, A. L., Lombart, M., Brunet-Lecompte, P., Arnaud, J., Richard, M. J., & Galan, P. (1997). Effect of a two-year supplementation with low doses of antioxidant vitamins and/or minerals in elderly subjects on levels of nutrients and antioxidant defense parameters. *Journal of the American College of Nutrition, 16*(4), 357–365.

Glaister, J. A. (1994). Projective drawings: Helping adult survivors of childhood abuse recognize boundaries. *Journal of Psychosocial Nursing and Mental Health Services, 32*(10), 28–34.

Glaser, R., & Kiecolt-Glaser, J. (Eds.). (1994). *Handbook of human stress and immunity.* San Diego, CA: Academic Press.

Goddaer, J., & Abraham, I. L. (1994). Effects of relaxing music on agitation during meals among nursing home residents with severe cognitive impairment. *Archives of Psychiatric Nursing, 8*(3), 150–158.

Goldberg, B. (Ed.). (1993). *Alternative medicine: The definitive guide.* Tiburon, CA: Future Medicine Publishing.

Goldberg, N. (1986). *Writing down the bones: Freeing the writer within.* Boston: Shambhala.

Goldenberg, D. L. (1989). Treatment of fibromyalgia syndrome. *Rheumatic Disease Clinics of North America, 15*, 61–71.

Goldfried, M. R. (1977). The use of relaxation and cognitive relabeling as coping skills. In R. B. Stuart (Ed.), *Behavioral self management: Strategies, techniques, and outcomes* (pp. 82–116). New York: Brunner-Mazel.

Goldfried, M. R. (1980). Psychotherapy as coping skills training. In M. J. Mahoney (Ed.), *Psychotherapy process: Current issues and future direction* (pp. 89–119). New York: Plenum Press.

Goleman, D., & Gurin, J. (1993). *Mind body medicine.* New York: Consumer Reports Books.

Goleman, D, Kaufman, P., & Ray, M. (1992). *The creative spirit.* New York: Dutton.

Gong, Y. F., Huang, Z. J., Qiang, M. Y., et al. (1991). Suppression of radioactive strontium absorption by sodium alginate in animals and human subjects. *Biomedical and Environmental Sciences, 4*(3), 273–282.

Goode, H. F., Burns, E., & Walker, B. E. (1992). Vitamin C depletion and pressure sores in elderly patients with femoral neck fracture. *British Medical Journal, 305*(6859), 925–927.

Goodill, S. W. (1995). Dance movement therapy for adults with cystic fibrosis: Office of Alternative Medicine funded study. http://www.altmed.od.nih.gov/oam.cgi-bin/research/search_simple.cgi

Goodkin, D. E., Ransohoff, R. M., & Rudick, R. A. (1992). Experimental therapies for multiple sclerosis: Current status. *Cleveland Clinic Journal of Medicine, 59*, 63–74.

Goodman, M. T., Wilkens, L. R., Hankin, J. H., et al. (1997). Association of soy and fiber consumption with the risk of endometrial cancer. *American Journal of Epidemiology, 146*(4), 294–306.

Goodrick, G. K., Poston II, W. S. C., Kimball, K. T., Reeves, R. S., & Foreyt, J. P. (in press). Non-dieting vs. dieting treatment for overweight binge-eating women. *Journal of Consulting and Clinical Psychology.*

Gordon, J. S. (1996). *Manifesto for a new medicine.* Reading, MA: Addison Wesley.

Gordon, R. J., & Silverstein, G. (1998). Marketing channels for alternative health care. In R. J. Gordon, B. C. Nienstedt, & W. M. Gesler (Eds.), *Alternative therapies: Expanding options in health care* (pp. 87–103). New York: Springer Publishing Company.

Gordon, R. J., Meister, J. S., & Hughes, R. G. (1992). Accounting for shortages of rural physicians: Push and pull factors. In W. M. Gesler & T. C. Ricketts (Eds.), *Health in rural North America: The geography of health care services and delivery* (pp. 153–178). New Brunswick, NJ: Rutgers University Press.

Gorecki, D. K., Richardson, C. J., Wallace, S. M., & Pavlakadies, P. (1989). Dissolution rates in calcium carbonate tablets: A consideration in product selection. *Canadian Pharmacy Journal, 122,* 484–487.

Gorh, M., Ropcke, B., Pistor, K., & Eggers, C. (1997). Autogenic training in children and adolescents with type 1 diabetes mellitus. *Praxis Kinderpsychologie und Kinderpsychiatrie, 46*(4), 288–303.

Gossling, H. R., Bernstein, R. A., & Abbott, J. (1992). Treatment of ununited tibial fractures: A comparison of surgery and pulsed electromagnetic fields (PEMF). *Orthopedics, 17,* 711–719.

Gottliev, B. (1995). *New Choices in Natural Healing.* Emmaus, PA: Rodale Press.

Gould, K. L., Ornish, D., Scherwitz, L., et al. (1995). Changes in myocardial perfusion abnormalities by positron emission tomography after long-term intense risk factor modification. *Journal of the American Medical Association, 275*(18), 1402–1403.

Govindarajan, V. S., & Sathyanarayana, M. N. (1991). Capsicum—production, technology, chemistry, and quality. Part V. Impact on physiology, pharmacology, nutrition, and metabolism: Structure, pungency, pain and desensitization sequences. *Critical Reviews of Food Science and Nutrition, 29*(6), 435–474.

Grad, B. (1963). A telekinetic effect on plant growth. *International Journal of Parapsychology, 5*(2), 117–131.

Grad, B., Cadoret, R. F., & Paul, G. I. (1961). An unorthodox method of treatment of wound healing in mice. *International Journal of Parapsychology, 3*(2), 5–19.

Gradinger, G. (1995). Update from the American Board of Plastic Surgery. *Plastic Surgery News, 8*(3), 3.

Graham, I. M., Daly, L. E., Refsum, H. M., et al. (1997). Plasma homocysteine as a risk factor for vascular disease. *Journal of the American Medical Association, 277,* 1775–1881.

Grant, A. E. (1964). Massage With Ice (Cryokinetics) in the Treatment of Painful Conditions of Musculoskeletal System. *Archive of Physical Medicine, 45,* 233–238.

Grant, K. E., Chandler, R. M., Castle, A. L., & Ivy, J. L. (1997). Chromium and exercise training: Effect on obese women. *Medicine and Science in Sports and Exercise, 29*(8), 992–998.

Grassel, E. (1992). Effect of Ginkgo-biloba extract on mental performance. Double-blind study using computerized measurement conditions in patients with cerebral insufficiency. *Fortschr Med, 110*(5), 73–76.

Graves, C. (1998, June 29). Iron overload: More common than you think. *Nursing Spectrum,* p. 7.

Gray, H. (1966). *Anatomy of the human body, 28th edition.* Charles Mayo Goss, Editor. Philadelphia: Lea & Febiger.

Green, E. E., Parks, P. A., Guer, B. A., Fahrion, S. L., & Coyne, L. (1991). Anomalous electrostatic phenomena in exceptional subjects. *Subtle Energies, 2,* 69–94.

Green, H. (1986). *Fit for America. Health, fitness, sport, and American society.* New York: Pantheon.

Green, J. (1990). *The herbal medicine-maker's handbook: The art and science of herbal medicine-making as taught at the California school of herbal studies.* Forestville, CA: Wildlife & Green Publications.

Greene, E. (1994). Manual healing methods. In *Alternative Medicine: Expanding medical horizons, a report to the National Institutes of Health on alternative medical systems and practices in the United States.* NIH Publication No. 94-066. Washington, DC: U.S. Government Printing Office, pp. 124–129.

Greer, M. W., Young, J., Inayat, Q., Burgess, C., & Robertson, B. (1988). Development of a questionnaire measure of adjustment to cancer: The MAC scale. *Psychological Medicine, 18,* 203–209.

Greeske, K., & Polhmann, B. K. (1996). Horse chestnut seed extract—an effective therapy principle in general practice. Drug therapy of chronic venous insufficiency. *Fortschr Med, 114*(15), 196–200.

Gregoire, I., Kalogeropoulos, D., & Corcos, J. (1997). The effectiveness of a professionally led support group for men with prostate cancer. *Urological Nursing, 17*(2), 58–66.

Greisheimer, E., & Troyer, J. R. (1963). *Physiology and Anatomy with Practical Considerations* (pp. 408, 469–477). Philadelphia: J. B. Lippincott Co.

Grimble, R. F. (1997). Effect of antioxidative vitamins on immune function with clinical appliations. *Int Journal Vitamin Nutr Res, 67*(5), 312–320.

Grissom-Sandler, G., & Kullman, M. (1990). Stretch into a better shape: Reshaping traditional stretches with Aston-Patterning concepts. Author.

Groer, M., & Ohnesorge, C. (1993). Menstrual-cycle lengthening and reducion in premenstrual distress through guided imagery. *Journal of Holistic Nursing, 11*(3), 286–294.

Grover, K. (Ed.). (1989). *Fitness in American culture. Images of health, sport, and the body, 1830–1940.* University of Massachusetts Press: Amherst.

Gruber, B. L., Hersh, S. P., Hall, et al. (1993). Immunological responses of breast cancer patients to behavioral interventions. *Biofeedback and Self Regulation, 18*(1), 1–22.

Gruenfeld, D. H., & Wyer, R. S. (1992). Semantics and pragmatics of social influence: How affirmations and denials affect beliefs in referent propositions. *Journal of Personal and Social Psychology, 62*(1), 38–49.

Guenel, P., Raskmark, P., Anderson, J. B., & Lynge, E. (1993). Incidence of cancer in persons with occupational exposure to electromagnetic fields in Denmark. *British Journal of Industrial Medicine, 50,* 232–245.

Guided imagery proven a powerful adjunct to colorectal surgery. *Consult Magazine,* Vol. XV, no. 1. Winter 1996.

Guillaume, M., & Padioleau, F. (1994). Veinotonic effect, vascular protection, anti-inflammatory and free radical scavenging properties of horse chestnut extract. *Arzneimittelforschung, 44*(1), 25–35.

Gullette, E. C. D., Blumenthal, J. A., Babyak, M., et al. (1997). Effects of mental stress on myocardial ischemia during daily life. *Journal of the American Medical Association, 277*(20), 1521–1526.

Gunn, J. (1830). *Domestic medicine.* Knoxville, TN: Author.

Guttormsen, A. B., Ueland, P. M., Nesthus, I., et al. (1996). Determinants and vitamin responsiveness of intermediate hyper-homocysteinemia: The Hordaland Homocysteine Study. *Journal of Clinical Investigation, 98*(9), 2174–2183.

Guyton, A. C. (1956, 1986). *Textbook of medical physiology.* Philadelphia: W. B. Saunders Company.

Haase, J. E. (1997). Hopeful teenagers with cancer living courage. *Reflections, 1,* 25.

Haase, J., Halama, P., & Horr, R. (1996). Effectiveness of brief infusions with *Ginkgo biloba* Special Extract EGb 761 in dementia of the vascular and Alzheimer type. *Zeitschrift fur Gerontologie und Geriatrie, 29*(4), 301–309.

Habermann, E. (1968). Biochemistry, pharmacology and toxicology of honey bee venom. *Ergeb Physiol, 60,* 220–325.

Hafling, W. R. (1974). Hypnosis (Review). *Science World.*

Hagberg, J., Blair, S., Gordon, N., Ehsani, A., Kaplan, N., et al. (1996, February). Exercise training helps control blood pressure. *Current Comment.*

Hagerstrand, T. (1968). *Innovation diffusion as a spatial process.* Chicago: University of Chicago Press.

Hain, T. C. (1995). *T'ai Chi for balance disorders* (OAM research report). http://www.altmed.od. nih.gov/oam/.

Hall, N., Altman, F., & Blumenthal, S. (Eds.). (1996). *Mind-body interactions and disease.* Orlando, FL: Health Dateline Press.

Hall, N., Groppel, J., & Loehr, J. (1996). *Optimal health.* Niles, IL: Nightingale-Conant Corporation.

Hallberg, L., Rossander-Hulthen, L., Brune, M., & Gleerup, A. (1993). Inhibition of haem-iron absorption in man by calcium. *British Journal of Nutrition, 69*(2), 533–540.

Hallfrish, J., Singh, V. N., Muller, D. C., et al. (1994). High plasma vitamin C associated with high plasma HDL- and HD12 cholesterol. *American Journal of Clinical Nutrition, 60*(1), 100–105.

Halper, J. (1997). Guided imagery treatment for asthma. Research abstract, Office of Alternative Medicine, National Institutes of Health.

Hamadeh, M. J. (1992). The effect of dietary flaxseed on N-3 fatty acids, cholesterol profile and laxation in the young and institutitionalized elderly. Masters Thesis. University of Toronto.

Hammerschlag, C. A., & Silverman, H. D. (1997). *Healing ceremonies: Creating personal rituals for spiritual, emotional, physical, and mental health.* New York: Perigee.

Han, T. S., Schouten, J. S., Lean, M. E., & Seidell, J. C. (1997). The prevalence of low back pain and associations with body fatness, fat distribution and height. *Int Journal Obes Relat Metab Disord, 21*(7), 600–607.

Hanna, K. M., & Jacobs, P. (1993). The use of photography to explore the meaning of health among adolescents with cancer. *Issues in Comprehensive Pediatric Nursing, 16,* 155–164.

Hanna, T. (1980). A somatics interview with Judith Aston. *Somatics: Magazine Journal of the Bodily Arts and Sciences, 3*(1), 12.

Hannerz, J. (1997). Symptoms and diseases and smoking habits in female episodic cluster headache and migraine patients. *Cephalalgia, 17*(4), 499–500.

Hansen, G. V., Nielsen, L., Kluger, E., et al. (1996). Nutritional status of Danish rheumatoid arthritis patients and effects of a diet adjusted in energy intake, fish-meal, and antioxidants. *Scandinavian Journal of Rheumatology, 25*(5), 325–330.

Haraguchi, H., Ishikawa, H., Shirataki, N., & Fukuda, A. (1997). Antiperoxidative activity of neolignans from *Magnolia obovata. Journal Pharm Pharmacol, 49*(2), 209–212.

Haraguchi, H., Saito, T., Ishikawa, H., et al. (1996). Antiperoxidative components in Thymus vulgaris. *Planta Med, 62*(3), 217–221.

Hardin, D. S., Hebert, J. D., Bayden, T., et al. (1997). Treatment of childhood syndrome X. *Pediatrics, 199*(2 Pt 1), E5.

Hardy, J. E. (1996). *Mercury free: The wisdom behind the global consumer movement to ban "silver" dental fillings.* Glassboro, NJ: Gabriel Rose Press.

Hargrave, T. D., & Sells, J. N. (1997). The development of a forgiveness scale. *Journal of Marital and Family Therapy, 23*(1), 41–63.

Harper, B. (1994). *Gentle birth choices.* Rochester, VT: Inner Traditions.

Harreby, M., Hesselsoe, G., Kjer, J., & Neergaard, K. (1997). Low back pain and physical exercise in leisure time in 38-year-old men and women: A 25-year prospective cohort study of 640 school children. *European Spine Journal, 6*(3), 181–186.

Harris, L., & Associates, Inc. (1989). *The Prevention Index '89: Summary report.* Emmaus, PA: Rodale.

Harris, R. (1992). An introduction to manual lymph drainage: The Vodder Method. *Massage Therapy Journal, 31*(1), 55–66.

Harrison, P. A., Fulkerson, J. A., & Beebe, T. J. (1997). Multiple substance use among adolescent physical and sexual abuse victims. *Child Abuse and Neglect, 21*(6), 529–539.

Harwood, A. (1987). *RX Spiritist as needed.* Ithaca, NY: Cornell University Press.

Hasselmark, L., Malmgren, R., Zetterstrom, O., et al. (1993). Selenium supplementation in intrinsic asthma. *Allergy, 48,* 30–36.

Hatch, G. E. (1995). Asthma, inhaled oxidants and dietary antioxidants. *American Journal of Clinical Nutrition, 61,* 625S–630S.

Hatono, S. (1994). Role of garlic and disease prevention—preclinical Models. Designer Foods III Proceedings: May 23–25, 1994. Rutgers University, Cook College, New Brunswick, NJ.

Hauger, M. A., Kjeldsen-Kragh, J., Bjerve, K. S., Hostmark, A. T., & Fone, O. (1994). Changes in plasma phospholipid fatty acids and their relationship to disease activity in rheumatoid arthritis patients treated with a vegetarian diet. *British Journal of Nutrition, 72*(4), 555–566.

Hay, L. L. (1987). *You can heal your life* (p. 226). Santa Monica: Hay House.

Hay, L. L. (1988a). *Heal your body* (p. 83). Santa Monica: Hay House.

Hay, L. L. (1988b). *The AIDS book: Creating a positive approach* (p. 276). Santa Monica: Hay House.

Hayes, D. (1993). *Body trust: Undieting your way to health and happiness*. Billings, MT: Production West.

He, C. M., Hseu, S. S., Tsai, S. K., & Lee, T. Y. (1996). Effect of P-6 acupressure on prevention of nausea and vomiting after epidural morphine for post–cesarean section pain relief. *Acta Anaesthesiol Scand, 40*(3), 372–375.

He, J., Klag, M. J., Whelton, P. K., Chen, J. Y., Qian, M. C., & He, G. Q. (1995). Dietary macronutrients and blood pressure in southwestern China. *Journal of Hypertension, 13*(11), 1267–1274.

He, J., Klag, M. J., Whelton, P. K., et al. (1995). Oats and buckwheat intakes and cardioascular disease risk factors in an ethnic minority of China. *American Journal of Clinical Nutrition, 61*(2), 366–372.

Healthy People Progress Report: Cancer. (1994). U.S. Dept of Health and Human Services. Washington, D.C.

Heaney, R. (1986). Calcium bioavailability. *Cont Nutr, 11*(8), 1–2.

Heaney, R., Recker, R., & Weaver, C. (1990). Absorbability of calcium sources: The limited role of solubility. *Bone Tissue, 46*, 301–304.

Heaney, R., Weaver, C., & Fitzsimmons, M. (1991). Soybean phytate content: Effect on calcium absorption. *American Journal of Clinical Nutrition, 53*, 745–747.

Heber, L. (1993/April–June). Dance movement: A therapeutic program for psychiatric clients. *Perspectives in Psychiatric Care, 29*(2).

Heidt, P. (1981). Effect of Therapeutic Touch on the anxiety level of hospitalized patients. *Nursing Research, 30*(1), 32–37.

Heidt, P. (1990). Openness: A qualitative analysis of nurses' and patients' experiences of Therapeutic Touch. *Image: Journal of Nursing Scholarship, 22*(3), 180–186.

Heinerman, J. (1997). *The Health Benefits of Cayenne*. New Canaan: Keats Publishing Company.

Heller, J., & Henkin, W. A. (1986). *Bodywise*. Los Angeles: Jeremy P. Tarcher.

Helvie, C. (1981). *Community health nursing, theory and process*. New York: Harper and Row.

Helvie, C. (1991). *Community health nursing, theory and practice*. New York: Springer Publishing Company.

Helvie, C. O. (1995, Spring). A theory for alternative health practitioners. *Alternative Health Practitioner, 1*(1), 15–22.

Hemila, H. (1994). Does vitamin C alleviate the symptoms of the common cold?—a review of current evidence. *Scan Journal Infect Dis, 26*(1), 1–6.

Hemila, H. (1996). Vitamin C and common cold incidence: A review of studies with subjects under heavy physical stress. *International Journal of Sports Medicine, 17*(5), 379–383.

Hemila, H. (1997). Vitamin C intake and susceptibility to the common cold. *Brit Journal Nutr, 77*(1), 59–72.

Hemila, H., & Herman, Z. S. (1995). Vitamin C and the common cold: A retrospective analysis of Chalmers' review. *Journal of the American College of Nutrition, 14*(2), 116–123.

Hennig, B., & McClain, C. (1992). The function of zinc in atherosclerosis. *Nutr Rep, 10*, 81, 88.

Henry, L. L. (1995). Music therapy: a nursing intervention for the control of pain and anxiety in the ICU: A review of the research literature. *Dimensions of Crit Care Nsg, 14*(6), 295–304.

Herman, D. B., Susser, E. S., Struening, E. L., & Link, B. L. (1997). Adverse childhood experiences: Are they risk factors for adult homelessness? *American Journal of Public Health, 87*(2), 249–255.

Hernandez-Avila, M. (1991). Caffeine, alcohol intake, and risk of fractures in middle-aged women. *American Journal of Clinical Nutrition, 54*, 157–163.

Herzenberg, L. & L. (1997, March). N-acetylcysteine and HIV survival. *Medical Tribune, 20*: 25.

Heuser, G., & Vojdani, A. (1997). Enhancement of natural killer cell activity and T and B cell function by buffered vitamin C in patients exposed to toxic chemicals: The role of protein kinase-C. *Immunopharmacol Immunotoxicol, 19*(3), 291–312.

Hickie, I. B. (1995). Chronic Fatigue Syndrome: Current perspectives on evaluation and management. *Med Journal Australia, 163*, 314–318.

Hilgard & Hilgard (1975). *Hypnosis in the Relief of Pain*. Los Altos, CA: Kaufmann, Inc.

Hindmarch, I. (1986). Activate de l'extrait de ginkgo biloba sur la memoir a court term. *Presse Med, 15*(31), 1592–1594.

Hinds, S. (1997). Once upon a time . . . therapeutic stories as a psychiatric nursing intervention. *Journal Psychosocial Nursing and Mental Health Services*, 35(5), 46–47.

Hinds, T. S., West, W. L., & Knight, E. M. (1997). Carotenoids and retinoids: A review of research, clinical, and public health applications. *Journal Clin Pharmacol*, 37(7), 551–558.

Hobbs, L. M., Rayner, T. E., & Hower, P. R. (1996). Dietary fish oil prevents the development of renal damage in salt-loaded stroke-prone spontaneously hypertensive rats. *Clinical and Experimental Pharmacology and Physiology*, 23(6–7), 508–513.

Hodis, H. N., Mack, W. J., LaBree, L., Cashin-Hemphill, L., Sevanian, A., Johnson, R., & Azen, S. P. (1995). Serial coronary angiographic evidence that antioxidant vitamin estimated intake reduces progression of coronary artery atherosclerosis. *Journal of the American Medical Association*, 273, 1849–1854.

Hodis, H. N., Mack, W. J., Dunn, M., Liu, C., et al. (1997). Intermediate-density lipoproteins and progression of carotid arterial wall intima-meda thickness. *Circulation*, 95(8), 2022–2026.

Hoffer, A. (1989). *Orthomolecular medicine for physicians*. New Canaan, CT: Keats Publishing.

Hoffman, D. (1996). *The complete illustrated holistic herbal: A safe and practical guide to making and using herbal remedies*. New York: Barnes and Noble Books.

Holden-Lund, C. (1988). Effects of relaxation with guided imagery on surgical stress and wound healing. *Research in Nursing and Health*, 11, 235–244.

Holmes, E. (1938). *The science of mind*. New York: G. P. Putnam's Sons.

Holmes, E. (1949). *How to use the science of mind*. New York: G. P. Putnam's Sons.

Holmes, T., & Rahe, R. (1967). The social readjustment rating scale. *Journal of Psychosomatic Research*, 11, 213–218.

Holtzapfel, W. (1989). *Children's illnesses*. Spring Valley, NY: Mercury Press.

Homeopathic pharmacopoeia of the U.S. (1981).

Hong, G. X., Qin, W. C., & Huang, L. S. (1994). Memory-improving effect of aqueous exract of *Astragalus membranaceus*. *Chung Kuo Chung Yao Tsa Chih*, 19(11), 687–688.

Hopkins, C. (1996). *The principles of aromatherapy*. Thorsons.

Horan, P. (1992). *Empowerment through Reiki*. Wilmot, WI: Lotus Light Publications.

House, J. S., Landis, K. R., & Umberson, D. (1988, July 29). Social relationships and health. *Science*, 241, 540–545.

Hover-Kramer, D., et al. (1996). *Healing touch: A resource for health care professionals*. New York: Delmar Publishers.

Hu, Y., & Goldman, N. (1990, May). Mortality differentials by marital status: An international comparison. *Demography*, 27(2), 233–250.

Huang, H. (Trans.). (1974). *Ear acupuncture*. Emmaus, PA: Rodale Press.

Huang, H. C., Jan, T. R., & Yeh, S. F. (1992). Inhibitory effect of curcumin, an anti-inflammatory agent, on vascular smooth muscle cell proliferation. *European Journal of Pharmacology*, 221, 381–384.

Huang, L. C. (1996). *Auriculotherapy, diagnosis and treatment*. Bellaire, TX: Longevity Press.

Huang, Z., Hankinson, S. E., Colditz, G. A., et al. (1997). Dual effects of weight and weight gain on breast cancer risk. *Journal of the American Medical Association*, 278, 1407–1411.

Hubel, C. A., Kagan, V. E., Kisin, E. R., et al. (1997). Increased ascorbate radical formation and ascorbate depletion in plasma from women with preeclampsia: Implications for oxidative stress. *Free Radical Biology and Medicine*, 23(4), 597–609.

Hudak, D., Dale, A., Hudak, M., & DeGood, D. (1991). Effects of humorous stimuli and sense of humor on discomfort. *Psychological Reports*, 69(3), 779–786.

Huemer, R. P. (1986). *The roots of molecular medicine: A tribute to Linus Pauling*. New York: W. H. Freeman and Company.

Huemer, R. P. (1977). A theory of diagnosis for orthomolecular medicine. *Journal Theor Biol*, 67, 625–635; reprinted in *Advances* (1984), 1(3), 53–59.

Huk, I., Brovkorych, V., Nonobash, V. J., Weigel, G., Neumayer, C., Partyka, L., Patton, S., & Malinski, T. (1998). Bioflavonoid quercetin scavenges superoxide and increasing nitric oxide concentration in ischaemia-reperfusion injury: An experimental study. *Brit J Surgery*, 85(8), 1080–1085.

Humphrey, J. H., Agoestina, T., Wu, L., Usman, A., Nurachim, M., Subardja, D., Hidayat, S., Tielsch, J., West, K. P. Jr., & Sommer, A. (1996). Impact of neonatal vitamin A supplementation on infant morbidity and mortality. *Journal Pediatr, 128*(4), 489–496.

Hunt, C., Johnson, P., Herbel, J., et al. (1992). Effects of dietary zinc depletion on seminal volume and zinc loss, serum testosterone concentrations, and sperm morphology in young men. *American Journal of Clinical Nutrition, 56,* 148–157.

Hunyor, S. N., Henderson, R. J., Lai, S. K., Carter, N. L., Kobler, H., et al. (1997). Placebo-controlled biofeedback blood pressure effect in hypertensive humans. *Hypertension, 29*(6), 1225–1231.

Hyde, E. (1989). Acupressure therapy for morning sickness. A controlled clinical trial. *Journal of Nurse Midwifery, 34*(4), 171–178.

Ichibe, Y., & Ishikawa, S. (1996). Optic neuritis and vitamin C. *Nippon Ganka Gakkai Zasshi, 100*(5), 381–387.

Idle, N., Nelson, A. B., & Lau, B. H. (1997). Aged garlic extract and its constituents inhibit CU(2+)-induced oxidative modification of low density lipoprotein. *Planta Med, 63*(3), 263–264.

Ilacqua, G. E. (1994). Migraine headaches: Coping efficacy of guided imagery training. *Headache, 34*(2), 99–102.

Incao, P. (1997). Supporting children's health. *Alternative Medicine Digest, 19,* 54–59.

Ingham, E. (1938). *Stories the feet can tell.* Saint Petersburg, FL: Ingham.

Ingham, E. (1951). *Stories the feet have told.* Saint Petersburg, FL: Ingham.

Ingram, D., Sanders, K., Kolybaba, M., & Lopez, D. (1997). Case-control study of phyto-oestrogens and breast cancer. *Lancet, 350*(9083), 990–994.

Institute of Medicine, Division of health Sciences Policy and Division of Mental Health and Behavioral Medicine. (1989). Research Briefing: Behavioral influences on the immune system. Washington, DC: National Academy Press.

Ionescu-Tirgoviste, C. (1992). *Bazele teoretice ale acupuncturii* (Vol. si 2). Bucuresti: Ed. Athaeneum.

Ironson, G. A., Field, T., Scafidi, F., Kumar, M., Patarca, R., Price, A., Goncalves, A., Hashi-moto, M., Kumar, A., Burman, I., Tetenman, C., & Fletcher, M. (1993). Massage effects on cocaine-exposed preterm neonates. *Developmental and Behavioral Pediatrics, 14*(5).

Ironson, G., Field, T. M., Scafidi, F., Kumar, M., Patarca, R., Price, A., Goncalves, A., Hashimoto, M., Kumar, A., Burman, I., Tetenman, C., & Fletcher, M. A. (1996). Massage therapy is associated with enhancement of the immune system's cytotoxic capacity. *International Journal of Neuroscience, 84,* 205–218.

Irwin, M., Daniels, M., Bloom, E. T., Smith, R. L., & Weiner, H. (1987). Life events, depressive symptoms, and immune function. *American Journal of Psychiatry, 144,* 437–441.

Ishihara, N., Yuzawa, M., & Tamakoshi, A. (1997). Antioxidants and angiogenetic factor associated with age-related macular degeneration. *Nippon Ganka Gakkai Zasshi, 101*(3), 248–251.

Isler, H. (1982). Migraine treatment as a cause of chronic migraine. In F. C. Rose (Ed.), *Advances in migraine research and therapy* (pp. 159–164). New York: Raven Press.

Itil, T., & Martorano, D. (1995). Natural substances in psychiatry. *Ginkgo biloba* in dementia. *Psychopharmacology Bulletin, 31*(1), 147–158.

Ivanov, S. G., Smirnov, V. V., Solov'eva, F. V., Liashevskaia, S. P., & Selezneva, L. (1990). The magnetotherapy of hypertension patients. *Ter Arkh, 62*(9), 71–74.

Iversen, T., Flirgaard, K. M., Schriver, P., et al. (1997). The effect of NaO Li Su on memory functions and blood chemistry in elderly people. *Journal of Ethnopharmacology, 56*(2), 109–116.

Jacob, R. A., & Burri, B. J. (1996). Oxidative damage and defense. *American Journal of Clinical Nutrition, 63*(6), 985S–990S.

Jacobs, J., Jiménez, M., Gloyd, S., Gate, J., & Cruthers, D. (1994). A treatment of acute diarrhea with homeopathic medicine: A randomized clinical trial in Nicaragua. *Pediatrics, 93,* 719–725.

Jacobson, B. H., Chen, H. C., Cashel, C., & Guerrero, L. (1997). The effect of T'ai Chi Chuan training on balance, kinesthetic sense, and strength. *Percept Mot Skills, 84*(1), 27–33.

Jacobson, E. (1974). *Progressive relaxation.* Chicago: The University of Chicago Press, Midway Reprint.

Jacques, P. F., & Chylack, L. T. (1991). Epidemiologic evidence of a role for the antioxidant vitamins and carotenoids in cataract prevention. *American Journal of Clinical Nutrition, 53*(Suppl. 1), 352S–355S.

Jacques, P. F., & Taylor, A. (1997). Vitamin C and cataract risk in women. *American Journal of Clinical Nutrition, 59*(10), 200–242.

Jacques, P. F., Hartz, S. C., Chylack, L. T., et al. (1988). Nutritional status in persons with and without senile cataract: Blood vitamin and mineral levels. *American Journal of Clinical Nutrition, 48*(1), 152–158.

Jaeger, B., & Skootsky, S. A. (1987). Double-blind controlled study of different myofascial trigger point injection techniques. *Pain, 31*(Suppl.), S292.

Jain, S. C., & Talukdar, B. (1993). Evaluation of a yoga therapy program for patients with bronchial asthma. *Singapore Medical Journal, 34*(4), 306–308.

Jain, S. C., Uppal, A., Bhatnagar, S. O., & Talukdar, B. (1993). A study of response pattern of non-insulin dependent diabetics to yoga therapy. *Diabetes Res Clin Pract, 19*(1), 69–74.

Jameson, S. (1993). Zinc status in pregnancy: The effect of zinc therapy on perinatal mortality, prematurity and placental ablation. *Annals NY Academy Medicine, 678,* 178–192.

Janghorbani, M., Kasper, L., & Young, V. (1984). Dynamic of selenite metabolism in young men: Studies with the stable isotope tracer method. *American Journal of Clinical Nutrition, 40,* 208–218.

Janiszewski, M., Kronenberger, M., & Drozd, B. (1996). Studies on the use of music therapy as a form of breathing exercise in bronchial asthma. *Pol Merkuriusz Lek, 1*(1), 32–33.

Jankun, J. (1997, June 5). More than green tea and sympathy. *Nature, 56l.*

Janov, A. (1983). *Imprints: The lifelong effects of the birth experience.* New York: Coward McCann, Inc.

Jennings, L.C., & Dick, E.C. (1987). Transmission and control of rhinovirus colds. *Eur Journal Epidemiol, 3*(4), 327–335.

Jensen, B. (1995). *The science and practice of iridology* (Vol. 1). Escondido, CA: Author.

Jensen, C. B. (1997, August). Common paths in medical education: The training of allopaths, osteopaths, and naturopaths. *Alternative and Complementary Therapies,* pp. 276–280.

Jensen, C. D., Haskell, W., & Whittman, J. H. (1997). Long-term effects of water-soluble dietary fiber in the management of hypercholesterolemia in healthy men and women. *Am J Cardiology, 79*(1), 34–37.

Jerome, F. (1995). *Tooth truth: A patient's guide to metal-free dentistry.* San Diego: ProMotion Publishing.

Ji, B. T., Chow, W. H., Hsing, A. W., McLaughlin, J. K., et al. (1997). Green tea consumption and the risk of pancreatic and colorectal cancers. *International Journal of Cancer, 70*(3), 255–258.

Ji, L., Stratment, F., & Lardy, H. (1992). Antioxidant enzyme response to selenium deficiency in rat myocardium. *Journal of the American College of Nutrition, 11,* 79–86.

Jiansan, Y. (1988). *The way to locate acupoints.* Beijing: Foreign Language Press.

Jin, L., & Baillie, T. A. (1997). Metabolism of the chemoprotective agent diallyl sulfide to glutathione conjugates in rats. *Chem Res Toxicol, 10*(3), 318–327.

Jin, P. (1992). Efficacy of Tai Chi, brisk walking, meditation, and reading in reducing mental and emotional stress. *Journal of Psychosomatic Research, 36*(4), 361–370.

John, E. (1997). Sunlight may guard against breast cancer. Paper presented to a scientific meeting of breast cancer oncologists, Washington, DC: November 3.

Johnson, D. H. (1989). Presence. In R. Carlson & B. Shield (Eds.), *Healers on healing* (pp. 131–134). Los Angeles: Jeremy P. Tarcher.

Jonas, W. B., & Jacobs, J. (1996). *Healing with Homeopathy, The Complete Guide.* New York: Warner.

Jones, A. (1996). Not to worry. *Psychology & Health Update, 16*(2), 5.

Jones, F. P. (1965, May). Method for changing stereotyped response patterns by the inhibition of certain postural sets. *Psychological Review, 72,* 3.

Jones, F. P. (1997). *Freedom to change.* First published as *Body Awareness in Action.* Endorsement by Sherrington, (pp. 90). London, England: Mouritz.

Joshi, L. N., Joshi, V. D., & Gokhale, L. V. (1992). Effect of short term Pranayam practice on breathing rate and ventilatory functions of lung. *Indian Journal Physiol Pharmacol, 36*(2), 105–108.

Juhan, D. (1987). *Job's Body.* Barrytown, NY: Station Hill Press, Inc.

Justice, B. (1997). Imagery/support and immune function in breast cancer. Results of grant R21 RR9505, Office of Alternative Medicine on the world wide web at http://altmed.od.nih.gov/oam/gi-bin/research-simple.cgi

Kabat-Zinn, J. (1990). *Full catastrophe living: Using the wisdom of your body and mind to face stress, pain and illness.* New York: Delacorte.

Kabat-Zinn, J. (1993). Mindfulness meditation: Health benefits of an ancient Buddhist practice. In D. Goleman & J. Gurin (Eds.), *Mind/Body medicine* (pp. 259–275). Yonkers, NY: Consumer Reports Books, Chapter 15.

Kabat-Zinn, J. (1994). *Wherever you go, there you are: Mindful meditation in everyday life.* New York: Hyperion.

Kabat-Zinn, J., Lipworth, L., & Burney, R. (1985). The clinical use of mindfulness meditation for the self-regulation of chronic pain. *Journal of Behavioral Medicine, 8*(2), 163–191.

Kabat-Zinn, J., Massion, A., Kristeller, J., Peterson, L. G., Fletcher, K. E., Pbert, L., Lenderking, W. R., & Santorelli, S. F. (1992). Effectiveness of a meditation-based stress reduction program in the treatment of anxiety disorders. *American Journal of Psychiatry, 149*, 936–943.

Kamen-Siegel, L., Rodin, J., Seligman, M. E. P., & Dwyer, J. (1991). Explanatory style and cell-mediated immunity in elderly men and women. *Health Psychology, 10*(4), 229–235.

Kamenetz, H. L. (1980). History of massage. In J. B. Rogoff (Ed.), *Manipulation, traction and massage* (pp. 1–44). Baltimore: Williams & Wilkins.

Kaminski, J., & Hall, W. (1996). The effect of soothing music on neonatal behavioral states in the hospital newborn nursery. *Neonatal Network—Journal of Neonatal Nursing, 15*(1), 45–54.

Kanfer, F. H., & Busemeyer, J. R. (1982). The use of problem solving and decision making in behavior therapy. *Clinical Psychology Review, 2*, 239–266.

Kang, J. X., & Leaf, A. (1996). The cardiac antiarrhythmic effects of polyunsaturated fatty acid. *Lipids, 31*, A41–A44.

Kang, J. Y., Yeoh, K. G., Chia, H. P., et al. (1995). Chili-protective factor against peptic ulcer? *Digestive Diseases and Sciences, 40*(3), 576–579.

Kano, S. (1989). *Making peace with food: Freeing yourself from the diet/weight obsession.* New York: Harper and Row.

Kanowski, S., Herrmann, W. M., Stephan, K., et al. (1996). Proof of efficacy of the *Ginkgo biloba* special extract EGb 761 in outpatients suffering from mild to moderate primary degenerative dementia of the Alzheimer type or multi-infarct dementia. *Pharmacopsychiatry, 29*(2), 47–56.

Kapit, W., & Elson, L. M. (1977). *The Anatomy Coloring Book* (pp. 67–69). New York: Canfield Press/Barnes & Noble.

Kaptchuk. *The web that has no weaver— understanding Chinese medicine.*

Karling, K. (1954). Per Henrik Ling and Swedish Medical Gymnastics. *Physiotherapy, 40*, 335–338.

Katiyar, S. K., Korman, N. J., Mukhtar, H., & Agarwal, R. (1997). Protective effects of silymarin against photocarcinogenesis in a mouse skin model. *Journal of the National Cancer Institute, 89*(8), 556–566.

Kaufman, M. (1971). *Homeopathy in America.* Baltimore: Johns Hopkins University Press.

Kawachi, I., Colditz, G. A., Stampfer, M. J., et al. (1995). Prospective study of shift work and risk of coronary heart disease in women. *Circulation, 92*(11), 3178–3182.

Kawachi, I., Sparrow, D., Spiro, A., et al. (1996). A prospective study of anger and coronary heart disease. The Normative Aging Study. *Circulation, 94*(9), 2090–2095.

Kawada, T., et al. (1986). Effects of capsaicin on lipid metabolism in rats fed a high fat diet. *Journal of Nutrition, 116*, 1271–1278.

Keen, C., Taubeneck, M., Daston, G., et al. (1993). Primary and secondary zinc deficiency as factors underlying abnormal CNS development. *Ann NY Acad Med, 678*, 37–47.

Kefu, W., Delong, W., Xiaoyin, Y., Wenge, M., Yantao, F., Yanhui, Z., & Xinhua, G. (1982). *Anatomical atlas of Chinese acupuncture point.* Jinan, China: Shandong Science and Technology Press.

Keli, S. O., Hertog, M. G., Feskens, E. J., & Kromhout, D. (1996). Dietary flavonoids, antioxidant vitamins, and incidence of stroke: The Zutphen study. *Archives of Internal Medicine, 156*(6), 637–642.

Keller, E. (1991). *The complete guide to aromatherapy, self help with essential oils.* Germany.

Keller, E., & Bzdek, V. M. (1986). Effects of Therapeutic Touch on tension headache pain. *Nursing Research, 35*(2), 101–106.

Keller, V. E. (1995). Management of nausea and vomiting in children. *Journal of Pediatric Nursing, 19*(5), 280–286.

Kellert, S., & Wilson, E. (Eds.). (1993). *The biophilia hypothesis.* Washington, DC: Island Press.

Kelley, C. D. (1997). Understanding Syndrome X. *Clinician Reviews, 7*(10), 55–65, 69–76, 78–80.

Kelly, S. *Imagine yourself well.* New York: Da Capo Press.

Keltner, D., & Bonanno, G. A. (1997). A study of laughter and dissociation: Distinct correlates of laughter and smiling during bereavement. *Journal of Personal and Social Psycology, 73*(4), 687–702.

Kemeny, M., & Solomon, G. (1993). Psychoneuroimmunology, *Seminar on PNI.* Esalen Institute, Big Sur, California.

Kendler, B. S. (1997). Recent nutritional approaches to the prevention and therapy of cardiovascular disease. *Prog Cardio-vasc Nurs, 12*(3), 3–23.

Kendrick, J. S., Atrash, H. K., Strauss, L. T., et al. (1997). Vaginal douching and the risk of ectopic pregnancy among black women. *American Journal of Obstetrics and Gynecology, 176*, 991–997.

Kennedy, A. R. (1995). The evidence for soybean products as cancer preventive agents. *Journal of Nutrition, 125*(3 Suppl.), 733S–743S.

Kennell, J., Klaus, M., et al. Continuous emotional support during labor in a US hospital. *Journal of the American Medical Association*, May 1, 1991; Vol. 265; No. 17, 2197–2201.

Kents, V. V., & Mavrodii, V. M. (1995). Decimeter-wave physiotherapy in viral hepatitis. *Lik Sprava, 9*(12), 140–144.

Kern, P. A. (1997). A prudent and practical approach to the treatment of obesity. *Journal of the Arkansas Medical Society, 94*(5), 191–197.

Kesselring, A. (1994). Foot reflex zone massage. *Schweizerische Medizinische Wochenschrift Supplementum, 62*, 88–93.

Kessler, R., & Whalen, T. (1998). Hypnosis in surgery. In R. Temes (Ed.), *Hypnosis and medicine.* New York: Churchhill Livingston.

Key, T. J., Rhorogood, M., Appleby, P. N., & Burr, M. L. (1996). Dietary habits and mortality in 11,000 vegetarians and health-conscious people: Results of a 17-year follow-up. *Brit Med Journal, 313*(7060), 775–779.

Key, T. J., Silcocks, P. B., Davey, G. K., et al. (1997). A case-control study of diet and prostate cancer. *British Journal of Cancer, 76*(5), 678–687.

Khan, B. SA., Abraham, A., & Leelamma, S. (1996). Biochemical response in rats to the addition of curry leaf (*Murraya koenigii*) and mustard seeds (*Brassica juncea*) to the diet. *Plant Foods for Human Nutrition, 49*(4), 295–299.

Kiecolt-Glaser, J. K., & Glaser, R. (1988). Psychological influences of immunity: Implications for AIDS. *American Psychologist, 43*, 892–898.

Kiecolt-Glaser, J. K., Fisher, L. D., Ogrocki, P., Stout, J. C., Speicher, C. E., & Glaser, R. (1987, Jan/Feb). Marital quality, marital disruption and immune function. *Psychosomatic Medicine, 49*(1), 13–34.

Kiecolt-Glaser, J. K., Glaser, R., Cacioppo, J. T., MacCallum, R. C., Snydersmith, M., Kim, C., & Malarkey, W. B. (1997). Marital conflict in older adults: Endocrinological and immunological correlates. *Psychosomatic Medicine, 59*(4), 339–349.

Kilborn, P. T. (1998, March 21). Nashville clinic offers case study of chronic gap in black and white health. *New York Times*, p. A6.

King, A. C., Oman, R. F., Brassington, M. A., Beiwise, D. L., & Haskell, W. L. (1997). Moderate-intensity exercise and self-rated quality of sleep in older adults: A randomized controlled trial. *The Journal of the American Medical Association, 277*(1), 32–37.

King, D. E., & Bushwick, B. (1994, October). Beliefs and attitudes of hospital inpatients about faith healing and prayer. *Journal of Family Practice, 39*(4), 349–352.

King, L. (1984). Central place theory. In G. I. Tappan (Ed.), *Scientific geography series*, Vol. 1. Beverly Hills: Sage Publications.

Kiremidjian-Schumacher, L., & Stotzky, G. (1987). Selenium and immune responses. *Environmental Research, 42,* 277–303.

Kirkaldy-Willis, W. H., & Cassidy, J. D. (1985). Spinal manipulation in the treatment of lower back pain. *Canadian Family Physician, 31,* 535–540.

Kirshbaum, M. (1996). Using massage in the relief of lymphoedema. *Professional Nurse, 11*(4), 230–232.

Kishikawa, M., & Sakae, M. (1997). Herbal medicine and the study of aging in senescence-accelerated mice(SAMP1TA/Ngs). *Exp Gerontol, 32*(1–2), 229–242.

Kjeldsen-Kragh, J., Haugen, M., Borchgrevink, C. F., & Forre, O. (1994). Vegetarian diet for patients with rheumatoid arthritis—status: two years after introduction of the diet. *Clinical Rheumatology, 13*(3), 475–482.

Klaus, M. H., Kennell, J. H., & Klaus, P. H. (1993). *Mothering the mother.* Reading, MA: Addison-Wesley.

Kleifield, E. I., Wagner, S., & Halmi, K. A. (1996). Cognitive-behavioral treatment of anorexia nervosa. *Psychiatr Clin North Am, 19*(4), 715–737.

Kleijnen, J., Knipschild, P., & ter Riet, G. (1991, February 9). Clinical trials in homoeopathy. *British Medical Journal.*

Kleinman, A., Eisenberg, L., & Good, B. (1978). Culture, illness, and care. *Annals of Internal Medicine, 88,* 251–258.

Kligman, E. W. (1998). Medical education: Changes and responses. In R. J. Gordon, B. C. Nienstedt, & W. M. Gesler (Eds.), *Alternative therapies: Expanding options in health care* (pp. 199–218). New York: Springer.

Kluft, E. S. (Ed.). (1993). *Expressive and functional therapies in the treatment of multiple personality disorders.* Springfield, IL: Charles C. Thomas.

Knaster, M. (1991). A new dimension in intensive care: Premature infants grow with massage, Dr. Tiffany Field's research. *Massage Therapy Journal, 30*(3), 50–60.

Knaster, M. (1994). Dr. Tiffany Field: Researching massage as real therapy. *Massage Therapy Journal, 33*(3), 56–113.

Knaster, M. (1996). *Discovering the body's wisdom: A comprehensive guide to more than fifty mind-body practices that can relieve pain, reduce stress, and foster health, spiritual growth, and inner peace.* New York: Bantam Books, pp. 167–169.

Knaster, M. (1996). *Discovering the body's wisdom: A comprehensive guide to more than fifty mind-body practices that can relieve pain, reduce stress, and foster health, spiritual growth, and inner peace.* New York: Bantam Books.

Knaster, M. (1998). Tiffany Field Provides Proof Positive Scientifically. *Massage Therapy Journal, 37*(1), 84–88.

Knekt, P., Jarvinen, R., Seppanen, R., et al. (1997). Dietary flavonoids and the risk of lung cancer and other malignant neoplasms. *American Journal of Epidemiology, 146*(3), 223–230.

Knekt, P., Reunanen, A., Jarvinen, R., et al. (1994). Antioxidant vitamin intake and coronary mortality in a longitudinal population study. *American Journal of Epidemiology, 139,* 1180–1189.

Knight, D. C., & Eden, J. A. (1996). A review of the clinical effects of phytoestrogens. *Obste Gynecol, 87*(5, Pt. 2), 897–904.

Koenig, H. G., Hays, J. C., George, L. K., et al. (1997). Modeling the cross-sectional relationships between religion, physical health, social support, and depressive symptoms. *Am Journal Geriatr Psychiatry, 5*(2), 131–144.

Koening, H. G., Larson, D. B., & Matthews, D. A. (1996). Religion and psychotherapy with older adults. *Journal of Geriatric Psychiatry, 29,* 155–184.

Koes, B. W., Bouter, L. M., & van Mameren, H. (1992). Randomised clinical trial of manipulative therapy and physiotherapy for persistent back and neck complaints: Results of one-year follow-up. *BMJ, 304,* 601–605.

Koffler, M., & Kisch, E. S. (1996). Starvation diet and very-low-calorie diets may induce insulin resistance and overt diabetes mellitus. *Journal of Diabetes Complications, 10*(2), 109–112.

Kohen, Dp. P., & Wynne, E. (1997). Applying hypnosis in a preschool family asthma education program: Uses of storytelling, imagery, and relaxation. *American Journal of Clinical Hypnosis, 39*(3), 169–181.

Kokjohn, K., Schmid, D. M., Triano, J. J., & Brennan, P. C. (1992). The effect of spinal manipulation on pain and prostaglandin levels in women with primary dysmenorrhea. *Journal Manipulative Physiol Ther, 15,* 279–285.

Kolata, G. (1996). On fringes of health care, untested therapies thrive. *New York Times*, June 17, 1996: A1, B6.

Kolcaba, K. (1995). Comfort as process and product, merged in holistic nursing art. *Journal of Holistic Nursing, 13*(2), 117–131.

Kolcaba, K. (1997). Spreading comfort around the world. *Reflections, 23*(2), 12–13.

Koller, L., Exon, J., Talcott, P., et al. (1986). Immune responses in rats supplemented with Selenium. *Clinical and Experimental Immunology, 63*, 570–576.

Komatireddy, G. R., Leitch, R. W., Cella, K., et al. (1997). Efficacy of low load resistive muscle training in patients with rheumatoid arthritis functional class II and III. *Journal of Rheumatology, 24*(8), 1531–1539.

Kong, X. T., Fang, H. T., Jiang, G. Q., Zhai, S. Z., O'Connell, D. L., & Brewster, D. R. (1993). Treatment of acute bronchiolitis with Chinese herbs. *Archives of Disease in Childhood, 68*(4), 468–471.

Koniak-Griffin, D. (1994). Aerobic exercise, psychological well-being, and physical discomforts during adolescent pregnancy. *Research in Nursing and Health, 17*(4), 253–263.

Kopelman, L., & Moskop, J. (1981). The holistic health movement: A survey and critique. *Journal of Medicine and Philosophy, 8*, 209–235.

Kotchoubey, B., Schneider, D., Schleichert, H., et al. (1996). Self-regulation of slow cortical potentials in epilepsy: A retrial with analysis of influencing factors. *Epilepsy Research, 25*(3), 269–276.

Kovac, F. M., Abraira, V., Pozo, F., Kleinbaum, D. G., Beltran, J., et al. (1997). Local and remote sustained trigger point therapy for exacerbations of chronic low back pain. A randomized, double-blind, controlled, multicenter trial. *Spine, 22*(7), 786–797.

Krajcovicova-Kudlackova, M., Simoncic, R., Bederova, A., et al. (1994). Lipid and pro-oxidative and antioxidative parameters in the blood of vegetarians. *Bratislavske LeKarske Listy, 95*(8), 344–348.

Krajcovicova-Kudlackova, M., Simoncic, R., Bederova, A., et al. (1996). Lipid and antioxidant blood levels in vegetarians. *Nahrung, 40*(1), 17–20.

Kraus, G. A., Pratt, D., Tossberg, J., & Carpenter, S. (1990). Antiretroviral activity of synthetic hypericin and related analogs. *Biochemical and Biophysical Research Communication, 172*(1), 149–153.

Kreiger, D. (1979). *The therapeutic touch.* Englewood Cliffs, NJ: Prentice Hall.

Kreiger, D. (1993). *Accepting your power to heal.* Santa Fe, NM: Bear & Co.

Kremer, J. M., & Bigaouette, J. (1996). Nutrient intake of patients with rheumatoid arthritis is deficient in pyridoxine, zinc, copper and magnesium. *Journal of Rheumatology, 23*(6), 990–994.

Krieger, D. (1972). The response of in-vivo human hemoglobin to an active healing therapy by direct laying on of hands. *Human Dimensions, 1*, 12–15.

Krieger, D. (1973). The relationship of touch with intent to help or heal subjects; in-vivo hemoglobin values: A study of personalized interaction. In *Proceedings of the Ninth American Nurses' Association Nursing Research Conference* (pp 39–58). Kansas City: American Nurses' Association.

Krieger, D. (1976). Healing by the "laying-on" of hands as a facilitator of bioenergetic change: The response of in-vivo human hemoglobin. *International Journal of Psychoenergetic Systems, 1*(2), 121–129.

Krieger, D. (1979). *The therapeutic touch: How to use your hands to help or to heal.* Englewood Cliffs, NJ: Prentice-Hall.

Krieger, D. (1981). *Foundations for holistic health nursing practices: The Renaissance nurse.* Philadelphia: J. B. Lippincott.

Krieger, D. (1987). *Living the Therapeutic Touch: Healing as a lifestyle.* New York: Dodd, Mead & Co.

Krieger, D. (1993). *Accepting Your Power to Heal, the Personal Practice of Therapeutic Touch.* Santa Fe, NM: Bear & Company.

Krieger, D. (1997). *Therapeutic Touch Inner Workbook.* Santa Fe, NM: Bear & Company.

Krishna, G. G. (1994). Role of potassium in the pathogenesis of hypertension. *American Journal of Medical Science, 307*(Suppl. 1), S21–S25.

Kroll, D. (Nov. 1995). Acupressure Therapy for Tension Headaches. *Alternative and Complementary Therapies.*

Kropp, P., Gerber, W. D., Keinath-Specht, A., et al. (1997). Behavioral treatment in migraine. Cognitive-behavioral therapy and blood-volume-pulse biofeedback: A cross-over study with a two-year follow-up. *Functional Neurology*, *12*(1), 17–24.

Kugler, J., Seelbach, H., & Kruskemper, G. M. (1994). Effects of rehabilitation exercise programmers on anxiety and depression in coronary patients: A meta-analysis. *British Journal of Clinical Psychology*, *33*(3), 401–410.

Kuhn, O. (1953). Echinacea and phagocytosis. *Arzneimittel-Forschung*, *3*, 194–200.

Kuligowski, J., & Halperin, K. (1992). Stainless steel cookware as a significant source of nickel, chromium and iron. *Archives of Environmental Contamination and Toxicology*, *23*, 211–215.

Kunidev, L. A. (1979). Therapeutic massage. *Medicine*, p. 216.

Kunz, D. (1985). *Spiritual aspects of the healing arts*. Wheaton, IL: The Theosophical Publishing House.

Kunz, K., & Kunz, B. (1985). *Hand and Foot Reflexology, A Self-Help Guide*. New York: Simon & Schuster.

Kunz, K., & Kunz, B. (1985). *Hand Reflexology Workbook*. Albuquerque, NM: RRP Press.

Kunz, K., & Kunz, B. (1993). *The Complete Guide to Foot Reflexology* (Revised). Albuquerque, NM: RRP Press.

Kunz, K., & Kunz, B. (1997). *The parent's guide to reflexology*. New York: Harmony House.

Kunz, K., & Kunz, B. (1987, Jan./Feb./Mar.). The Paralysis Report. *Reflexions*, *8*(1), 1.

Kuo, S., Shankel, D. M., Telikepalli, H., & Mitscher, L. A. (1992). *Glycyrrhiza glabra* extract as an effector of interception in Escherichia coli K12+. *Mutation Research*, *282*(2), 93–98.

Kurosawa, M., Lundeberg, T., Agren, G., Lund, I., & Uvnas-Moberg, K. (1995). Massage-like stroking of the abdomen lowers blood pressure in anesthetized rats: Influence of oxytocin. *Journal of the Autonomic Nervous System*, *56*(1–2), 26–30.

Kurz, I. (1996). *Textbook of Dr. Vodder's Manual Lymph Drainage*, vol. 3: Treatment Manual, 3rd ed. Portland, OR: Medicina Biologica.

Kurz, I. (1997). *Textbook of Dr. Vodder's Manual Lymph Drainage*, vol. 2: Therapy, 5th ed. Portland, OR: Medicina Biologica.

Kurzer, M. S., Lampe, J. W., Martini, M. C., & Adlercreutz, H. (1995). Fecal lignan and isolfavonoid excretion in premenopausal women consuming flaxseed powder. *Cancer Epidemiology, Biomarkers and Prevention*, *4*(4), 353–358.

Kushi, L. H., Fee, R. M., Sellers, T. A., et al. (1996). Intake of vitamins A,C, and E and post menopausal breast cancer: The Iowa Women's Health Study. *American Journal of Epidemiology*, *144*(2), 165–174.

Kushi, L. H., Folsom, A. R., Prineas, R. J., et al. (1996). Dietary antioxidant vitamins and death from coronary heart disease in postmenopausal women. *New England Journal of Medicine*, *334*(18), 1156–1162.

Kushi, L. H., Lenart, E. B., & Willett, W. D. (1995). Health implications of Mediterranean diets in light of contemporary knowledge: 2. Meat, wine, fats, and oils. *American Journal of Clinical Nutrition*, *61*(Suppl. 6), 1416S–1427S.

Kynast-Gales, S. A., & Massey, L. K. (1994). Effect of caffeine on circadian excretion of urinary calcium and magnesium. *Journal of the American College of Nutrition*, *13*(5), 467–472.

Labott, S., Ahleman, S., Wolever, M., & Martin, R. (1990). The physiological and psychological effects of the expression and inhibition of emotion. *Behavioral Medicine*, *16*(4), 182–189.

Lachman, M. E., Weaver, S. L., Bandura, M., et al. (1992). Improving memory and control beliefs through cognitive restructuring and self-generated strategies. *Journal of Gerontology*, *47*(5), 293–299.

Lai, J. S., Lan, C., Wong, M. K., & Teng, S. H. (1995). Two-year trends in cardiorespiratory function among old Tai Chi Chuan practitioners. *Journal of the American Geriatrics Society*, *43*(11), 1222–1227.

LaLonde, C., Nayak, U., Hennigan, J., & Demling, R. H. (1997). Excessive liver oxidant stress causes mortality injury combined with endotoxin and is prevented with antioxidants. *Journal Burn Care Rehabil*, *18*(3), 187–192.

Lam, R. W., Zis, A. P., Grewal, A., Delgado, P. L., Charney, D. S., & Krystal, J. H. (1996). Effects of rapid tryptophan depletion in patients with seasonal affective disorder in remission after light therapy. *Archives of General Psychiatry*, *53*, 41–44.

Lama Surya Das. (1997). *Awakening the Buddha within*. N.Y. Broadway.

Lambert, R., & Lambert, N. (1995). The effects of humor on secretory immunoglobulin A levels in school-aged children. *Pediatric Nursing, 21*(1), 16–19.

Lambert, S. A. (1996). The effects of hypnosis/ guided imagery on the postoperative course of children. *Journal of Developmental and Behavioral Pediatrics, 17*(5), 307–310.

Lampertico, M., Comis, S., et al. (1993). Italian multicenter study on the efficacy of Coenzyme Q10 as an adjuvant therapy in heart failure. *Clinical Investigator, 71*, S129–S133.

Lan, C., Lai, J. S., Wong, M. K., & Yu, M. L. (1996). Cardiorespiratory function, flexibility, and body composition among geriatric Tai Chi Chuan practitioners. *Arch Phys Med Rehabil, 77*(6), 612–616.

Land, D. (1994). Extended bed rest can be harmful to pregnant women. *Nurs Dimensions* (Fall), 7–8.

Landis, R., & Khalsa, K. P. (1997). *Herbal defense*. New York: Warner.

Landon, R. A., & Young, E. A. (1993). The role of magnesium in regulation of lung function. *J Am Dietetic Assoc, 93*(6), 674–677.

Lane, C. A., & Davis, A. W. (1985). Implementation: We Can Weekend in the rural setting . . . Retreat for cancer families. *Cancer Nursing, 8*, 323–328.

Langer, E. J., & Rodin, J. (1976). The effects of choice and enhanced personal responsibility for the aged. *Journal of Personality and Social Psychology, 34*, 191–198.

Lanthony, P., & Cosson, J. P. (1988). The course of color vision in early diabetic retinopathy treated with *Ginkgo biloba* extract: A preliminary double-blind versus placebo study. *Journal Fr Ophtalmol, 11*(10), 671–674.

Larkin, K. T., & Zayfert, C. (1996). Anger management training with mild essential hypertensive patients. *Journal Behav Med, 19*(5), 415–433.

Larsson, M., Rossander-Hulthen, L., Sandstrom, B., & Sandberg, A. S. (1996). Improved zinc and iron absorption from breakfast meals containing malted oats with reduced phytate content. *British Journal of Nutrition, 76*(5), 677–688.

Laumer, U., Bauer, M., Fichter, M., & Milz, H. (1997). Therapeutic effects of the Feldenkrais method "awareness through movement" in patients with eating disorders. *Psychother Psychosom Med Psychol, 47*(5), 170–180.

Lawless, J. (1995). *The illustrated encyclopedia of essential oils: The complete guide to the use of oils in aromatherapy and herbalism*. Element.

Lawrence, R., Rosch, P. J., & Plowden, J. (1998). *Magnet therapy*. Rocklin: Prima Press.

Lazar, J. (1996). Mind body medicine in primary care. *Primary Care, 23*(1), 169–182.

Le Bars, P. L., Katz, M. M., Berman, N., et al. (1997). A placebo-controlled, double-blind, randomized trial of an extract of *Ginkgo biloba* for dementia. *Journal of the American Medical Association, 278*(16), 712–718.

Le Marchand, L., Hankin, J. H., Wilkens, L. R., et al. (1997). Dietary fiber and colorectal cancer risk. *Epidemiology, 8*(6), 658–665.

Lee, D., Prasad, A., Hydrick-Adair, C., et al. (1993). Homeostasis of zinc in marginal human zinc deficiency: Role of absorption and endogenous excretion of zinc. *Journal of Laboratory and Clinical Medicine, 122*, 549–556.

Lefcourt, H., Davidson-Katz, K., & Kueneman, K. (1990). Humor and immune-system functioning. *Humor: International Journal of Humor Research, 3*(3), 305–321.

Lehrer, P. M., Carr, R., Sargunarai, D., & Woolfolk, R. L. (1993). Differential effects of stress management therapies in behavioral medicine. In P. M. Lehrer & R. L. Woolfolk (Eds.), *Principles and practice of stress management* (2nd. ed., pp. 571–605). New York: Guilford Press.

Leibowitz, J., & Connington, B. (1990). Judith's story. In *The Alexander technique* (pp. 3–8). New York: Harper & Row.

Leonardi, M. (1993). Treatment of fibercystic disease of the breast with myrtillus anthocyanins. Our experience. *Minerva Ginecologica, 45*(12), 617–621.

Leslie, C. (1977). Medical pluralism and legitimation in the Indian and Chinese medical systems. In D. Landy (Ed.), *Culture, disease, and healing: Studies in medical anthropology* (pp. 511–517). New York: MacMillan.

Leslie, C., & Young, A. Editors. (1992). *Paths to Asian medical knowledge*. Berkeley, CA: University of California Press.

Leste, A., & Rust, J. (1984). Effects of dance on anxiety. *Percept Mot Skills, 58*(3), 767–772.

Levander, O. A., & Beck, M. A. (1997). Insights from Coxsackie-induced Myocarditis in Mice Deficient in Selenium or Vitamin E. *Biological Trace Element Research*, *56*(1), 5–22.

Leventhal, L. J., Boyce, E. G., & Zurier, R. B. (1994). Treatment of rheumatoid arthritis with gammalinolenic acid. *Annals of Internal Medicine*, *119*(9), 867–873.

Leventhal, L. J., Boyce, E. G., & Zurier, R. B. (1994). Treatment of rheumatoid arthritis with blackcurrant seed oil. *British Journal of Rheumatology*, *33*(9), 847–852.

Levi, L. (1965). The urinary output of adrenalin and noradrenalin during pleasant and unpleasant emotional states. *Psychosomatic Medicine*, *27*, 403–419.

Levine, S. (1991). *Guided meditations, explorations and healings*. New York: Anchor Books/Doubleday.

Levy, F., Pines Fried, J., & Leventhal, F. (Eds.). (1995). *Dance and other expressive arts therapies: When words are not enough*. New York: Routledge.

Levy, S., Herberman, R., Lippman, M., & D'Angelo, T. (1987). Correlation of stress factors with sustained depression of natural killer cell activity and predicted prognosis in patients with breast cancer. *Journal of Clinical Oncology*, *5*, 348–353.

Lewin, G., & Popove, I. (1994). Antioxidant effects of aqueous garlic extract: Inhibition of Cu2+-initiated oxidation of low density lipoproteins. *Arheim Forsch*, *44*, 604–607.

Lewis, P. (1993). *Creative transformation: The healing power of the arts*. Wilmette, IL: Chiron.

Lewit, J. (1979). The needle effect in the relief of myofascial pain. *Pain*, *6*, 83–90.

Li, K. H., Xin, Y. L., Gu, Y., Xu, B., Fan, D., & Ni, B. (1997). Effects of direct current on dog liver: Possible mechanisms for tumor electrochemical treatment. *Bioelectromagnetics*, *18*, 2–7.

Liang, B., Chung, S., Araghiniknam, M., et al. (1996). Vitamins and immunomodulation in AIDS. *Nutrition*, *12*(1), 1–7.

Liang, W. (1996). An Exploration of the Clinical Indications of Foot Reflexology—A Retrospective Analysis of Its Clinical Application to 8,096 Cases, 1996 China Reflexology Symposium Report, Beijing, China Reflexology Association, pp. 140–143.

Liangyue, D., Yijun, G., Shuhui, H., Xiaoping, J., Yang, L., Rufen, W., Wenjing, W., Xuetai, W., Hengze, X., Xiuling, X., & Jiuling, Y. (1987). *Chinese acupuncture and maxibustion*. Beijing: Foreign Languages Press.

Lidell, L. (1984). *The book of massage, the complete step-by-step guide to Eastern and Western techniques*. New York: Simon and Schuster.

Lim, J. H., Wen, T. C., Matsuda, S., et al. (1997). Protection of ischemic hippocampal neurons by ginsenoside Rb1, a main ingredient of ginseng root. *Neurosci Res*, *28*(3), 191–200.

Lin, C. C., Lu, J. M., Yang, J. J., et al. (1996). Anti-inflammatory and radical scavenge effects of Arctium lappa. *American Journal of Chinese Medicine*, *24*(2), 127–137.

Lincoln, N. B., Flannaghan, T., Sutcliffe, L., & Rother, L. (1997). Evaluation of cognitive behavioural treatment for depression after stroke: A pilot study. *Clin Rehabil*, *11*(2), 114–122.

Lindbohm, M. L., Hietanen, M., Kyyronen, P., et al. (1992). Magnetic fields of video display terminals and spontaneous abortion. *American Journal of Epidemiology*, *136*, 9.

Linde, K., Ramirez, G., Mulrow, C. D., et al. (1996). St. John's wort for depression—an overview and metaanalysis of randomized clinical trials. *British Medical Journal, 313*(7052).

Lindenbaum, J., Rosenberg, I. H., Wilson, P. W., et al. (1994). Prevalence of cobalamin deficiency in the Framingham elderly population. *American Journal of Clinical Nutrition*, *60*(1), 12–14.

Lindquist, T. L., Beilin, L. J., & Knulman, M. W. (1997). Influence of lifestyle, coping, and job stress on blood pressure in men and women. *Hypertension*, *29*(1, part 1), 1–7.

Linehan, M. M., Tutek, D. A., Heard, H. L., & Armstrong, H. E. (1994). Interpersonal outcome of cognitive behavioral treatment for chronically suicidal borderline patients. *Am Journal Psychiatry*, *151*(12), 1771–1776.

Linn, D. (1995). *Sacred space*. Ballantine Books.

Lipchik, G., & LeResche, L. (1994). Panel on women and pain. American Psychological Associations conference. Psychosocial and behavioral factors in women's health. Washington, D. C., May 11–14.

Lipton & Bryan. (1989). *The Therapeutic Art of Polarity: Introduction & Reference Manual*. Atlanta, GA: J Hanson.

Liskin, J. (1996). *Moving Medicine: The life and work of Milton Trager, MD*. Barrytown, NY: Station Hill Press, Inc.

Liu, W. H., Song, Z. H., & Du, N. Q. (1994). Study of treatment on acquired infantile mental retardation with traditional Chinese and Western medicine. *Chung Kuo Chung Hsi I Chieh Ho Tsa Chih, 14*(12), 730–732.

Ljunggren, A. E., Weber, H., Kogstad, O., Thom, E., & Kirkesola, G. (1997). Effect of exercise on sick leave due to low back pain. A randomized, comparative, long-term study. *Spine, 22*(14), 1610–1636.

Lloyd, H. M., Green, M. W., & Rogers, P. J. (1994). Mood and cognitive performance effects of isocaloric lunches differing in fat and carbohydrate content. *Physiology and Behavior, 56*, 51–57.

Lo, S. Y. (1996). Anomalous state of ice. *Modern Physics Letters B, 10*(19), 909–919.

Lo, S. Y., Lo, A., Chong, L., Tianzhang, L., Hua, L., et al. (1996). Physical Properties of water with Ie Structures. *Modern Physics Letters B, 10*(19), 921–930.

Locke, S., & Colligan, D. (1986). *The healer within: The new medicine of mind and body*. New York: Penguin Books USA, Inc.

Loehr, J. E. (1983). *Toughness training for life*. New York: Plume Penguin.

Logan, S. (1997). Home visiting reduces the rates of childhood injuries. *Child: Care, Health and Development, 23*(1), 101–102.

London, R. S., Murphy, L., Kitlowski, K. E., & Reynolds, M. A. (1987). Efficacy of alpha-tocopherol in the treatment of premenstrual syndrome. *Journal Reprod Med, 32*(6), 400–404.

London, R. S., Sundaram, G. S., Murphy, L., & Goldstein, P. J. (1983). The effect of alpha-tocopherol on premenstrual symptomatology: A double-blind study. *Journal of the American College of Nutrition, 2*(2), 115–122.

Look, M. P., Rockstroh, J. K., Rao, G. S., Kreuzer, K. A., Spengler, U., & Sauerbruch, T. (1997). Serum Selenium Versus Lymphocyte Suibsets and Markers of Disease Progression and Inflammatory Response in Human Immunodeficiency Virus-1 Infection. *Biological Trace Element Research, 56*, 31–41.

Look, M. P., Rokstroh, J. K., Rao, G. S., et al. (1997). Serum selenium, plasma glutathione (GSH) and erythrocyte glutathione peroxidase (GSH-Px)-levels in asymptomatic versus symptomatic human immunodeficiency virus-l (HIV-l)-infection. *European Journal of Clinical Nutrition, 51*(4), 266–272.

Loomis, D. P., & Savitz. (1995). Magnetic field ˙ʌposure in relation to leukemia and brain cancer mortality among electric utility workers. *American Journal of Epidemiology, 141*, 2.

Loomis, D. P., Savitz, D. A., & Ananth, C. V. (1994). Breast cancer mortality among female electrical workers in the United States. *Journal of the National Cancer Institute, 86*, 12.

Lopez, L. R., Frati Munari, A. C., Hernandez Dominguez, B. C., et al. (1996). Monounsaturated fatty acid (avocado) rich diet for mild hypercholesterolemia. *Archives of Medical Research, 27*(4), 519–523.

Lorscheider, F. L., Viing, M. J., & Summers, A. D. (1995). Mercury exposure from "silver" tooth fillings: Emerging evidence questions a traditional dental paradigm. *Federation of American Societies for Experimental Biology Journal, 9*, 504–508.

Losonczy, K. G., Harris, T. B., & Havlik, R. J. (1996). Vitamin E and vitamin C supplement use and risk of all-cause and coronary heart disease mortality in older persons: The Established Populations for Epidemiologic Studies of the Elderly. *American Journal of Clinical Nutrition, 64*(2), 190–196.

Lotan, R. (1997). Roles of retinoids and their nuclear receptors in the development and prevention of upper aerodigestive tract cancers. *Environ Health Perspec, 105*(Suppl. 4), 985–988.

Low, J. (1988, October-November). The modern body therapies. *Massage Magazine, 16*, 48–50, 52, 54–55.

Lowen, A. (1971). *Language of the body*. New York: Collier.

Ludianskii, E. A. (1990). Dissociated symptoms of the progressive course of brain injury. *Zh Nevropatol Psikhiatr Im S S Korsakova, 90*(7), 53–55.

Ludington, S. (1977). Effects of extra tactile stimulation upon vaginally and cesearean born infants. *Proceedings of the 5th Annual Nursing Research Forum*: 57–71.

Luettig, B., Steinmuller, C., Gifford, G. E., et al. (1989). Macrophage activation by the polysaccharide arabinogalactan isolated from plant cell cultures of Echinacea purpurea. *Journal of the National Cancer Institute, 81*(9), 669–675.

Luthe, W. (Ed.). (1969). *Autogenic therapy*, six vols. New York: Grune & Stratton.

Macdonald, R. (1997). *The use of the voice*. London, England: Bookcraft Ltd.

Machover, I., Drake, A., & Drake, J. (1993). *The Alexander Technique Birth Book*. New York: Sterling Publishing Company.

Macrae, J. (1994). *Therapeutic touch: A practical guide*. New York: Albert A. Knopf.

Macrae, J. (1987). *Therapeutic touch: A practical guide*. New York: Alfred A. Knopf.

Macrae, J. (1988). *Therapeutic touch: A practical guide*. New York: Knopf.

Mada, Z., Abel, R., Samish, S., & Arad, J. (1988). Gluocose-lowering effect of fenugreek in non-insulin dependent diabetics. *European Journal of Clinical Nutrition, 42*, 51–54.

Madanmohna, TDP, Balakumar, B., Nambinarayanan, T. K., Thakur, S., Krishnamurthy, N., & Chandrabose, A. (1992). *Indian J Physiol Pharmacol, 36*(4), 229–233.

Mader, F. H. (1990). Treatment of hyperlipidaemia with garlic-powder tablets. *Arzneimittel-Forschung (Drug Research), 40*(10), 3–8.

Mahoney, M. J. (1974). *Cognition and behavior modification*. Cambridge: Ballinger Publishing Co.

Mailhot, C. B. (1996). The operating room of the future. *Nurs Manage, 27*(12), 28E.

Maitra, I., Marocci, L., Droy-Lefaix, M. T., & Packer, L. (1995). Peroxyl radical scavenging activity of *Ginkgo biloba* extract EGb 761. *Biochemical Pharmacology, 49*(11), 1649–1655.

Malinski, V. (1993). Therapeutic Touch: A View from Rogerian nursing science. *Visions: The Journal of Rogerian Nursing Science, 1*, 45–54.

Malvy, D. J., Arnaud, J., Burtschy, B., et al. (1997). Antioxidant micronutrients and childhood malignancy during oncological treatment. *Med Pediatr Oncol, 29*(3), 213–217.

MANA *Information Packet for Aspiring Midwives.*

Manaka. *A layman's guide to acupuncture.*

Mandarino, J. V., Waziri, R., & Wallace, R. (1997). Anger expression correlates with platelet aggregation. *Behav Med, 22*(4), 174–177.

Manderino, M. A., & Berkey, N. (1997). Verbal abuse of staff nurses by physicians. *Journal of Professional Nursing, 13*(1), 48–55.

Mangels, A. R., et al. (1993). Carotenoid content of fruits and vegetables: An evaluation of analytic data. *Journal Am Diet Assoc, 93*, 284–286.

Mangrum, A., & Bakris, G. L. (1997). Predictors of renal and cardiovascular mortality in patients with non-insulin-dependent diabetes: A brief overview of microalbuminuria and insulin resistance. *Journal of Diabetes Complications, 11*(6), 352–357.

Manson, J. E., Nathan, D. M., Krolewski, A. S., et al. (1992). A prospective study of exercise and incidence of diabetes among US male physicians. *Journal of the American Medical Association, 268*(1), 63–67.

Manson, J. E., Willett, W. C., Stampfer, M. J., et al. (1994). Vegetable and fruit consumption and incidence of stroke in women. 34th Annual Conference on Cardiovascular Disease Epidemiology and Prevention. March 16–17, Tampa, Florida.

Manson, J. E., Willett, W. C., Stampper, M. J., Colditz, G. A., Speizer, F. E., & Hennekens, C. H. (1994). Vegetable and fruit consumption and incidence of stroke in women. *Circulation, 89*(2), 678.

Manyam, B. (1996). *Method of evaluating Ayurvedic drug in Parkinsonism*. U.S. Office of Alternative Medicine, http://www.altmed.od.nih.gov/oam.cgi-bin/research/search_simple.cgi

Manyande, A., Berg, S., Gettins, D., Stanford, S. C., Mazhero, S., Marks, D. F., & Salmon, P. (1995). Preoperative rehearsal of active coping imagery influences subjective and hormonal responses to abdominal surgery. *Psychosomatic Medicine, 57*(2), 177–182.

Marabini, S., Ciabatta, P. G., Polli, G., et al. (1991). Beneficial effects of intranasal applications of capsaicin in patients with vasomotor rhinitis. *Eur Arch Otorhinolaryngol, 248*(4), 191–194.

Marean, M., Cumming, C. E., Fox, E. E., & Cumming, D. C. (1995). Fluid intake in women with premenstrual syndrome. *Women Health, 23*(3), 75–78.

Mares-Perlman, J. A. (1995). Serum antioxidants and age-related macular degeneration in a population-based case-control study. *Archives of Opthalmology*, *113*(2), 1518–1523.

Mares-Perlman, J. A., Klein, R., Klein, B. E., et al. (1996). Association of zinc and antioxidant nutrients with age-related maculopathy. *Archives of Opthalmology*, *114*, 991–997.

Marini, A., Agosti, M., Motta, G., & Mosca, F. (1996). Effects of a dietary and environmental prevention programme on the incidence of allergic symptoms in high atopic risk infants: Three years' follow-up. *Acta Paediatr*, Supple 4l4: 1-21.

Marion Merrell Dow, Managed care digest. (1995). Kansas City, MO: Marion Merrell Dow.

Mark, D. (1994). Help for an ailing heart: Look on the bright side. Press Release, Duke University, April 16.

Markham, U. *Hypnosis*. Charles E. Tuttle.

Markov, M. S., et al. (1994). Static Magnetic Field Modulation of Myosin Phosphorylation: Calcium Dependence in Two Enzyme Preparations. *Bioelectrochemistry and Bioenergetics*, *35*, 57.

Marshall, C. M. (1971). The Use of Ice Cube Massage for the Relief of Chronic Pain Following Herpes Ophthalmicus. *Physiotherapy*, *57*, 374.

Martin-Moreno, J. M., Willett, W. C., Gorgojo, L., et al. (1994). Dietary fat, olive oil intake and breast cancer risk. *International Journal of Cancer*, *58*(6), 774–780.

Martin, A., Foxall, T., Blumberg, J. B., & Meydani, M. (1997). Vitamin E inhibits low-density lipoprotein-induced adhesion of monocytes to human aortic endothelial cells in vitro. *Arteriosclerosis, Thrombosis and Vascular Biology, 17*(3), 429–436.

Martin, A., Wu, D., Baur, W., Meydani, S. N., Blumberg, J. B., & Meydani, M. (1996). Effect of vitamin E on human aortic endothelial cell responses to oxidative injury. *Free Radical Biological Medicine, 21*(4), 505–511.

Martin, J. E., & Dubbert, P. M. (1982). Exercise applications and promotion in behavioral medicine: Current status and future directions. *Journal of Consulting and Clinical Psychology*, *5*(6), 1004–1017.

Martin, L., Edworthy, S. M., MacIntosh, B., et al. (1993). Is exercise helpful in the treatment of fibromyalgia? *Arthritis Rheumatism*, *36*(Suppl.), S251.

Martinez, M. E., Giovannucii, E., Spiegelman, D., et al. (1997). Leisure-time physical activity, body size, and colon cancer in women. *Journal of the National Cancer Institute*, *89*(13), 948–955.

Massey, L., & Berg, L. (1985). The effect of dietary caffeine on urinary excretion of calcium, magnesium, phosphorus, sodium, potassium, chloride and zinc in healthy males. *Nutrition Research*, *5*, 1281–1284.

Masunaga, S., with Ohashi, W. (1977). *Zen Shiatsu, how to harmonize yin and yang for better health.* Japan Publications.

Matkovic, V., et al. (1995). Urinary calcium, sodium, and bone mass of young females. *American Journal of Clinical Nutrition*, *62*, 417–425.

Matthew, N. T. (1993). Chronic refractory headache. *Neurology*, *43*(Suppl. 3), S26–S33.

Matthews, D. (1997). Religion and spirituality in primary care. *Mind/Body Medicine*, *2*(1), 9–19.

Maugars, U., Berthelot, J. M., Lalande, S., et al. (1996). Osteoporotic fractures revealing anorexia nervosa in five females. *Revue du Rhumatisme* (English Edition), *63*(3), 201–206.

Maultsby, M. C. (1984). *Rational behavior therapy*. Englewood Cliffs, NJ: Prentice-Hall.

Maxwell, N. (1990). *Witch-Doctor's Apprentice. Hunting for medicinal plants in the Amazon.* New York: Citadel Press.

Mazariegos-Ramos, E., Guerrero-Romero, F., Rodriguez-Moran, M., et al. (1995). Consumption of soft drinks with phosphoric acid as a risk factor for the development of hypocalcemia in children: A case-control study. *Journal of Pediatrics*, *126*(6), 940–942.

McAdam, P., Lewis, K., Helzlsouer, C., et al. (1985). Absorption of selenite and L-selenomethionine in healthy young men using a selenium tracer. *Fed Proc*, *44*, 1671.

McAlindon, T. E. (1997). Nutrition: Risk factors for osteoarthritis. *Annals of Rheumatic Disease, 56*(7), 397–400.

McAlindon, T. E., Felson, D. T., Zhang, Y., et al. (1995). Effects of a modified based exercise on cardiorespiratory fitness, psychological state and health status of persons with rheumatoid arthritis. *American Journal Phys Med Rehabil*, *74*(1), 19–27.

McAllindon, T., Zhang, Y., Hannan, M., et al. (1996). Are risk factors for patellofemoral and tibiofemoral knee osteoarthritis different? *Journal of Rheumatology, 23*(2), 332–337.

McCarty, M. F. (1996). Magnesium taurate and fish oil for prevention of migraine. *Medical Hypotheses, 47*(6), 461–466.

McCauley, J., Kern, D. E., Kolodner, K., et al. (1997). Clinical characteristics of women with a history of childhood abuse: Unhealed wounds. *Journal of the American Medical Association, 277*(1), 1362–1368.

McClain, C., Stuart, M., Vivian, B., et al. (1992). Zinc status before and after zinc supplementation of eating disorder patients. *Journal Am Col N, 11*, 694–700.

McClure, V. (1989). *Infant Massage: A Handbook for Loving Parents.* revised, New York: Bantam Books.

McDaniel, H. R., Combs, C., & McDaniel, R. (1990). An increase in circulating monocyte/macrophages is induced by oral acdmannan (ACE-M) in HIV-l patients. *American Journal of Clinical Pathology, 94*, 516–517.

McDermott, J. H., Riedlinger, J. E., & Chapman, E. (1995). What pharmacists should understand about homeopathic remedies. *American Journal of Health-Systems Pharmacists, 52*(21), 2442–2445.

McDougall, J. M. (1985). *McDougall's Medicine.* Piscataway, NJ: New Century.

McDougall, M. (1993). *The New McDougall Cookbook.* New York: Dutton.

McGrady, A. (1996). *Biofeedback assisted relaxation in control of insulin dependent diabetes.* Grant number R21 RR09418, Office of Alternative Medicine, National Institutes of Health. http://www.altmed.od.nih.gov/oam/cgi-bin/research/search_simple.cgi.

McGuire, M. B. (1988). *Ritual healing in suburban America.* New Brunswick, NJ: Rutgers University Press.

McKinney, C. H., Antoni, M. H., Kumar, M., et al. (1997). Effects of guided imagery and music (GIM) therapy on mood and cortisol in healthy adults. *Health Psychology, 16*(4), 390–400.

McLellan, A. T., Grossman, D. S., Blaine, J. D., & Haverkos, H. W. (1993). Acupuncture treatment for drug abuse: A technical review. *Journal of Substance Abuse Treatment, 10*(6), 569–576.

McNeely, D. A. (1987). *Touching: Body therapy and depth psychology.* Ontario: Inner City Books.

McPartland, J. M., & Mitchell, J. A. (1997). Caffeine and chronic back pain. *Arch Phys Med Rehabil, 78*(1), 61–63.

Meade, T. W., Dyer, S., Browne, W., et al. (1990). Low back pain of mechanical origin: Randomized comparison of chiropractic and hospital outpatient treatment. *BMJ, 300*, 1431–1437.

Meehan, T. C. (1993). Therapeutic Touch and postoperative pain: A Rogerian research study. *Nursing Science Quarterly, 6*(2), 69–78.

Mehl, L. (1994). Hypnosis and conversion of breech vertex to presentation. *Archives of Family Medicine, 3*(10), 881–887.

Mehl-Madrona, L. (1997). *Coyote medicine.* New York: Scribners.

Meichenbaum, D. (1975). A cognitive-behavior modification approach to assessment. In M. Hersen & A. Bellack (Eds.), *Behavioral assessment. A practical handbook* (pp. 143–171). New York: Pergamon Press.

Meichenbaum, D. (1977). *Cognitive behavior modification. An integrated approach.* New York: Plenum Press.

Meleis, A. (1991). *Theoretical nursing: Development and progress.* Philadelphia: J. B. Lippincott.

Mellin, L., Croughan-Minihane, M., & Dickey, L. (1997). The Solution Method: 2-year trends in weight, blood pressure, exercise, depression, and functioning of adults trained in development skills. *Journal of the American Dietetic Association, 97*(10), 1133–1138.

Melzack, R., & Bentley, K. C. (1983). Relief of Dental Pain by Ice Massage of Either Hand or the Contralateral Arm. *Canadian Dental Association, 49*, 257–260.

Melzack, R., & Wall, P. D. (1973/82). *The challenge of pain.* New York: Basic Books, Inc.

Melzack, R., Guite, S. M., & Gonshor, A. (Jan 1980). Relief of Dental Pain By Ice Massage of the Hand. *Canadian Medical Association, 122*, 189–191.

Melzack, R., Jeans, M. E., Stratford, J. G., et al. (1980). Ice Massage and Transcutaneous Electrical Stimulation: Comparison of Treatment for Low Back Pain. *Pain, 9*, 209–217.

The Merck Manual of Diagnosis and Therapy, 14th Edition. (1985). Rahway, NJ: Merck Sharp & Dohme Research Laboratories.

Meruelo, D., Lavie, G., & Lavie, D. (1988). Therapeutic agents with dramatic anti-retroviral activity and little toxicity at effective doses: aromatic polycyclicciones hypericin and pseudohypericin. *Proceedings of the National Academy of Sciences of the United States of America, 85*(14), 5230–5234.

Metori, K., Furutsu, M., & Takahashi, S. (1997). The preventive effect of ginseng with du-zhong leaf on protein metabolism in aging. *Biol Pharm Bull, 20*(3), 237–242.

Metz, J. A. (1993). Lifestyle factors related to bone mineral density of young adult women. *Dissertation Abstracts International,* University of North Carolina at Chapel Hill, #54-04B, page 1899.

Meunier, P. (1996). Prevention of hip fractures by correcting calcium and vitamin D insufficiencies in elderly people. *Scandinavian Journal of Rheumatology*(Suppl. 103), 75–78.

Meydani, S. N., Meydani, M., Blumberg, J. B., et al. (1997). Vitamin E supplementation and in vivo immune response in healthy elderly subjects: A randomized controlled trial. *Journal of the American Medical Association, 277,* 1380–1386.

Meyer, F. (1994). Ischemic heart disease incidence and mortality in relation to vitamin supplement use in a cohort of 2,226 men. Presented at the American Heart Association's 34th Annual Conference on Cardiovascular Disease Epidemiology and Prevention, March 16–19, Tampa, Florida.

Meyer, H. E., Pedersen, J. I., Loken, E. G., & Tverdal, A. (1997). Dietary factors and the incidence of hip fracture in middle-aged Norwegians: A prospective study. *American Journal of Epidemiology, 145*(2), 117–123.

Meyer, H. E., Tverdal, A., Henriksen, C., et al. (1996). Risk factors of femoral neck fractures in Oslo. *Tidsskrift for Den Norske Laegeforening, 116*(22), 2656–2659.

Meyers, A. R. (1994). *Course syllabus: Public health perspectives on alternative and complementary health care.* Boston: School of Public Health, Boston University School of Medicine.

Miasnikov, I. G. (1992). Magnetotherapy of initial manifestations of cerebrovascular disorders in hypertension. *Zh Nevropatol Psikhiatr Im S S Korsakova, 92*(1), 63–67.

Michaud, T., Brenna, D., et al. (1995). Aquarunning and gains in cardiorespiratory fitness. *Journal Strength and Conditioning, 9*(2), 73–84.

Michel, A., Kolhmann, T., & Raspe, H. (1997). The association between clinical findings on physical examination and self-reported severity in back pain. Results of a population-based study. *Spine, 22*(3), 296–303.

Micozzi, M. (1996). *Fundamentals of complementary and alternative health care.* New York: Churchill Livingstone.

Micozzi, M. (1996). Point of view—The need to teach alternative medicine. *Chronicle of Higher Education.* August 16, A48.

Migration and Homing of Lymphoid Cells, Volume I. (1988). Alan J. Hubbard, Editor. Boca Raton, FL: CRC Press, Inc.

Milberger, S., Biederman, J., Faraone, S. V., et al. (1996). Is maternal smoking during pregnancy a risk factor for attention deficit hyperactivity disorder in children? *American Journal of Psychiatry, 153*(9), 11138–1142.

Miles, R. B. (1998, November–December). Medical care at a crossroads. *At Work.*

Miles, R. B. (1998, Spring). Organizing collaborative practices. *Alternative Health Practitioner.*

Miller, B. (1987, January 14). Learning the touch. *Physical Therapy Forum, 6*(2), 1, 3–4.

Miller, B. (1992). Alternative somatic therapies. In *Conservative Care of Low Back Pain.* William & Wilkins.

Miller, C. H., Zhong, Z., Hamilton, S. M., & Teel, R. W. (1993). Effects of capsaicin on liver microsomal metabolism of the tobacco-specific nitrosamine NNK. *Cancer Letter, 75*(1), 45–52.

Miller, J. J., Fletcher, K., & Kabat-Zinn, J. (1995). Three-year follow-up and clinical implications of a mindfulness meditation-based stress reduction intervention in the treatment of anxiety disorders. *General Hospital Psychiatry, 17*(3), 192–200.

Miller, L. G., & Murray, W. J. (1997). Herbal instruction in united states pharmacy schools. *American Journal of Pharmaceutical Education, 61*(2), 160–162.

Miller, M. (1996). Diet and psychological health. *Altern Ther Health Med, 2*(5), 40–48.

Miller, W. L. (1992). Routine, ceremony, or drama: An exploratory field study of the primary care clinical encounter. *Journal of Family Practice, 34*(3), 289–296.

Millham, S. (1996). Increased incidence of cancer in a cohort of office workers exposed to strong magnetic fields. *Am Journal Ind Med, 30*(6), 702–704.

Mills, E. M. (1994). The effect of low-density aerobic exercise on muscle strength, flexibility, and balance among sedentary elderly persons. *Nursing Research, 43* (July/August), 207–211.

Milner, J. (1994). Role of garlic and disease prevention—preclinical Models. Designer Foods III Proceedings: May 23–25, 1994. Rutgers University, Cook College, New Brunswick, NJ.

Milner, J. A. (1996). Garlic: Its anticarcinogenic and antitumorigenic properties. *Nutr Rev, 54*(11 Pt 2), S82–S86.

Mittleman, M. S., Ferris, S. H., Shulman, E., et al. (1996). A family intervention to delay nursing home placement of patients with Alzheimer's disease. A randomized controlled trial. *Journal of the American Medical Association, 276*(21), 1725–1731.

Mock, V., Dow, K. H., Measres, C. J., et al. (1997). Effects of exercise on fatigue, physical functioning and emotional distress during radiation therapy for breast cancer. *Oncology Nursing Forum, 24*(6), 991–1000.

Moerman, C. J. (1993). Dietary sugar intake in the etiology of biliary tract cancer. *International Journal of Epidemiology, 22,* 207–214.

Moisan, P. A., Sanders-Phillips, K., & Moisan, P. M. (1997). Ethnic differences in circumstances of abuse and symptoms of depression and anger among sexually abused black and Latino boys. *Child Abuse Negl, 21*(5), 473–488.

Moller, S. E. (1992). Serotonin, carbohydrates, and atypical depression. *Pharmacology and Toxicology, 71*(Suppl. 1), 61–71.

Molodofsky, H., et al. (1975). Musculoskeletal Symptoms and Non-REM sleep disturbance in patients with "Fibrositis Syndrome" and healthy subjects. *Psychosomatic Medicine, 37,* 341–351.

Monmaney, T. (1998, August 31). Remedy's U.S. sales zoom, but quality control lags. *Los Angeles Times,* pp. A1, A10–A11.

Moody, L. E., Fraser, M., & Yarandi, H. (1993). Effects of guided imagery in patients with

chronic bronchitis and emphysema. *Clinical Nursing Research, 2*(4), 478–486.

Moody, R. *Reunions.* Fawcett.

Moon, T. E., Levine, N., Cartmel, B., & Bangert, J. L. (1997). Retinoids in prevention of skin cancer. *Cancer Lett, 114*(1–2), 203–205.

Moore, K. L. (1980). *Clinically oriented anatomy.* Baltimore: Williams & Wilkins.

Moore, L. E., & Wiesner, S. L. (1996). Hypnotically-induced vasodilation in the treatment of repetitive strain injuries. *American Journal of Clin Hypnosis, 39*(2), 97–104.

Morcos, N. C. (1997). Modulation of lipid profile by fish oil and garlic combination. *Journal Natl Med Assoc, 89*(10), 673–678.

Mori, T. A., Vandongen, R., Beilin, L. J., Burke, V., Morris, J., & Ritchie, J. (1994). Effects of varying dietary fat, fish and fish oils on blood lipids in a randomized controlled trial in men at risk of heart disease. *American Journal of Clinical Nutrition, 59,* 1060–1068.

Moriguchi, T., Saito, H., & Nishiyama, N. (1997). Anti-ageing effect of aged garlic extract in the inbred brain atrophy mouse model. *Clin Exp Pharmacol Physiol, 24*(3–4), 235–242.

Morris, M. C., Sacks, F., & Rosner, B. (1993). Does fish oil lower blood pressure? A meta-analysis of controlled trials. *Circulation, 88,* 523–533.

Morris, P. A. (1994). Superkids: Short-term group therapy for children with abusive backgrounds. *Journal Child Adolescent Psychiatric Nursing, 7*(1), 25–31.

Morrison, R. (1993). *Desktop Guide to Keynotes and Confirmatory Symptoms.* Albany, CA: Hahnemann Clinic Publishing.

Morse, G. G. (1997). Effect of positive reframing and social support on perception of perimenstrual changes among women with premenstrual syndrome. *Health Care Women Int, 18*(2), 175–193.

Mortensen, S. A. (1993). Prospectives on therapy of cardiovascular disease with coenzyme Q10 (ubiquinone). *Clin Investig, 71,* S116–S123.

Mosby's Medical, Nursing, & Allied Health Dictionary. (1994). St Louis: Mosby.

Moser, D. K., Dracup, K., Woo, M. A., & Stevenson, L. W. (1997). Voluntary control of vascular tone by using skin-temperature biofeedback-relaxation in patients with advanced heart failure. *Altern Ther Health Med*, *3*(1), 51–59.

Moss, D. P. (Ed.). (1995). Biofeedback therapy: An exposition. *Biofeedback*, *23*, 12–14.

Mossad, S. B., Macknin, M. L., Medendorp, S. V., & Mason, P. (1996). Zinc gluconate lozenges for treating the common cold. *Annals of International Medicine*, *125*(2), 81–88.

Mowrey, D. (1986). *The scientific validation of herbal medicine*. New Canaan, CT: Keats Publishing, Inc.

Mowry, D. B. (1993). Echinacea. In *Herbal tonic therapies* (pp. 40–46). New Canaan, CT: Keats.

Mowry, D. B. (1993). Ginkgo. *Herbal tonic therapies* (pp. 166–179). New Canaan, CT: Keats.

Mowry, D. B. (1993). Ginseng. In *Herbal tonic therapies* (pp. 46–52). New Canaan, CT: Keats.

Moyer, D. M., DiPietro, L. O., Berkowitz, R. I., & Stunkard, A. J. (1997). Childhood sexual abuse and precursors of binge eating in an adolescent female population. *International Journal of Eating Disorders*, *21*(1), 23–30.

Muehsam, D. J., Markov, M. S., Muehsan, P. A., Pilla, A., Ronger, S., & Wu, I. (1993). Static magnetic field modulation of myosin phosphorylation: Preliminary experiment. *Subtle Energies*, *4*, 1–16.

Mulroy, E. A. (1997). Building a neighborhood network: Interorganizational collaboration to prevent child abuse and neglect. *Soc Work*, *42*(3), 255–264.

Munck, A., & Guyre, P. M. (1991). Glucocorticoids and immune function. In R. Ader, D. L. Felton, & N. Cohen (Eds.), *Psychoneuroimmunology* (2nd ed., pp. 447–474). New York: Academic Press.

Murat, F. (1981). *Bee pollen miracle food*, 28th ed. Miami: F. Murat Co.

Murphy, J. J., Heptinstall, S., & Mitchell, J. R. (1988). Randomised double-blind placebo-controlled trial of feverfew in migraine prevention. *Lancet*, *2*(8604), 189–192.

Murphy, M. *The future of the body*.

Murphy, R. (1993). *The Homeopathic Medical Repertory*. Pagosa Springs: Hahnemann Academy of North America.

Murray, J. T. (1994). Are botanical medicines useful in diabetes? *American Journal of Natural Medicine*, *1*(3), 5–7.

Murray, M. (1994). Dietary and life-style factors in treating asthma, hay fever and allergies. *Natural Alternatives to Over-the-Counter and Prescription Drugs*. New York: William Morrow and Company, Inc. pp. 91–99.

Murray, M. (1994). Magnesium therapy in new-onset atrial fibrillation. *American Journal of Natural Medicine*, *1*(2), 16.

Murray, M. (1995). PCO sources: Grape seed vs. pine bark. *American Journal of Natural Medicine*, *2*(1), 6–9.

Murray, M. (1995). Ruscus extract improves microvascular permeability. *American Journal of Natural Medicine*, *2*(1), 26–27.

Murray, M. T. (1994). Do headache medicine cause chronic headaches? *American Journal of Natural Medicine*, *1*(2), 5–7.

Murray, M. T. (1995). Echinacea: Pharmacology and clinical applications. *American Journal of Natural Medicine*, *2*(1), 18–24.

Music Therapy Program, California State University (1997), http://www.csun.edu/-hcmus006/Music Therapy/html1#2.

Naeser. Acupuncture in America. *New England Journal of Medicine*.

Naganawa, R., Iwata, N., Ishikawa, K., et al. (1996). Inhibition of microbial growth by ajoene, a sulfur-containing compound derived from garlic. *Applied Environmental Microbiology*, *62*(11), 4238–4242.

Nakagawa, K. (1976). Magnetic field deficiency syndrome. *Japanese Medical Journal*, No. 2745.

Nakamura, T., Nishiyama, S., Furagolshi-Suginohara, Y., et al. (1993). Mild-to-moderate zinc-deficiency in short children: Effects of zinc supplementation on linear growth velocity. *Journal of Pediatrics*, *123*, 65–69.

Nakao, M., Nomura, S., Shimosawa, T., Yoshiuchi, K., Kumano, H., et al. (1997). Clinical effects of blood pressure biofeedback treatment on hypertension by auto-shaping. *Psychosomatic Medicine*, *59*(3), 331–338.

Namikowski, T. (1981). *The complete book of Shiatsu therapy*. Japan Publications.

National Association for Music Therapy (1997), http://www.namt.com/NAMT.html.

National Center for Homeopathy. (703) 548-7790.

National Conference on Medical and Nursing Education in Complementary Medicine. (1997, June

5–7). Blue ribbon panel preamble and recommendations. Bethesda, MD: Author.

National Institute of Nursing Research. (1994, June). National Nursing Research Agenda: Volume 6. *Symptom management: Acute Pain* (NIH Publication No. 94-2421). Bethesda, MD: National Institutes of Health, U.S. Public Health Service, U.S. Department of Health and Human Services.

National Institutes of Health. (1995). NIH Consensus Statement: Physical Activity and Cardiovascular Health. U.S. Department of Health and Human Services, Public Health Service, Bethesa, MD.

National Institutes of Health. (1996). Technology assessment panel on integration of behavioral and relaxation approaches into the treatment of chronic pain and insomnia. *Journal of the American Medical Association, 276*, 313–318.

National Institutes of Health. (1997). National Center for Complementary and Alternative Medicine [on line]. Available: http://altmed.od.nih.gov/nccam

Nebbe, L. (1995). *Nature as a guide: Nature in counseling, therapy and education* 2nd ed. Minneapolis, MN: Educational Media.

Nebeling, L. C., Forman, M. R., Graubard, B. I., & Snyder, R. A. (1997). Changes in carotenoid intake in the United States: The 1987 and 1992 National Health Interview Surveys. *Journal of the American Dietetic Association, 97*(9), 991–996.

Ness, A. R., Chee, D., & Elliott, P. (1997). Vitamin C and blood pressure—an overview. *Journal of Human Hypertenstion, 11*(6), 343–350.

Newman, M. A. (1994). *Health as expanding consciousness* (2nd ed.). New York: National League for Nursing Press.

Nichols, D. S. (1997). Balance retraining after stroke using force platform biofeedback. *Phys Ther, 77*(5), 553–558.

Nichols, M. G. (1850). *Experience in water-cure: A familiar exposition of the principles and results of water treatment in the cure of acute and chronic diseases, illustrated by numerous cases in the practice of the author; with an explanation of water-cure processes, advice on diet and regimen, and particular directions to women in the treatment of female diseases, water treatment in childbirth and the diseases of infancy.* New York: Fowler and Wells.

Nichols, P. A. (1988). *Homeopathy and the medical profession.* New York: Croom Helm.

Nieman, D. C. (1986). *The Sports Medicine Fitness Course.* Palo Alto, CA: Bull.

Nieman, D. C. (1989). Exercise and the mind. *Women's Sports and Fitness,* September, pp. 55–57.

Nilsson, N., Christensen, H. W., & Hartvigsen, J. (1997). The effect of spinal manipulation in the treatment of cervicogenic headache. *Journal Manipulative Physiol Ther, 20*(5), 326–330.

Nishino, H., Kitagawa, K., Fujiki, H., & Iwashima, A. (1986). Berberine sulfate inhibits tumor-promoting activity of teleocidin in two-stage carcinogenesis on mouse skin. *Oncology, 43*(2), 131–134.

Nishiyama, N., Moriguchi, T., & Saito, H. (1997). Beneficial effects of aged garlic extract on learning and memory impairment in the senescence-accelerated mouse. *Exp Gerontol, 32*(1–2), 149–160.

Noen-Hoeksema, S., Seligman, M. E. P., & Girgus, J. S. (1992). Predictors and consequences of childhood depressive symptoms: A 5-year longitudinal study. *Journal of Abnormal Psychology, 101*(3), 405–422.

Nogier, P. (1983). *From auriculotherapy to auriculomedicine.* Moulins-les-Metz, France: Maisonnueve.

Nogier, P., & Nogier, R. (1985). *The man in the ear.* Moulins-les-Metz, France: Maisonnueve.

Nordenström, B. E. W. (1983). *Biologically Closed Electric Circuits: Clinical, Experimental and Theoretical Evidence for an Additional Circulatory System.* Stockholm: Nordic Medical Publications.

Nordenström, B., Näslund, I., Nordenström, J., & Wersäll, P. (1994). Proceeding of the IABC International Association for Biologically Closed Electric Circuits (BCEC) in Medicine and Biology. *The European Journal of Surgery* supplement 574.

Nordfors, M., & Hartvig, P. (1997). St. John's wort against depression in favour again. *Lakartidningen, 94*(25), 2365–2367.

Noreau, L., Martineau, H., Roy, L., & Belzile, M. (1995). Effects of a modified dance-based exercise on cardiorespiratory fitness, psychological state and health status of persons with rheumatoid arthritis. *Am Journal Phys Med Rehabil,* *74*(1), 19–27.

Nuckolls, C. H., Cassel, J., & Kaplan, B. H. (1972). Psychosocial assets, life crisis, and the prognosis of pregnancy. *American Journal of Epidemiology, 95,* 431–441.

Nygard, O., Refsum, H., Ueland, P. M., et al. (1997). Coffee consumption and plasma total homocysteine: The Hordaland Homocysteine Study. *American Journal of Clinical Nutrition, 65*(1), 136–143.

O'Connor & Bensky. *Acupunture—A comprehensive text.*

O'Connor, B. B. (1995). *Healing traditions: Alternative medicine and the health professions.* Philadelphia: University of Pennsylvania Press.

O'Connor, P. J., Bryant, C. X., Veltri, J. P., & Gebhardt, S. M. (1993). State anxiety and ambulatory blood pressure following resistance exercise in females. *Med Sci Sports Exerc, 25*(4), 516–521.

O'Dell, N. E., & Cook, P. A. (1997). *Stopping hyperactivity, A New Solution.* Garden City Park, NY: Avery Publishing.

O'Leary, A., Shoor, S., Kate, L., & Holman, H. R. (1988). A cognitive-behavioral treatment for rheumatoid arthritis. *Health Psychology, 7*(6), 527–544.

Oakley, L. D. (1994, Fall). Striving for 'Sugar 'n Spice' may produce depression in some women. *Nursing Dimension,* p. 5.

Odeh, M. (1992). The role of zinc in acquired immunodeficiency syndrome. *Journal Int Med, 231,* 463–469.

Ody, P. (1993). *The complete medicinal herbal.* London: Dorling Kindersley.

Ody, P. l. (1993). *Herbal first aid. The Complete Medicinal Herbal.* New York: Dorling Kindersley.

Ohashi, W. (1976). *Do it yourself Shiatsu.* New York: Penguin.

Okun, B. F. (1987). *Effective helping: Interviewing and counseling techniques.* Monterey, CA: Brooks/Cole.

Oleson, T. (1996). *Auriculotherapy manual* 2nd edition. Los Angeles, CA: Health Care Alternatives.

Oleson, T., & Flocco, W. (1993). Randomized controlled study of premenstrual symptoms treated with ear, hand and foot reflexology. *Obstet Gynecol, 82*(6), 906–911.

Oleson, T., Kroening, R., & Bresler, D. (1980). An experimental evaluation of auricular diagnosis: The somatic mapping of musculoskeletal pain at ear acupuncture points. *Pain, 8,* 217–229.

Olmsted, L., Schrauzer, G. N., Flores-Arce, M., & Dowd, J. (1989). Selenium supplementation of symptomatic human immunodeficiency virus infected patients. *Biological Trace Element Research, 25,* 89–96.

Olson, M., Sneed, N., LaVia, M., Virella, G., Bonadonna, R., & Michel, Y. (1997). Stress-Induced Immunosuppression and Therapeutic Touch. *Alternative Therapies in Health and Medicine,* March, *3*(2), 68–73.

Olszewski, W. L. (1985). *Peripheral lymph: Formation and immune function.* Boca Raton, FL: CRC Press, Inc.

Orekhov, A. N., & Grunwald, J. (1997). Effects of garlic on atherosclerosis. *Nutrition, 13*(7–8), 656–663.

Ornstein, R., & Sobel, D. (1988). *The healing brain.* New York: Simon & Schuster.

Ornstein, R., & Sobel, D. (1989). *Healthy pleasures.* Reading, MA: Addison-Wesley.

Osawa, K. (1996, September 16). Eucalyptus extract may prevent cavities. *Press Digest.*

Osborn, A. (1998). The regional distribution of alternative health care. In R. J. Gordon, B. C. Nienstedt, & W. M. Gesler (Eds.), *Alternative therapies: Expanding options in health care* (pp. 105–116). New York: Springer Publishing Company.

Ostrom, B. (1997). Esalen massage: Bodywork with a place in history. *Massage Magazine, 66,* 29.

Ouimette, P. C., Finney, J. W., & Moose, R. H. (1997). Twelve-step and cognitive-behavioral treatment for substance abuse: A comparison of treatment effectiveness. *Journal of Consulting and Clinical Psychology, 65,* 230–240.

Ouseley, S. G. J. (1949). *Colour meditations: A course of instructions and exercises in developing colour consciousness.* Essex, England: L. N. Fowler & Co.

Overgaard, J., Gonzalez, D. G., Hulshof, M. C. C. M., Arcangeli, G., Dahl, O., Mella, O., & Bentzen, S. M. (1996). Hyperthermia as an adjuvant to radiation therapy of recurrent or metastatic malignant melanoma: A multicentre randomized trial by the European Society for Hyperthermic Oncology. *International Journal Hyperthermia, 12,* 3–20.

Overholser, L. C., & Moody, R. A. (1988). Lymphatic massage and recent scientific discoveries. *Massage Therapy Journal, 27*(3), 55–58.

Owen, M. D. (1971). Insect venoms: Identification of dopamine and noradrenaline in wasp and bee stings. *Experiencia, 27,* 544–546.

Oz, M. C., Lemole, E. J., Oz, L. L, Whitworth, G. C., & Lemole, M. (1996). Treating CAD with cardiac surgery combined with complementary therapy. *Medscapes Women's Health, 1*(10), 2–17.

Palevitch, D., & Craker, L. E. (1995). Nutritional and medical importance of red pepper (Capsicum ssp.). *Journal Herbs, Spices and Medicinal Plants, 3*(2), 67–70.

Panizzi, L., Flamini, G., Cioni, P. L., & Morelli, I. (1993). Composition and antimicrobial properties of essential oils of four Mediterranean Lamiaceae. *Journal of Ethnopharmacology, 39*(3), 167–170.

Panjwani, U., Selvamurthy, W., Singh, S. H., et al. (1996). Effect of Sahaja yoga practice on seizure control and EEG changes in patients with epilepsy. *Indian Journal Med Res, 103,* 165–172.

Panos, M. B., & Heimlich, J. (1980). *Homeopathic medicine at home.* J. P. Tarcher/Putnam, New York.

Papadopulos-Eleopulos, E. (1988). Reappraisal of AIDS—is the oxidation induced by the risk factors the primary cause? *Medical Hypothesis, 25,* 151–162.

Papageorgiou, A. C., Macfarlane, G. J., Thomas, E., Croft, P. R., Jayson, M. I., & Silman, A. J. (1997). Psychosocial factors in the workplace—do they predict new episodes of low back pain? Evidence from the South Manchester Back Pain Study. *Spine, 22*(10), 1137–1142.

Papapanou, P. N. (1996). Periodontal diseases: Epidemiology. *Annals of Periodontology, 1*(1), 1–36.

Parish, E. S. (1997). Folate and neural tube birth defects. *Medical Bulletin, 27*(1), 4.

Parivar, F., Low, R. K., & Stoller, M. L. (1996). The influence of diet on urinary stone disease. *Journal of Urol, 155*(2), 432–440.

Partinen, M. (1997). Sleep disorder related to Parkinson's disease. *Journal of Neurology, 244*(Suppl. 1), S3–S6.

Pasche, B., Erman, M., Hayduk, R., et al. (1996). Effects of low energy emission therapy in chronic psychophysiological insomnia. *Sleep, 19*(4), 327–336.

Pascual-Leone, A., et al. (1996). Rapid-rate transcranial magnetic stimulation of left dorsolateral prefrontal cortex in drug-resistant depression. *Lancet, 348,* 233–237.

Patankar, S. K., Ferrara, A., Levy, J. R., et al. (1997). Biofeedback in colorectal practice: A multicenter, statewide, three-year experience. *Disease of the Colon and Rectum, 40*(7), 827–831.

Patten, C. A., Gillin, J. C., Farkas, A. J., et al. (1997). Depressive symptoms in California adolescents: Family structure and parental support. *Journal of Adolescent Health, 20*(4), 271–278.

Pauletto, P., Puato, M., Angeli, M. T., et al. (1996). Blood pressure, serum lipids, and fatty acids in populations on a lake-fish diet or on a vegetarian diet in Tanzania. *Lipids, 31,* S309–S312.

Pauling, L. (1968). Orthomolecular psychiatry. *Science, 160,* 265–271.

Payer, J. (1988). *Medicine and culture.* New York: Penguin.

Payne, H. (Ed.). (1992). *Dance/movement therapy: Theory and practice.* London and New York: Tavistock/Routledge.

Pellegrino, M. J., Van Fossen, D., Gordon, C., Ryan, J. M., & Waylonis, G. W. (1989). Prevalence of mitral valve prolapse in primary fibromyalgia: A pilot investigation. *Archives of Physical Medical Rehabilitation, 70,* 541–543.

Pennebaker, J. W. (1989). Confession, inhibition, and disease. In L. Berkowitz (Ed.), *Advances in experimental social psychology* (Vol. 22, pp. 211–244). New York: Academic Press.

Pennebaker, J. W., & Beall, S. K. (1986). Confronting a traumatic event: Toward an understanding of inhibition and disease. *Journal of Abnormal Psychology, 95,* 274–281.

Pennebaker, J. W., & O'Heeron, R. (1984). Confiding in others and illness rates among spouses of suicide and accidental-death victims. *Journal of Abnormal Psychology, 93,* 473–476.

Pennebaker, J. W., Kiecolt-Glaser, J. K., & Glaser, R. (1988). Disclosure of traumas and immune function: Health implications for psychotherapy. *Journal of Clinical and Consulting Psychology*, *63*, 787–792.

Pereira, M. A., Grubbs, C. J., Barnes, L. H., et al. (1996). Effects of phytochemicals, curcumin and quercetin, upon azoxymethane-induced colon cancer and 7,12-dimethylbenz(a)anthracene-induced mammary cancer in rats. *Carcinogenesis*, *17*(6), 1305–1311.

Peretz, A., Neve, J., & Famaey, J. (1991). Selenium in rheumatic diseases. *Seminars in Arthritis and Rheumatism*, *20*, 305–316.

Periquet, B. A., Jammes, N. M., Lambert, W. E., et al. (1995). Micronutrient levels in HIV-1-infected children. *AIDS*, *9*(8), 887–893.

Perlman, S. G., Connell, K. J., Clark, A., et al. (1990). Dance-based aerobic exercise for rheumatoid arthritis. *Arthritis Care Research*, *3*(1), 29–35.

Perls, F. *In and out the garbage pail*.

Perrig, W. J., Perrig, P., & Stahelin, H. B. (1997). The relation between antioxidants and memory performance in the old and very old. *Journal of the American Geriatrics Society*, *45*(6), 718–724.

Perrone, B., Stockel, H. H., & Krueger, V. (1989). *Medicine women, curanderas, and women doctors*. Norman, OK: University of Oklahoma Press.

Pert, C. (1997). *Molecules of Emotion why you feel the way you feel*. New York: Scribner.

Petajan, J. H., Gappmaier, E., White, A. T., et al. (1996). Impact of aerobic training on fitness and quality of life in multiple sclerosis. *Ann Neurol*, *39*(4), 432–441.

Peters, E. M., Goetzsche, J. M., Grobbelaar, B., & Noakes, T. D. (1993). Vitamin C supplementation reduces the incidence of postrace symptoms of upper-respiratory-tract infection in ultramarathon runners. *American Journal of Clinical Nutrition*, *57*, 170–174.

Peters, J. M., Preston-Martin, S., London, S. J., Bowman, J. D., Buckley, J. D., & Thomas, D. C. (1994). Processed meats and risk of childhood leukemia. *Cancer Causes Control*, *5*(2), 195–202.

Peterson, G., & Mehl, L. (1981). *Pregnancy as healing*. Berkeley, CA: Mindbody Press.

Petitto, J. M. (1997). UF researchers: Stress can hasten progression of HIV. Press Release, University of Florida, August 7th., Fax: (352) 392-9220.

Petrie, K. J., Booth, R. J., Pennebaker, J. W., Davison, K. P., & Thomas, M. (1995). Disclosure of trauma and immune response to Hepatitis B vaccination program. *Journal of Consulting and Clinical Psychology*, *63*, 787–792.

Pettegrew, J. W., Klunk, W. E., Panchalingam, K., et al. (1995). Clinical and neurochemical effects of acetyl-L-carnitine in Alzheimer's disease. *Neurobiology of Aging*, *16*(1), 1–4.

Pezzuto, J. (1994). Science says mom was right: Eat vegetables and fruit. *UIC News Tips*. The University of Illinois at Chicago, Office of Public Affairs, 601 South Morgan Street, Chicago, IL 60607-7126.

Phytochemicals for cancer protection. (1995). *American Institute for Cancer Research Newsletter*, *46*, 11.

Piaget, J. (1963). *The child's conception of the world*. Totowa, NJ: Littlefield, Adams & Co.

Picozzi, M. (1996, March). A retail buyer's guide to supplements: Understanding what to expect from different sales channels can streamline buying and increase customer services. *Natural Foods Merchandiser*, *17*(3), 120.

Pienta, K. J., Naik, H., Alchtar, A., et al. (1995). Inhibition of spontaneous metastasis in rat prostate cancer model by oral administration of modified citrus pectin. *Journal of the National Cancer Institute*, *87*(5), 348–353.

Pierce, E. F., & Pate, D. W., (1994). Mood alterations in older adults following acute exercise. *Perceptual Motor Skills*, *79*(1), 191–194.

Pierson, H. (1994). Designer Foods III: Phytochemicals in Garlic, Soy, and Licorice: Research Update and Implications. Conference Proceedings, May 23–25, 1994, Cook College, Rutgers, the State University, New Brunswick, NJ.

Pierson, H. (1994). Role of licorice extract in human disease and prevention. *Designer Foods III Proceedings* Cook College, Rutgers University, New Brunswick, NJ.

Pikalov, A. A., & Kharin, V. V. (1994). Use of spinal manipulative therapy in the treatment of duodenal ulcer. *Journal Manipulative Physiol Ther*, *17*, 310–313.

Pilla, A. A. (1993). State of the art in electromagnetic therapeutics. In M. Blank (Ed.), *Electricity and magnetism in biology and medicine.* San Francisco: San Francisco Press Inc.

Pincomb, G. A., Lovallo, W. R., McKey, R. N., et al. (1996). Acute blood pressure elevations with caffeine in men with borderline systemic hypertension. *American Journal of Cardiology, 77,* 270–274.

Pinto, J. T., Qiao, C., Xing, J., et al. (1997). Effects of garlic thioallyl derivatives on growth, glutathione concentration, and polyamine formation of human prostate carcinoma cells in culture. *American Journal of Clinical Nutrition, 66*(2), 398–405.

Pizzorno, J. E., Jr. (1996). *Total wellness.* Rocklin, CA: Prima Publishing.

Pizzorno, J. E., Jr., & Murray, M. T. (1990). *The encyclopedia of natural medicine.* Rocklin, CA: Prima Publishing.

Pizzorno, J. E., Jr., & Murray, M. T. (1996). *A textbook of natural medicine* vol 1 & 2. Bastyr University Publications, Bothell, WA.

Plotkin, M. (1993). *Tales of a shaman's apprentice: An ethnobotanist searches for new medicines in the Amazon rainforest.* New York: Viking.

The Politics of Alternative Medicine. Plenary Session of the Third Annual International Congress of Alternative and Complementary Therapies, September 7, 1997, Foundation for the Advancement of Innovative Medicine, Suffern, New York, 1997.

Polivy, J., & Herman, C. P. (1992). Undieting: A program to help people stop dieting. *International Journal of Eating Disorders, 11,* 261–268.

Pompei, R., Flore, O., Marccialis, M. A., et al. (1979). Glycyrrhizic acid inhibits virus growth and inactivates virus particles. *Nature, 281*(5733), 689–690.

Pool-Zobel, B. L., Bub, A., Muller, H., et al. (1997). Consumption of vegetables reduces genetic damage in humans: First results of a human intervention trial with carotenoid-rich foods. *Carcinogenesis, 18*(9), 1847–1850.

Popov, I., Blumstein, A., & Lewin, G. (1994). Antioxidant effects of aqueous garlic extract. Direct detection using the photo-chemiluminescence. *Arzheim Forsch, 44,* 602–604.

Porkert. *Chinese medicine.*

Potter, J. D. (1996). Nutrition and colorectal cancer. *Cancer Causes and Control, 7*(1), 127–146.

Powers, P. S., Tyson, I. B., Stevens, B. A., & Heal, A. V. (1995). Total body potassium and serum potassium among eating disorder patients. *International Journal of Eating Disorders, 18*(3), 269–276.

Powers, W. (1993). *Yuwipi.* Lincoln: University of Nebraska Press.

Prasad, A. (1993). Essentiality and toxicity of zinc. *Sc Journal Work E, 19*(Suppl.), 134–136.

Preuss, H. G. (1997). Effects of glucose/insulin perturbations on aging and chronic disorders of aging: The evidence. *Journal of the American College of Nutrition, 16*(5), 397–403.

Price, S., & Price, L. (1995). *Aromatherapy for Health Professionals.* London: Churchill Livingstone, 298.

Principles of physiology. (1990). St. Louis: C.V. Mosby.

Propst, L. R., Ostrom, R., Watkins, P., Dean, T., & Mashburn, D. (1992). Comparative efficacy of religious and nonreligious cognitive-behavioral therapy for the treatment of clinical depression in religious individuals. *Journal of Consulting and Clinical Psychology, 60,* 94–103.

Province, M. A., Hadley, E. C., Hornbrook, M. C., et al. (1995). The effects of exercise on falls in elderly patients. A preplanned meta-analysis of the FICSIT Trials. Frailty and Injuries: Cooperative Studies of Intervention Techniques. *Journal of the American Medical Association, 273*(17), 1341–1347.

Prudden, B. (1980). *Pain erasure the Bonnie Prudden way.* New York: Ballantine.

Prudden, B. (1985). *Myotherapy, Bonnie Prudden's complete guide to pain-free living.* New York: Ballantine.

Pub. L. No. 103-417, 108 *Stat.* 4325, 21 *U.S.C.* §§ 301 et seq. (1994).

Puntila, E., Roger, H., Lakka, T., et al. (1997). Physical activity in adolescence and bone density in peri- and postmenopausal women: A population-based study. *Bone, 21*(4), 363–367.

Purpura, M., & Henry, M. (1997). Stress and bowel pain. Hippocrates (October), 5.

Quang, S. X. (1985). *Applied Chinese acupuncture for clinical practitioners.* Jinan, China: Shandong Science and Technology Press.

Quicksilver Associates. (1994, 1996). *The mercury in your mouth: The truth about "silver" dental fillings.* New York: Quicksilver Press.

Quinn, J. (1992). Holding sacred space: The nurse as healing environment. *Holistic Nursing Practice, 6*(4), 26–36.

Quinn, J. F. (1982). The effects of Therapeutic Touch done without physical contact on state anxiety of hospitalized cardiovascular patients. *Dissertation Abstracts International, 43, 1797B. (University Microfilms No. 8226788)*

Quinn, J., & Strelkauskas, A. J. (1993). Psychoimmunologic effects of therapeutic touch on practitioners and recently bereaved recipients: A pilot study. *Advances in Nursing Science, 25*(4), 13–26.

Racagni, G., Brunello, N., & Paoletti, R. (1986). Neuromediator changes during cerebral aging. The effect of ginkgo biloba extract. *Presse Med, 15*(31), 1488–1490.

Rademacher, W. (1991). *Lay ministry: A theological, spiritual & pastoral handbook* (p. 274). New York: Crossroad.

Raglin, J. S., Turner, P. E., & Eksten, F. (1993). State anxiety and blood pressure following 30 minutes of leg ergometry or weight training. *Med Sci Sports Exerc, 25*(9), 1044–1048.

Ragneskog, H., Brane, G., Karlsson, I., & Kihlgren, M. (1996). Influence of dinner music on food intake and symptoms common in dementia. *Scand Journal Caring Sci, 10*(1), 11–17.

Ragneskog, H., Kihlgren, M., Karlsson, I., & Norberg, A. (1996). Dinner music for demented patients: Analysis of video-recorded observations. *Clinical Nursing Research, 5*(3), 262–277.

Rahman, M. M., Mahalanabis, D., Alvarez, J. O., Wahed, M. A., Islam, M. A., Habte, D., & Khaled, M. A. (1996). Acute respiratory infections prevent improvment of vitamin A status in young infants supplemented with vitamin A. *Journal of Nutrition, 126*(3), 628–633.

Ramanoelina, A. R., Terrom, G. P., Bianchini, J. P., & Coulanges, P. (1987). Antibacterial action of essential oils extracted from Madagascar plants. *Archives of the Institute of Pasteur Madagascar, 53*(1), 217–226.

Ramodan, N. M., Halvorson, H., & Vonde-Linde, A. (1989). Low brain magnesium in migraine. *Headache, 29*, 590–593.

Ramsey, P. W. (1992). The effect of community support groups on psychosocial adjustment, uncertainty, and hopelessness in persons infected with HIV. *SEARC? Improved Nursing Care Through Research, 15*, 6.

Ramsey, T. (1992). *Baby's First Massage* Program, Dayton, OH: Self Published.

Randolf, N. (1993). Addiction disorders. *American Review for Psychiatric and Mental Health Nursing Certification.* Springhouse, PA: Springhouse Corporation, p. 81.

Randolph, L., Seidman, B., & Pasko, T. (1996). *Physician Characteristics and Distribution in the U.S..* Chicago: American Medical Association.

Rangavajhyala, N., Shahani, K. M., Sridevi, G., & Srikumaran, S. (1997). Nonlipopolysaccharide components of Lactobacillus acid-ophilus stimulates the production of interleukin-1 alpha and tumor necrosis factor-alpha by murine macrophages. *Nutrition in Cancer, 28*(2), 130–134.

Rapkin, D. A., Straubing, M., & Holroyd, J. C. (1991). Guided imagery, hypnosis and recovery from head and neck cancer surgery: An exploratory study. *International Journal of Clinical and Experimental Hypnosis, 39*(4), 215–226.

Rapoport, A. M., et al. (1985). Analgesic-rebound headache: Theoretical and practical implications. *Cephalgia, 5*(Suppl. 3), 448–449.

Rattan, V., Thind, S. K., Jethi, R. K., & Nath, R. (1993). Intestinal absorption of calcium and oxalate in magnesium-deficient rats. *Magnesium Research, 6*(1), 3–10.

Ray, B. (1983). *The Reiki factor.* St. Petersburg, FL: Radiance Associates.

Reaven, P., Grasse, B., & Barnett, J. (1996). Effect of antioxidants alone and in combination with monounsaturated fatty acid-enriched diets on lipoprotein oxidation. *Arteriosclerosis, Thrombosis and Vascular Biology, 16*(12), 1465–1472.

Recker, R. R. (1985). Calcium absorption and achlorhydria. *New England Journal of Medicine, 313*, 70–74.

Redd, W. H. (1994). Behavioral interventions for cancer treatment side effects. *Acta Oncologica, 33*, 113–117.

Redwood, D. (1996). Chiropractic. In M. Micozzi (Ed.), *Fundamentals of complementary and alternative medicine* (pp. 91–110). New York: Churchill Livingstone.

Reed, J. C. (1996). Review of acute and chronic pain published studies. *Journal of Alternative and Complementary Medicine, 2*(1), 129–144.

Reid, M., & Hammersley, R. (1995). Effects of carbohydrate intake on subsequent food intake and mood state. *Physiology and Behavior, 58,* 421–427.

Reilly, D. T., Taylor, M. A., et al. (1986). Is homeopathy a placebo response? Controlled trial of homeopathic potency, with pollen in hayfever as model. *Lancet, 2*(8512), 881–886.

Reilly, D. T., Taylor, M. A., et al. (1994). Is evidence for homeopathy reproducible? *Lancet, 344,* 1601–1606.

Rein, G., Atkinson, M., & McCraty, R. (1995). The physiological and psychological effects of compassion and anger. *Journal of Advancement in Medicine, 8*(2), 87–103.

Reis, E., Goepp, J., Katz, S., & Santosham, M. (1994). Barriers to use of oral rehydration therapy. *Pediatrics, 93,* 708–711.

Reis, J. G. (1995, June 26). A Parkinson's primer. *Nursing Spectrum,* 12–14.

Reiser, S. S. (1997). The Alexander technique: Stress reduction and optimal psychophysical functioning. Oral presentation: Sixth International Montreux Congress on Stress. Bon Port, Switzerland. Reprinted in *The Alexander Technique Published Research.* North American Society of Teachers of the Alexander Technique.

Rejeski, W. J., Thompson, A., Brubaker, P. H., & Miller, H. S. (1992). Acute exercise: Buffering psychosocial stress responses in women. *Health Psychology, 11*(6), 355–362.

Remen, R. N. (1989). The search for healing. In R. Carlson & B. Shield (Eds.), *Healers on healing* (pp. 91–98). Los Angeles: Jeremy P. Tarcher.

Ren, S., & Lien, E. J. (1997). *Natural products and their derivatives as cancer chemopreventive agents.* Progress in Drug Research Volume 48. E. Jucker (Ed.). Basel, Switzerland: Birkhauser Verlag, pp. 147–170.

Report of the US Preventive Services Task Force. (1996). *Guide To Clinical Preventive Services* (2nd. ed). Baltimore: Williams & Wilkins.

Revillard, J. P., Vincent, C. M. A., Favier, A. E., et al. (1992). Lipid peroxidation in human immunodeficiency virus infection. *Journal Acquired Immunodeficiency Syndrome, 5,* 637–638.

Rhiner, M., Ferrell, B. R., Ferrell, B. A., & Grant, M. M. (1993). A structured nondrug intervention program for cancer pain. *Cancer Practice, 1,* 137–143.

Rhodes, J., Zheng, B., & Lifely, M. R. (1992). Inhibition of specific T-cell activation by monosaccharides is through their reactivity as aldehydes. *Immunology, 75*(4), 626–631.

Ricchini, W. (1997, January). Zinc helps resolve cold symptoms. *Advance for Nse Pract, 10.*

Rice, R. (1977). Neurophysiological development in premature infants following stimulation. *Developmental Psychology, 13*(1), 69–76.

Richards, P. S., & Potts, R. W. (1995). Using spiritual interventions in psychotherapy: Practices, successes, failures, and ethical concerns of Mormon psychotherapists. *Professional Psychology: Research and Practice, 26,* 163–170.

Richardson, M. A., et al. (1997). Coping, life attitudes, and immune responses to imagery and group support after breast cancer treatment. *Alternative Therapies, 3*(5), 62.

Richardson, N. (1987). Aston-Patterning. *Physical Therapy Forum, 6*(43), 1, 3.

Richer, S. (1996). Multicenter ophthalmic and nutritional age-related macular degneration study: 2. Antioxidant intervention and conclusions. *Journal of the American Optometric Association, 67*(1), 30–49.

Riddle, D. (1989). Psychosocial support groups for people with HIV infection and AIDS. *Holistic Nurse Practitioner, 3,* 52–62.

Rieger, N. A., Wattchow, D. A., Sarre, R. G., et al. (1997). Prospective trial of pelvic floor retraining in patients with fecal incontinence. *Dis Colon Rectum, 40*(7), 821–826.

Riehl, J., & Roy, C. (1990). *Conceptual models for nursing practice.* Norwalk, CT: Appleton-Century-Crofts.

Riggs, D. R., DeHaven, J. I., & Lamm, D. L. (1997). Allium sativum (garlic) treatment for murine transitional cell carcinoma. *Cancer, 79*(10), 1987–1994.

Rime, B. (1995, September). Social sharing of emotional experiences. Paper presented at the Metroplex mini-conference of social psychology, Dallas, Texas.

Rimm, E. B., Stampfer, M. J., Ascherio, A., et al. (1996). Vitamin E consumption and the risk of coronary heart disease in men. *Journal of the American Medical Association, 275*(6), 447–45l.

Risch, H. A., Jain, M., Marrett, L. D., et al. (1994). Dietary fat intake and risk of epithelial ovarian cancer. *Journal of the National Cancer Institute*, *86*, 1409–1415.

Riskind, J. H., Wheeler, D. J., & Picerno, M. R. (1997). Using mental imagery with subclinical OCD to "freeze" contamination in place: Evidence for looming vulnerability theory. *Behav Res Ther*, *35*(8), 757–768.

Risse, G., Numbers, R., & Leavitt, J. (Eds.). (1977). *Medicine without doctors. Home health care in American history*. New York: Science History Publications.

Robbins, J. (1987). *Diet for a New America: How Your Food Choices Affect your Health, Happiness, and the Future of Life on Earth*. Walpole, NJ: Stillpoint Publishing.

Robbins, P. R., & Tanck, R. H. (1997). Anger and depressed affect: Interindividual and intraindividual perspectives. *Journal Psychol*, *131*(5), 489–500.

Robin, A. L., Siegel, P. T., & Moye, A. (1995). Family versus individual therapy for anorexia: Impact on family conflict. *International Journal of Eating Disorders*, *17*(4), 313–322.

Robinson, L. S. (1995). *The Effects of Therapeutic Touch on the Grief Experience*. (Doctoral dissertation, University of Alabama at Birmingham.) Available from University microfilms.

Rock, C. L., & Vasantharajan, S. (1995). Vitamin status of eating disorder patients: Relationship to clinical indices and effect of treatment. *International Journal of Eating Disorders*, *18*(3), 257–262.

Rock, C. L., Dechert, R. E., Khilnani, R., et al. (1997). Carotenoids and antioxidant vitamins in patients after burn injury. *Journal Burn Care Rehabil*, *18*(3), 269–278.

Rodin, J. (1986). Aging and health: Effects of the sense of control. *Science*, *233*, 1271–1276.

Rodriguez, C. M., & Green, A. J. (1997). Parenting stress and anger expression as predictors of child abuse potential. *Child Abuse and Neglect*, *21*(4), 367–377.

Rodriguez, N., Ryan, S. W., Vande Kemp, H., & Foy, D. W. (1997). Posttraumatic stress disorder in adult female survivors of childhood sexual abuse: A comparison study. *Journal of Consulting and Clinical Psychology*, *65*(1), 53–59.

Rogers, M. E. (1970). *An introduction to the theoretical basis of nursing*. Philadelphia: F. A. Davis.

Rolf, I. (1977). *Rolfing: The integration of human structures*. New York: Harper and Row Publishers.

Rolf, I. (1978). *Rolfing and physical reality*. Healing Arts Press.

Romans, S. E., Martin, J. L., & Morris, E. M. (1997). Risk factors for adolescent pregnancy: How important is child sexual abuse? *New Zealand Medical Journal*, *110*(1037), 30–33.

Rooks, D. S., Kiel, D. P., Parsons, C., & Hayes, W. C. (1997). Self-paced resistance training and walking exercise in community-dwelling older adults: Effects on neuromotor performance. *Journal Gerontol A Biol Sci Med Sci*, *52*(3), M161–M168.

Rosal, M. C., Ockene, I. S., Ockene, J. K., et al. (1997). A longitudinal study of students' depression at one medical school. *Academic Medicine*, *72*(6), 542–546.

Rosch, P. J. (1988). Electromagnetic waves and neurobehavioral function: Comments from clinical medicine. In M. E. O'Connor & R. H. Lovely (Eds.), *Electromagnetic fields and neurobehavioral function*. New York: Alan R. Liss.

Rosch, P. J. (1994). Stress and Subtle Energy Medicine. *Stress Medicine*, *10*, 1–3.

Rosch, P. J. (1998). In Nordenström B. E. W., *Exploring BCEC-systems*, 98–112. Stockholm: Nordic Medical Publications.

Rosenfeld, J. P., Cha, G., Blair, T., & Gotlib, I. H. (1995). Operant (biofeedback) control of left-right frontal alpha power differences: Potential neurotherapy for affective disorders. *Biofeedback Self Regul*, *20*(3), 241–258.

Rosengren, A., & Wilhelmsen, L. (1997). Physical activity protects against coronary death and deaths from all causes in middle-aged men. Evidence from a 20-year follow-up of the primary prevention study in Goetborg. *Ann Epidemiol*, *7*(1), 69–75.

Rosenstein, D. L., Elin, R. J., Hosseini, J. M., et al. (1994). Magnesium measures across the menstrual cycle in premenstrual syndrome. *Biological Psychiatry*, *35*(8), 557–561.

Ross, J. (1983). Traditional Chinese medicine and gynecology, part 2. *Journal of Chinese Medicine*, *12*, 8–19.

Ross, M. F. (1996, November 12). Heart patients who exercise have lower levels of harmful hormones. Press Release, University of Florida Health Science Center, Gainesville.

Ross, M. F. (1996). UF researchers describe link between chronic pain and depression. Health Sciences Center Communications. University of Florida, Gainesville, 32610-0253.

Ross, M. F. (1997). UF researchers hope to shed light on questions brewing over caffeine consumption. Press release, the University of Florida, Gainesville, August 28, (352) 392-2621.

Ross, M. L. (1997). UF Researchers study link between emotions, heart disease. *Vital Signs*, January 7, p. 14.

Rossbach, S. (1983). *Feng Shui: The Chinese art of placement*. New York: E. P. Dutton.

Rossbach, S., & Yun, L. (1994). *Living color: Master Lin Yun's guide to Feng Shui and the art of color*. New York: Kodansha International.

Rossbach. (1987). *Interior design with Feng Shui* (with Lin Yun). New York: E. P. Dutton.

Rossbach. (1994). *Living Color* (Master Lin Yun's Guide to Feng Shui and the Art of Color). Kodansha International.

Rossi, E. L. (1992). *The psychobiology of mind-body healing: New concepts of therapeutic hypnosis*. New York: W. W. Norton & Company, Inc.

Rossi, E. *Mind Body Therapy*. New York: W. W. Norton and Company.

Rossman, M. L. (1989). *Healing yourself, A step-by-step program for better health through imagery*. New York: Pocket Books.

Rowe, J. W., & Kahn, R. L. (1987). Human aging: Usual and successful. *Science, 237*, 143–149.

Rowe, K. S., & Rowe, K. J. (19994). Synthetic food coloring and behavior: a dose response effect in a double-blind, placebo-controlled, repeated-measures study. *Journal Pediatr, 125*(5), 691–698.

Rozen, F., Yang, X. F., Huynh, H., & Pollak, M. K. (1997). Antiproliferative action of vitamin D-related compounds and insulin-like growth factor-binding protein 5 accumulation. *Journal of the National Cancer Institute, 89*, 652–656.

Rubenfeld, I. (1992). Gestalt Therapy and the Bodymind: An Overview of the Rubenfeld Synergy™ Method. In Nevins (Ed.), *Gestalt Therapy: Perspectives and Applications*. New York: Gardner Press, 147–177.

Ruff, A., Kavanaugh-McHugh, E., Perlman, E., Hutton, N., Modlin, J., & Rowe, S. (1991). Selenium deficiency and cardiomyopathy in acquired immunodeficiency syndrome. *Journal Parenteral Enteral Nutrition, 15*, 347–349.

Rush, D., Wilson, P. lW. & Jacques, P. (1996). Relation of dietary intake and serum levels of vitamin D to progression of osteoarthritis of the knee among participants in the Framingham Study. *Annals of Internal Medicine, 125*(5), 353–359.

Rushford, N., & Ostermeyer, A. (1997). Body image disturbances and their change with video-feedback in anorexia nervosa. *Behav Res Ther, 35*(5), 389–398.

Rusk, T., & Read, R. (1984). *I want to change but I don't know how!* Los Angeles, CA: Price/Stern/Sloan.

Russell, C. (1993). *The master trend: How the baby boom generation is remaking America*. New York: Plenum Press.

Sabate, J., Fraser, G. E., Burke, K., et al. (1993). Effects of walnuts on serum lipid levels and blood pressure in normal men. *New England Journal of Medicine, 328*(9), 603–607.

Sabo, C. E., & Michael, S. R. (1996). The influence of personal message with music on anxiety and side effects associated with chemotherapy. *Cancer Nursing, 19*(4), 283–289.

Sacks, F. M., Hebert, P., Appel, L. J., et al. (1994). The effect of fish oil on blood pressure and high-density lipoprotein-cholesterol levels in phase I of the Trials of Hypertension Prevention. *Journal Hypertension, 12*(Suppl. 7), S23–S31.

Sahakian, V., Rouse, D., Sipes, S., Rose, N., & Niebyl, J. (1991). Vitamin B6 is effective therapy for nausea and vomiting of pregnancy: A randomized, double-blind placebo-controlled study. *Obstetrics and Gynecology, 78*(1), 33–36.

Sakagami, H., Satoh, K., Makino, Y., et al. (1997). Effect of alpha-tocopherol on cytotoxicty induced by UV irradiation and antioxidants. *Anticancer Research, 17*(3C), 2079–2082.

Sakai, M. (1996). A clinical study of autogenic training-based behavioral treatment for panic disorder. *Pukuoka Igaku Zasshi, 87*(3), 77–84.

Sale, D. M. (1995). *Overview of Legislative Developments Concerning Alternative Health Care in the United States* (John E. Fetzer Institute).

Salmeron, J., Manson, J. E., Stampfer, M. J., et al. (1997). Dietary fiber, glycemic load, and risk of non-insulin-dependent diabetes mellitus in women. *Journal of the American Medical Association, 277*(6), 472–477.

Salonen, J., Salonen, R., Seppanen, K., et al. (1991). Effects of antioxidant supplementation on platelet function: A randomized pair-matched, placebo-controlled, double-blind trial in men with low antioxidant status. *American Journal of Clinical Nutrition, 53*, 1222–1229.

Salvati, G., Genovesi, G., Marcellini, L., et al. (1996). Effects of *Panax ginseng C.A. Meyer* saponins on male fertility. *Panminerva Med, 38*(4), 249–254.

Samarel, N. (1992). The experience of receiving Therapeutic Touch. *Journal of Advanced Nursing, 17*(6), 651–657.

Samborski, W., Stratz, T., Schochat, T., Mennet, P., & Muller, W. (1996, May-June). Biochemical changes in fibromyalgia. *Z Rheumatology, 55*(3), 168–173.

Sanchez, V. C., Lewinsohn, P. M., & Larson, D. W. (1980). Assertion training: Effectiveness in the treatment of depression. *J Clin Psychol, 36*(2), 526–529.

Sandstead, H. (1991). Zinc deficiency: A public health problem? *Am Journal Dis Ch, 145*, 853–959.

Sandstead, H. H. (1995). Requirements and toxicity of essential trace elements, illustrated by zinc and copper. *American Journal of Clinical Nutrition, 61*(3 Suppl.), 621S–624S.

Sandyk, R. (1996). Reversal of acute Parkinson syndrome associated with multiple sclerosis by application of weak electromagnetic fields. *Int J Neurosci, 86*, 33–45.

Sandyk, R. (1996). Electromagnetic fields for treatment of multiple sclerosis (editorial). *Int J Neurosci, 79*, 1–4.

Sandyk, R. (1997). Resolution of sleep paralysis by weak electromagnetic fields in a patient with multiple sclerosis. *International Journal of Neurosciences, 90*(3–4), 145–157.

Sandyk, R. (1997). Treatment with weak electromagnetic fields restores dream recall in a parkinsonian patient. *International Journal of Neurosciences, 90*(1–2), 75–86.

Sano, M., Ernesto, C., Thomas, R. G., et al. (1997). A controlled trial of selegiline, alpha-tocopherol, or both as treatment for Alzheimer's disease. *New England Journal of Medicine, 336*, 1216–1222.

Sappington, A., Pharr, R., Tunstall, A., Rickert, E. (1997). Relationships among child abuse, date abuse, and psychological problems. *Journal Clin Psychol, 53*(4), 319–329.

Sartori, S., & Poirrier, R. (1996). Seasonal affective syndrome and phototherapy: Theoretical concepts and clinical applications. *Encephale, 22*(1), 7–16.

Satorelli, S. F. (1996). Mindfulness and mastery in the workplace: 21 ways to reduce stress during the workday. In A. Kotler (Ed.), *Engaged Buddhist reader*. Parallax Press.

Savage, P. (1996). Snoezelen for confused older people: Some concerns. *Elder Care, 8*(6), 20–21.

Savary, L., & Berne, P. (1988). *Kything: The Art of Spiritual Presence*. NJ, Paulist Press.

Sayegh, R., Schiff, I., Wurtman, J., et al. (1995). The effect of a carbohydrate-rich beverage on mood, appetite, and cognitive function in women with premenstrual syndrome. *Obstetrics and Gynecology, 86*(Pat 1), 520–528.

Scalzo, R. (1994). *Naturopathic handbook of herbal formulas: A practical and concise herb user's guide*. Durango, CO: Kivaki Press.

Schachter, M. B. (1996). Overview, historical background and current status of EDTA chelation therapy for atherosclerosis. *Journal of Advancement in Medicine, 9*(3), 159–177.

Schambelan, M. (1994). Licorice ingestion and blood pressure regulating hormones. *Steroids, 59*(2), 127–130.

Schaub, B. (1995, Spring). Alternative health and spiritual practices. *Alternative Health Practitioner, 1*(1), 35–38.

Scheer, S. J., & Mital, A. (1997). Ergonomics. *Archives of Phys Med Rehabil, 78*(3 Suppl.), S36–S45.

Scheffer, M. (1996). *Mastering Bach flower therapies: A guide to diagnosis and treatment*. Rochester, VT: Healing Arts Press.

Scheider, W. L., Hershey, L. A., Vena, J. E., et al. (1997). Dietary antioxidants and other dietary factors in the etiology of Parkinson's disease. *Movement Disorders, 12*(2), 190–196.

Schell, F. J., Allolio, B., & Schonecke, O. W. (1994). Physiological and psychological effects of Hatha-Yoga exercise in healthy women. *Int Journal Psychosom, 41*(1–4), 46–52.

Schlesinger, L., Arevalo, M., Arredondo, S., et al. (1992). Effect of a zinc-fortified formulat on immunocompetence and growth of malnourished infants. *American Journal Clin N, 56*, 491–498.

Schneider, C. J., & Wilson, E. S. (1985). *Foundations of biofeedback practice*. Wheat Ridge, CO: A publication of the Biofeedback Society of America.

Schneider, D. (1998). Demand for alternative therapies: The case of childbirth. In R. J. Gordon, B. C. Nienstedt, & W. M. Gesler (Eds.), *Alternative therapies: Expanding options in health care* (pp. 117–128). New York: Springer Publishing Company.

Schneider, J. A., & Agras, W. S. (1985). A cognitive behavioural group treatment of bulimia. *Br Journal Psychiatry, 146*, 66–69.

Scholl, T. O., Hediger, M. L., Bendich, A., et al. (1997). Use of multivitamin/mineral prenatal supplements: Influence on the outcome of pregnancy. *American Journal of Epidemiology, 146*(2), 134–141.

Scholmerich, J., Freudemann, A., Kottgen, E., et al. (1987). Bioavailability of zinc from zinc-histidine complexes. *Journal Clin Nutr, 45*, 1480–1486.

Scholmerich, J., Krauss, E., Wietholtz, H., et al. (1987). Bioavailability of zinc from zinc-histidine complexes: 2. Studies on patients with liver cirrhosis and the influence of time application. *American Journal of Clinical Nutrition, 45*, 1487–1491.

Schorr, J. A. (1993). Music and pattern change in chronic pain. *Advances in Nursing Science, 15*(4), 27–36.

Schrauzer, G. N., & Sacher, J. (1994). Selenium in the maintenance and therapy of HIV-infected patients. *Chemico-Biological Interactions, 91*, 199–205.

Schrauzer, G. N., & Sacher, J. (1995). Selenium in the maintenance and therapy of HIV-infected patients. *Chemico-Biological Interactions, 94*(2), 167.

Schubert, H., & Halama, P. (1993). Depressive episode primarily unresponsive to therapy in elderly patients: Efficacy of Ginkgo biloba (Egb 761) in combination with antidepressants. *Geriatr Forsch, 3*, 45–53.

Schultes, R. E., & Raffauf, R. F. (1990). *Medicinal and toxic plants of the Northwest Amazonia*. Portland, OR: Dioscorides Press.

Schultz, J. H., & Luthe, W. (1959). *Autogenic training*. New York: Grune & Stratton.

Schulz, K., & Schulz, H. (1992). Overview of psychoneuroimmunological stress- and intervention studies in humans with emphasis on the uses of immunological parameters. *Psycho-Oncology, 1*, 51–70.

Schutz, W. *Joy*.

Schwartz, M. S. & Associate. (1995). *Biofeedback: A practitioner's guide* (2nd ed.). New York: Guilford Press.

Schwartzman, R. A., & Cidlowski, J. A. (1993). Apoptosis: The biochemistry and molecular biology of programmed cell death. *Endocrine Reviews, 14*(2), 133–145.

Schwitters, B., & Masquelier, J. (1993). *OPC in practice: Bioflavanols and their application*. Rome: Alfa Omega.

Schwontkowski, D. (1995). *Herbs of the Amazon: Traditional and common uses*. Salt Lake City: SSBT Publishing.

Schwyzer, R. U. (1991). Multiple sclerosis: Prevention of serious illness—vision of a desired future for newly ascertained patients. *Medical Hypotheses, 37*, 115–118.

Seale, D. R., Silverman, H. G., Reiling, M. J., & Davy, K. P. (1997). Effect of regular aerobic exercise on elevated blood pressure in postmenopausal women. *American Journal of Cardiology, 80*(1), 49–55.

Seddon, J. M., Ajani, U. A., Sperduto, R. D., et al. (1994). Dietary carotenoids, vitamins A, C, and E, and advanced age-related macular degeneration. *Journal of the American Medical Association, 272*, 1413–1420.

See Pub. L. No. 104-191 (Aug. 21, 1996), 110 *Stat.* 2016; Colloquy between Senators William Cohen and Orrin Hatch, 142:50 *Cong. Rec.* S3569 (Apr. 18, 1996); "Report on H.R. 3103, Health Insurance Portability and Accountability Act of 1996," 142:115 *Cong. Rec.* H9537-38 (July 31, 1996).

See, D. M., Broumand, N., Sahl, L., & Tilles, J. G. (1997). In vitro effects of echinacea and ginseng on natural killer and antibody-dependent cell cytotoxicity in health subjects and chronic fatigue syndrome or acquired immunodeficiency syndrome patients. *Immunopharmacology*, *35*(3), 229–235.

Seedon, J. M., Christen, W. G., Manson, J. E., et al. (1994). The use of vitamin supplements and the risk of cataract among US male physicians. *American Journal of Public Health*, *84*, 788–792.

Seegenschmiedt, H. M., Fessenden, P., & Vernon, C. C. (1995). *Thermo-Radiotherapy and Thermo-Chemotherapy*. Springer, U.K.

Seeley, R., Stephens, T., & Tate, P. (1995). *Anatomy and physiology* (3rd ed., pp. 280–306). Baltimore, MD: Mosby.

Seelig, M. S. (1994). Consequences of magnesium deficiency on the enhancement of stress reactions: Preventive and therapeutic implications, a review. *Journal of the American College of Nutrition*, *13*(5), 429–446.

Selhub, J., Jacques, P. F., Bostom, A. G., et al. (1995). Association between plasma homocysteine concentrations and extracranial carotid-artery stenosis. *New England Journal of Medicine*, *332*, 286–291.

Sellmayer, A., Witzgall, H., Lorenz, R., & Weber, P. C. (1995). Effects of dietary fish oil on ventricular premature complexes. *American Journal of Cardiology*, *76*, 974.

Selye, H. (1956). *The stress of life*. New York: McGraw Hill.

Selye, H. (1978). *The stress of life*. New York: McGraw-Hill.

Sempertegui, F., Estrella, B., Correa, E., Aguirre, L., Saa, B., Torres, M., Navarrete, F., Alarcon, C., Carrion, J., Rodriguez, G., & Griffiths, J. K. (1996). Effects of short-term zinc supplementation on cellular immunity, respiratory symptoms, and growth of malnourished Equadorian children. *Eur Journal Clin Nutr*, *50*(1), 42–46.

Sen, C. K., Atalay, M., Agren, J., Laaksonen, D. E., Roy, S., & Hanninen, O. (1997). Fish oil and vitamin E supplementation in oxidative stress at rest and after physical exercise. *Journal of Applied Physiology*, *83*(1), 189–195.

Serfaty, D., & Magneron, A. C. (1997). Premenstrual syndrome in France. Epidemiology and therapeutic effectiveness of 1000 mg of micronized purified flavonoid fraction in 1473 gynecological patients. *Contracept Fertil Sex*, *25*(1), 85–90.

Serlin, I. (1993). Root images of healing in dance therapy. *American Journal of Dance Therapy*, *15*(2), Fall/Winter, 65–76.

Serraino, M., & Thompson, L. (1992). The effect of flaxseed supplementation on the initiation and promotional stages of mammary tumorigenesis. *Nutr Cancer*, *17*, 153–159.

Shafarman, S. (1997). *Awareness heals*. Addison-Wesley Publishing Co.: New York, California, Ontario, England, Amsterdam, Bonn, Sydney, Singapore, Tokyo, Madrid, San Juan, Paris, Seoul, Milan, Mexico City, Taipei

Shaffer, H. J., LaSilva, T. A., & Stein, J. P. (1997). Comparing hatha yoga with dynamic group psychotherapy for enhancing methadone maintenance treatment: A randomized clinical trial. *Alternative Therapies in Health Med*, *3*(4), 57–66.

Shafranske, E. P., & Malony, H. N. (1990). Clinical psychologists' religious and spiritual orientations and their practice of psychotherapy. *Psychotherapy*, *27*, 72–78.

Shames, K. H. (1996). *Creative imagery in nursing*. New York: Delmar Publishers.

Shankel, D. M., Kuo, S., Haines, C., & Mitscher, L. A. (1993). Extracellular interception of mutagens. *Basic Life Sciences*, *61*, 65–74.

Shanmugasundaram, E. R., & Shanmugasundaram, K. R. (1986). An Indian herbal formula (SKV) for controlling voluntary ethanol intake in rats with chronic alcoholism. *Journal of Ethnopharmacology*, *17*(2), 171–182.

Shanmugasundaram, K. R., Ramanujam, S., & Shanmugasundaram, E. R. (1994). Amrita-Bindu—a salt-spice-herbal health food supplement for the prevention of nitrosamine induced depletion of antioxidants. *Journal of Ethnopharmacology*, *42*(2), 83–93.

Shannahoff-Khalsa, D. S., & Beckett, L. R. (1996). Clinical case report: Efficacy of yogic techniques in the treatment of obsessive compulsive disorders. *International Journal of Neurosciences*, *85*(1–2), 1–17.

Shannahoff-Khalsa, D. S., & Kennedy, B. (1993). The effects of unlateral forced breathing on the heart. *International Journal of Neuroscience*, *73*(1–2), 47–60.

Shannon, K. (1986). SKIP: (Sick Kids Need Involved People) . . . Family learning retreat camp. *Caring*, *5*, 48–50.

Shapiro, A., & Morris, L. (1978). *Placebo effects in medical and psychological therapies: Handbook of psychotherapy and behavior change.* New York: Wiley.

Shapiro, D., Goldstein, I. B., & Jamner, L. D. (1996). Effects of cynical hostility, anger out, anxiety, and defensiveness on ambulatory blood pressure in black and white college students. *Psychosom Med, 58*(4), 354–364.

Shapiro, J. A., Koepsell, T. D., Voigt, L. F., et al. (1996). Diet and rheumatoid arthritis in women: A possible protective effect of fish consumption. *Epidemiology, 7*(3), 256–263.

Sharma, K. K. (1977). Antihyperglycemic effect of onion: Effect on fasting blood sugar and induced hyperglycemia in man. *Indian Journal of Medical Research, 65*, 422–429.

Sharma, R. D., Raghuram, T. C., & Rao, N. S. (1990). Effect of fenugreek seeds on blood glucose and serum lipids in type 1 diabetes. *European Journal of Clinical Nutrition, 44*, 301–306.

Shealy, C., Cady, R. K., Wilkie, R. G., Cox, R. H., Liss, S., & Closson, W. (1989). Depression: A diagnostic neurochemical profile and therapy with cranial electrical stimulation (CES). *Journal of Neurological and Orthopaedic Medicine and Surgery, 10*(4), 319–321.

Shealy, C., Cady, K., & Cox, R. H. (1995). Pain, stress and depression: Psychoneurophysiology and therapy. *Stress Medicine, 11*, 75–77.

Shealy, C. N. (1995). A Review of Dehydroepiandrosterone (DHEA). *Integrative Physiological and Behavioral Science, 30*(4), 308–313.

Shealy, C. N. (1993, March). Microwave Resonance Therapy: Innovations from the Ukraine. *Greene County Medical Bulletin, XLVII*(3), 15–17.

Shealy, C. N., & Borgmeyer, V. (1997). Decompression, reduction and stabilization of the lumbar spine: A cost-effective treatment for lumbosacral pain. *American Journal of Pain Management, 7*(2), 63–65.

Shealy, C. N., Myss, C. M., Cady, R. K., Dudley, L., & Cox, R. (1995). Electrical Stimulation Raises DHEA and Improves Diabetic Neuropathy. *Stress Medicine, 11*, 215–217.

Sheehan, M. P., & Atherton, D. J. (1994). One-year follow up of children treated with Chinese medicinal herbs for atopic eczema. *British Journal of Dermatology, 130*(4), 488–493.

Sheela, C. G., & Augusti, K. T. (1992). Antidiabetic effects of S-allyl cysteine suphoxide isolated from garlic (Allum sativum, Linn.). *Indian Journal Exp Biol, 30*, 523–526.

Shelhav-Silberbush, C. (1986). The Feldenkrais Method, for Children With Cerebral Palsy, p. 116. MS Thesis, Boston University School of Education, Boston MA, USA. Published by Feldenkrais Resources, PO Box 2067, Berkeley, CA 94702: 1-800-765-1907.

Sheng, C. (1986). The treatment of urogenital diseases by acupuncture. *Journal of Chinese Medicine, 22*, 3–12.

Shew, J. (1845). *Hydropathy, or, the water cure: Its principles, modes of treatment.* New York: Wiley and Putnam.

Shimade, H., Tyler, V. E., & McLaughlin, J. L. (1997). Biologically active acylglycerides from the berries of saw-palmetto (*Serenoa repens*). *Journal of Natural Products, 60*(4), 417–418.

Shipman, M. K., Boniface, D. R., Tefft, M. E., & McCloghry, F. (1997). Antenatal perineal massage and subsequent perineal outcomes: A randomised controlled trial. *British Journal of Obstetrics and Gynecology, 104*(7), 787–791.

Shukla, A., Rasik, A. M., & Patnaik, G. K. (1997). Depletion of reduced glutathione, ascorbic acid, vitamin E and antioxidant defence enzymes in a healing cutaneous wound. *Free Radical Research, 26*(2), 93–101.

Sidney, S. (1996). Television viewing and cardiovascular risk factors in young adults: The CARDIA study. *Annals of Epidemiology, 6*(2), 154–159.

Siegman, A. W., & Snow, S. C. (1997). The outward expression of anger, the inward experience of anger and CVR: The role of vocal expression. *Journal Behav Med, 20*(1), 29–45.

Sigounas, G., Hooker, J. L., Li, W., et al. (1997). S-allylmercapto-cysteine, a stable thioallyl compound, induces apoptosis in erythroleukamia cell lines. *Nutr Cancer, 28*(2), 153–159.

Silagy, C., & Neil, A. (1994). Garlic as a lipid lowering agent-a meta-analysis. *Journal Royal Coll Phys Lond, 28*, 39–45.

Silman, A. J., O'Neill, T. W., Cooper, C., et al. (1997). Influence of physical activity on vertebral deformity in men and women: Results from the European Vertebral Osteoporosis Study. *Journal Bone Miner Res, 12*(5), 813–819.

Simington, J. A., & Laing, G. P. (1993). Effects of therapeutic touch on anxiety in the institutionalized elderly. *Clinical Nursing Research, 2*(4), 438–450.

Simon, G. A., Schmid, P., Reifenrath, W. G., et al. (1994). Wound healing after laser injury to the skin—the effect of occlusion and vitamin E. *Journal Pharm Sci, 83*(8), 1101–1106.

Simon, R. (1997). Listening hands: An interview with Ilana Rubenfeld. *Family Therapy* Networker, *21*(5), 62–73.

Simons, D. J. (1937). A note on the effect of heat and cold upon certain symptoms of multiple sclerosis. *Bulletin of the Neurological Institute, 6*, 385–386.

Sims, S. (1986). Slow stroke back massage for cancer patients. *Nursing Times, 82*, 4750.

Singer, J. L. (1974). *Imagery and daydream methods in psychotherapy and behavior modification.* New York: Academic Press.

Singer, P. (1977). Introduction: From anthropology and medicine to "therapy" and neo-colonialism. In P. Singer (Ed.), *Traditional healing: New science or new colonialism* (pp. 1–25). London: Conch Magazine Limited.

Singer, P., Rubinstein, A., Askanazi, J., et al. (1992). Clinical and immunologic effects of lipid-based parenteral nutrition in AIDS. *Journal Parenteral Enteral Nutrition, 16*, 165–167.

Singer, S. R., & Grismaijer, S. (1995). *Dressed to kill: The link between breast cancer and bras.* Garden City Park: Avery.

Singh, K., Zaldi, S., Ralsuddin, S., et al. (1992). Effect of zinc on immune function and host resistance against infection and tumor challenge. *Immunoh Im, 14*, 813–840.

Singh, N. A., Clements, K. M., & Fiatarone, M. A. (1997). A randomized controlled trial of progressive resistance training in depressed elders. *Journal Gerontol A Biol Sci Med Sci, 52*(1), M27–35.

Singh, R. B., Niaz, M. A., Rastogi, S. S., & Rastogi, S. (1996). Usefulness of anti-oxidant vitamins in suspected acute myocardial infarction (the Indian experiment of infarct survival-3). *American Journal of Cardiology, 77*(4), 232–236.

Singh, R. B., Rastogi, S. S., Ghosh, S., & Niag, M. A. (1994). Dietary and serum magnesium levels in patients with acute myocardial infec-tion, coronary artery disease and noncardiac diagnoses. *J Am Coll Nutr, 13*(2), 116–117.

Sirica, C. M. (Ed.). (1996). *Osteopathic Medicine: Past, Present, and Future.* New York: Josiah Macy Jr. Foundation.

Sivam, G. P., Lampe, J. W., Ulness, B., et al. (1997). Helicobacter pylori—in vitro susceptibility to garlic (Allium sativum) extract. *Nutrition and Cancer, 27*(2), 118–121.

Skaggs, R. (1997a). The Bonny method of guided imagery and music in the treatment of terminal illness: A private practice setting. *Music Therapy Perspectives, 15*(1), 39–44.

Skaggs, R. (1997b). *Finishing strong: Treating chemical addictions with music and imagery.* St. Louis: MMB Music, Inc.

Skaper, S. D., Fabris, M., Ferrari, V., et al. (1997). Quercetin protects cutaneous tissue-associated cell types including sensory neurons from oxidative stress induced by glutathione depletion: Cooperative effects of ascorbic acid. *Free Radical Biology and Medicine, 22*(4), 669–678.

Slater, V. (1996). Healing touch. In M. Micozzi (Ed.), *Fundamentals of complementary and alternative medicine* (pp. 121–136). New York: Churchill Livingstone, Inc.

Slater, V. E. (1995a). Toward an understanding of energetic healing, Part 1: Energetic structures. *Journal of Holistic Nursing, 13*(3), 209–224.

Slater, V. E. (1995b). Toward an understanding of energetic healing, Part 2: Energetic processes. *Journal of Holistic Nursing, 13*(3), 225–238.

Slattery, M. L., Benson, J., Berry, T. D., et al. (1997a). Dietary sugar and colon cancer. *Cancer Epidemiol Biomarksers Prev, 6*(9), 677–685.

Slattery, M. L., Potter, J. D., Coates, A., et al. (1997). Plant foods and colon cancer: An assessment of specific foods and their related nutrients. *Cancer Causes Control, 8*(4), 575–590.

Smilkstein, G. (1986). A commentary on psychosocial risk and obstetrical risk scoring.

Smilkstein, G., Helsper-Lucas, A., Ashworth, C., Montano, D., & Pagel, M. (1984). Predicting pregnancy complications: An application of the biopsychosocial model. *Social Sciences and Medicine, 18*, 15–321.

Smilkstein, G., Pagel, M., & Regen, H. (1985). *Risk assessment for pregnancy: Biopsychosocial evaluation.* (Report to the Family Health Foundation, Grant. No. 63-3335). Seattle: Department of Family Practice, University of Washington.

Smith, K. T., Heaney, R. P., Flora, L., & Hinders, S. (1987). Calcium absorption from calcium citrate-malate. *Calcified Tissue International, 41*, 351–352.

Smith, M. J. (1972). Paranormal effects on enzyme activity. *Human Dimensions, 1*, 15–19.

Smith, N. M., Floyd, M. R., Scogin, F., & Jamison, C. S. (1997). Three-year follow-up bibliotherapy for depression. *Journal of Consulting and Clinical Psychology, 65*(2), 324–327.

Smith, S. R., Klotman, P. E., & Svetkey, L. P. (1992). Potassium chloride lowers blood pressure and causes natriuresis in older patients with hypertension. *Journal of the American Society of Nephrology, 2*(8), 1302–1309.

Smith, W. P., Compton, W. C., & West, W. B. (1995). Meditation as an adjunct to a happiness enhancement program. *Journal of Clinical Psychology, 52*(2), 269–273.

Snodderly, D. M. (1995). Evidence for protection against age-related macular degeneration by carotenoids and antioxidant vitamins. *American Journal of Clinical Nutrition, 62*(Suppl. 6), 1448S–1461S.

Snow, L. F. (1993). *Walkin' on medicine.* Boulder, CO: Westview Press.

Snowdon, D. A., Gross, M. D., & Butler, S. M. (1996). Antioxidants and reduced functional capacity in the elderly: Findings from the Nun Study. *Journal of Gerontol, 51*(1), M10–M16.

Snyder, J. (1991). Use and misuse of oral therapy for diarrhea: Comparison of U.S. practices with American Academy of Pediatrics recommendations. *Pediatrics, 87*, 28–33.

Sobel, D. (1993). Mind matters, money matters: The cost of effectiveness of behavioral medicine. Mental medicine update special report.

Society for Clinical & Experimental Hypnosis (SCEH). Liverpool, NY.

Sodi Pallares, D. (1997). Magnetotherapy of metastatic cancer. Proceedings of The Ninth International Montreux Congress on Stress. Montreux: Biotonus Press.

Solberg, E. E., Halvorsen, R., Sundgot-Borgen, J., Ingjer, F., & Holen, A. (1995). Meditation: A modulator of the immune response to physical stress? A brief report. *British Journal of Sports Medicine, 29*(4), 255–257.

Solomon, G. (1985). The emerging field of psychoneuroimmunology. *Advances, 2*(1), 6–19.

Solomon, G. (1987). Psychoneuroimmunologic approaches to research on AIDS. *Annals of the New York Academy of Science, 494*, 628–636.

Solomon, G. (1987). Psychoneuroimmunology: Interactions between central nervous system and immune system. *Journal of Neuroscience Research, 18*, 1–9.

Solomon, G., & Moos, R. (1964). Emotions, immunity, and disease: A speculative theoretical integration. *Archives of General Psychiatry, 11*, 657–674.

Solomons, N., Juswigg, T., & Pineda, O. (1984). Bioavailability of oral zinc from the sulfate salt and the gluconate chelate in humans: A comparative study. *Federal Proceedings, 43*, 850.

Somerville, R. (1997). *Flower remedies. The alternative advisor.* New York: Time-Life Books.

Somerville, R. (1997). Qigong. In *Alternative health advisor.* New York: Time-Life Books.

Sonenklar, N. Z. (1995). Acupuncture point treatment for attention deficit hyperactivity disorder. Grant number R21 RR09463, Office of Alternative Medicine. http://altmed.od.nih/gov/oam

Song, Z., Johnasen, H. K., Faber, V., et al. (1997). Ginseng treatment reduces bacterial load and lung pathology in chronic *Pseudomonas aeruginosa* pneumonia in rats. *Antimicrobial Agents and Chemotherapy, 41*(5), 961–964.

Sotaniemi, E. A., et al. (1995). Ginseng and the management of non-insulin-dependent (Type II) diabetes. *Diabetes Care, 18*, 1373.

Soutar, A., Seaton, A., & Brown, K. (1997). Bronchial reactivity and dietary antioxidants. *Thorax, 52*(2), 166–170.

Spear, W. (1995). *Feng Shui made easy.* San Francisco: Harper.

Specter, R. E. (1996). *Cultural diversity in health and illness* (4th ed.). Stamford, CT: Appleton & Lange.

Spencer, H., Norris, C., & Williams, D. (1994). Inhibitory effects of zinc on magnesium balance and magnesium absorption in man. *Journal of the American College of Nutrition, 13*(5), 479–484.

Sperduto, R. D., Hu, T. S., Milton, R. C., et al. (1993). The Linxian cataract studied. Two nutrition intervention trials. *Archives of Opthalmology, 111*(9), 1246–1253.

Spicer, J., & Chamberlain, K. (1996). Cynical hostility, anger, and resting blood pressure. *Journal of Psychosomatic Research*, 40(4), 359–368.

Spiegel, D. (1994). Health caring, psychosocial support for patients with cancer. *Cancer*(Supplement, August 15), 74(4), 1453–1457.

Spiegel, D., Bloom, H. C., Kraemer, J. R., & Grottheil, E. (1989, October 14). Effect of psychosocial treatment on survival of patients with metastatic breast cancer. *Lancet*, 2(8668), 888–901.

Spink, Jan. 1993. *Developmental riding therapy.* Tucson, AZ: Therapy Skill Builders.

Squires, S. (1996, September–October). The new medicine. *Modern Maturity*, p. 69.

Srivastava, Y., et al. (1993). Antidiabetic and adaptogenic properties of Momordica charantia extract: An experimental and clinical evaluation. *Phytotherapy Res*, 7, 285–289.

Stabile, A., Pesaresi, M., Stabile, A., et al. (1991). Immunodeficiency and plasma zinc levels in children with Down's syndrome: A long-term follow-up of oral zinc supplementation. *Clinical Immunology Immunopathology*, 58, 207–216.

Staehelin, H. (1997). Dietary therapy for Alzheimer's disease. Research paper presented at the World Congress of Gerontology in Adelaide, Australia, August 18–22.

Stamler, J., Ruth, K. J., Lui, K., & Shekelle, R. B. (1994). Dietary antioxidants and blood pressure change in the Western Electric Study, Presented at the 34th Annual Conference on Cardio vascular Disease Epidemiology and Prevention. Tampa, FL, March 16 and 17.

Stampfer, M. J., Krauss, R. M., Ma, J., et al. (1997). A prospective study of triglyceride level, low-density lipoprotein particle diameter, and risk of myocardial infarction. *Journal of the American Medical Association*, 276(11), 882–888.

Stander, V., Piercy, F. P., Mackinnon, D., & Helmeke, K. (1994). Spirituality, religion and family therapy: Competing or complementary worlds? *Journal of Family Therapy*, 22, 27–41.

Standley, J. M., & Moore, R. S. (1995). Therapeutic effects of music and mother's voice on premature infants. *Pediatr Nurs*, 21(6), 509–512.

Stanford Research Institute. (1960). *Chiropractic in California.* Los Angeles: The Haynes Foundation.

Stanton-Jones, K. (1992). *An introduction to dance movement therapy in psychiatry.* London and New York: Routledge.

Starr, P. (1982). *The social transformation of American medicine.* New York: Basic Books.

Steege, J. F., & Blumenthal, J. A. (1993). The effects of aerobic exercise on premenstraul symptoms in middle-aged women: A preliminary study. *Journal of Psychosomatic Research*, 37(2), 127–133.

Stein, D. (1990). *All women are healers.* Freedom, CA: Crossing Press.

Stein, D. (1995). *Essential Reiki.* Freedom, CA: The Crossing Press, Inc.

Stein, D., Ed. (1991). *The Goddess Celebrates: An Anthology of Women's Rituals.* Freedom, CA: The Crossing Press.

Steiner, R. (1989). *Spiritual science and medicine.* Blauvelt, NY: Steinerbooks. (Original work published in 1948)

Stephens, N. G., Parsons, A., Schofield, P. M., et al. (1996). Randomized controlled trial of vitamin E in patients with coronary disease: Cambridge Heart Antioxidant Study. *Lancet*, 347(9004), 781–786.

Stephenson, J. (Nov. 1955). A review of investigations into the action of substances in dilutions greater than 1 x 10 to the 24. *Journal American Inst Homeop*, 48, 327–335.

Sternfield, B., Quesenberry, C. P., Jr., Eskenazi, B., & Newman, L. A. (1995). Exercise and pregnancy outcomes. *Med Sci Sports Exerc*, 27, 634–640.

Stewart, A. (1987). Clinical and biochemical effects of nutritional supplementation on the premenstrual syndrome. *Journal Reprod Med*, 32(6), 435–441.

Stewart, A. C., & Thomas, S. E. (1995). Hypnotherapy as a treatment for atopic dermatitis in adults and children. *Br Journal Dermatol*, 132(5), 778–783.

Stillerman, E. (1996). *The encyclopedia of bodywork from accupressure to zone therapy.* New York: Facts on File.

Stoff, J., & Pellegrino, C. (1992). *Chronic fatigue syndrome: The hidden epidemic.* New York: Harper Perennial.

Stoll, B. A. (1997). Macronutrient supplements may reduce breast cancer risk: How, when and which? *European Journal of Clinical Nutrition*, 51(9), 573–577.

Stone, J. (1996). *Complementary medicine and the law.* New York: Oxford University Press.

Stone, R. (1985). *Health building: The conscious art of living well*. Sebastopol, CA: CRCS Publications.

Stone, R. (1986). *Polarity Therapy, Vol I*. Sebastopol, CA: CRCS Publications.

Stone, R. (1987). *Polarity Therapy, Vol II*. Sebastopol, CA: CRCS Publications.

Storr, A. (1992). *Music and the mind*. New York: Ballentine Books.

Störtebecker, P. (1985). *Mercury poisoning from dental amalgam—a hazard to human brain*. Stockholm: Störtebecker Foundation for Research.

Stress free exercise. (1985). *New Body, 4*(5).

Strong, G. A. *Does mercury from dental amalgams influence systemic health?* Billings, MO: Strong Health Publications.

Su, Z. Z., He, Y. Y., & Chen, G. (1993). Clinical and experimental study on effects of man-shen-ling oral liquid in the treatment of 100 cases of chronic nephritis. *Chung Kuo Chung Hsi I Chieh Ho Tsa Chih, 13*(5), 269–272.

Suadicani, P., Hein, H., & Gyntelberg, F. (1992). Serum selenium concentration and risk of ischaemic heart disease in a prospective cohort study of 3000 males. *Atherosclerosis, 96*, 33–42.

Sucov, J. L. (1994). Aromatherapy makes scents. Healthy mind healthy body. *Oxford Health Plans Quarterly Magazine, 1*(3), 3.

Sun, P., Li, L., & Si, M. (1992). Comparison between acupuncture and epidural anesthesia in appendectomy. *Chen Tza Yen Chiu, 17*(2), 87–89.

Sunshine, W., Field, T. M., Schanberg, S., Quintino, O., Kilmer, T., Fierro, K., Burman, I., Hashimoto, M., McBride, C., & Henteleff, T. (1996). Massage therapy and transcutaneous electrical stimulation effects on fibromyalgia. *Journal of Clinical Rheumatology, 2*, 18–22.

Sutcher, H. (1997). Hypnosis as adjunctive therapy for multiple sclerosis: A progress report. *American Journal of Clinical Hypnosis, 39*(4), 283–290.

Swanson, C. A., Coates, R. J., Malone, K. E., et al. (1997). Alcohol consumption and breast cancer risk among women under age 45 years. *Epidemiology, 8*, 231–237.

Swanson, D. R. (1988). Migraine and magnesium: Eleven neglected conditions. *Perspectives in Biological Medicine, 31*, 526–527.

Swanston-Flatt, S. K., Day, C., Bailey, C. J., & Flatt, P. R. (1989). Evaluation of traditional plant treatments for diabetes: Studies in streptozotocin diabetic mice. *Acta Diabetol Lat, 26*(1), 51–55.

Sweet route to heading off colon cancer. (1993). *Science News, 144*, 207.

Swinson, R. P., Soulios, C., Cox, B. J., et al. (1992). Brief treatment of emergency room patients with panic attacks. *American Journal of Psychiatry, 149*(7), 944–946.

Szabo, R. M. (1988). *Nerve Compression Syndromes: Diagnosis and treatment*. Slack, Inc.

Tabak, N., Bergman, R., & Alpert, R. (1996). The mirror as a therapeutic tool for patients with dementia. *International Journal of Nursing Practice, 2*(3), 155–159.

Taillandier, J., Ammar, A., Rabourdin, J. P., et al. (1986). Treatment of cerebral aging disorders with *Ginkgo biloba* extract. A longitudinal multicenter double-blind drug vs. placebo study. *Press Medicale, 15*(31), 1583–1587.

Tamborini, A., & Taurelle, R. (1993). Value of standardized *Ginkgo biloba* extract (EGb 761) in the management of congestive symptoms of premenstrual syndrome. *Rev Fr Gynecol Obstet, 88*(7–9), 447–457.

Tandan, R., Lewis, G. A., Krusinski, P. B., et al. (1992). Topical capsaicin in painful diabetic neuropathy. Controlled study with long-term follow-up. *Diabetes Care, 15*(1), 8–14.

Tang, A. M., Graham, N. M., Kirby, A. J., et al. (1993). Dietary micronutrient intake and risk of progression to acquired immuno-deficiency syndrome (AIDS) in human immunodeficiency virus type 1 (HIV-1)-infected homosexual men. *American Journal of Epidemiology, 138*(11), 937–951.

Tappan, F. (1988). *Healing massage techniques: Holistic, classic, and emerging methods* (2nd ed., pp. 299–300). Norwalk, CT: Appleton & Lange.

Tavola, T., Gala, C., Conte, G., & Invernizzi, G. (1992). Traditional Chinese acupuncture in tension-type headache: A controlled study. *Pain, 48*(3), 325–329.

Taylor, A. G. (1998). Complementary/alternative therapies in the treatment of pain. In J. Spencer & J. Jacobs (Eds.), *Complementary medicine: An evidence-based approach*. Baltimore: Mosby Year Book, 282–339.

Taylor, D. H., & Ricketts, T. C. (1993). Helping nurse-midwives provide obstetrical care in rural North Carolina. *American Journal of Public Health*, 83, 904–905.

Taylor, E. W., Nadimpalli, R. G., & Ramanathan, C. S. (1997). Genomic structures of viral agents in relation to the biosynthesis of seleno-proteins. *Biological Trace Element Research*, 56(1), 63–92.

Taylor, J. (1988). *The complete guide to mercury toxicity from dental fillings*. San Diego: Scripps Publishing.

Teeguarden, I. M. (1979). *The Acupressure Way of Health: Jin Shin Do*. Japan Publications, Tokyo, New York.

Teeguarden, I. M. (1985, August). Acupressure in the Classroom. *East West Journal*.

Teeguarden, I. M. (1987). *The Joy of Feeling: Bodymind Acupressure*. Japan Publications, Tokyo, New York.

Teeguarden, I. M. (1989). The Jin Shin Do™ Story. The Jin Shin Do Foundation.

Teeguarden, I. M. (1996). *The complete guide to acupressure*. Japan Publications, Tokyo, New York.

Telle, S., Narendran, S., Raghuraj, P.l, Nagarathna, R., & Nagendra, H. R. (1997). Comparison of changes in autonomic and respiratory parameters of girls after yoga and games at a community home. *Percept Mot Skills*, 84(1), 251–257.

Thal, L. J., Carta, A., Clarke, W. R., et al. (1996). A l-year multicenter placebo-controlled study of acetyl-L-carnitine in patients with Alzheimer's disease. *Neurology*, 47(3), 705–711.

Thayer, R. E., Newman, J. R., & McClain, T. M. (1994). Self-regulation of mood: Strategies for changing a bad mood, raising energy, and reducing tension. *Journal of Personal and Social Psychology*, 67(5), 910–925.

Therapeutic Touch Teaching Guidelines: Beginner's Level Krieger/Kunz Method published by Nurse Healers-Professional Associates, Inc. 1992.

Thomas, C. (Ed.). (1985). *Taber's cyclopedic medical dictionary* (pp. 926, 1087, 603). Philadelphia: F. A. Davis Company.

Thomas, C. L. (1996). *Taber's cyclopedic dictionary* (18th ed.). Philadelphia: F. A. Davis.

Thomas, S. P., & Droppleman, P. (1997). Channeling nurses' anger into positive interventions. *Nurs Forum*, 32(2), 13–21.

Thomas, W. (1994). *The Eden Alternative: Nature hope and nursing home*. Sherburne, NY: The Eden Alternative.

Thompson, L. U., Rickard, S. E., Orcheson, L. J., & Seidel, M. M. (1996). Flaxseed and its lignan and oil components reduce mammary tumor growth at a late stage of carcinogenesis. *Carcinogenesis*, 17(6), 1373–1376.

Thompson, L. U., Seidl, M. M., Rickard, S. E., et al. (1996). Antitumorigenic effect of a mammalian lignan precursor from flaxseed. *Nutrition in Cancer*, 26(2), 159–165.

Thompson, N. J., Potter, J. S., Sanderson, C. A., & Maibach, E. W. (1997). The relationship of sexual abuse and HIV risk behaviors among heterosexual adult female STD patients. *Child Abuse Negl*, 21(2), 149–156.

Thune, I., Brenn, T., & Lund, E. (1997). Physical activity and the risk of breast cancer. *New England Journal of Medicine*, 336(18), 1269–1274.

Thys-Jacobs, S., Ceccarelli, S., Bierman, A., et al. (1989). Calcium supplementation in premenstrual syndrome: A randomized crossover trial. *Journal General Intern Med*, 4(3), 183–189.

Tierra, M. (1988). *Planetary herbology*. Santa Fe, NM: Lotus Press.

Tiller, W., McCraty, R., & Atkinson, M. (1996). Cardiac coherence: A new, non-invasive measure of autonomic nervous system order. *Alternative Therapies*, 2(1), 87–103.

Tillotson, A. (1996, September 24). Migraines. *Paracelsus mailing list*. (AlanT3@aol.com).

Ting, H. H., Timini, F. K., Boles, K. S., et al. (1996). Vitamin C improves endothelium-dependent vasodilation in patients with non-insulin-dependent diabetes mellitus. *Journal of Clinical Investigation*, 97(1), 22–28.

Tiwari, M. (1995). *Ayurveda: A life of balance*. Rochester, VT: Healing Arts Press.

Tollan, A., Oian, P., Fadnes, H. O., & Maltau, J. M. (1993). Evidence for altered transcapillary fluid balance in women with the premenstrual syndrome. *Acta Obstet Gynecol Scan*, 72(4), 238–242.

Toors, F. A. (1992). Chewing gum and dental health. Literature review. *Rev. Belge. Med. Dent.*, 47(3), 67–92.

Tope, D. M., Hann, D. M., & Pinkson, B. (1943). Massage therapy: An old intervention comes of age. *Quality of Life—A Nursing Challenge, 3,* 14–18.

Tortora, G. J., & Anagnostakos, N. P. (1990). *Principles of anatomy and physiology, 6th edition.* New York: Harper & Row.

Trachtenberg. *Acupuncture Consensus Development Conference.*

Trager, M., (with Guadagno, C.) (1987). *Trager Mentastics: Movement as a way to agelessness.* Barrytown, NY: Station Hill Press, Inc.

Tragini, E., et al. (1985). Evidence from two classic irritation tests for an anti-inflammatory action of a natural extract, echinacin B. *Food and Chemical Tox, 23*(2), 317–319.

Trall, R. T. (1850). *Hydropathic encyclopedia: A system of hydropathy and hygiene in eight parts: Designed as a guide to families and students, and a text-book for physicians,* 2 vols. New York: Fowler and Wells.

Transformation-Oriented Bodywork Network, P.O. Box 24967, San Jose, CA 95154, ph: (408) 371-6716.

Transformational Bodywork. 44800 Fish Rock Road, Gualala, CA 95445, ph: (707) 884-3138.

Travell, J. G., & Simon, D. G. (1992). *Myofascial pain and dysfunction: The trigger point manual.* Baltimore: Williams & Wilkins.

Travell, J. G., & Simons, D. (1983). *Myofascial Pain and Dysfunction: The Trigger Point Manual* Vol I & II. Baltimore: Williams and Wilkins.

Treasure, J., Todd, G., Brolly, M., et al. (1995). A pilot study of a randomised trial of cognitive analytical therapy vs educational behavioral therapy for adult anorexia nervosa. *Behavior Research and Therapy, 33*(4), 363–367.

Tribole, E., & Resch, E. (1995). *Intuitive eating: A recovery book for the chronic dieter.* New York: St. Martin's Press.

Trice, A., & Price, J. (1986). Joking under the drill: A validity study of the Coping Humor Scale. *Journal of Social Behavior and Personality, 1*(2), 265–266.

Trichopoulou, A., Katsouyanni, K., Stuver, S., et al. (1995). Consumption of olive oil and specific food groups in relation to breast cancer risk in Greece. *Journal of the National Cancer Institute, 87*(2), 110–116.

Troisi, R. J., Speizer, F. E., Willett, W. C., et al. (1995). Menopause, postmenopausal estrogen preparations and the risk of adult-onset asthma.

A prospective cohort study. *American Journal of Respiratory and Critical Care Medicine, 152*(4 Pt 1), 1183–1188.

Troisi, R. J., Willett, W. C., Weiss, S. T., et al. (1995). A prospective study of diet and adult-onset asthma. *American Journal of Respiratory and Critical Care Medicine, 151*(5), 1401–1408.

Troop, N. A., & Treasure, J. L. (1997). Setting the scene for eating disorders, II. Childhood helplessness and mastery. *Psychological Medicine, 27*(3), 531–538.

Trosko, J. E. (1996). Role of low-level ionizing radiation in multi-step carcinogenic process. *Health Physics, 70*(6), 812–822.

Trotter, R., & Chavira, J. (1997). *Curanderismo: Mexican-American Folk Healing* (2nd ed.). Athens, GA: University of Georgia Press.

Tuburan, R. (1993). Interview with Hildegard Wittlinger. *Massage Therapy Journal, 32*(2), 46–53.

Tucker, K. L., Selhub, J., Wilson, P. W., & Rosenberg, I. H. (1996). Dietary intake pattern relates to plasma folate and homocysteine concentrations in the Framingham Heart Study. *Journal of Nutrition, 126*(12), 3025–3031.

Tulloch, I., Smellie, W. S., & Buck, A. C. (1994). Evening primrose oil reduces urinary calcium excretion in both normal and hypercalciuric rats. *Urological Research, 22*(4), 227–230.

Tuomainen, T. P., Punnonen, K., Nyyssonen, K., Salonen, J. T. (1998). Association between body iron stores and the risk of acute myocardial infarction in men. *Circulation, 97,* 1461–1466.

Tureanu, V., & Tureanu, L. (1994). *Acupunctură in obstetrica si ginecologie.* Bucuresti: Ed. All.

Turner, R. P., Lukoff, D., Barnhouse, R. T., & Lu, F. G. (1995). Religious or spiritual problem: A culturally sensitive diagnostic category in the DSM-IV. *Journal of Nervous and Mental Disease, 183,* 435–444.

21 *U.S.C.* § 321(g)(1)(B).

211 N.E.2d 253 (1965), *cert. denied,* 383 U.S. 946 (1966).

Tyler, V. (1994). *Herbs of choice: The therapeutic use of phytomedicinals.* New York: Pharmaceutical Products Press.

Tyler, V. E. (1996). What pharmacists should know about herbal remedies. *Journal of the American Pharmaceutical Association, NS36*(1), 29–37.

Tyson, P. D. (1996). Biodesensitization: Biofeedback-control systematic desensitization of the stress response to infant crying. *Biofeedback and Self Regulation, 21*(3), 273–290.

U.S. Bureau of the Census. (1984). *Statistical Abstract of the United States: 1984*. Washington, DC: U.S. Government Printing Office.

U.S. Bureau of the Census. (1996). *Statistical Abstract of the United States: 1996*. Washington, DC: U.S. Government Printing Office.

U.S. Bureau of the Census. (1996a). Resident population by age and state: 1995. In *Statistical abstract of the U.S.* (116th ed.). Washington, DC: U.S. Government Printing Office.

U.S. Bureau of the Census. (1996b, February). Current population reports, population projections of the U.S. by age, sex, race, and Hispanic origin: 1995–2050 (Series #P25-1130). Washington, DC: U.S. Government Printing Office.

U.S. Department of Agriculture. (1995). Continuing Survey of Food Intake of Individuals, 1989–1991. Unpublished data.

Ullman, D. (1991). *Discovering homeopathy: Medicine for the 21st century*. Berkeley, CA: North Atlantic Books.

Ullman, D. (1996). *The consumer's guide to homeopathy*. New York: Jeremy Tarcher/Putnam.

United States v. Rutherford, 438 F. Supp. 1287 (W.D. Okla. 1977), *remanded*, 582 F.2d 1234 (10th Cir. 1978), *rev'd*, 442 U.S. 544 (1979), *on remand*, 616 F.2d 455 (10th Cir. 1980), *cert. denied*, 449 U.S. 937 (1980), *later proceeding*, 806 F.2d 1455 (10th Cir. Okla. 1986). Compare *Rutherford* with Andrews v. Ballard, 498 F. Supp. 1038 (S.D. Tex. 1980); *but see* United States v. Burzynski Cancer Research Institute, et al., 819 F.2d 1301, 1313 (5th Cir. 1987) (rejecting, based on *Rutherford*, patients' claim of a constitutional right to obtain a specific cancer treatment), *reh'g denied en banc*, 829 F.2d 1124 (5th Cir. 1987), *cert. denied*, 484 U.S. 1065 (1988).

United States Department of Agriculture/Human Nutrition Information Service. (1990). *Dietary Fiber*.

Upledger, J. E. (1978). Relationship of craniosacral examination findings in grade school children with developmental problems. *Journal of the American Osteopathic Association, 77*, 760–776.

Upledger, J. E. (1983). Craniosacral function in brain dysfunction. *Osteopathic Annals, 11*, 318–324.

Upledger, J. E. (1995). Research and observations support the existence of a craniosacral system. *Alternative Medicine Journal, 2*, 31–43.

Upledger, J. E. Cranial therapy proves successful with some LDD children. Advocate. 1980.

Upledger, J. E., & Vredevoogd, J. D. (1983). *CranioSacral Therapy*. Seattle: Eastland Press.

Utne, L. (1995, August). Holistic health online. *New Age Journal*, 78–80.

Valat, J. P., Goupille, P., & Vedere, V. (1997). Low back pain: Risk factors for chronicity. *Revue du Rhumatisme* (English Edition), *64*(3), 189–194.

Van Den Broucke, C. O., & Lemli, J. A. (1983). Spasmolytic activity of the flavonoids from *Thymus vulgaris*. *Pharm Weekly, 5*(1), 9–14.

Van Deusen, J., & Harlowe, D. (1987). The efficacy of the ROM Dance Program for adults with rheumatoid arthritis. *American Journal Occupational Therapy, 41*(2), 90–95.

van Dulmen, A. M., Fennis, J. F., & Bleijenberg, F. (1996). Cognitive-behavioral group therapy for irritable bowel syndrome: Effects and long-term follow-up. *Psychosomatic Medicine, 58*(5), 508–514.

Van Why, R. P. (1992). A brief history and exhortation concerning massage therapy in America. *Massage Therapy Journal, 31*(1), 42–48.

Varela, P., Marcos, A., & Navarro, M. (1992). Zinc status in anorexia nervosa. *Annals of Nutrition and Metabolism, 36*, 197–202.

Vaya, J., Belinky, P. A., & Aviram, M. (1997). Antioxidant constituents from licorice roots: Isolation, structure elucidation and anti-oxidative capacity toward LDL oxidation. *Free Radical Biology and Medicine, 23*(2), 302–313.

Vernon, C. C., Hand, J. W., Field, S. B., Machin, D., Whaley, J. B., Vanderzee, J., Vanputten, W. L. J., Vanrhoon, G. C., Vandijk, J. D. P., Gonzalez, D. G., Liu, F. F., Goodman, P., & Sherar, M. (1996). Radiotherapy with or without hyperthermia in the treatment of superficial localized breast cancer—results from five randomized controlled trials. *International Journal of Radiation Oncology Biology Physics, 35*, 731–744.

Verri, A. P., Verticale, M. S., Vallero, E., et al. (1997). Television and eating disorders. Study of adolescent eating behavior. *Minerva Pediatrica, 49*(6), 235–243.

Vick, J. A., & Shipman, W. H. (1972). Effects of whole bee venom and its fractions (apamin and melittin) on plasma cortisol levels in the dog. *Toxicon, 10,* 377–380.

Visudhiphan, S., et al. (1982). The relationship between high fibrinolytic activity and daily capsicum ingestion in Thasis. *American Journal of Clinical Nutrition, 35,* 1452–1458.

Vitale, S., West, S., Hallfrisch, J., et al. (1993). Plasma antioxidants and risk of cortical and nuclear cataract. *Epidemiology, 4,* 195–203.

Vitamin E stabilizes ferritin: New insights into iron-ascorbate interactions. (1987). *Nutrition Reviews, 45,* 217–219.

Vlajinac, H. D. (1997). Caffeine and low-birth-weight babies. *American Journal of Epidemiology, 145,* 335–338.

Vogel, V. J. (1977). *American Indian medicine.* Norman, OK: University of Oklahoma Press.

Von Rohr, I., & Von Rohr, W. (1992). *Harmony is the healer.* Rockport, MA: Element.

Vredevoogd, J. D., & Upledger, J. E. (1979). Management of autogenic headache. *Osteopathic Annals.*

Wacker, A., & Hilbig, A. (1978). Virus inhibition by *Echinacea purpurea. Planta Medica, 33,* 89–102.

Wadsworth, C. (1988). *Manual examination and treatment of the spine and extremities.* Baltimore, MD: Williams & Wilkins.

Wager, S. (1996). *A doctor's guide to therapeutic touch.* New York: Berkley Publishing.

Walco, G. A., Varni, J. W., & Ilowite, N. T. (1992). Cognitive-behavioral pain management in children with juvenile rheumatoid arthritis. *Pediatrics, 89*(6), 1075–1079.

Walker, M. (1994). *The chelation answer: How to prevent hardening of the arteries and rejuvenate your cardiovascular system.* Dunwoody, GA: Second Opinion Publishing.

Walker, S. R. (1995). *Intercessory prayer.* http://www.altmed.od.nih.gov/gov/oam.cgi-bin/research/search_simple.cgi

Walsh-Burke, K. (1992). Family communication and coping with cancer: Impact of the We Can Weekend. *Journal of Psychosocial Oncology, 10,* 63–81.

Wardle, J. (1995). Cholesterol and psychological well-being. *Journal of Psychosomatic Research, 39,* 549–562.

Wardwell, W. I. (1988). Chiropractors: Evolution to acceptance. In N. Gevitz (Ed.), *Other healers: Unorthodox medicine in America* (pp. 157–191). Baltimore: The Johns Hopkins University Press.

Warshafsky, S., Kamer, R. S., & Sivak, S. L. (1993). Effect of garlic on total serum cholesterol. *Annals of Internal Medicine, 119,* 599–605.

Watanabe, Y., Halberg, F., Cornelissen, G., et al. (1996). Chronobiometric assessment of autogenic training effects upon blood pressure and heart rate. *Percept Mot Skills, 83*(3), 1395–1410.

Waters, B. (1995). *Massage during pregnancy.* Research Triangle Publishing.

Watrous, I. S. (1992). The Trager Approach: An effective tool for physical therapy. *Physical Therapy Forum,* April 10, 22–25.

Watson, C. W. (1959). Effects of lowering of body temperature on the symptoms of multiple sclerosis. *New England Journal of Medicine, 261,* 1253–1259.

Watson, J. (1988). *Nursing: Human science and human care: A theory of nursing.* New York: National League for Nursing Press.

Weber, R. (1986). *Dialogues with Scientists and Sages: The Search for Unity.* New York and London: Routledge & Kegan Paul.

Weber, S. (1996). The effects of relaxation exercises on anxiety levels in psychiatric inpatients. *Journal of Holistic Nursing, 14*(3), 196–205.

Weil, A. (1995). *Health and healing.* Boston: Houghton Mifflin.

Weil, A. (1995). *Natural health, natural medicine.* Boston: Houghton Mifflin.

Weil, A. (1995). *Spontaneous healing.* New York: Knopf.

Weil, A. (1997, December). New hope for infertility. *Self-Healing, 1,* 6.

Weinberger, M. W., & Ostergard, D. R. (1996). Stress incontinence: Complications of surgery. *Obstet and Gynecol, 87,* 50.

Weinrich, S. P., & Weinrich, M. C. (1990). The effect of massage on pain in cancer patients. *Applied Nursing Research, 3,* 140–145.

Weisbord, M. (1997). *Asthma: Breathe again naturally and reclaim your life.* New York: St. Martin's Press.

Weiss, B. *Many lives many masters.* New York: Simon and Schuster.

Weiss, B. *Through time into healing.* New York: Simon and Schuster.

Weiss, H. B., & Kemble, H. R. (1967). *The great American water-cure craze: A history of hydropathy in the United States.* Trenton, NJ: Past Times Press.

Welch, L. (1997). *Qi Gong.* http:/www.shiatsu.org/html/article

Welihinda, J., et al. (1982). The insulin-releasing activity of the tropical plant Momordica charantia. *Acta Biol Med Germ, 41,* 1229–1240.

Wenneberg, S. R., Schneider, R. H., Walton, K. G., et al. (1994). Interpersonal outcome of cognitive behavioral treatment for chronically suicidal borderline patients. *American Journal of Psychiatry, 151*(2), 1771–1776.

Wenneberg, S. R., Schneider, R. H., Walton, K. G., Maclean, C. R., Levitsky, D. K., et al (1997). A controlled study of the effects of Transcendental Meditation program on cardiovascular reactivity and ambulatory blood pressure. *International Journal of Neurosciences, 89*(1), 15–28.

Werbach, M. R. (1996). *Nutritional influences on illness* Second Edition. Tarzana, CA: Third Line Press.

Werbach, M. R., & Murray, M. T. (1994). *Botanical influences on illness.* Tarzana, CA: Third Line Press.

West, S., Vitale, S., Hallfrisch, J., et al. (1994). *Archives of Opthalmology, 112,* 222–227.

Westman, J. C. (1997). Reducing governmental interventions in families by licensing parents. *Child Psychiatry Hum Dev, 27*(3), 193–205.

Wetzel, M., & Eisenberg, D. (1997). A survey in courses involving alternative medicine in U. S. and Canadian Medical Schools. Presented by the Association of American Medical Colleges at the Center of Alternative Medicine Research at Beth Israel Deaconess Medical Center, Boston.

Wetzel, M., & Eisenberg, D. (1997, November). A survey in courses involving alternative medicine in U.S. and Canadian medical schools. Presented by the Association of American Medical Colleges at the Center of Alternative Medicine Research at Beth Israel Deaconess Medical Center, Boston.

Wharton, R., & Lewith, G. (1986, June 7). Complementary medicine and the general practitioner. *British Medical Journal, 292*(6534) 1498–1500.

Whelton, P. K., He, J., Culter, J. A., et al. (1997). Effects of oral potassium on blood pressure. Metanalysis of randomized controlled clinical trials. *Journal of the American Medical Association, 277*(20), 1624–1632.

Whiffen, V. E., & Clark, S. E. (1997). Does victimization account for sex differences in depressive symptoms? *British Journal of Clinical Psychology, 36*(Part 2), 185–193.

White, C. L., LeFort, S. M., Amsel, R., & Jeans, M. E. (1997). Predictors of the development of chronic pain. *Res Nurs Health, 20*(4), 309–318.

White, P. D., & Fulcher, K. Y. (1997). Effect of exercise on Chronic Fatigue Syndrome. *British Medical Journal, 314*(1), 647–652.

White-Traut, R., & Carrier-Goldman, M. (1988). Premature infant massage: Is it safe? *Pediatric Nursing, 14*(4).

White-Traut, R., Nelson, M., Burns, K., & Cunningham, N. (1994). Environmental influences on the developing premature infant: Theoretical issues and applications to practice. *JOGNN, 23*(5), 393–401.

Whiteman, M. C., Deary, I. J., Lee, A. J., & Fowkes, F. G. (1997). Submissiveness and protection from coronary heart disease in the general population: Edinburgh Artery Study. *Lancet, 350*(9077), 541–545.

Whiting, S. J., Wood, R., & Kim, K. (1997). Pharmacology update: Calcium supplementation. *Journal American Academy of Nurse Practitioners, 9*(4), 187–192.

Whorton, J. (1982). *Crusaders for fitness.* Princeton, NJ: Princeton University Press.

Whyte, F., & Smith, L. (1997). A literature review of adolescence and cancer. *Eur Journal Cancer Care, 6*(2), 137–146.

Wigmore Publications, Ltd. (1993). *Bach flower essences for the family: An introduction to the basic principles and standards of the Bach flower essences and a guide to their use.* Oxfordshire, England.

Wijayakusuma, H. (1986). *The acupuncture bee venom therapy.* Sri Lanka:

Wilke, W. S. (1995). Treatment of "resistant" fibromyalgia. *Rheumatic Disease Clinics of North America, 21*(1), 247–246.

Willett, W. C. (1992). Folic acid and neural tube defect: Can't we come to closure? *American Journal of Public Health, 82*(5), 666–668.

Williams, R., Haney, T., Lee, K., Kong, Y., Blumenthal, J., & Whalen, R. (1980). Type A behavior, hostility, and coronary atherosclerosis. *Psychosomatic Medicine, 42*, 539–549.

Wilson, R. (1995). *A Complete Guide to Understanding & Using Aromatherapy.* Garden City Park: Avery Publishing.

Wilson, R. (1995). *A complete guide to understanding and using aromatherapy for vibrant health and beauty.* Avery.

Winslow, E. H., & Jacobson, A. F. (1997). Nondrug therapies help patients with insomnia. *AJN, 97*(6), 23.

Winters, J. C., Sobel, J. S., Gronier, K. H., et al. (1997). Comparison of physiotherapy, manipulation, and corticosteroid injection for treating shoulder complaints in general practice: Randomised, single blind study. *British Medical Journal, 314*, 1320–1325.

Wirth, D. (1990). The effect of non-contact Therapeutic Touch on the healing rate of full thickness dermal wounds. *Subtle Energies, 1*(1), 1–20.

Wirth, D. P., Richardson, J. T., Eidelman, W. S., & O'Malloy, A. C. (1993). Full thickness dermal wounds treated with non-contact Therapeutic Touch: A replication and extension. *Complementary Therapies in Medicine, 1*, 127–132.

Wise, B. (1989). Comparison of immune response to mirth and to distress in women at risk for recurrent breast cancer. *Dissertation Abstracts International, 49*(7), 2918.

Witt, J. S., Longnecker, M. P., Bird, C. L., et al. (1996). Relation of vegetable, fruit, and grain consumption to colorectal adenomatous polyps. *American Journal of Epidemiology, 144*(11), 1015–1025.

Witt, P. (1986). An additional tool in the treatment of chronic spinal pain and dysfunction. *Whirlpool, Summer*, 24–26.

Witt, P. L., & MacKinnon, J. (1986). Trager psychophysical integration: A method to improve chest mobility of patients with chronic lung disease. *Physical Therapy, 66*(2), 214–217.

Witt, P. L., & Parr, C. A. (1988). Effectiveness of Trager psychophysical integration in promoting trunk mobility in a child with cerebral palsy: A case report. *Physical and Occupational Therapy Pediatrics, 8*(4), 75–94.

Wittlinger, H. and G. (1995). *Textbook of Dr. Vodder's Manual Lymph Drainage,* vol. 1: Basic Course, 5th ed. Portland, OR: Medicina Biologica, 1995.

Wolf, S. L., Barnhart, H. X., Ellison, G. L., & Coogler, C. E. (1997). The effect of Tai Chi Quan and computerized balance training on postural stability in older subjects. *Physical Therapy, 77*(4), 371–381.

Wolfe, F., Smythe, H. A., Yunus, M. B., Bennett, R. M., Bombardier, C., Goldenberg, D. L., et al. (1973). American College of Rheumatology 1990 criteria for the classification of fibromyalgia. (report of the Multicenter Criteria Committee). *Arthritis Rheumatism, 33*, 160–172.

Wolffers, I., & de Moree, S. (1994). Use of alternative treatments by HIV-positive and AIDS patients in The Netherlands. *Ned Tijdschr Geneesd, 138*(6), 307–310.

Wolfson, L., Whiple, R., Derby, C., et al. (1996). Balance and strength training in older adults: Intervention gains and Tai Chi maintenance. *Journal of the American Geriatrics Society, 44*(5), 498–506.

Wolin, S., & Bennett, L. (1984, September). Family rituals. *Family Process, 23*, 403.

Wolinsky, S. (1991). *Trances people live.* Falls Village, CT: The Bramble Co.

Wolpe, P. R. (1994). The dynamics of heresy in a profession. *Social Science and Medicine, 39*(9), 1133–1148.

Wood, R. J., & Zheng, J. (1995). Calcium supplementation reduces intestinal zinc absorption and balance in humans. *FASEB Journal, 9*, 283.

Woods, D. L., Craven, R., & Whitney, J. (1996). The effect of Therapeutic Touch on disruptive behaviors of individuals with dementia of the Alzheimer type. *Alternative Therapies in Health and Medicine,* July, *2*(4), 95.

Woods, N. F., Lentz, M., Mitchell, E. S., et al. (1997). PMS after 40: Persistence of a stress-related symptom pattern. *Research in Nursing and Health, 20*(4), 329–340.

Wooten, J. (1996). WebWatch. *Alternative and Complementary Therapies, 2*, 59.

Wooten, J. (1996). WebWatch. *Alternative and Complementary Therapies, 2*, 121–122.

Wooten, J. (1996). WebWatch. *Alternative and Complementary Therapies, 2*, 337–338.

World Health Organization. (1984). *A manual for the treatment of acute diarrhea for use by physi-*

cians and other senior health workers. Switzerland: Author.

World Health Organization. (1985). *Report on second WHO regional working group on the standardization auricular acupuncture nomenclature.* Hong Kong: WHO.

World Health Organization. (1987). *Report on third WHO regional working group on the standardization of auricular acupuncture nomenclature.* Seoul, Korea: WHO.

World Health Organization. (1990). *Report on the WHO working group meeting on auricular acupuncture nomenclature.* Lyon, France: WHO.

Worwood, S. (1995). *Essential aromatherapy: A pocket guide to essential oils and aromatherapy.* New World Library.

Worwood, V. A. (1991). *The Complete Book of Essential Oils & Aromatherapy.* San Rafael, CA: New World Library.

Wright, K. P., Badia, P., Myers, B. L., et al. (1997). Caffeine and light effects on nighttime melatonin and temperature levels in sleep-deprived humans. *Brain Research, 747*(1), 78–84.

Wu, A. H., Yu, M. C., & Mack, T. M. (1997). Smoking, alcohol use, dietary factors and risk of small intestinal adenocarcinoma. *International Journal of Cancer, 70*(5), 512–517.

Wu, A. H., Ziegler, R. G., Horn-Ross, P. L., et al. (1996). Tofu and risk of breast cancer in Asian-Americans. *Cancer Epidemiol Biomarkers Prev, 5*(11), 901–906.

Wunderlich, R. Jr. (1995). *Natural Alternatives to Antibiotics.* New Canaan, CT: Keats Publishing.

Wunderlich, R. Jr. (1997). *The Candida-Yeast Syndrome.* New Canaan, CT: Keats Publishing.

Wunderlich, R. Jr. (1997). *Will the Real Doctor Please Stand Up?* To be published.

Wyshak, G., & Frisch, R. E. (1994). Carbonated beverages, dietary calcium, the dietary calcium/phosphorous ratio in girls and boys. *Journal of Adol Health, 15*(3), 210–215.

Xin, Y. L. (1995). *Electrochemical treatment of cancer.* Beijing, China: People's Health Publications.

Xin, Y. L., Xue, F., Ge, B., Zhao, F., Shi, B., & Zhang, W. (1997). Electrochemical treatment of lung cancer. *Bioelectromagnetics, 18*, 8–13.

Yamashiki, M., Nishimura, A., Suzuki, H., Sakaguchi, S., & Kosaka, Y. (1997). Effects of the Japanese herbal medicine Sho-saiko-to (TJ-9) on

in vitro interleukin-10 production by peripheral blood mononuclear cells of patients with chronic hepatitis C. *Hepatology, 25*(6), 1390–1397.

Yang, X., Liu, X., Luo, H., & Jia, Y. (1994). Clinical observation on needling extrachannel points in treating mental depression. *Journal Trad Chin Med, 14*(1), 14–18.

Yao, X. J., Wainberg, M. A., & Parniak, M. A. (1992). Mechanism of inhibition of HIV-1 infection in vitro by purified extract of Prunella vulgaris. *Virology, 187*(1), 56–62.

Yasgur, J. (1994). *A dictionary of homeopathic medical terminology.* Greenville, PA: Van Hoy Publishers.

Yates, J. (1990). *A physician's guide to therapeutic massage.* Vancouver: Massage Therapists Association of British Columbia.

Yeoh, K. G., Kang, J. Y., Yap, I., et al. (1995). Chili protects against aspirin-induced gastroduodenal mucosal injury in humans. *Digestive Diseases and Sciences, 40*(3), 580–583.

Yesalis, C. E. III, Wallace, R. B., Fisher, W. P., & Tokheim, R. (1980). Does chiropractic utilization substitute for less available medical services? *American Journal of Public Health, 70*(4), 415–417.

Yo, A. (1997). Diet and stomach cancer in Korea. *International Journal of Cancer* (Suppl. 10), 7–9.

Yoirich, N. (1959). *Curative properties of honey and bee venom.* Moscow.

Yong, L. C., Brown, C. C., Schatzkin, A., et al. (1997). Intakes of vitamins E, C, and A and risk of lung cancer. The NHANES I epidemiologic followup study. First National Health and Nutrition Examination Survey. *American Journal of Epidemiology, 146*(3), 231–243.

Young. (1990). *The art of polarity therapy: A practitioner's perspective.* Devon, England: Prism Press.

Your aching back: how to prevent and treat back pain. (1983, September). *Bestways,* 52–55.

Yu, P., Li, F., Wei, X., Su, R., & Fu. (1991). Treatment of essential hypertension with auriculacupressure. *Journal of Traditional Chinese Medicine, 11*(1), 17–21.

Yu, S-Y., Li, W. G., Zhu, J., Yu, W. P., & Hou, C. (1989). Chemoprevention trial of human hepatitis with selenium supplementation in China. *Biological Trace Element Research, 20*, 15–22.

Yuan, J. M., Wang, Q. S., Ross, R., et al. (1995). Diet and breast cancer in Shanghai and Tianjin, China. *Brit Journal Cancer, 71*(6), 1353–1358.

Yun, L. Temple News Tibetan Tantric Buddhism Black Sect Feng Shui 2959 Russell Street, Berkeley, CA 94705.

Zachariae, R., Oster, H., Bjerring, P., & Kragballe, K. (1996). Effects of psychologic intervention on psoriasis: A preliminary report. *Journal Am Acad Dermatol, 34*(6), 1008–1015.

Zamarra, J. W., Schneider, R. H., Besseghini, I., et al. (1996). Usefulness of the transcendental meditation program in the treatment of patients with coronary artery disease. *American Journal of Cardiology, 77*(10), 867–870.

Zani, F., Cuzzoni, M. T., Daglia, M., et al. (1993). Inhibition of mutagenicity in Salmonella typhimurium by Glycyrrhiza glabra extract, glycyrrhizinc acid, 18 alph- and 18 beta-glycyrrhetinic acids. *Planta Med, 59*(6), 502–507.

Zanolla, R., Mizeglio, C., & Balzarini, A. (1984). Evaluation of the results of three different methods of post-mastectomy lymphedema treatment. *Journal Surg Oncol, 26*, 210–213.

Zava, D. T., Blen, M., & Duwe, G. (1997). Estrogenic activity of natural and synthetic estrogens in human breast cancer cells in culture. *Environ Health Perspect, 105*(Suppl. 3), 637–645.

Zazzo, J. F., Lafont, A., Darwiche, E., et al. (1988). Is non-onstructive myocardiopathy (NOMC) in AIDS selenium-deficiency related? In J. Neve & A. Favier (Eds.), *Selenium in biology and medicine* (pp. 281–282). Berlin, NY: W. de Gruyter & Co.

Zee-Cheng, R. K. (1992). Shi-quan-da-bu-tang (ten significant tonic decoction, SQT). A potent Chinese biological response modifier in cancer immunotherapy, potentiation and detoxifier of anti-cancer drugs. *Methods Findings in Experimental Clinical Pharmacology, 14*(9), 725–736.

Zeller, J., McCain, N., & Swanson, B. (1996). Psychoneuroimmunology: An emerging framework for nursing research. *Journal of Advanced Nursing, 23*, 657–664.

Zhang, M. J., Wang, Q. F., Gao, L. X., et al. (1992). Comparative observation of the changes in serum lipid peroxides influenced by the supplementation of vitamin E in burn patients and healthy controls. *Burns, 18*(1), 19–21.

Zhang, Z. M., Shi, B. J., & Fan, R. (1995). Clinical observation on child aplastic anemia treated with integrated Chinese and Western medicine. *Chung Kuo Chung Hsi 1 Chieh Ho Tsa Chih, 15*(12), 713–715.

Zheng, W., Kushi, L. H., Potter, J. D., et al. (1995b). Dietary intake of energy and animal foods and endometrial cancer incidence. The Iowa women's health study. *American Journal of Epidemiology, 142*(4), 388–394.

Zheng, W., Sellers, T. A., Doyle, T. J., et al. (1995a). Retinol, antioxidant vitamins, and cancers of the upper digestive tract in a prospective cohort study of postmenopausal women. *American Journal of Epidemiology, 142*(9), 955–960.

Zhou, J., & Zhou, S. (1990). Treatment of orthostatic dysregulation by the principle of bu-shen yi-qi. *Chung Hsi I Chieh Ho Tsa Chih, 10*(5), 280–282.

Zhu, B-Q, & Parmley, W. W. (1990) Modification of experimental and clinical atherosclerosis by dietary fish oil. *American Heart Journal, 119*(1), 168–178.

Ziegler, J. (1994). Just the flax, ma'am: Researchers testing linseed. *Journal of the National Cancer Institute, 86*(23), 1746–1748.

Ziegler, J. (1995). It's not easy being green: Chlorophyll being tested. *Journal of the National Cancer Institute, 87*(1), 11.

Ziff, S. *Silver dental fillings, the toxic time bomb, can the mercury in your dental fillings poison you?* Santa Fe: Aurora Press.

Ziff, S., & Ziff, M. F. *Dentistry without mercury.* Orlando, FL: Bio-Probe.

Zimmerman, L., Nieveen, J., Barnason, S., & Schmaderer, M. (1996). The effects of music interventions on postoperative pain and sleep in coronary artery bypass graft (CABG) patients. *Sch Inq Nurs Pract, 10*(2), 153–157.

Zola, I. K. (1972). Studying the decision to see a doctor. In Z. Lipowski (Ed.), *Advances in Psychosomatic Medicine* v. 8 (pp. 216–236). Basel: Karger.

Zucav, G. *Seat of the soul.* Simon and Schuster.

SUBJECT INDEX

Abdominal/pelvic pain, effects of Therapeutic Touch, 497

Absorption of bioavailability of food/minerals, 33–34

Abuse, childhood physical or sexual, 111–112

Academy for Guided Imagery, 411, 412

Accessing stored body memories in Centropic Integration, 334

Access to complementary practice, federal role in regulating, 89–91

Access to complementary practice, state legislation for, 91–93

Access to health care services, 23, 43–45

Accreditation/licensure for acupuncture, 282

Acetyl-L-carnitine, impact on Alzheimer's symptoms, 124

Acidosis, effects on seizure threshold, 416

Activity increase, effects on back pain, 143–144

Acupressure
  effects on blood pressure, 201
  effects on morning sickness, 216–217
  effects on nausea and vomiting, 219
  effects on postoperative pain, 225–226
  and Jin Shin Do, 412–414
  points in Centropic Integration, 332, 334

Acupuncture
  and Chinese medicine, 281–288
  and color therapies, 310
  effects on attention deficit hyperactive disorder (ADHD), 140
  effects on depression, 169
  effects on headache pain, 226

effects on mental retardation in infants, 216

effects on multiple sclerosis (MS) symptoms, 217

energetic structures of, 283

gynecological illness case study, 287

impact on anemia, 126

and Jin Shin Do, 412–414

rank in U.S. health care system, 23

treatment of addiction, 289–291

Acupuncture points, electrical properties of, 32–33

Acute heart attacks, effects of polyunsaturated fatty acids, 260

Acute otitis media, homeopathic treatments, 256

Adaptation of an individual, 7–9

Adaptogens, 249, 266

Addiction, treatments of, 288–291

Adrenal gland health, herbal medicine therapies, 384–385

Advanced practice nurses and anthroposophically extended medicine, 301

Advertising/commercialization of medical treatment, 21

Aerobic exercise
  effects on anxiety and panic, 132
  effects on depression, 171
  effects on heart and blood vessels, 193
  effects on multiple sclerosis (MS) symptoms, 217–218
  in health and fitness, 363–365

Aesculus hippocastanum, 266–267

Affirmations, 215, 291

CONTRIBUTOR INDEX

⑤ Springer Publishing Company

Complementary / Alternative Therapies in Nursing, 3rd Edition

Mariah Snyder, PhD, RN, FAAN
Ruth Lindquist, PhD, RN

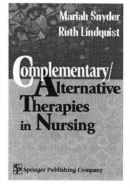

This book offers a systematic approach to a wide range of complementary/alternative therapies that can be used independently by nurses. Each of the 28 chapters describes a different therapy and follows a standard format: definition, review of current research, description of uses and techniques, precautions, and a list of questions for further research.

Many of these therapies such as massage and application of heat and cold have traditionally been part of nursing practice, while others such as imagery, meditation, and biofeedback are interventions that nurses can use to enrich their practice. Students and clinicians in all specialty areas of nursing will find this a straightforward and practical resource.

Contents: Progressive Muscle Relaxation, *M. Snyder* • Breathing, *J. Wang and M. Snyder* • Exercise, *D. Treat-Jacobson and D.L. Mark* • Tai Chi/Movement Therapy, *K. Shaller* • Therapeutic Touch, *E. Egan* • Massage, *M. Snyder and W. Cheng* • Biofeedback, *M. Good* • Application of Heat and Cold, *S. Ridgeway, et al.* • Imagery, *J. Post-White* • Meditation, *M.J. Kreitzer* • Aromatherapy, *K. James* • Purposeful Touch, *M. Snyder and Y. Nojima* • Presence, *S. Moch and C. Schaefer* • Active Listening, *M. Ryden* • Positioning, *M.F. Tracy* • Sensation Information, *J.B. Ruiz-Bueno* • Journal Writing, *M. Snyder* • Reminiscence, *M. Snyder* • Storytelling, *P. Dicke* • Validation Therapy, *L. Taft* • Music Therapy, *L. Chlan* • Prayer, *M. Gustafson* • Humor, *K. Smith* • Pet Therapy, *K. James* • Contracting, *R. Lindquist* • Groups, *M. Kaas and M.F. Richie* • Family Support, *M. Mirr* • Advocacy, *M. Nelson*

1998   384pp.   0-8261-1169-6   hardcover   www.springerpub.com

536 Broadway, New York, NY 10012-3955 • (212) 431-4370 • Fax (212) 941-7842

Wellness Practitioner
Concepts, Theory, Research, Strategies, and Programs, 2nd Edition
Carolyn Chambers Clark, EdD, RN, FAAN

Now in a second edition, this is a comprehensive resource on health maintenance, disease prevention, and alternative health practices. The author explores conceptual bases and practical techniques for a wide range of programs, activities, and therapies that promote wellness. Topics include relaxation and stress management, nutrition, exercise, herbal remedies, massage, imagery, affirmations, reflexology, aromatherapy, natural healing, and self care measures for conditions ranging from hay fever to multiple sclerosis.

Environmental influences and community wellness are each addressed in a separate chapter. Learning exercises are included with each chapter to facilitate integration of the material. A useful resource for nurses, physicians, and other health professionals — both traditional and alternative.

Partial Contents:
- Introduction to Wellness Theory
- Beginning to Move Toward Wellness
- Positive Relationship Building
- Stress Management
- Nutritional Wellness
- Exercise and Movement
- Self-Care, Touch, and Wellness
- Environmental Wellness
- Community Wellness Programs
- Research and Wellness Theory
- Appendix: Resources/ Index

1996   368pp .   0-8261-5151-5   hardcover   www.springerpub.com

536 Broadway, New York, NY 10012-3955 • (212) 431-4370 • Fax (212) 941-7842

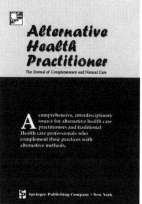